Handbook of
GROWTH FACTORS
Volume III: Hematopoietic Growth Factors And Cytokines

Handbook of Growth Factors
Enrique Pimentel, M.D.

Volume I
General Basic Aspects
Regulation of Cell Functions
Growth Factor Receptors
Postreceptor Mechanisms of Growth Factor Action
Cyclic Nucleotides
Guanosine Triphosphate-Binding Proteins
The Calcium-Calmodulin System
Phosphoinositide Metabolism
Protein Phosphorylation
Proto-Oncogene and Onco-Suppressor Gene Expression
Role of Growth Factors in Neoplastic Processes

Volume II
Peptide Growth Factors
Insulin
Insulin-Like Growth Factors
Epidermal Growth Factor
Fibroblast Growth Factors
Neurotrophic Growth Factors
Organ-Specific Growth Factors
Cell-Specific Growth Factors
Transforming Growth Factors
Regulatory Peptides with Growth Factor-Like Properties

Volume III
Hematopoietic Growth Factors and Cytokines
Hematopoietic Growth Factors
Interleukins and Cytokines
Colony-Stimulating Factors
Interferons
Tumor Necrosis Factors
Erythropoietic Growth Factors
Platelet-Derived Growth Factor
Transferrins

Handbook of GROWTH FACTORS
Volume III: Hematopoietic Growth Factors and Cytokines

Enrique Pimentel, M.D.
National Center of Genetics
Institute of Experimental Medicine
Central University of Venezuela
Caracas, Venezuela

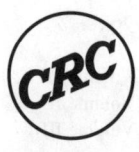

CRC Press
Boca Raton   Ann Arbor   London   Tokyo

Library of Congress Cataloging-in-Publication Data

Pimentel, Enrique.
   Handbook of growth factors.
   Includes bibliographical references and index.
   Contents: v. 1. General basic aspects. —
v. 2. Peptide growth factors — v. 3. Hematopoietic
growth factors and cytokines.
   1. Growth factors. I. Title. [DNLM: 1. Growth
Substances. QU 100 P644h 1994]
   QP552.G76P56   1994   612.6   93-40108

   This book contains information obtained from authentic and highly regarded sources. Reprinted material is quoted with permission, and sources are indicated. A wide variety of references are listed. Reasonable efforts have been made to publish reliable data and information, but the author and the publisher cannot assume responsibility for the validity of all materials or for the consequences of their use.

   Neither this book nor any part may be reproduced or transmitted in any form or by any means, electronic or mechanical, including photocopying, microfilming, and recording, or by any information storage or retrieval system, without prior permission in writing from the publisher.

   CRC Press, Inc.'s consent does not extend to copying for general distribution, for promotion, for creating new works, or for resale. Specific permission must be obtained in writing from CRC Press for such copying.

   Direct all inquiries to CRC Press, Inc., 2000 Corporate Blvd., N.W., Boca Raton, Florida 33431.

© 1994 by CRC Press, Inc.

No claim to original U.S. Government works
International Standard Book Number 0-8493-2505-6 (Volume I)
International Standard Book Number 0-8493-2506-4 (Volume II)
International Standard Book Number 0-8493-2507-2 (Volume III)
Library of Congress Card Number 93-40108

Printed in the United States of America 1 2 3 4 5 6 7 8 9 0
Printed on acid-free paper

CONTENTS

Chapter 1
Hematopoietic Growth Factors
- I. Introduction 1
- II. Hematopoiesis 1
  - A. Control of Hematopoietic Processes 1
  - B. Regulation of Hematopoiesis By Growth Factors 2
  - C. Gene Expression in Hematopoiesis 4
- III. Hematopoietic Growth Factors 4
  - A. Pluripotent HGFs 5
    - 1. Hemopoietins 5
    - 2. Stem Cell Growth Factor 5
    - 3. Other Pluripotent HGFs 7
  - B. Colony-Stimulating Factors 7
  - C. Cytokines 9
  - D. Hematopoietic Inhibiting Factors 13
    - 1. T-Cell-Derived Growth Inhibitors 13
    - 2. Oncostatin M 13
    - 3. Murine Growth Inhibitory Factor 14
    - 4. Leukocyte Inhibitory Factor 14
    - 5. Macrophage-Derived Growth Inhibitor 14
  - E. Role of HGFs in Neoplastic Processes 14
  - F. HGFs and Oncogene-Induced Transformation 15
- IV. Proto-Oncogene and Tumor Suppressor Gene Expression in Hematopoietic Cells ... 16
  - A. Expression of the c-*myc* Gene 16
  - B. Expression of the c-*fos* Gene 17
  - C. Expression of the c-*myb* Gene 17
  - D. Expression of the *vav* Gene 17
  - E. Proto-Oncogene Expression in the Induced Differentiation of Hematopoietic Neoplastic Cells 17
- References 18

Chapter 2
Interleukins and Cytokines
- I. Introduction 35
- II. Interleukin 1 36
  - A. Biological Effects of IL-1 36
    - 1. Effects of IL-1 on Hematopoietic Cells 36
    - 2. Effects of IL-1 on the Digestive Tract 38
    - 3. Effects of IL-1 on Bone, Cartilage and Connective Tissue 38
    - 4. Effects of IL-1 on Vascular Cells 40
    - 5. Effects of IL-1 on the Skin 40
    - 6. Effects of IL-1 on the Endocrine System and the Gonads 40
    - 7. Effects of IL-1 on Neural Tissues 41
  - B. IL-1 Structure and the IL-1 Gene 41
    - 1. IL-1α and IL-1β 41
    - 2. Human IL-1α and IL-1β Genes and Their Products 42
    - 3. Rodent IL-1 Genes and Their Products 42
    - 4. Secretion of IL-1α and IL-1β and Binding to the IL-1 Receptor 42
    - 5. Biological Activities of IL-1α and IL-1β 43
    - 6. IL-1-Related Proteins 43
  - C. IL-1 Production and Secretion 43
    - 1. Production of IL-1 by Malignant Cells 44
    - 2. Regulation of IL-1 Production and Secretion 45
    - 3. Mechanisms of Regulation of IL-1 Production and Secretion 45

- D. IL-1 Inhibitors 46
  1. Urine-Derived Inhibitors of IL-1 46
  2. α-Melanocyte-Stimulating Hormone 46
  3. Protein p15E 47
  4. IL-1 Receptor Antagonist 47
- E. IL-1 Receptors 47
  1. Classes of Surface IL-1 Receptors 47
  2. Expression of IL-1 Receptors on the Cell Surface 48
  3. Nuclear IL-1 Receptors 48
  4. Bacterial IL-1 Receptors 48
- F. Postreceptor Mechanisms of Action of IL-1 49
  1. Production of Cyclic Nucleotides 49
  2. Changes in Ion Fluxes 49
  3. Production of Polyamines 49
  4. Production of Prostaglandins 50
  5. Protein Phosphorylation 50
  6. Phosphoinositide Metabolism 50
  7. Protein Synthesis 51
  8. Gene Expression 51
  9. Proto-Oncogene Expression 51
- G. Effects of IL-1 on the Proliferation and Differentiation of Normal and Neoplastic Cells 52

III. Interleukin 2 53
- A. Biological Effects of IL-2 53
  1. Effects of IL-2 on T Lymphocytes 53
  2. Effects of IL-2 on NK and Large Granular Lymphocytes 54
  3. Interaction of IL-2 With Other Lymphokines 54
  4. Abrogation of IL-2 Requirement by Oncoproteins 55
  5. Effects of IL-2 on B Lymphocytes 55
  6. Effects of IL-2 on Monocytes 55
  7. Effects of IL-2 on Myelopoiesis 55
  8. Effects of IL-2 on Endocrine Cells 55
- B. The Human T-Cell Antigen Receptor Complex 56
  1. T Lymphocyte Subsets 56
  2. Structure of the T-Cell Antigen Receptor 57
  3. The T3 Molecule 58
  4. The T-Cell Activating Protein 58
  5. Activation of the T-Cell Receptor Complex 58
  6. T-Cell Receptor Gene Rearrangements 58
  7. Role of the T-Cell Antigen Receptor Complex and IL-2 in Activation of T Cells 59
- C. Structure of IL-2 60
- D. The IL-2 Gene 60
  1. Transcriptional Expression of the IL-2 Gene 60
  2. Homologies of the Flanking Regions of the IL-2 Gene 61
- E. Production of IL-2 61
  1. Role of Calcium Ions and Phosphoinositide Turnover 62
  2. IL-1 and Phorbol Esters 62
  3. Steroid Hormones 62
  4. Platelet-Activating Factor 62
  5. Age-Related Changes in IL-2 Secretion and Action 62
  6. Constitutive Production of IL-2 63
  7. Serum Inhibitors of IL-2 63
- F. The IL-2 Receptor 63
  1. The IL-2 Receptor α-Chain 64
  2. The IL-2 Receptor β-Chain 64

        3. Phosphorylation of the IL-2 Receptor 65
    G. Expression of the IL-2 Receptor 66
        1. Factors Involved in the Induction of IL-2 Receptors 66
        2. Low-Affinity IL-2 Receptors 67
        3. Expression of IL-2 Receptors in Non-T Cells 67
        4. Internalization and Degradation of the IL-2 Receptor 67
        5. Soluble IL-2 Receptors 67
    H. Regulation of IL-2 Receptor Expression 68
        1. Inducers of IL-2 Receptors 68
        2. Inhibitors of IL-2 Receptor Expression 68
        3. Regulatory Mechanisms of IL-2 Receptor Expression 68
    I. IL-2 Receptor in Leukemia and Lymphoma Cells 69
        1. Adult T-Cell Leukemia and HTLV-I-Infected Cells 69
        2. T-Cell Chronic Lymphocytic Leukemia 69
        3. B-Cell Leukemias and Other Leukemias 69
        4. Hodgkin's and Non-Hodgkin's Lymphoma 70
        5. Chronic Myelogenous Leukemia 70
        6. Role of IL-2 in the Proliferation of Leukemic Cells 70
        7. Mechanisms of IL-2 Receptor Expression in Leukemic Cells 70
        8. Significance of Altered IL-2 Receptor Expression 70
    J. Postreceptor Mechanisms of Action of IL-2 71
        1. Production of cAMP 71
        2. GTP Binding and Hydrolysis 71
        3. Phosphoinositide Metabolism, Calcium Influx, and Protein Kinase C Activity ... 71
        4. Monovalent Ion Transport 72
        5. Polyamine Synthesis 72
        6. Pteridine Synthesis 72
        7. Protein Phosphorylation 73
        8. Induction of Gene Expression 74
        9. IL-2-Induced Proto-Oncogene Expression 74
        10. Induction of DNA Synthesis 75
    K. IL-2 and the IL-2 Receptor Functions in Neoplastic Cells 76
        1. Adult T-Cell Leukemia 76
        2. Other Hematologic Diseases 77
        3. Solid Tumors 77
    L. IL-2 and the Acquired Immune Deficiency Syndrome 77
    M. IL-2 as an Agent for Cancer Treatment 79
    N. Alterations of IL-2 in Nonmalignant Diseases 79
IV. Interleukin 3 80
    A. Biological Effects of IL-3 80
    B. IL-3 Structure and the IL-3 Gene 82
        1. Regulation of IL-3 Gene Expression 82
        2. IL-3-Like Proteins 82
        3. Homology Between IL-3 and HTLV Sequences 83
    C. IL-3 Receptors 83
    D. Post-receptor Mechanisms of Action of IL-3 84
        1. Phosphoinositide Metabolism 84
        2. Protein Phosphorylation 84
    E. IL-3 Requirement and Oncogene Expression 85
    F. Influence of IL-3 in Proto-Oncogene Expression 86
    G. Role of IL-3 in Neoplastic Processes 86
    H. IL-3-Induced Neoplastic Transformation 86
V. B-Cell Growth Factors 87
    A. Regulation of B-Cell Differentiation and Proliferation 87
    B. Effect of BCGFs on Proto-Oncogene Expression 88
    C. Production of BCGFs by Neoplastic Cells 89

    D. Actions of BCGFs on Neoplastic and Immortalized Cells 89
    E. Neuroleukin 89
  VI. Interleukin 4 89
    A. The IL-4 Gene and IL-4 Structure 90
    B. Biological Effects of IL-4 90
    C. The IL-4 Receptor 92
    D. Postreceptor Mechanisms of Action of IL-4 92
    E. Role of IL-4 in Neoplastic Processes 93
  VII. Interleukin 5 93
    A. The IL-5 Gene and IL-5 Structure 93
    B. The IL-5 Receptor 94
    C. Postreceptor Mechanisms of Action of IL-5 94
  VIII. Interleukin 6 94
    A. Biological Effects of IL-6 95
    B. IL-6 Gene and the Structure of IL-6 96
    C. Production of IL-6 96
    D. The IL-6 Receptor 98
    E. Postreceptor Mechanisms of Action of IL-6 98
    F. Role of IL-6 in Neoplasia 99
  IX. Interleukin 7 99
    A. IL-7 Gene and the Structure of IL-7 99
    B. Biological Effects of IL-7 100
    C. The IL-7 Receptor 100
    D. Postreceptor Mechanisms of IL-7 Action 100
    E. Role of IL-7 in Neoplasia 100
  X. Interleukin 8 100
    A. Production and Biological Effects of IL-8 101
    B. The IL-8 Gene and IL-8 Structure 101
    C. The IL-8 Receptor 101
    D. Postreceptor Mechanisms of Action of IL-8 101
    E. Role of IL-8 in Neoplasia 102
  XI. Interleukin 9 102
  XII. Interleukin 10 102
  XIII. Interleukin 11 103
  XIV. Interleukin 12 103
  XV. Interleukin 13 104
  XVI. Leukemia Inhibitory Factor 104
    A. The LIF Gene and LIF Structure 105
    B. Cellular Mechanisms of LIF Action 105
    C. Biological Properties of LIF 105
References 105

Chapter 3
Colony-Stimulating Factors
  I. Introduction 177
  II. Colony-Stimulating Factor 1 177
    A. Biological Effects of CSF-1 177
    B. CSF-1 Structure and the CSF-1 Gene 177
    C. Production of CSF-1 178
      1. Regulation of CSF-1 Production 179
      2. Genetic Deficiency of CSF-1 179
    D. The CSF-1 Receptor 179
      1. The CSF-1 Receptor and the v-Fms and c-Fms Proteins 180
      2. The Human c-*fms*/CSF-1 Receptor Gene 181
      3. Expression of the c-*fms*/CSF-1 Receptor Gene 181
      4. Phosphorylation and Internalization of the CSF-1 Receptor 182

     5. Expression of c-*fms* Transcripts in Neoplastic Cells 182
     6. Growth Factor Independence of v-*fms*-Transformed Cells 182
     7. Tumor Promoters, Differentiation Inducers, and c-*fms*/CSF-1
        Receptor Expression 182
   E. Postreceptor Mechanisms of Action of CSF-1 183
   F. Regulation of Gene Expression by CSF-1 183
   G. CSF-1 and Proto-Oncogene Expression 183
   H. Role of CSF-1 in Neoplastic Processes 184
III. Colony-Stimulating Factor 2 185
   A. Biological Effects of CSF-2 185
   B. CSF-2 Structure and the CSF-2 Gene 186
   C. Production of CSF-2 187
   D. The CSF-2 Receptor 187
   E. Postreceptor Mechanism of Action of CSF-2 188
   F. Role of CSF-2 in Neoplastic Processes 188
   G. CSF-2 and Proto-Oncogene Expression 189
   H. Influence of Viral Oncogenes on CSF-2 Expression 190
   I. Production of CSF-2 by Tumor Cells 190
   J. Oncogenic Potential of the Cloned CSF-2 Gene 190
   K. CSF-2 as an Agent for the Treatment of Cancer and AIDS 191
IV. Colony-Stimulating Factor 3 191
   A. Biological Effects of CSF-3 191
   B. CSF-3 Structure and the CSF-3 Gene 192
   C. Production of CSF-3 193
   D. The CSF-3 Receptor 193
   E. Postreceptor Mechanism of Action of CSF-3 194
   F. Effects of *In Vivo* Administration of CSF-3 194
   G. Role of CSF-3 in Neoplastic Processes 195
V. Megakaryocyte Colony-Stimulating Factors 196
   A. Megakaryocyte Colony-Stimulating Factor 196
   B. Thrombocytopoiesis-Stimulating Factor 197
VI. Macrophage-Derived Growth Factors 197
   A. Macrophage Colony-Stimulating Activity 197
   B. Macrophage-Derived Growth Factor 197
   C. Macrophage-Activating Factors 197
   D. Macrophage Migration Factors 198
   E. Macrophage Proinflammatory Proteins 198
References 198

Chapter 4
Interferons

I. Introduction 221
II. Regulation of Interferon Production 221
III. Interferon Structure and the Interferon Genes 222
IV. Interferon Receptors 223
V. Postreceptor Mechanisms of Interferon Action 223
VI. Effects of Interferon on Gene Expression 224
   A. Proto-Oncogene and Tumor Suppressor Gene Expression 225
VII. Effects of Interferon on Cell Proliferation and Cell Differentiation 227
VIII. Role of Interferons in Neoplastic Processes 228
   A. Interferon-Induced Differentiation of Neoplastic Cells 229
   B. Cytostatic and Tumoricidal Effects of Interferon 229
   C. Interferon-Induced Reversion of the Transformed Phenotype 230
   D. Effect of Interferon on Oncogene-Transformed Cells 230
   E. Oncosuppressor Activity of Interferons 230
References 231

Chapter 5
Tumor Necrosis Factors
    I. Introduction 241
   II. Tumor Necrosis Factor β 242
       A. Structure of TNF-β and the TNF-β Gene 242
       B. Functions of TNF-β 242
       C. Antineoplastic Effects of TNF-β 242
  III. Tumor Necrosis Factor α 243
       A. Production of TNF-α 243
       B. TNF-α Structure and the TNF-α Gene 244
       C. The TNF-α Receptor 245
           1. Structure and Function of the TNF-α Receptor 246
           2. Molecular Heterogeneity of the TNF-α Receptor 246
           3. Regulation of TNF-α Receptor Expression 247
           4. TNF-α Inhibitors 247
       D. Postreceptor Mechanisms of Action of TNF-α 247
           1. Production of cAMP and cGMP 248
           2. Production of Prostaglandins 248
           3. Production of Polyamines 248
           4. Membrane GTP Binding and GTPase Activity 248
           5. Intracellular Calcium 248
           6. Phospholipid and Sphingolipid Metabolism 248
           7. Protein Phosphorylation 249
           8. Transcriptional Effects 249
           9. Effect of TNF-α on Proto-Oncogene Expression 249
          10. Cytotoxic Effects of TNF-α 250
          11. TNF-α-Induced Proteins 250
          12. Effects of TNF-α on DNA Synthesis 250
       E. Physiologic Effects of TNF-α 250
           1. Hematopoietic, Immune, and Inflammatory Processes 251
           2. Blood Vessels and Blood Coagulation 252
           3. Bone, Cartilage, and Muscle 253
           4. Endocrine and Reproductive Systems 253
       F. TNF-α as a Growth Factor 254
       G. Growth-Inhibiting and Cell-Killing Effects of TNF-α 254
       H. Cachectin-Related Activities of TNF-α 255
           1. Role of TNF-α in Infectious Diseases 255
           2. Role of TNF-α in Cancer-Associated Cachexia 256
       I. Effects of TNF-α on Tumor Cell Growth 256
           1. Tumor Regression by TNF-α Treatment 256
           2. Mechanisms of the Antineoplastic Effects of TNF-α 257
           3. Sensitivity of Tumor Cells to TNF-α 258
           4. Undesirable and Dangerous Effects of TNF-α 258
           5. Combination of TNF-α with Other Agents 259
           6. Tumor-Promoting Effects of TNF-α 259
           7. Differentiation-Inducing Effects of TNFs on Tumor Cells 260
  IV. Tumor Migration Inhibiting Factor 260
   V. Tumor-Killing Factor 260
References 261

Chapter 6
Erythropoietic Growth Factors
    I. Introduction 279
   II. Erythroid-Potentiating Activity 279
  III. Erythroid Burst-Promoting Activity 280

IV. Erythropoietin 281
　　　A. Origin and Synthesis of Erythropoietin 281
　　　B. Biological Effects of Erythropoietin 281
　　　C. Structure of Erythropoietin and the Erythropoietin Gene 282
　　　D. The Erythropoietin Receptor 282
　　　E. Postreceptor Mechanisms of Action of Erythropoietin 283
　　　F. Erythropoietin and Neoplastic Transformation 284
　V. Erythroid Differentiation Factor 285
References 286

Chapter 7
Platelet-Derived Growth Factor
　I. Introduction 293
　II. Structure of PDGF and the PDGF Genes 293
　　　A. The PDGF Genes 293
　　　B. Molecular Forms of PDGF 293
　III. Production of PDGF and PDGF-Like Polypeptides 294
　IV. Functions of PDGF 296
　V. The PDGF Receptor 297
　　　A. The PDGF Receptor Gene 298
　　　B. Biosynthesis and Structure of the PDGF Receptor 298
　　　C. Molecular Forms of the PDGF Receptor 298
　　　D. Phosphorylation of the PDGF Receptor 299
　　　E. Regulation of PDGF Receptor Expression 300
　　　F. Internalization and Processing of the PDGF Receptor 300
　VI. Transductional Mechanisms of PDGF Action 300
　　　A. Ras Proteins 300
　　　B. Protein Phosphorylation 301
　　　C. Phosphoinositide Metabolism and Translocation of Ca^{2+} 301
　　　D. Na^+/H^+ Antiport and Cytoplasmic Alkalinization 303
　　　E. Arachidonic Acid and Prostacyclin 303
　　　F. Modulation of Cellular Responses to PDGF 303
　VII. Effects of PDGF on EGF Action 303
　VIII. Posttransductional Mechanisms of Action of PDGF 304
　　　A. Protein Phosphorylation 304
　　　B. Cytoskeletal Changes 304
　　　C. RNA and Protein Synthesis 304
　　　D. Proto-Oncogene Expression 305
　IX. Role of PDGF in Mitogenic Processes 306
　X. PDGF and the Sis Oncoprotein 307
　　　A. Comparative Structures of PDGF and v-Sis 308
　　　B. The c-*sis* Proto-Oncogene 308
　　　C. Sis-Induced Transformation 309
　XI. PDGF and PDGF-Like Factors in Relation to Neoplasia 310
　　　A. PDGF-Induced Neoplastic Transformation 310
　　　B. Role of PDGF and PDGF-Like Factors in Neoplastic Diseases 310
　　　C. Production of PDGF and PDGF-Like Proteins by Transformed Cells ...311
　　　　　1. Human Osteosarcoma Cells 311
　　　　　2. Human Neural Tumors 312
　　　　　3. Other Human Tumors 313
　　　　　4. Embryonal Carcinoma Cells 313
　　　　　5. Virus-Transformed Cells 313
　　　D. Role of Proto-Oncogenes in v-*Sis*-Induced Transformation 314
　　　E. Role of PDGF in Oncogene-Induced Transformation 314
　XII. Non-PDGF-Like Factors Produced by Platelets 314
References 314

Chapter 8
Transferrins
- I. Introduction ... 335
- II. Structure and Synthesis of Transferrins ... 335
  - A. Human Transferrin ... 335
  - B. Rat Transferrin ... 336
  - C. Transferrins and the B-Lym-1 Protein ... 336
  - D. Lactotransferrin ... 337
  - E. Melanotransferrin ... 337
  - F. Hormonal Regulation of Transferrin Gene Expression ... 337
- III. The Transferrin Receptor ... 337
  - A. The Transferrin Receptor Gene ... 338
  - B. Structure of the Transferrin Receptor ... 338
  - C. Posttranslational Modification of the Transferrin Receptor ... 338
  - D. Transferrin Receptor Expression ... 339
    1. Regulation of Transferrin Receptor Expression ... 339
    2. Mechanism of Regulation of Transferrin Receptor mRNA ... 340
    3. Internalization of the Transferrin Receptor ... 341
  - E. Transferrin Receptors in Normal and Neoplastic Cells ... 342
    1. Testicular Transferrin Receptors ... 342
    2. Placental Transferrin Receptors ... 342
    3. Transferrin Receptors in Lymphocyte Activation ... 342
    4. Effect of Antitransferrin Receptor Antibodies ... 342
    5. Transferrin Receptors in Neoplastic Cells ... 343
    6. Neoplastic Cell Differentiation and Transferrin Receptor Expression ... 343
- IV. Effects of Transferrin on Cell Proliferation and Differentiation ... 344
  - A. Mechanisms of the Growth-Promoting Action of Transferrin ... 344
  - B. Tumor-Promoting Effects of Transferrin ... 344

References ... 344
Index ... 353

THE AUTHOR

Enrique Pimentel, M.D., is Professor of General Pathology and Pathophysiology at the School of Medicine, Central University of Venezuela, Caracas. He was formerly Director of the Institute of Experimental Medicine at the same university and founded and directed the National Center of Genetics in Venezuela.

Born on April 7, 1928, in Caracas, Venezuela, he obtained an M.D. degree from the Universities of Madrid, Spain, and Caracas, Venezuela, in 1953. He is President of the National Academy of Medicine in Venezuela and an honorary, corresponding, or active member of 32 national and international scientific academies and societies. He is an active member of the New York Academy of Sciences and Vice President of the International Academy of Tumor Marker Oncology (IATMO). He has received several decorations in his own country and the Grosse Verdienstrkreuz (Great Cross to the Merit) of the Federal Republic of Germany. In 1982 he received the National Award of Science in Venezuela. On many occasions Dr. Pimentel has been invited to give lectures and seminars at universities and other scientific institutions in North America and Europe.

Dr. Pimentel is the author of more than 100 papers and co-author of seven books on topics related to endocrinology, genetics, and oncology. In addition, he is the author of *Hormones, Growth Factors, and Oncogenes* and *Oncogenes* (first edition in one volume, second edition in two volumes) published by CRC Press. He is editor of the bimonthly journal Critical Reviews in Oncogenesis.

Chapter 1

Hematopoietic Growth Factors

I. INTRODUCTION

Normal cells circulating in the blood are relatively short-lived and need to be replaced constantly throughout life. A constant supply of mature blood cells is required to replace those lost through damage or senescence. The scale of this requirement is astonishingly large: in normal human adults about 3×10^6 red blood cells reach the end of their life span every second, and a slightly smaller number of white blood cells are similarly lost.[1] The process of blood cell formation (hematopoiesis or hemopoiesis) is not only enormous in scale but is also very complex, since cells of different hematopoietic lineages, each with multiple maturation stages, are apparently admixed at random within the bone marrow — the main site where hematopoiesis occurs in adult animals. Normal hematopoiesis must fulfill the maintenance of a dynamic equilibrium, constantly replacing mature blood cells lost through apoptosis (active cell death) or damage. The hematopoietic tissues must also respond in a rapid and controlled manner to acute challenges such as infection and hemorrhage.[2]

The normal site of hematopoiesis changes during development from the yolk sac to the liver to the bone marrow.[3] All blood cells originate from a small common population of multipotential stem cells with immortal characteristics associated with an extensive capacity for self-generation. Derangements of hematopoiesis may result in life-threatening diseases such as anemias, leukemias, and lymphomas.[4] Leukemias and lymphomas are clonal malignancies originated by deregulation of the maturation and proliferation of the respective blood cell precursors in the marrow and lymphoid organs. Leukemic blasts may be independent clones maintained by hematopoietic stem cells.[5] However, under normal conditions the hematopoietic system functions with remarkable fidelity as a consequence of regulation by an overlapping and precise system of control mechanisms.[6-9]

II. HEMATOPOIESIS

Maintenance of normal hematopoiesis requires a delicate balance between self-renewal and differentiation. These two processes depend on the presence of stem cells, which are characterized by a high capacity for self-renewal and by the potential to produce a differentiated progeny.[10] In contrast to the stem cells of the epidermis, hematopoietic stem cells are pluripotential and can give rise to more than one type of differentiated cell. Clinical and experimental observations indicate that all types of blood cells (erythrocytes, granulocytes, monocytes, lymphocytes, and megakaryocytes) originate from common stem cells (Figure 1). On this basis, the hematopoietic system may be divided into three compartments: (1) multipotential hematopoietic stem cells that possess extensive capabilities to give rise to new hematopoietic stem cells (self-renewal) and generate primitive progenitors that are programmed to differentiate (commitment); (2) progenitor cells committed to differentiation in a single specific lineage (erythropoiesis, granulopoiesis, or megakaryopoiesis); and (3) mature cells such as erythrocytes and granulocytes, which have lost the ability to proliferate.[11] However, fully differentiated hematic cells such as peripheral blood lymphocytes may be induced to grow when exposed to appropriate mitogens, including foreign substances such as plant lectins.

A. CONTROL OF HEMATOPOIETIC PROCESSES

The mechanisms involved in the control of hematopoiesis are only partially understood. It has been postulated that no humoral control would exist for the commitment of undifferentiated stem cells in one of the several lineages, and that this process is controlled by either stochastic or deterministic phenomena of an unknown nature. A stochastic model for multipotent hematopoietic progenitor cell differentiation proposes that there is a fixed probability that a progenitor with a potential for differentiation along a particular lineage maintains the potential in each cell division in each daughter cell, and this differentiation process of each lineage would proceed independently.[12] There is evidence that single murine hematopoietic progenitor cells can proliferate in the absence of any colony-stimulating factor (CSF) and serum.[13] In normal steady-state hematopoiesis the great majority of stem cells are at a quiescent (G_0) state, serving as a reserve from which the system may be replenished if it becomes depleted.[14] Only cells of the

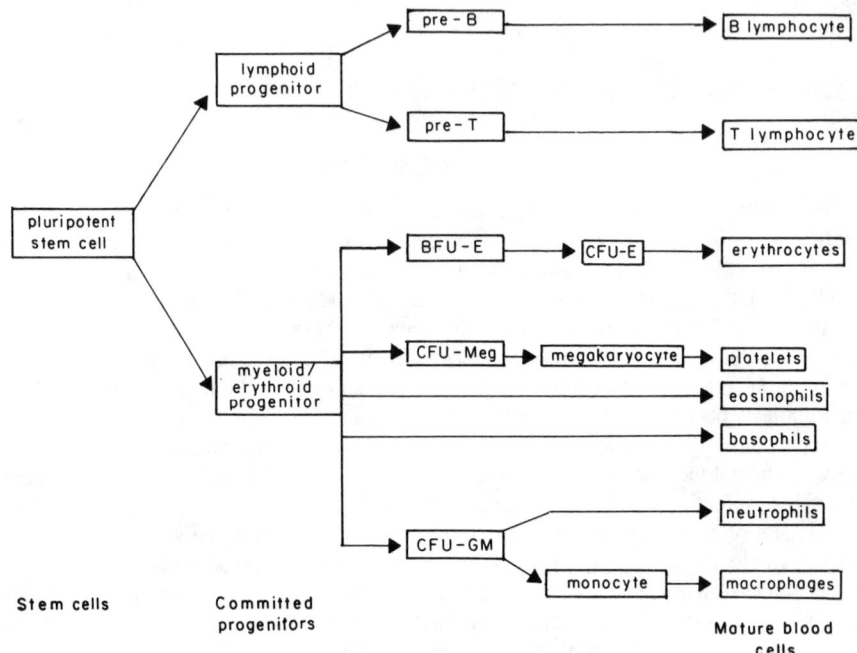

Figure 1.1 Stages of normal erythroid differentiation.

second compartment, i.e., progenitor cells committed to differentiation in a single lineage, would respond to humoral regulators represented by the hematopoietic growth factors (HGFs).[15] Hematopoietic cells may rapidly die in the absence of appropriate HGFs, and the HGFs, in particular the CSFs, are involved not only in stimulating the proliferation and differentiation of hematopoietic progenitors, but are also capable of promoting cell survival by suppressing apoptosis.[16]

B. REGULATION OF HEMATOPOIESIS BY GROWTH FACTORS

Endogenous regulation of the growth and differentiation of the different hematopoietic cell lineages depends, at least in part, on the action of signal molecules represented by the HGFs. An interplay between the hematopoietic progenitor cells and the bone marrow stroma is of essential importance for the action of both stimulatory and inhibitory factors involved in the regulation of hematopoiesis within the marrow microenvironment. A single cell appears to be capable of reconstituting the hematopoietic cells and their associated marrow microenvironment.[17] Two distinct subsets of pluripotent cells are present in human fetal bone marrow, one ($CD34^+$, $HLA-DR^+$, $CD38^-$) that can differentiate into all hematopoietic lineages, and another more primitive subset ($CD34^+$, $HLA-DR^-$, $CD38^-$) that can differentiate into hematopoietic precursors and stromal cells capable of supporting the differentiation of these precursors. Thus, in the early development of the hematopoietic system, common stem cells first generate stromal cells which give rise to a specific microenvironment which then induces the common stem cells to differentiate into hematopoietic stem cells. The structure and function of HGFs have been reviewed in many articles,[18-34] and is the subject of a book.[35]

In early studies, hematopoietic progenitors were exposed *in vitro* to different conditioned media that would provide the necessary HGFs. More recently, the characterization of HGFs has experienced a marked expansion with the availability of recombinant substances with specific HGF properties. The response of a hematopoietic progenitor to a given HGF may result in either its division or differentiation, depending in part on the physiological conditions and the stage of differentiation achieved by the cell. A given HGF, such as erythropoietin, may be capable of inducing two signals — one for proliferation and the other for differentiation — and the two signals are not necessarily linked in the progenitors.[36] The HGFs may act according to a hierarchical model of differentiation in which progenitor cells proceed sequentially through a program involving changes in growth factor sensitivity.[37] Not only progenitors located in the bone marrow, but also myeloid progenitors circulating in the peripheral blood may undergo this differentiation process. Specific combinations of different HGFs may be required for an optimal clonal proliferation of primitive myeloid bone marrow cells *in vitro* and probably also *in vivo*.[38]

Multiple HGFs with partially overlapping functions may operate both independently and in combination to regulate early stages of hematopoiesis.[39] Both stimulatory and inhibitory circuits operate in these regulatory processes.[40] Whether HGFs act on hematopoietic stem cells in a hierarchical or a synergistic manner is still a subject of controversy.[41] Moreover, the precise role of each known HGF on hematopoiesis as it occurs *in vivo* is not clear. Available evidence may not support the concept that hematopoiesis is totally controlled by circulating humoral factors, since some of the HGFs thus far identified are not found at detectable levels in the serum, even following perturbations that lead to increased myelopoiesis.[42] Considerable evidence exists suggesting that hematopoietic proliferation, at least at the stem-cell level, is locally controlled inside the bone marrow. The factors involved in this local control are unknown, but there is evidence suggesting that they may be replaced by rather unspecific stimuli. Tumor-promoting phorbol esters not only enhance the effects of a pluripotent HGF on mouse hematopoietic stem cells *in vitro*, but can also promote the survival and proliferation of colony-forming units even under serum-free conditions.[43,44]

The HGFs can be broadly classified into two groups: multilineage HGFs and lineage-specific HGFs. Multilineage HGFs are able to stimulate the growth of more than one lineage of hematopoietic cells.[45,46] CSF-2 and IL-3 (multi-CSF) are multilineage CSFs, capable of supporting the proliferation of a broad variety of hematopoietic cell types. CSF-3 would be capable of stimulating the growth of multipotential hematopoietic precursors.[47] However, CSF-3, as a single agent, does not appear to be able to support the growth of multipotential progenitors but may act synergistically with IL-3 to shorten the G_0 period of stem cells.[48] A recently developed methodology for the purification and abundant recovery of early hematopoietic progenitors from normal human adult peripheral blood may contribute to a better knowledge of factors specifically involved in the regulation of hematopoiesis.[49] Using this method, it has been shown that pure hematopoietic progenitors require for their proliferation, in addition to IL-3, CSF-2, and erythropoietin, the permissive effect of basic FGF. This factor influences early- and late-stage hematopoietic cell progenitors and exhibits synergistic activity with HGFs.[50] The leukemia inhibitory factor (LIF) is also capable, along with IL-6 and CSF-3, to regulate early hematopoietic stem cells.[51] LIF is as effective as IL-6 and CSF-3 in the enhancement of IL-3-dependent colony formation of primitive blast colony-forming cells. It is thus clear that multiple cytokines and HGFs are required for the regulation of early hematopoiesis. The action of multilineage HGFs/CSFs may be exerted, at least in part, through a common intracellular pathway involving protein kinase C activation.[52]

In addition to the HGFs, many other hormones and growth factors may be involved in the control of hematopoiesis. IGF-I and its receptor are required for the proliferation of hematopoietic cells.[53] The hepatocyte growth factor (HCGF) is a synergistic factor for the growth of hematopoietic progenitor cells.[54] There is evidence of the existence of HGFs which remain only partially identified.[55] A factor derived from the KPB-M15 human myeloid leukemia cell line, and capable of supporting the survival and proliferation of early primitive progenitor cells of both granulocyte and erythroid lineages, may be represented by a 25-kDa glycoprotein.[56] An unidentified factor produced by PHA-stimulated human peripheral blood mononuclear cells can induce human myelomonocytic leukemia cell line RC-2A to differentiate toward macrophages.[57] A normal myeloid regulatory protein, MGI-2, with no CSF or IL-3 activity, can induce the differentiation of normal myeloid precursors through binding to specific receptors on the cell surface.[58] However, MGI-2 is probably identical to IL-6. Some of the known and unknown HGFs may not be specific for blood cells, but may be involved in the control of growth and differentiation of other types of cells or tissues. An unidentified growth factor activity contained in serum-free supernatants of human peripheral blood mononuclear cell cultures can stimulate DNA synthesis of human hematopoietic and nonhematopoietic tumor cells.[59]

Significant structural homologies exist among different types of HGFs, especially at their amino-terminal regions, but the possible functional meaning of these homologies is unknown.[60] In addition to their essential role in the regulation of hematopoiesis, some HGFs are able to stimulate the growth of clonogenic cells from nonhematopoietic cell lines *in vitro*. IL-3, CSF-2, and CSF-3 can stimulate the growth of human colon adenocarcinoma cell lines HTB-38, CCL 187, and WiDr (CCL 218).[61] The biological significance of this heterologous regulation is unknown. HGFs may stimulate some consensus biochemical and molecular events regardless of the specificity detailed by unique ligand and receptor structures.[62] Stimulation of the phosphorylation of cellular proteins on tyrosine and nontyrosine residues plays a central role in the mechanisms of action of HGFs. These changes may lead to changes in many cellular functions, including gene expression.

C. GENE EXPRESSION IN HEMATOPOIESIS

Regulation of hematopoietic processes by HGFs is effected, in part, through the expression of specific genes, which include homeobox-containing genes (*HOX* genes) as well as proto-oncogenes and tumor suppressor genes. Several *HOX* genes are selectively expressed in hematopoietic blast cells. A lineage- and stage-specific expression of *HOX*1 genes occurs in the human hematopoietic system.[63,64] Modulation of the expression of *HOX*2 genes can alter the phenotype of human hematopoietic cell lines.[65]

Activation of specific proto-oncogenes may play a role in normal hematopoiesis.[66] Proto-oncogene expression in bone marrow can be studied by *in situ* hybridization methods with radiolabeled probes.[67] Proto-oncogenes encoding tyrosine kinases or nuclear proteins have an important role in the regulation of hematopoietic cell functions.[68] High-level expression of c-*myc*, c-*myb*, c-*fes*, and other genes is observed in early precursors of the myeloid, erythroid, and megakaryocytic lineages (myeloblasts, promyelocytes, basophilic erythroblasts, and megakaryoblasts). Expression of c-*myc* and c-*myb*, but not c-*fes*, decreases in advanced stages of maturation of the myeloid lineage. No expression of c-*myc*, c-*myb*, and c-*fes* is detected in erythroblasts beyond the basophilic stage, whereas mature megakaryocytes exhibited high levels of mRNA for all three proto-oncogenes. These results suggest that c-*myc* and c-*myb* expression is related to the proliferation of myeloid and erythroid precursors, whereas c-*fes* expression is restricted to myeloid differentiation. In another study, low levels of expression of c-*myc*, c-*myb*, c-*fes*, and c-*raf* genes were observed in normal human bone marrow.[69] Whereas the c-*fos* gene was expressed at high levels in these cells, no expression of c-*sis* was detected. Proto-oncogenes encoding tyrosine kinases are actively expressed in hematopoietic cells.[70] Expression of oncosuppressor genes may also be regulated in hematopoiesis. The differential activation or inactivation of proto-oncogenes and oncosuppressor genes in hematopoietic cells is associated, at least in part, with the regulatory action exerted by endogenous hormones and growth factors in hematopoietic processes.

III. HEMATOPOIETIC GROWTH FACTORS

Hematopoietic growth factors (HGFs) are crucially involved in the regulation of hematopoiesis. In contrast to other growth factors, HGFs are strictly required, not only for the proliferation and differentiation of the target cells, but also for their survival. In the absence of particular HGFs, cultured hematopoietic cells die at a constant rate, but addition of the specific factor prevents cell death and allows the rapid proliferation of the progenitor cells to continue.

Production and secretion of HGFs in the intact animal occurs in a highly regulated microenvironment. Interaction between the different cell types that form the marrow microenvironment is most important for the regulation of hematopoiesis. Cells that supply HGFs in the bone marrow have not been completely characterized, but include endothelial cells, fibroblasts, macrophages, and lymphocytes. The microenvironment required for normal hematopoiesis is provided in part by bone marrow stromal cells, which can produce factors involved in the complex hematopoietic processes. Formation and maintenance of a layer of stromal cells is absolutely required for the occurrence of hematopoiesis in long-term cultures *in vitro*. Growth factors such as IGF-I are produced by marrow stromal cells.[71] Thymic stroma produces a growth factor, called thymic stroma-derived T-cell growth factor, which can induce the proliferation of immature thymocytes by synergy with various cytokines.[72]

Mesenchymal cells can support hematopoiesis in coculture systems *in vitro* by substituting for some of the regulatory functions characteristic of marrow stroma cells.[73] The IL-3-dependent, multipotent hematopoietic cell line FDCP-mix, cultured in the presence of IL-3 but in the absence of stromal cells, has a characteristic blast morphology; in the absence of IL-3 the cells die unless they are cocultured with marrow stromal cells or 3T3 cells. In the latter case they attach, proliferate, and differentiate on both normal and irradiated Swiss 3T3 cell layers without the addition of IL-3.[74] At the initial attachment sites of FDCP-mix and 3T3 cells, cellular recognition is mediated by the formation of microvillus cytoplasmic projections and extracellular matrix. These areas may be sites of membrane-bound adhesional molecules involved in the functional regulation of interacting cells. Specific HGFs may participate in such regulatory processes. IL-1 has been shown to induce stromal cells from the bone marrow, including endothelial cells and fibroblasts, to produce multilineage HGFs.[75] Stimulation with IL-1 increases the expression of genes for GM-CSF/CSF-2, G-CSF, and BSF-2/IL-6 by cells such as the ST-1 human stromal fibroblastoid cell line.[76]

Expression of genes related to HGF production can be studied in intact animals by stimulation with i.v. injection of bacterial endotoxin or LPS.[77] Whereas the genes encoding some HGFs remain silent in both the LPS-treated and untreated animals, other HGF genes show an increased rate of expression after the stimulation, and still other genes are constitutively expressed at similar levels in both the untreated and treated animals. Regulation of hematopoiesis within the bone marrow microenvironment may require the expression of particular genes by stromal cells, including proto-oncogenes. IL-1α and TNF-α induce the transcriptional expression of the c-*abl* gene in cultured human bone marrow stromal cells, suggesting that the c-Abl tyrosine kinase may have an important role in the regulation of hematopoiesis by HGFs.[78]

HGFs are produced by cells from tissues other than bone marrow *in vivo* as well as by certain cell lines maintained *in vitro*. Normal human mesothelial cells and human malignant mesothelioma cell lines can produce HGFs.[79] Mesothelial cells are the major cavity-lining cells in vertebrates, covering the large surface areas of the pleura, pericardium, and peritoneum, where they may serve as a first-line barrier to infection. Exposure of normal mesothelial cells to inflammatory mediators such as LPS and TNF-α increases the levels of mRNAs for HGFs such as CSFs and IL-1. Malignant mesothelioma cells may exhibit aberrant gene expression for multiple HGFs.

HGFs are released by human T cell lines grown in long-term culture under the stimulus of the T cell growth factor, IL-2.[80] EBV-negative human lymphoma cell lines produce HGFs, and some of these lines are able to function as feeder cells to promote colony formation by growth factor-dependent cell lines.[81] Cell lines that display feeder cell function release activities into supernatants able to replace their cellular source, and some of these endogenously produced growth-promoting activities can be replaced by known HGFs. Constitutive production of HGFs such as IL-1 by human leukemia cells may induce endothelial cells to overproduce CSFs, thus contributing to the unrestricted growth of leukemic cells.[82] Constitutive production of CSF-1 and TGF-β, but not other CSFs or interleukins, was observed in adherent layers from normal and chronic phase CML bone marrows.[83] However, expression of IL-1α, IL-1β, CSF-3, and IL-6 could be induced by exposure of the stromal cells to specific cytokines.

Growth and differentiation of hematopoietic cells induced by HGFs are mediated by their binding to specific receptors on the cell surface.[84,85] A hierarchical modulation in the expression of HGF receptors may determine the final effects of the different types of HGFs.[86] The cellular receptors for HGFs are labile and are continuously synthesized and degraded. Several of the HGFs can exist and function in a membrane-bound form and, conversely, several of the HGF receptors can exist as soluble molecules that retain ligand-binding activity.[87] The HGFs enhance the functional activity of mature cells and upregulate the levels of expression of receptors for HGFs that are required during differentiation as well as for the functioning of the differentiated cells.[88]

A. PLURIPOTENT HGFs

Certain humoral factors are able to stimulate the proliferation and differentiation of cells that possess the capability to form more than one blood cell type. These factors are designated multilineage growth factors, in contradistinction to lineage-specific growth factors which act at later stages, controlling cells already committed to form a particular type of cell.[89,90] Synergistic interaction between lineage-specific and multilineage growth factors is important for the regulation of hematopoiesis. Two distinct multilineage HGFs are represented by different types of molecules, termed hematopoietin 1 and hematopoietin 2, which display distinct biological properties.[91,92] Other pluripotent HGFs have been identified recently.

1. Hemopoietins

A pluripotent HGF, termed hemopoietin 1 or pluripoietin, was purified from a serum-free medium conditioned by the human urinary bladder carcinoma cell line HBT 5637. It appears to be represented by two molecular species of polypeptides with similar size and different charges that act on primitive hematopoietic cells, generating cells bearing receptors for CSF-1.[93,94] Similar or identical factors have been detected in the cell line HBT 5637.[95-97] Such factors have functions additional to that of stimulating the development of primitive multipotent bone marrow cells, and are able to cooperate with IL-2 in promoting the activity of lymphocyte subpopulations to develop NK cells.[98] This effect of hemopoietin 1 may be due to a rapid induction of IL-2 receptors in the lymphoid cells. Serological analysis using a monoclonal antibody against purified recombinant IL-1α and amino acid sequencing data demonstrated conclusively that hemopoietin 1 and IL-1α are identical molecules.[99,100] The activity previously designated as hemopoietin 2 is identical to IL-3.[101]

2. Stem Cell Growth Factor

An important advance in the knowledge of HGFs acting on very primitive, pluripotent hematopoietic progenitors has been the identification, cloning, and characterization of the stem cell growth factor (SCGF or SCF).[102,103] The SCGF is identical with the mast cell growth factor (MCGF). SCGF/SCF/MCGF was isolated from several sources, including Buffalo rat liver-conditioned medium, and was identified as the product encoded by the Steel *(Sl)* locus of the mouse.[104-110] The structure and functional expression of rat and human SCGF have been reported and the SCGF gene was mapped to human chromosome region 12q22.[111] The 142 amino-terminal residues of the murine SCGF protein are sufficient for biological activity.[112] SCGF acts on primitive hematopoietic stem cells by itself and also is a potent synergistic factor in combination with IL-3 or IL-1α.[113] Administration of SCGF to rats as a single i.v. injection causes a dose-dependent neutrophilia and lymphocytosis, as well as the appearance of immature myeloid cells and occasional blast cells in the circulation.[114] SCGF is involved in expanding the growth of mast cell populations.[115] It also functions as a chemoattractant for both mucosal and connective tissue-type mast cells.[116] Administration of SCGF to mice and rats promotes the development of connective tissue-type mast cells.[117] In combination with other HGFS, SCGF may have a role in human erythropoiesis and megakaryopoiesis.[118]

SCGF is the physiologic ligand of the product of the c-*kit* proto-oncogene, the c-Kit protein, which is a transmembrane receptor with tyrosine kinase activity.[119,120] Binding of SCGF to the c-Kit receptor on the cell surface induces dimerization and tyrosine phosphorylation of the receptor, which may lead to cellular proliferation.[121,122] SCGF binding to its receptor on the surface of intact cells induces circular actin reorganization and chemotaxis. A set of substrates is phosphorylated by activation of the c-Kit kinase.[123] The product of a proto-oncogene, *vav*, is a protein of 95 kDa (Vav), which may be a substrate for c-Kit protein kinase-induced tyrosine phosphorylation.[124]

The c-Kit receptor and its ligand have an important role in the survival and proliferation of primitive hematopoietic cells, but additional mechanisms are required for the proper development of these processes.[125] Only about 4% of low-density normal human bone marrow cells express the c-Kit/SCGF receptor protein. These cells are recognized by the monoclonal antibody YB5.B8, which binds to the extracellular domain of the c-Kit protein.[126] Human marrow cells positive for c-Kit express the CD33 and/or CD34 antigens and include early hematopoietic progenitors, multipotential and lineage-restricted progenitors, and developing mast cells. SCGF induces the proliferation and maturation of normal mast cells both *in vitro* and *in vivo*. Intradermal administration of SCGF to mice results in dermal mast cell activation and a mast cell-dependent acute inflammatory response.[127]

Cloning and functional analysis of the mouse c-*kit* promoter have been reported.[128] Transcripts of the c-*kit* gene are expressed in human and murine hematopoietic cells at early stages of erythroid and myeloid differentiation, but are not expressed in lymphoid lineages.[129] The c-Kit protein kinase may be involved, however, in regulating the proliferation of early pre-B cells.[130] Expression of c-Kit mRNA and protein in mast cells and stem cell progenitors is downregulated by IL-3, CSF-2, and erythropoietin.[131]

The c-*kit* gene is identical to the mouse dominant white spotting *W* locus, which has pleiotropic effects on the development of hematopoietic, melanocyte, and germ-cell lineages. Mutation of a homologous rat gene, *Ws*, is associated with anemia and deficiency in mast cells and melanocytes.[132] Expression of functional c-Kit receptors can rescue the genetic defect of *W* mutant mast cells.[133] Piebaldism, a human autosomal dominant genetic disease characterized by the presence of congenital patches of skin and hair from which melanocytes are completely absent, is the human homologue to dominant white spotting of the mouse and is associated with c-*kit* gene mutation.[134] SCGF is a survival factor for melanoblasts, but is not required for the early migration and initial differentiation of these cells.[135]

The c-Kit protein and its ligand, SCGF, may have an important role in gonadal development and function. The c-*kit* gene is expressed in germ cells of the mouse testis and SCGF mRNA is expressed in Sertoli cells.[136] SCGF expression in primary cultures of Sertoli cells is enhanced by treatment with cAMP analogs. Sertoli cells have a central role in the maintenance and normal function of the germinal epithelium. SCGF and the c-Kit receptor may be involved in oocyte growth and in facilitating the proliferation and/or differentiation of type A spermatogonia.[137] Mice homozygous for the viable Steel-Dickie mutation of the *Sl* locus, which encodes the SCGF, are sterile and severely anemic.[138] The SCGF/Steel factor is essential for the survival, but not the growth, of murine primordial germ cells in culture.[139,140]

The c-Kit/SCGF receptor and its ligand may have an important role in hematopoietic malignancies as well as in other types of human cancers. In several human AML cell lines, there is an association between proliferative potential and c-Kit protein expression.[141] The c-Kit protein is expressed on blast cells from most patients with ANLL and CML in blast crisis, but is absent on blastcells from patients with ALL expressing the T-lineage, B-lineage, or common ALL phenotypes.[142] Fresh human AML blast cells frequently express c-*kit* mRNA and respond in culture to SCGF with increases in self-renewal and terminal divisions.[143-145] The most obvious effects are seen when SCGF is combined with either IL-3 or

CSF-3. The response of AML cell lines to SCGF mirrors their expression of c-*kit*. Cells negative for c-*kit* expression do not respond to SCGF. Human SCGF stimulates growth of a human glioblastoma cell line that expresses the c-*kit* gene.[146] Coexpression of the SCGF and c-*kit* genes is found in the majority of small-cell lung cancers, suggesting an autocrine mechanism for these tumors.[147,148] The c-Kit receptor and its ligand may be involved in the growth control of mammary epithelium.[149] A decreased expression of the c-Kit receptor precedes the development of human breast cancer and is maintained in primary and metastatic breast cancer lesions.

3. Other Pluripotent HGFs

Growth factors capable of stimulating the proliferation of multipotential hematopoietic stem cells and progenitor cells have been isolated and purified from pokeweed mitogen-stimulated mouse spleen conditioned medium.[150] Two protein species of 24,000 and 19,000 Da, respectively, were identified in the purified factor, but the biological significance of these proteins, as well as their relation to other multipotential HGFs, is unclear. SCGF, produced by the KPB-M15 myeloid leukemia cell line and placenta, was characterized as a protein of 20 kDa.[151] SCGF shows diverse biological activities, including erythroid burst-promoting activity and granulocyte-macrophage colony potentiation.

B. COLONY-STIMULATING FACTORS

The biological activity of a diversity of glycoproteins with HGF activity is associated with their ability to stimulate cultured nonlymphoid clonogenic hematopoietic progenitors (bone marrow stem cells) to form clusters or colonies of differentiated cells in semisolid medium. For this reason these factors are called colony-stimulating factors (CSFs) or myeloid growth factors.[1,152-164] The colonies formed by CSF-stimulated precursor cells are constituted by authentic clones in which immature cells give rise to cells exhibiting morphological and functional characteristics of terminal differentiation. The CSFs are HGFs that stimulate the formation of neutrophils, eosinophils, basophils, and monocytes from marrow progenitor cells. However, CSFs exert important physiologic actions, not only on the proliferation of bone marrow progenitor cells, but also on the effector functions of mature blood cells including granulocytes and macrophages. While CSFs secreted by bone marrow cells, including endothelial cells and fibroblasts, serve to stimulate the proliferation and differentiation of myeloid progenitor cells, CSFs present in peripheral tissue sites such as areas of local infection would be involved in the activation of mature myeloid cell function.

CSFs are produced by mitogen-activated T lymphocytes as well as by a variety of other cell types including fibroblasts, macrophages, and endothelial cells. Uteroferrin, a 35-kDa glycoprotein induced in the uterus by treatment with progesterone, has colony-forming-unit (CFU) activity for committed erythroid and granulocyte-monocyte/macrophage cell lines.[165] Astrocytes, which may play a central role in the regulation of immune-mediated processes in the central nervous system, express transcripts encoding CSFs.[166] In the absence of exogenous activation stimuli, T lymphocytes and monocytes may not express transcripts for CSFs.[167] Certain tumor cell lines produce high amounts of CSF, and some of these lines are characterized by the simultaneous production of two different types of CSFs.[168] Thus, tumor cell lines have been exploited for the isolation and purification of CSFs and other types of HGFs. Normal human mesothelial cells and human malignant mesothelioma cell lines produce CSFs either spontaneously or upon stimulation with inflammatory mediators such as LPS and TNF-α.[79] EGF is an essential cofactor for the production of CSFs by normal and malignant human mesothelial cells. Expression of CSFs by human leukemic cells is partially regulated at a posttranscriptional level.[169]

Antigenical or biochemical markers can be used in certain cases for studying the effects of HGFs in responsive cells. Another approach to this purpose is represented by the measurement of specific receptors in cells incubated with putative HGFs. All CSFs exert their biological effects upon binding to specific, high-affinity receptors expressed on the surface responsive cells. The *in vitro* systems used to study the effects of CSFs usually contain serum, which has substances capable of modulating CSF activity. The assay of purified CSFs may be improved by using a serum-free methylcellulose medium that is able to support the growth of colonies derived from primitive erythroid and nonerythroid progenitors in the same cultures.[170,171] Unfortunately, some CSFs remain poorly characterized. The use of modern high-resolution purification procedures may contribute to the characterization of such CSFs and to the definition of their respective physiological roles.[172]

Recombinant human CSFs have been used to study the effects of CSFs on enriched population of human hematopoietic cells after a single pulse stimulation.[173] CSFs are classified according to the types of mature blood cells found in the resulting colonies. A number of CSFs can stimulate the proliferation of committed progenitors of the granulocyte-macrophage lineage. The macrophage CSF (M-CSF) or colony-stimulating factor-1 (CSF-1) stimulates the proliferation of progenitors committed to the macrophage lineage, while the granulocyte CSF (G-CSF), also termed colony-stimulating factor-3 (CSF-3),[159] stimulates the growth of progenitors committed to the granulocyte lineage. Another HGF, the granulocyte-macrophage CSF (GM-CSF) or colony-stimulating factor-2 (CSF-2), is capable of stimulating the proliferation of both the macrophage and granulocyte lineages. CSF-1 and CSF-2 may act independently, influencing the proliferative capacity of a single bone marrow progenitor cell population.[174] The actions of CSF-1 and CSF-2 on marrow progenitors are probably not redundant but may account for the heterogeneity existing in macrophage cell populations.[175] Alveolar macrophages which express a characteristic macrophage phenotype are not only able to proliferate but also have two potential fates: in the presence of CSF-2 they proliferate and continue to maintain their phenotype, whereas in the presence of CSF-1 they proliferate and develop into peritoneal macrophage-like cells.[176] These results suggest that one of the mechanisms controlling macrophage heterogeneity is based on the type of CSF.

IL-3 possesses CSF activity and is also known as multilineage CSF (multi-CSF). It supports the multilineage proliferation *in vitro* of early hematopoietic lineage cells which differentiate into mature cells of several lineages and is an obligatory HGF for growth factor-dependent hematopoietic cell lines. IL-3, CSF-2, and CSF-3 may stimulate the growth of distinct populations of granulocyte-macrophage colony-forming cells.[177] A megakaryocyte colony-stimulating factor (MK-CSF) is apparently identical to IL-3.[178] Stimulation of tyrosine phosphorylation of distinct sets of proteins may be a common cellular mechanism of action of interleukins and CSFs, including IL-2, IL-3, IL-4, and CSF-2.[179]

The CSFs do not generally act as isolated agents with each one controlling a specific step of hematopoiesis in a given cell type, but complex additive or synergistic interactions occur between the biological effects of different types of CSFs. Additive effects on the production of neutrophilia have been observed in rats injected with a mixture of IL-3 and CSF-3.[180] However, the hematopoietic cell populations upon which CSFs exert their physiological actions may be partially different. Distinct populations of granulocyte-macrophage colony-forming cells exist that respond to CSF-2, CSF-3, and IL-3.[177] CSF-2 and CSF-3 may interact synergistically, and this action is a direct effect on progenitor cells not stimulated by CSF-2 or CSF-3 alone.

The factors responsible for the regulation of CSF production and secretion *in vivo* are only partially known. Regulation of CSF biosynthesis takes place mainly at the level of transcription, and there is evidence that the different genes can be selectively induced by specific stimuli *in vitro*.[181] In suspensions of freshly isolated human blood monocytes, the T cell-derived factor IL-3 induces expression of the CSF-1 gene at the mRNA level as well as secretion of CSF-1, but has much less effect on expression of the CSF-3 gene. In contrast, LPS induces expression of the CSF-3 gene and secretion of CSF-3, but has a considerably lesser effect on expression of the CSF-1 gene. The interleukin IL-4, produced by T lymphocytes, stimulates the accumulation of CSF-1 and CSF-3 transcripts in human monocytes.[182] Complex interactions between different CSFs may be of utmost importance for the control of normal hematopoietic processes in the intact animal.[183,184] Bacterial endotoxin, IL-1, and TNF-α stimulate the expression of transcripts for several types of CSFs in endothelial cells, acting through independent pathways.[185] IL-1α and TNF-α induce *in vivo* CSF activity in mice in a dose- and time-dependent fashion.[186]

The growth-stimulatory action of CSFs on hematopoietic cells may be counterbalanced by factors with growth-inhibitory properties. TGF-β is a potent inhibitor of hematopoiesis *in vitro* and may have a critical role in balancing the function of the hematopoietic system *in vivo*. TGF-β is able to suppress the proliferation of hematopoietic stem and progenitor cells stimulated by CSFs.[187-190]

The role of CSFs in leukemogenic processes is little known, but appears to be a very complex one. The blasts of the majority of AML patients do not express CSF-2 and CSF-3 transcripts, but in some cases an altered pattern of CSF expression is detected, including abnormally large CSF mRNAs.[191] Most leukemic cells require an exogenous supply of particular CSFs, but in certain cases the leukemic cells may be able to partially supply their own growth factors.[192,193] In general, CSFs are active growth factors for human AML cells and their effects are frequently additive in promoting maximum colony size *in vitro*.

HGFs can regulate the growth and differentiation not only of normal hematopoietic cells but also of myeloid leukemic cells.[194] CSF-2 and CSF-3 induce differentiation of HL-60 human myeloid leukemia cells with suppression of clonogenicity.[195] However, the presence of the receptor for an HGF in a leukemic cell clone does not ensure a biological response. Combined treatment of specific HGFs with other types of differentiation inducers may be more effective than treatment with single HGFs. Biological response modifiers used for the treatment of leukemias may act, at least in part, through the induction of CSFs which can induce terminal differentiation of malignant hematopoietic progenitor cells.[196]

CSFs have found clinical application as agents with potentially beneficial properties for the therapy of selected hematologic diseases as well as in AIDS patients and cancer patients after intensive chemotherapy.[197] CSFs may have considerable promise for therapy of bone marrow failure states and can accelerate bone marrow engraftment as a result of their effect on stem cells. Recombinant CSFs have protective and reconstitutive properties in mice against the lethal effects of irradiation and the alkylating agent, cyclophosphamide, which is used for the treatment of human cancer.[198] However, caution should be exerted with the use of CSFs for therapeutic purposes. CSF-2 and CSF-3, in some cases, can stimulate the *in vitro* growth of blast cells from AML patients, and a striking synergism for stimulation of these cells may be observed when both factors are used together.[199]

C. CYTOKINES

Lymphocytes and other types of blood cells would be derived from a common progenitor, but it is not known whether there is a common progenitor for T and B lymphocytes or whether they directly descend from pluripotent lymphohematopoietic stem cells.[200] In any case, there is clear evidence that the differentiation and proliferation of cells committed to the lymphoid-cell lineage depends on the presence of specific humoral factors. Soluble proteins elaborated by lymphocytes and transmitting signals for the growth and differentiation of various cell types and for regulation of immune responses are called lymphokines.[201-205] The term lymphokine was originally introduced to designate nonantibody protein mediators of cellular immunity produced by activated lymphocytes. The similar monocyte products were termed monokines. Since neither the origin of lymphokines and monokines nor their effects are restricted to lymphoid cells and monocytic cells, the generic name cytokines may be conveniently applied to these extracellular mediators.[206-210] Endothelial cells and fibroblasts also produce similar cytokines, and there is evidence that cytokines may display some hormonal activities.[211] The cytokines are involved in important metabolic and endocrine functions.[212] The general biological importance of cytokines is indicated by the fact that cells producing certain types of cytokines are present even in invertebrates.[213]

The presence of cytokines in biological samples can be detected by different types of assays, including assays using monoclonal antibodies.[214] Activation of CD28, a 44-kDa glycoprotein expressed as a homodimer on the surface of a major subset of human T cells, results in the induction of multiple cytokine genes and the subsequent secretion of different types of cytokines by the activated cells.[215] In addition to lymphocytes, cytokines are produced by many other types of cells, including endothelial cells, marrow stromal cells, and fibroblasts. High levels of cytokine-encoding transcripts are present in different tissues from normal individuals, suggesting that cytokines may function in consort as regulators of cellular growth and function in normal tissues.[216] Cytokines produced by the vascular endothelium have an important role in mediating inflammatory reactions to noxious agents.[217] Recent evidence indicates that NGF can stimulate human B and T lymphocytes, inducing their growth and differentiation, and may thus be considered as an immunoregulatory cytokine.[218]

The mechanisms of cytokines signal transduction are similar to those of hormones and their physiologic actions may extend beyond the immune system. Reproductive functions, especially those related to the ovary, may be importantly influenced by cytokines locally produced by resident cells including macrophages, granulocytes, and lymphocytes.[219] The cytokines show considerable overlap in their effects on lymphoid, myeloid, and connective tissue target cells. Agents that can be considered as cytokines include the interleukins (ILs), the colony-stimulating factors (CSFs), the interferons (IFNs), and the tumor-necrosis factors (TNFs). The patterns of protein induction resulting from treating cells such as human fibroblasts with different cytokines (IFN-α, IFN-γ, IL-1α, IL-1β, and TNF-α) exhibit striking similarities.[220] The inclusion of these factors under the generic name of cytokines seems thus justified.

The cytokines are importantly involved in the regulation of both the generation and function of lymphocytes. In general, for stem cells, renewal and differentiation are incompatible alternatives, and differentiation is usually associated with progressive limitation in the proliferative capacity of the cell lineage. A terminally differentiated cell is usually a "dead cell" in relation to its inability to reproduce. However, this general concept does not appear to hold for lymphopoiesis.[14] Cells phenotypically recognized as differentiated T lymphocytes can be maintained in long-term culture provided the specific growth factor, IL-2, is included in the medium. A clone of differentiated B cells, capable of synthesizing a particular Ig species, may be expanded by cell proliferation *in vivo* under the appropriate antigenic stimulus. Both T and B lymphocytes are differentiated cells that maintain their capacity for proliferation after specific stimulation.

Lymphocyte mitogenic and activating factors such as lymphokines and interleukins were first identified in the supernatants of human lymphocyte cultures.[221,222] A number of factors have been classified in the category of lymphokines or interleukins.[223-226] According to their origin and functions, as well as to the assay systems used for their identification, these factors have been frequently designated and classified in confusing manners.[227] Soluble mediators required for optimal stimulation of T cell mitogenesis are IL-1 and IL-2.[228,229] IL-6 may also be an essential factor in T cell activation, but activation of human T lymphocytes by IL-1 and IL-6 appears to be due to the effects of these two interleukins on the production of and response to IL-2. Thus, IL-2 is a second messenger in the cascade of events triggered by the interaction of human T lymphocytes by IL-1 and IL-6.[230,231] Other interleukins may be produced thereafter in an orderly fashion, according to the cellular system and the physiologic conditions. IL-2, IL-4, and IL-5 are sequentially produced in mitogen-stimulated murine spleen cell cultures.[232] The cytokines were discovered through different means since they are frequently involved in multiple functions in many different organs and tissues, which resulted in designating the same substance by different names, according to the type of cell where its action was initially detected. Synonyms of cytokines and CSFs are listed in Table 1.

The number of known cytokines and interleukins has been increasing in the last few years, and there is evidence for the existence of more of these agents. Genes for putative cytokines have been isolated from stimulated lymphocytes. The gene for a protein, termed LD78, was isolated from PMA-stimulated human tonsillar lymphocytes by differential hybridization.[233] The LD78 protein is composed of 92 amino acids, and the LD78 gene exhibits homology in its 5' region with the genes for IL-2 and IFN-γ. Transcripts of the LD78 gene were detected in fresh samples of cells from patients with ANLL as well as in leukemic cell lines, but the normal function of the LD78 protein is unknown. LD78 may be the human counterpart of a macrophage inflammatory protein (MIP) that has been isolated from mouse peritoneal macrophages stimulated with endotoxin.

The existence of additional members of the cytokine family is also suggested by the detection and characterization of proteins that may function as receptors for unidentified cytokines. The human c-*mpl* proto-oncogene, which is the normal counterpart of the v-*mpl* oncogene contained in the myeloproliferative leukemia virus (MPLV), may encode a receptor subunit for a receptor subunit of a member of the cytokine receptor superfamily.[234] The putative c-Mpl cytokine receptor is a transmembrane protein which contains no consensus sequence for tyrosine kinase activity in its cytoplasmic domain. The murine c-*mpl* gene is transcribed in adult mouse spleen and bone marrow and its c-Mpl product transduces a proliferative signal.[235] The c-*mpl* gene is localized on chromosome 1p34 and is actively expressed in human hematopoietic cells.[236] The normal ligand of the c-Mpl receptor is unknown.

Complex endogenous and exogenous factors are involved in the regulation of lymphokine synthesis and secretion, including dietary influences.[237] Cytokines may play a role in the important bidirectional interactions that occur between nutrition, immune responses, and infectious diseases. Both the effects of nutrients on the pathogenesis of infectious, inflammatory, and neoplastic diseases and the effects of these diseases on nutrient status may be mediated, for the most important part, through cytokines.

Analysis of long-term T-cell clones indicates the existence of subsets of murine T helper (Th) cells that can be identified on the basis of their cytokine secretion profiles and their relative stage of development.[238] Th1 lines secrete IL-2, IL-3, IFN-γ, TNF-α, and CSF-2; whereas Th2 lines secrete IL-3, IL-4, IL-5, IL-6, IL-10, and CSF-2. The production of specific lymphokines may be differentially regulated in individual cells of a given clone, which would allow them to play partially independent roles in the host immune response.[239] However, the study of cytokine gene expression in a panel of 116 short-term murine T-lymphocyte clones, derived by single-cell micromanipulation from allogeneic mixed leukocyte cultures, showed that lymphokine production is randomly assorted among the T-cell clones and that there is no intrinsic preclusion of the expression of any combination of the cytokine production.[240]

Lymphokines are non-Ig peptide factors secreted by lymphocytes, whereas the monokines are produced and secreted by monocyte macrophages. Human monocyte subsets may exhibit a differential ability to release monokines after appropriate stimulation.[241] Both lymphokines and monokines are also produced by a wide variety of nonhematopoietic tissues — including epidermal, fibroblast, mesangial, and neural tissues — which justifies the use of the term cytokines for their designation. Cytokines are involved in immunologic and inflammatory reactions and may participate in the afferent or efferent aspects of these reactions. Important obstacles for the characterization of cytokines reside in the facts that a single cytokine may have a multiplicity of biological effects and, conversely, a number of cytokines may exert the same effect in a given bioassay. A comprehensive program was designed to isolate human cytokine genes and investigate their relative induction, as well as to analyze cytokine activities in cell culture, animal tumor models, and human clinical trials.[242]

Table 1 **Synonyms of Cytokines and Colony-Stimulating Factors**

Factor	Synonym
IL-1	Osteoclast-activating factor (OAF)
	Lymphocyte-activating factor (LAF)
	Hepatocyte-stimulating factor (HSF)
	Fibroblast-activating factor (FAF)
	B-cell-activating factor (BAF)
	Tumor inhibitory factor 2 (TIF-2)
	Keratinocyte-derived T-cell growth factor (KD-TCGF)
IL-2	T-cell growth factor (TCGF)
	T-cell mitogenic factor (TCMF)
IL-3	Hematopoietin 2
	Multipotential colony-stimulating factor (multi-CSF)
	Multilineage colony-stimulating activity (multi-CSA)
	Mast cell growth factor (MCGF)
	Erythroid burst-promoting activity (BPA-E)
IL-4	B-cell growth factor I (BCGF-I)
	B-cell stimulatory factor 1 (BSF-1)
IL-5	B-cell growth factor II (BCGF-II)
	Eosinophil colony-stimulating factor (Eo-CSF)
	Immunoglobulin A-enhancing factor (IgA-EF)
	T-cell replacing factor (TCRF)
IL-6	B-cell stimulatory factor 2 (BSF-2)
	B-cell hybridoma growth factor (BCHGF)
	Interferon β_2 (IFN-β_2)
	T-cell activating factor (TAF)
IL-7	Lymphopoietin 1 (LP-1)
	Pre-B-cell growth factor (pre-BCGF)
IL-8	Monocyte-derived neutrophil chemotactic factor (MDNCF)
	Granulocyte chemotactic factor (GCF)
	Neutrophil-activating peptide 1 (NAP-1)
	Leukocyte adhesion inhibitor (LAI)
	T-lymphocyte chemotactic factor (TLCF)
IL-9	T-cell growth factor III (TCGF-III)
	Factor P40
	Megakaryoblast growth factor (MKBGF)
	Mast cell growth enhancing activity (MEA or MCGEA)
IL-10	Cytokine synthesis inhibitory factor (CSIF)
IL-11	Stromal cell-derived cytokine (SCDC)
IL-12	Natural killer cell stimulating factor (NKCSF or NKSF)
	Cytotoxic lymphocyte maturation factor (CLMF)
TNF-α	Cachectin
TNF-β	Lymphotoxin
LIF	Differentiation-inducing factor (DIF)
	Differentiation-inducing activity (DIA)
	D factor
	Human interleukin for DA cells (HILDA)
	Hepatocyte stimulating factor III (HSF-III)
	Cholinergic neuronal differentiation factor (CNDF)
CSF-1	Macrophage colony-stimulating factor (M-CSF)
CSF-2	Granulocyte-macrophage colony-stimulating factor (GM-CSF)
CSF-3	Granulocyte colony-stimulating factor (G-CSF)

Accumulation of mononuclear cells at sites of antigenic challenge is partially mediated by the local production of lymphokines and monokines by activated mononuclear cells. IL-1 and TNF-α produced by monocytes stimulate T-cell colony formation by human peripheral blood lymphocytes.[243] Chemotactic factors for lymphocytes produced by mononuclear cells include IL-2 and IL-1 as well as another factor, the lymphocyte chemotactic factor. The latter is a protein of approximate 14,500 Da and is different from IL-1 and IL-2.[244] A human macrophage-derived factor that *in vitro* possesses chemotactic activity and *in vivo* induces granulocytosis upon systemic injection and skin reaction upon local injection in experimental animals may mediate effects similar to those of IL-1.[245] This factor is a 6.5-kDa protein which shows no homology with other known growth factors, but possesses an amino-terminal stretch of sequence which is identical to that derived from a cDNA clone isolated from mitogen-stimulated human leukocytes. Mast-cell and T-cell growth factor activities distinct from IL-2 and IL-3 have been identified and partially purified from the supernatant of an activated murine helper T-cell line.[246]

Synergistic and antagonistic actions occurring between different lymphokines are of crucial importance for the development of immune reactions to exogenous and endogenous agents. Interaction between monocytes and T lymphocytes is critical in the generation of an immune response. Monocytes present antigen to T cells in the context of class II MHC molecules and also augment the T-cell proliferative response by the release of soluble factors such as IL-1. Activated T lymphocytes, in turn, secrete factors which induce monocyte cytotoxic activities. TNF-α, TNF-β, and IFN-γ have been named lymphotoxins because they are secreted by activated lymphocytes and can display cytostatic properties for cells such as normal human keratinocytes.[247] T-cell-derived lymphokines such as IFN-γ and IL-2 may act in a sequential fashion on monocytes to amplify the immune response by establishing a positive feedback circuit.[248] In some cases immune reactions may result in tissue damage or destruction, especially during autoimmune processes. For example, destruction of the β cells in the pancreatic islets of Langerhans, leading to development of type I (insulin-dependent) diabetes mellitus, may result from a synergistic interaction of various cytokines (IL-2, IFN-γ, TNF-α, TNF-β, and IL-1) produced by the infiltrating lymphocytes, macrophages/monocytes, and NK cells in lesions of insulitis.[249]

Neovascularization is associated with chronic inflammatory lesions and requires endothelial cell proliferation. The combined effects of cytokines such as IFN-γ, IL-1, and TNF-α are of great importance in the regulation of local vascular proliferation.[250] Studies on human umbilical-vein endothelial cells performed *in vitro* indicate that low concentrations of IFN-γ stimulate cell proliferation, whereas IL-1 and TNF-α markedly inhibit the proliferation induced by a specific factor, the endothelial cell growth factor (ECGF).

The cellular effects of cytokines are initiated by their initial binding to specific receptors on the cell surface. Many cytokine receptors are members of the hematopoietin/cytokine receptor superfamily.[251] Members of this family include the receptors for IL-2, IL-3, IL-4, IL-5, IL-6, IL-7, IL-9, CSF-2, CSF-3, LIF, and erythropoietin, as well as the receptors for growth hormone, prolactin, and the ciliary neurotrophic factor (CNTF). The c-Mpl oncoprotein is also a member of this receptor superfamily. The receptors of this superfamily are transmembrane single-chain polypeptides which are characterized by the presence of highly conserved cysteine residues and a single WSXWS motif within a less well-conserved stretch of approximately 200 amino acids. This basic unit is duplicated in some members of the receptor superfamily, whereas other members contain Ig-like domains or fibronectin type III domains. Although these receptors do not possess intrinsic tyrosine kinase activity, their actions are frequently associated with the rapid phosphorylation of cellular proteins on tyrosine residues, suggesting that they can secondarily activate tyrosine kinases. Substrates of these kinases include, in addition to the receptors themselves, the PI 3-kinase, the 120-kDa GAP protein involved in Ras signal transduction, and the Raf-1 serine/threonine kinase.

The cellular responses to cytokines may be associated with changes in proto-oncogene expression.[252] Complex interactions between cytokines and their effector cells may play a central role in oncogenesis as well as in the development of immune responses against tumors.[253,254] The cytokines may act as autocrine growth factors in cancer. Tumor cells may stimulate lymphokine-activated killer (LAK) cells to release factors that may be cytotoxic for tumor targets, including IFN-γ and TNF-α.[255] Human monocyte macrophages selectively recognize and bind to cells expressing a tumorigenic phenotype.[256] Such binding probably represents a key step in the selective killing of tumor cells when it is followed by the secretion of lytic mediators. The tumoricidal activity of monocytes-macrophages would be capable, at least in some cases, of inhibiting the spreading and metastasization of tumor cells.

Cytokines may be useful for the treatment of human malignancies. Adoptive immunotherapy using IL-2 alone or in combination with LAK cells may result in regression of metastatic cancer in murine tumors, and a similar approach has given promising results for the treatment of selected types of human tumors. Preincubation of tumor cell lines with cytokines such as IFN-γ and TNF-α enhances the susceptibility to lysis of the tumor cells by infiltrating lymphocytes.[257] Local production of cytokines by lymphocytes infiltrating the tumor may prepare the tumor cells for lysis by cytotoxic effector T cells.

D. HEMATOPOIETIC INHIBITING FACTORS

Both stimulatory and inhibitory circuits operate in the complex regulation of hematopoiesis. The growth-stimulating effects of HGFs such as the CSFs and some lymphokines are counterbalanced by factors that act as inhibitors or suppressors of hematopoietic progenitor cell proliferation.[258] The lymphokines may not only have growth-stimulating effects but may also partly function as inhibitors of hematopoietic cell proliferation.[259] The name restrictins has been proposed to designate cytokines that minimize the options available for the hematopoietic cell and thereby determine its growth and differentiation.[260] Lymphotoxin and IFN-γ are factors with well-known growth-inhibiting properties, but other factors with similar properties may exist. Natural killer (NK) cells, which are morphologically represented by large granular lymphocytes, may be involved either directly or via unidentified humoral factors in the homeostasis and regulation of stem-cell growth and differentiation, exerting inhibitory effects on colony-forming units (CFUs) *in vitro* and *in vivo*.[261] Many negative regulators of hematopoietic cell growth remain poorly characterized.

TGF-β plays a critical role in hematopoiesis by acting as a potent negative regulator of early, but not late, blood cell proliferation and differentiation.[187,262] It inhibits CSF-1-dependent macrophage precursor proliferation *in vitro* in a dose-dependent manner.[263] The transition of pre-B cells to mature, functional B cells is inhibited by TGF-β.[264] An inhibitor of megakaryocyte colony formation, stored in the α granules of platelets, is identical to TGF-β.[265] The growth of differentiated-arrested, growth factor-dependent and growth-factor-independent leukemic myelomonocytic cells, but not those of leukemias blocked late in their lineage, is inhibited by TGF-β.[262] Both TGF-$β_1$ and TGF-$β_2$ inhibit CSF-2- and IL-3-induced proliferation and colony growth in soft agar of normal bone marrow cells and their leukemic counterparts.[188] However, not all of the effects of TGF-β on hematopoietic cells are growth inhibitory. Although TGF-β exerts an inhibitory effect on the development of erythroid and multilineage colony-forming cells, the growth of cells from the granulocyte-macrophage lineage may be enhanced by TGF-β.[189] The growth-inhibitory effects of TGF-β on primitive hematopoietic progenitor cells may be abrogated by IL-6 and CSF-3.

1. T-Cell-Derived Growth Inhibitors

An inhibitory lymphokine, the colony-inhibiting lymphokine (CIL), produced by a T-cell hybridoma human cell line, exerts a potent inhibitory effect on the growth of bone marrow progenitor cells.[266] It is possible that growth inhibitory factors such as CIL play a role in the pathogenesis of some cases of human diseases, including aplastic anemia.

A growth-inhibitory factor represented by a suppressor lymphokine produced by T-leukemia cell lines, called T-leukemia-derived suppressor lymphokine (TLSL), is similar but distinct to CIL.[267] TLSL is a protein of 80 kDa capable of inhibiting DNA synthesis, cell proliferation, and colony formation in a variety of malignant hematopoietic cell lines as well as in normal myelomonocytic progenitor cells from bone marrow and peripheral blood. Target cell lines of B-cell origin (Burkitt's lymphomas) are more sensitive to TLSL than granulocytic, monocytic, erythroid, and T-cell lines. TLSL is not directly cytotoxic against neoplastic cells, but has cytostatic effects, and cell death occurs *in vitro* subsequent to several days of TLSL-induced proliferative arrest. Maximal inhibition of proliferation occurs earlier and is not accompanied by a great loss of cell viability.

Two growth-inhibitory factors are produced by the human T-cell-derived CD1+/CD8+ clone, GI-CO-T-9.[268] These inhibitors are proteins apparently not related to known factors such as TNFs, IFNs, or ILs. Factors with growth-inhibitory activity may be produced *in vivo* in patients with T-cell leukemia. Marrow leukemic T lymphoblasts from a patient with T-cell acute leukemia associated with severe leukopenia produced, when stimulated *in vitro* with PHA, an inhibitory activity for myeloid progenitor cells.[269] These results suggest that leukemic cells may exert *in vivo* a regulatory action on hematopoietic progenitor cells.

2. Oncostatin M

Oncostatin M is a cytokine produced by the U-937 human histiocytic lymphoma cell line after simulation with phorbol ester.[270] Oncostatin M shows reversible growth-inhibitory properties to A375 melanoma cells and other types of tumor cells. A similar or identical factor is produced by normal macrophages and activated human T cells.[271] The cDNA and genomic cloning, sequence analysis, and functional expression in heterologous cells of oncostatin M have been reported.[272] Oncostatin M is a single-chain polypeptide of 28 kDa. Binding sites for oncostatin M are present in a diversity of human and nonhuman tumor cell lines as well as in normal blood cells.[273] Subsequent to binding, the factor is internalized and degraded. Available evidence suggests that oncostatin M is a growth regulator.

Oncostatin M is a multifunctional cytokine and is a naturally occurring mitogen for rabbit vascular smooth-muscle cells.[274] It may function as a growth factor for AIDS-associated Kaposi's sarcoma cells.[275,276] Oncostatin M is structurally related to LIF and IL-6, and its physiological effects are mediated by the gp130 IL-6 signal transducer.[277,278] Oncostatin M is internalized and degraded subsequent to binding. It is able to regulate the expression of proto-oncogenes such as c-*myc,* c-*jun,* and *egr*-1.[279] Tyrosine phosphorylation is involved in the mitogenic mechanisms of oncostatin M.

3. Murine Growth Inhibitory Factor
A growth inhibitory factor, GI, was detected in the conditioned medium of differentiation inducer-resistant murine myelocytic leukemia M1 cells, clone R-1.[280] The GI factor is capable of inhibiting the growth of other murine leukemia cells (WEHI-3B D$^+$ and J774.1) but does not affect the growth of monocytic (U-937 and THP-1) or myeloid (KG-1, ML-1, and HL-60) human leukemia cell lines or the growth of normal peritoneal macrophages. These results indicate that GI inhibits the growth of mouse monocytic leukemia cells in intermediate stages of differentiation.

4. Leukocyte Inhibitory Factor
A lymphokine, termed leukocyte inhibitory factor (LIF), was initially defined by its ability to inhibit the random migration of neutrophils. However, LIF has other functions, including effects on phagocytosis and cell-mediated killing of bacteria.[281] In addition, highly purified LIF induces a significant neutrophil-mediated, antibody-dependent cellular cytotoxicity, which suggests a role for LIF in neutrophil-mediated tumor immunity.[282] The ability of LIF to activate polymorphonucleated neutrophils is dependent on the availability of extracellular calcium.[283] LIF is discussed in detail at the end of Chapter 2.

5. Macrophage-Derived Growth Inhibitor
Macrophages from a variety of animal species synthesize a growth inhibitor which specifically acts on spleen CFUs.[284] The inhibitor, produced by human blood macrophages, is active against mouse cells. The macrophage-derived inhibitor of the growth of hematopoietic stem cells, termed stem-cell inhibitor (SCI), has been purified to homogeneity.[285] SCI acts in a reversible manner and is identical to a cytokine called macrophage inflammatory protein-1α (MIP-1α) and to the CFU-S inhibitory activity obtained from primary cultures of normal bone marrow cells.

E. ROLE OF HGFs IN NEOPLASTIC PROCESSES
Cancer is frequently associated with hematopoietic alterations, which may be either a consequence of malnutrition and treatment or a direct effect of the tumor on hematopoietic processes.[286] The possible role of HGFs in hematologic malignancies is unknown, but it has been recognized that HGFs and other related factors such as the cytokines are importantly involved in oncogenic processes,[287] including those affecting the hematopoietic system.[288] Tumor cells may be sensitive to the growth-inhibitory action of cytokines in the early stages of tumor progression, but may become resistant in the more advanced stages of tumorigenesis, which may facilitate the production of metastasis. A "multicytokine-resistant" phenotype may allow metastatically competent melanoma cells to proliferate in the foreign environment of the dermal mesenchyme as well as in distant organ mesenchymes.[289] At least in the initial stages of tumorigenesis, some growth factors may be useful for the management of malignant diseases, including hematopoietic neoplasms such as adult acute leukemia.[290]

Autocrine mechanisms involving growth factors may have a role in leukemic hematopoiesis.[291] However, in general, hematologic neoplasms are not associated with autocrine mechanisms involving unregulated production of HGFs by the malignant cells themselves. To the contrary, HGFs are usually mandatory for the proliferation of leukemic cell clones.[292] Most frequently, human leukemic cells fail to proliferate autonomously *in vitro* and require the presence of specific HGFs.[293-295] Human leukemic blast cells may respond *in vitro* to specific HGFs or combinations of HGFs,[296,297] and different combinations of HGFs may display synergistic or antagonistic effects on the growth of leukemic cells *in vitro*. Whereas some combinations have stimulatory effects on the growth of human leukemic cells, other combinations are growth inhibitory.[298,299] The fact that the cells from some hematopoietic neoplasms, such as precursor B-cell ALL, do not respond *in vitro* to known HGFs suggests the possible existence of HGFs not identified as yet.[300] However, autostimulatory mechanisms may occur in some leukemias and lymphomas, and may show heterogeneity within clones derived from a single disease, which indicates that they can arise by independent genetic events.[301] Cytokines may act as autocrine growth factors in some types of normal cells and may have a similar role in malignant diseases.[252]

The HGFs may be useful for the treatment of cancer patients. Myelosuppression is recognized as the main limiting factor in cancer chemotherapy, and recombinant HGFs may be used to reduce this complication and to improve the quality of life of patients receiving chemotherapy.[302] Moreover, HGFs are capable of inducing, in some cases, the differentiation of leukemic cells.[303,304] The clinical application of particular types of HGFs for the treatment of hematologic diseases, including different forms of leukemia and other neoplasms characterized by specific blocks in the processes of cellular differentiation, has been proposed.[305] However, the growth-promoting effects of certain HGFs may counterbalance or even surpasses their differentiation-inducing properties, rendering difficult the clinical use of HGFs for the treatment of human hematologic malignancies.[306] Caution should be used in clinical trials involving administration of HGFs since there is evidence that, at least in some cases, an exaggerated endogenous production of a HGF may favor the proliferation of neoplastic cells or may even induce the malignant transformation of normal cells. Expression of a HGF cDNA in a factor-dependent cell clone may result in autonomous growth and tumorigenicity.[307] The use of HGFs for the treatment of human hematologic neoplasms is further complicated by the fact that tumor cells may exhibit, in contrast to the normal hematopoietic progenitor cells, a markedly hetcrogeneous differentiation response to different types of HGFs when used either alone or in combination.[308] Some leukemic progenitors act as normal progenitors when exposed to HGFs.[309] Different leukemic patients may exhibit different responses to a particular HGF or to combinations of different HGFs.[310,311] Thus, the heterogeneity of tumor cells in different patients, or even in a given patient, is also reflected in their response to HGFs. Moreover, although the human leukemic cells may react to HGFs, they are usually inert in their capacity to undergo maturation. In a study on the effects of CSF-2 and CSF-3 on marrow cells from AML patients it was concluded that, whereas some leukemic cells may become morphologically differentiated in suspension culture, this may occur both with and without the addition of the CSFs.[312] Thus, evidence for a differentiation-inducing effect of CSFs was not definite. In general, the results of studies performed by various investigators do not provide much encouragement for the clinical use of HGFs to treat leukemic patients. The mechanisms of the heterogeneous response of leukemic cells to HGFs are not understood, but they may reflect cellular alterations as a consequence of malignant transformation. Such alterations may occur at the receptor or postreceptor levels, or both.

F. HGFs AND ONCOGENE-INDUCED TRANSFORMATION

Infection of multilineage hematopoietic cells with retroviruses may result in deregulated production of HGFs. Transformed mast cell lines derived from A-MuLV-infected cells present in murine multilineage colonies exhibited expression of multiple HGF genes, including the genes coding for IL-3, CSF-2, IL-6, and a pre-B-cell stimulatory factor.[313] Thus, expression of a variety of HGF genes may be coordinately upregulated in A-MuLV-transformed mast cells.

Expression of an oncoprotein in hematopoietic cells may alter their requirement for specific HGFs, but the exogenous supply of specific HGFs may still be required. Infection of long-term mouse marrow cultures with a molecular recombinant of RSV and M-MuLV which expressed high levels of the v-Src oncoprotein leads to increased capacity for self-renewal *in vitro*, but in the absence of stroma the cells required the exogenous supply of hemopoietin for continuous proliferation.[314] Moreover, although the balance between self-renewal, differentiation, and development was disturbed in the hematopoietic cells expressing the v-Src oncoprotein, injection of the cells into irradiated mice did not lead to the development of leukemia, indicating that the host regulatory mechanisms were sufficient to impose a restraint on unlimited growth of these cells.

Immature hematopoietic cells or mature blood cells infected with acute retroviruses, or transfected with cloned viral oncogenes, may exhibit strikingly altered responses to HGFs. For example, the infection of a murine helper/inducer T-cell clone (D10.G4) with K-MuSV, which carries the v-K-*ras* oncogene, resulted in altered mitotic responses to certain cytokines (IL-1, Il-2, and BSF-1/IL-4), as compared to the uninfected parental clone.[315] However, the infected cells remained dependent on exogenous growth factors for continued growth in culture.

IV. PROTO-ONCOGENE AND TUMOR SUPPRESSOR GENE EXPRESSION IN HEMATOPOIETIC CELLS

The relationships between HGFs produced by different blood cells (B-lymphocytes, T-lymphocytes, and macrophages) and the functions of proto-oncogene and tumor suppressor gene protein products are little understood. Tyrosine kinases related to the Src oncoprotein may function as signaling components in blood cells.[316] Distinct tyrosine kinase activities are expressed in B and T lymphocytes, and this expression may be related either to cell differentiation along different lymphocytic pathways or to lymphocyte activation in response to different stimuli.[317] It is interesting to look for possible relationships between these kinase activities and similar activities present in members of the Src superfamily of proteins. Nuclear oncoproteins have an important role in hematopoiesis and in the signaling mechanisms of mature blood cells. Hematopoietic progenitor cells (CD34+) express the highest levels of c-Myb and c-Myc protein, whereas c-Fos protein levels in CD34+ progenitor cells are similar to the levels of c-Fos in mature monocytes and granulocytes.[318] Granulocytes are the only hematopoietic cells which do not express detectable levels of c-Myb and c-Myc. The role of tumor suppressor gene products in normal hematopoietic processes is little understood. The p53 protein is not expressed in proliferating hematopoietic precursor cells, but its expression increases in the nonproliferative mature cells of all lineages, including B and T cells, monocytes, and granulocytes.[319] These changes suggest that p53 may play a role in hematopoietic cell differentiation, possibly by inhibition of cell proliferation.

A. EXPRESSION OF THE C-*MYC* GENE

Activation of resting lymphocytes by mitogens is associated with sequential changes in proto-oncogene expression.[320,321] In resting cultured mouse lymphocytes, the levels of c-*myc* mRNA are almost undetectable, but are induced 20-fold between 1 and 2 h after the addition of the T-cell-specific mitogen, concanavalin A, to the cell culture.[322] Similar results on c-*myc* induction are obtained with stimulation of mouse spleen cells by the B-cell-specific mitogen, LPS. Stimulation of human peripheral blood mononuclear cells with the T-cell mitogen PHA results in a definite increase in the level of expression of both c-*myc* and c-*myb* genes.[323,324] Antibody-induced activation of B lymphocytes is accompanied by a specific induction of c-*myc* expression in the early G₁ phase of the cell cycle, but BCGF is required for the entry of cells into the S phase of the cycle.[325] In addition to c-*myc*, the expression of genes encoding IL-2, the IL-2 receptor, and IFN-γ are rapidly stimulated in human peripheral blood T lymphocytes after stimulation with either PHA or PMA.[326] Expression of the putative proto-oncogene *bcl-2* is also enhanced after stimulation of B and T cells with mitogenic agents, including IL-2.[321] Induction of these genes occurs in the presence of cycloheximide, indicating that protein synthesis is not required for the induction. Moreover, the presence of IL-2 protein is not required for the transcriptional activation of either the c-*myc*, the IL-2 receptor, or the IFN-γ gene. In contrast, transferrin receptor gene transcription is initiated later in the course of T-cell activation and its expression requires *de novo* protein synthesis.[326]

Expression of the c-*myc* gene is regulated in normal human lymphocytes at several points in the cell cycle.[327] Peripheral blood mononuclear cells stimulated with PHA, phorbol ester (PMA), calcium ionophore (ionomycin), or the monoclonal antibody OKT3 (anti-antigen receptor complex) show marked increases in the levels of c-*myc* mRNA within 3 h. IL-2 has little effect on c-*myc* gene expression, but in combination with PHA it augments the levels of c-*myc* mRNA at 24 h, but not at 3 h. Adding inhibitors of lymphocyte proliferation to PHA-stimulated lymphocyte cultures reveals that cyclosporin A (a fungal metabolite that selectively inhibits T-cell proliferation), dexamethasone (a synthetic glucocorticoid), and the OKT11A antibody (which binds to the sheep erythrocyte receptor present on all human T cells) diminish levels of c-*myc* mRNA measured at 3 h and 24 h, whereas anti-Tac antibody (which binds to Il-2 receptors) inhibits at 24 h, but not at 3 h.[327] The IL-2-induced increase of c-*myc* gene transcriptional activity in human peripheral blood mononuclear cells was confirmed in an independent study.[328] Since binding of IL-2 to its receptor on T cells leads to activation of protein kinase C,[329,330] these results further suggest that protein kinase C may be involved in the regulation of c-*myc* gene expression in normal human cells.

Recombinant murine retroviruses expressing v-*myc* oncogenes abrogate the requirement for IL-2 or IL-3 in cell lines dependent from these factors.[331] The expression of c-*myc* induced by IL-3 is suppressed in the cells infected with the recombinant vector, but the mechanism of this phenomenon is unknown. The results suggest that the action of growth factors in their respective target cells may be mediated partially by their ability to induce c-*myc* gene expression.

B. EXPRESSION OF THE C-FOS GENE

Studies with *in situ* hybridization of cells from human and murine marrow indicate that the differentiation and maturation of normal erythroblasts, but not granulocytic and monocytic precursors, is associated with the expression of large amounts of c-*fos* mRNA.[332] Although the expression of c-*fos* is a common property of mature blood cells, in the mononuclear phagocyte lineage this expression is restricted to differentiated cells.[333] The levels of c-*fos* mRNA increase between 30 min and 1 h after the addition of PHA to human peripheral blood lymphocytes.[334] In general, c-*fos* expression correlates with signals that stimulate a G_0-to-G_1 cell cycle transition. A rapid increase in c-*fos* expression occurs during human monocyte differentiation induced by TPA in hematopoietic cell lines.[335] Expression of the c-*fos* gene occurs only when the cell lines are induced to enter the macrophage differentiation pathway, not when the cells differentiate to granulocytes. Expression of the c-*fms* proto-oncogene is also regulated during the differentiation of human monocytes.[336]

C. EXPRESSION OF THE C-MYB GENE

Altered expression of c-*myb* may have an important role in the control of blood cell proliferation and differentiation. Exposure of human peripheral blood mononuclear cells to a c-*myb*-specific antisense RNA oligomer before mitogen or antigen stimulation results in almost complete inhibition of endogenous c-*myb* mRNA and protein synthesis and blockade of T-cell proliferation.[337] The c-Myb protein is required for the transition through late G_1 or S phase of the cycle in stimulated lymphocytes. Downregulation of c-*myb* expression is a prerequisite for commitment of erythroid-cell differentiation induced by erythropoietin.[338] Study of MuLV-induced murine myeloid leukemia cell lines supports the concept that the c-*myb* gene is involved in the control of hematopoietic cell differentiation.[339]

D. EXPRESSION OF THE VAV GENE

The human *vav* gene, which was discovered through its oncogenic activation in esophageal carcinomas, is expressed exclusively in hematopoietic cells.[340,341] The *vav* proto-oncogene may be importantly involved in the signal transduction pathways that regulate the development and maintenance of the hematopoietic system.[342] The oncogenic potential of the *vav* gene is activated by deletion of the sequences encoding the amino-terminal region of its product.[343] The *vav* gene product is a protein of 95 kDa which contains helix-loop-helix (HLH) and leucine zipper motifs, as well as an SH2 region which is involved in mediating the interaction of Vav with tyrosine kinases in signaling processes such as the antigen-induced activation of B and T lymphocytes.[344-346] The structural features of the Vav protein suggest its direct function in linking cell-surface-generated signals to transcriptional control in the nucleus.

E. PROTO-ONCOGENE EXPRESSION IN THE INDUCED DIFFERENTIATION OF HEMATOPOIETIC NEOPLASTIC CELLS

Expression of c-*myc* and c-*myb* decreases when differentiation is induced in neoplastic human hemopoietic cell lines by treatment with various compounds such as calcitriol, DMSO, TPA, retinoic acid, or inhibitors of poly(ADP)-ribose polymerase.[347-355] The c-*myc* and c-*myb* proto-oncogenes are structurally related and their protein products are predominantly located in the nucleus.

Human promyelocytic leukemia cells HL-60 can be induced to differentiate *in vitro* along either the monocytic or the myeloid pathways, depending on the inducer used.[356] Induction of HL-60 cell differentiation by either TPA (monocyte pathway) or DMSO (myeloid pathway) is accompanied by a decrease in the rate of c-*myc* gene transcription.[353] Changes in c-*myc* gene expression in HL-60 cells induced to differentiate by treatment with DMSO could be caused by the simultaneously occurring inhibition of cell proliferation, since c-*myc* expression remains elevated in HL-60 growth-inhibited but undifferentiated cells.[352] In cultured mouse erythroleukemia (MEL) cells induced to differentiate into mature erythroid cells by DMSO, the level of c-*myc* mRNA decreases markedly after 2 h of treatment, then remains low until 12 h, but increases to pretreatment levels by 18 h.[357] Whereas the induced decline does not require new protein synthesis, the reappearance of c-*myc* mRNA is dependent on continued protein synthesis, suggesting the existence of both negative and positive regulatory mechanisms of c-*myc* expression. A cell cycle-dependent change in the levels of c-*myc* expression is observed in chemically induced differentiation of MEL cells.[358] Prior to inducer treatment, the level of c-*myc* mRNA is relatively constant throughout the cell cycle, but when the c-*myc* mRNA level is restored in inducer-treated cells it is more highly restricted to cells in the G_1 phase of the cycle. Thus, treatment with differentiation inducers may lead to a change in the cell-cycle regulation of c-*myc* gene transcriptional activity. A selective reduction of c-*myc* expression is also observed in Daudi cells (a line of lymphoblastoid cells derived from an

African Burkitt's lymphoma) under the influence of human IFN-β, and a close link would exist between reduction of c-*myc* expression and IFN-induced arrest of cells at the G_0/G_1 phase of the cell cycle.[359,360] IFN regulates c-*myc* expression in Daudi cells at the posttranscriptional level.

The levels of c-*myc* mRNA are regulated in human lymphocytes by modulators of cell proliferation.[327] In the Kr62 human leukemia cell line, hemin-mediated erythroid induction and cell proliferation are associated with changes in the expression of c-*abl* and c-*myc*.[361] In the murine myeloid leukemia cell line WEHI-3B, the expression of c-*myc* and c-*myb* decreases after the cells reach the monocyte stage of differentiation induced by treatment with CSF-3 plus a low concentration of actinomycin D.[362] Transcripts of other proto-oncogenes are either unaltered (c-*abl*, c-K-*ras*, and c-*fes*) or not detectable (c-*src*, c-*sis*, c-*mos*, c-*erb*-A, and c-*erb*-B) during the process of differentiation induced in the same cells. In contrast, there is a marked increase in the expression of c-*fos*, which is associated with monocyte differentiation. A similar increase in c-*fos* gene expression occurs when HL-60 human leukemia cells are induced to differentiate by treatment with TPA, but not when the induction is performed by treatment with calcitriol or retinoic acid, which indicates that c-*fos* expression is not an obligatory step in the differentiation of leukemic cells.[363] Moreover, HL-60 cell variants resistant to TPA can be induced to differentiate into macrophages in the absence of detectable changes in c-*fos* gene expression.[364] In quiescent, terminally differentiated macrophages, expression of c-*fos* is inducible by CSF-1.[363]

The F-MuLV is a replication-competent, chronic retrovirus capable of inducing acute nonlymphocytic leukemias in mice. F-MuLV-induced leukemias can be divided into two stages, based on the growth properties of the leukemia cells. In the early stage (stage I disease) of leukemia, the blast cells are unable to grow outside their normal hematopoietic environment (bone marrow or spleen), whereas in the late stage of leukemia (stage II disease), leukemia cells can grow at any site in the mouse and will form continuous cell lines *in vitro*. However, hematopoietic cells obtained from mice with stage I disease will grow as immortal cell lines if cultured in the presence of IL-3 or in a WEHI-3 cell-conditioned medium (WEHI-3 cells produce IL-3 constitutively).[365] Superinfection of F-MuLV-induced stage I disease cells with A-MuLV, which carries the v-*abl* oncogene, but not with H-MuSV, which carries the v-H-*ras* oncogene, determines IL-3 independency and proliferation in culture in the absence of exogenous growth factors.[366] Concomitant with the growth factor-independent growth, the A-MuLV-superinfected lines become tumorigenic in syngeneic mice. Neither A-MuLV- nor H-MuSV-infected normal mouse myeloid cell cultures produce growth factor-independent or tumorigenic cell lines. The molecular basis of these results is unclear. In particular, it is not known which factor induces IL-3 independence in the A-MuLV-infected cells. Analysis of these cells fails to support an autocrine model of tumorigenesis since the conditioned medium obtained from these cells does not support the growth of HGF-dependent cell lines. Moreover, no evidence of altered IL-3 gene transcription or rearranged IL-3 DNA sequences is found in such cells.[366] It would appear that instead of triggering the production of IL-3, action of the v-Abl protein makes IL-3 superfluous for the control of cell proliferation. A detailed discussion on the role of proto-oncogenes in cell proliferation and differentiation processes is contained in a book.[367]

REFERENCES

1. **Whetton, A.D. and Dexter, T.M.,** Myeloid haematopoietic growth factors, *Biochim. Biophys. Acta,* 989, 111, 1989.
2. **Daniel, C.P. and Dexter, T.M.,** The role of growth factors in haemopoietic development: clinical and biological implications, *Cancer Metast. Rev.,* 8, 253, 1989.
3. **Christensen, R.D.,** Hematopoiesis in the fetus and neonate, *Pediatr. Res.,* 26, 531, 1989.
4. **Sachs, L.,** The control of growth and differentiation in normal and leukemic blood cells, *Cancer,* 65, 2196, 1990.
5. **McCulloch, E.A., Minden, M.D., Miyauchi, J., Kelleher, C.A., and Wang, C.,** Stem cell renewal and differentiation in acute myeloblastic leukaemia, *J. Cell Sci.,* Suppl. 10, 267, 1988.
6. **Metcalf, D.,** The granulocyte-macrophage colony-stimulating factors, *Science,* 229, 16, 1985.
7. **Andreeff, M.,** Cell kinetics of leukemia, *Semin. Hematol.,* 23, 300, 1986.
8. **Sachs, L.,** The molecular control of blood cell development, *Science,* 238, 1374, 1987.
9. **Cronkite, E.P.,** Analytical review of structure and regulation of hemopoiesis, *Blood Cells,* 14, 313, 1988.
10. **Hall, P.A. and Watt, F.M.,** Stem cells: the generation and maintenance of cellular diversity, *Development,* 106, 619, 1989.

11. **Ogawa, M., Porter, P.N., and Nakahata, T.,** Renewal and commitment to differentiation of hemopoietic stem cells (an interpretative review), *Blood,* 61, 823, 1983.
12. **Tsuji, K. and Nakahata, T.,** Stochastic model for multipotent hemopoietic progenitor differentiation, *J. Cell. Physiol.,* 139, 647, 1989.
13. **Péléraux, A. and Eliason, J.F.,** Proliferation of single hemopoietic progenitor cells in the absence of colony-stimulating factors and serum, *Exp. Hematol.,* 17, 1032, 1989.
14. **McCulloch, E.A.,** Stem cells in normal and leukemic hemopoiesis, *Blood,* 62, 1, 1983.
15. **Golde, D.W. and Marks, P.A., Eds.,** *Normal and Neoplastic Hematopoiesis,* Alan R. Liss, New York, 1983.
16. **Williams, G.T., Smith, C.A., Spooncer, E., Dexter, T.M., and Taylor, D.R.,** Haemopoietic colony stimulating factors promote cell survival by suppressing apoptosis, *Nature,* 343, 76, 1990.
17. **Huang, S. and Terstappen, W.M.M.,** Formation of haematopoietic microenvironment and haematopoietic stem cells from single human bone marrow stem cells, *Nature,* 360, 745, 1992.
18. **Sachs, L.,** The molecular regulators of normal and leukaemic blood cells, *Proc. R. Soc. London,* B231, 289, 1987.
19. **Morstyn, G. and Burgess, A.W.,** Hemopoietic growth factors — a review, *Cancer Res.,* 48, 5624, 1988.
20. **Nicola, N.A.,** Hemopoietic cell growth factors and their receptors, *Annu. Rev. Biochem.,* 58, 45, 1989.
21. **Platzer, E.,** Human hemopoietic growth factors, *Eur. J. Haematol.,* 42, 1, 1989.
22. **Morse, E.E.,** Factors involved in the regulation of hematopoiesis, *Ann. Clin. Lab. Sci.,* 19, 65, 1989.
23. **Metcalf, D.,** The molecular control of cell division, differentiation commitment and maturation of haemopoietic cells, *Nature,* 339, 27, 1989.
24. **Pierce, J.H.,** Oncogenes, growth factors and hematopoietic cell transformation, *Biochim. Biophys. Acta,* 989, 179, 1989.
25. **Groopman, J.E., Molina, J.-M., and Scadden, D.T.,** Hematopoietic growth factors. Biology and clinical applications, *N. Engl. J. Med.,* 321, 1449, 1989.
26. **Golde, D.W.,** Hematopoietic growth factors — an overview, *Int. J. Cell Cloning,* 8(Suppl. 1), 4, 1990.
27. **Dexter, T.M., Heyworth, C.M., Spooncer, E., and Ponting, I.L.O.,** The role of growth factors in self-renewal and differentiation of haemopoietic stem cells, *Philos. Trans. R. Soc. London,* B327, 85, 1990.
28. **Devereux, S. and Linch, D.,** Haemopoietic growth factors, *Q. J. Med.,* 75, 537, 1990.
29. **Whetton, A.D.,** Regulation of haemopoietic cell development by growth factors, *Cell. Signal.,* 2, 323, 1990.
30. **Robinson, B.E. and Quesenberry, P.J.,** Hematopoietic growth factors — overview and clinical applications, *Am. J. Med. Sci.,* 300, 163, 1990; 300, 237, 1990; and 300, 311, 1990.
31. **Tabbara, I.A. and Robinson, B.E.,** Hematopoietic growth factors, *Anticancer Res.,* 11, 81, 1991.
32. **Olofsson, T.B.,** Growth regulation of hematopoietic cells — an overview, *Acta Oncol.,* 30, 889, 1991.
33. **Crosier, P.S. and Clark, S.C.,** Basic biology of hematopoietic growth factors, *Semin. Oncol.,* 18, 349, 1992.
34. **Sachs, L.,** The molecular control of hematopoiesis —from cloned development in culture to therapy in the clinic, *Int. J. Cell Cloning,* 10, 196, 1992.
35. **Mertelsmann, R. and Herrmann, F., Eds.,** *Hematopoietic Growth Factors in Clinical Applications,* Marcel Dekker, New York, 1990.
36. **Noguchi, T., Fukumoto, H., Mishina, Y., and Obinata, M.,** Differentiation of erythroid progenitor (CFU-E) cells from mouse fetal liver cells and murine erythroleukemia (TSA8) cells without proliferation, *Mol. Cell. Biol.,* 8, 2604, 1988.
37. **Caracciolo, D., Clark, S., and Rovera, G.,** Differential activity of recombinant colony-stimulating factors in supporting proliferation of human peripheral blood and bone marrow myeloid progenitors in culture, *Br. J. Haematol.,* 72, 306, 1989.
38. **Baltelmez, S.H., Bradley, T.R., Bertoncello, I., Mochizuki, D.Y., Tushinki, R.J., Stanley, E.R., Hapel, A.J., Young, I.G., Kriegler, A.B., and Hodgson, G.S.,** Interleukin 1 plus interleukin 3 plus colony-stimulating factor 1 are essential for clonal proliferation of primitive myeloid bone marrow cells, *Exp. Hematol.,* 17, 240, 1989.
39. **Leary, A.G., Zeng, H.Q., Clark, S.C., and Ogawa, M.,** Growth factor requirements for survival in G_0 and entry into the cell cycle of primitive human hematopoietic progenitors, *Proc. Natl. Acad. Sci. U.S.A.,* 89, 4013, 1992.

40. Pantel, K. and Nakeff, A., Lymphoid cell regulation of hematopoiesis, *Int. J. Cell Cloning,* 7, 2, 1989.
41. Quesenberry, P.J., Synergistic hematopoietic growth factors, *Int. J. Cell Cloning,* 4, 3, 1986.
42. Eaves, A.C. and Eaves, C.J., Maintenance and proliferation control of primitive hemopoietic progenitors in long-term cultures of human marrow cells, *Blood Cells,* 14, 355, 1988.
43. Hogans, B.B. and Spivak, J.L., Tumor-promoting phorbol esters stimulate the proliferation of interleukin-3 dependent cells, *J. Cell. Physiol.,* 137, 346, 1988.
44. Spivak, J.L., Hogans, B.B., and Stuart, R.K., Tumor-promoting phorbol esters support the in vitro proliferation of murine pluripotent hematopoietic stem cells, *J. Clin. Invest.,* 83, 100, 1989.
45. Clark-Lewis, I., Kent, S.B.H., and Schrader, J.W., Purification to apparent homogeneity of a factor stimulating the growth of multiple lineages of hemopoietic cells, *J. Biol. Chem.,* 259, 7488, 1984.
46. Platzer, E., Welte, K., Gabrilove, J.L., Lu, L., Harris, P., Mertelsmann, R., and Moore, M.A.S., Biological activities of a human pluripotent hemopoietic colony stimulating factor on normal and leukemic cells, *J. Exp. Med.,* 162, 1788, 1985.
47. Suda, T., Suda, J., Kajigawa, S., Nagata, S., Asano, S., Saito, M., and Miura, Y., Effects of recombinant murine granulocyte colony-stimulating factor on granulocyte-macrophage and blast colony formation, *Exp. Hematol.,* 15, 958, 1987.
48. Ikebuchi, K., Clark, S.C., Ihle, J.N., Souza, L.M., and Ogawa, M., Granulocyte colony-stimulating factor enhances interleukin 3-dependent proliferation of multipotential hemopoietic progenitors, *Proc. Natl. Acad. Sci. U.S.A.,* 85, 3445, 1988.
49. Gabbianelli, M., Sargiacomo, M., Pelosi, E., Testa, U., Isacchi, G., and Peschle, C., "Pure" human hematopoietic progenitors: permissive action of basic fibroblast growth factor, *Science,* 249, 1561, 1990.
50. Gallicchio, V.S., Hughes, N.K., Hulette, B.C., Della Puca, R., and Noblitt, L., Basic fibroblast growth factor (B-FGF) induces early- (CFU-s) and late-stage hematopoietic progenitor cell colony formation (CFU-gm, CFU-meg, and BFU-e) by synergizing with GM-CSF, Meg-CSF, and erythropoietin, and is a radioprotective agent in vitro, *Int. J. Cell Cloning,* 9, 220, 1991.
51. Leary, A.G., Wong, G.G., Clark, S.C., Smith, A.G., and Ogawa, M., Leukemia inhibitory factor differentiation-inhibiting activity/human interleukin for DA cells augments proliferation of human hematopoietic stem cells, *Blood,* 75, 1960, 1990.
52. Colon-Otero, G., Sando, J.J., Sims, J.L., McGrath, E., Jensen, D.E., and Quesenberry, P.J., Inhibition of hemopoietic growth factor-induced proliferation by adenosine diphosphate-ribosylation inhibitors, *Blood,* 70, 686, 1987.
53. Reiss, K., Porcu, P., Sell, C., Pietrzkowski, Z., and Baserga, R., The insulin-like growth factor-1 receptor is required for the proliferation of hematopoietic cells, *Oncogene,* 7, 2243, 1992.
54. Kmiecik, T.E., Keller, J.R., Rosen, E., and Vande Woude, G.F., Hepatocyte growth factor is a synergistic factor for the growth of hematopoietic progenitor cells, *Blood,* 80, 2454, 1992.
55. Li, C.L. and Johnson, G.R., Stimulation of multipotential, erythroid and other murine haematopoietic progenitor cells by adherent cell lines in the absence of detectable multi-CSF (IL-3), *Nature,* 316, 633, 1985.
56. Hiraoka, A., Ohkubo, T., and Fukuda, M., Further characterization of the biological properties of human hematopoietic survival and growth factor, *Exp. Cell Biol.,* 57, 27, 1989.
57. Lyons, A.B. and Ashman, L.K., Studies on the differentiation of the human myelomonocytic cell line RC-2A in response to lymphocyte-derived factors, *Leukemia Res.,* 11, 797, 1987.
58. Lotem, J. and Sachs, L., Regulation of cell-surface receptors for hematopoietic differentiation-inducing protein MGI-2 on normal and leukemic myeloid cells, *Int. J. Cancer,* 40, 532, 1987.
59. Sandru, G., Veraguth, P., and Stadler, B.M., Stimulation of tumor cell growth in humans by a mononuclear cell-derived factor, *Cancer Res.,* 48, 5411, 1988.
60. Schrader, J.W., Ziltener, H.J., and Leslie, K.B., Structural homologies among the hemopoietins, *Proc. Natl. Acad. Sci. U.S.A.,* 83, 2458, 1986.
61. Berdel, W.E., Danhauser-Riedl, S., Steinhauser, G., and Winton, E.F., Various human hematopoietic growth factors (interleukin-3, GM-CSF, G-CSF) stimulate clonal growth of nonhematopoietic tumor cells, *Blood,* 73, 80, 1989.
62. Farrar, W.L., Evans, S.W., Harel-Bellan, A., and Ferris, D.K., Molecular events associated with the action of haemopoietic growth factors, *J. Cell Sci.,* Suppl. 10, 243, 1988.
63. Vieille-Grosjean, I., Roullot, V., and Courtois, G., Lineage- and stage-specific expression of HOX-1 genes in the human hematopoietic system, *Biochem. Biophys. Res. Commun.,* 183, 1124, 1992.

64. **Vielle-Grosjean, I., Roullot, V., and Courtois, G.,** Identification of homeobox-containing genes expressed in hematopoietic blast cells, *Biochem. Biophys. Res. Commun.,* 185, 785, 1992.
65. **Shen, W.-F., Detmer, K., Mathews, C.H.E., Hack, F.M., Morgan, D.A., Largman, C., and Lawrence, H.J.,** Modulation of homeobox gene expression alters the phenotype of human hematopoietic cell lines, *EMBO J.,* 11, 983, 1992.
66. **Rowley, P.T. and Skuse, G.R.,** Oncogene expression in myelopoiesis, *Int. J. Cell Cloning,* 5, 255, 1987.
67. **Emilia, G., Donelli, A., Ferrari, S., Torelli, U., Selleri, L., Zucchini, P., Moretti, L., Venturelli, D., Ceccherelli, G., and Torelli, G.,** Cellular levels of mRNA from c-*myc,* c-*myb* and c-*fes onc*-genes in normal myeloid and erythroid precursors of human bone marrow: an *in situ* hybridization study, *Br. J. Haematol.,* 62, 287, 1986.
68. **Punt, C.J.A.,** Regulation of hematopoietic cell function by protein tyrosine kinase-encoding oncogenes, a review, *Leukemia Res.,* 16, 551, 1992.
69. **Evinger-Hodges, M.J., Dicke, K.A., Gutterman, J.U., and Blick, M.,** Proto-oncogene expression in human normal bone marrow, *Leukemia,* 1, 597, 1987.
70. **Perlmutter, R.M., Marth, J.D., Ziegler, S.F., Garvin, A.M., Pawar, S., Cooke, M.P., and Abraham, K.M.,** Specialized protein tyrosine kinase proto-oncogenes in hematopoietic cells, *Biochim. Biophys. Acta,* 948, 1989.
71. **Abboud, S.L., Bethel, C.R., and Aron, D.C.,** Secretion of insulinlike growth factor-I and insulinlike growth factor-binding proteins by murine bone marrow stromal cells, *J. Clin. Invest.,* 88, 470, 1991.
72. **Mizushima, Y., Saitoh, M., Ogata, M., Kosaka, H., Tatsumi, Y., Kiyotaki, C., Hamaoka, T., and Fujiwara, H.,** Thymic stroma-derived T cell growth factor (TSTGF). IV. Capacity of TSTGF to promote the growth of L3T4- Lyt-2- thymocytes by synergy with phorbol myristate acetate or various IL, *J. Immunol.,* 142, 1195, 1989.
73. **Roberts, R.A., Spooncer, E., Parkinson, E.K., Lord, B.I., Allen, T.D., and Dexter, T.M.,** Metabolically inactive 3T3 cells can substitute for marrow stroma cells to promote the proliferation and development of multipotent haemopoietic stem cells, *J. Cell. Physiol.,* 132, 203, 1987.
74. **Yamazaki, K., Roberts, R.A., Spooncer, E., Dexter, T.M., and Allen, T.D.,** Cellular interactions between 3T3 cells and interleukin-3-dependent multipotent haemopoietic cells: a model system for stromal-cell-mediated haemopoieisis, *J. Cell. Physiol.,* 139, 301, 1989.
75. **Lee, M., Segal, G.M., and Bagby, G.C.,** Interleukin-1 induces human bone marrow-derived fibroblasts to produce multilineage hematopoietic growth factors, *Exp. Hematol.,* 15, 983, 1987.
76. **Yang, Y.-C., Tsai, S., Wong, G.G., and Clark, S.C.,** Interleukin-1 regulation of hematopoietic growth factor production by human stromal fibroblasts, *J. Cell. Physiol.,* 134, 292, 1988.
77. **Troutt, A.B. and Lee, F.,** Tissue distribution of murine hemopoietic growth factor mRNA production, *J. Cell. Physiol.,* 138, 38, 1989.
78. **Andrews, D.F., III, Nemunaitis, J.J., and Singer, J.W.,** Recombinant tumor necrosis factor α and interleukin 1 α increase expression of c-*abl* protooncogene mRNa in cultured human marrow stromal cells, *Proc. Natl. Acad. Sci. U.S.A.,* 86, 6788, 1989.
79. **Demetri, G.D., Zenzie, B.W., Rheinwald, J.G., and Griffin, J.D.,** Expression of colony-stimulating factor genes by normal human mesothelial cells and human malignant mesothelioma cell lines in vitro, *Blood,* 74, 940, 1989.
80. **Lanfrancone, L., Ferrero, D., Gallo, E., Foa, R., and Tarella, C.,** Release of hemopoietic factors by normal human T cell lines with either suppressor or helper activity, *J. Cell. Physiol.,* 122, 7, 1985.
81. **Tweeddale, M., Jamal, N., Nguyen, A., Wang, X.H., Minden, M.D., and Messner, H.A.,** Production of growth factors by malignant lymphoma cell lines, *Blood,* 74, 572, 1989.
82. **Griffin, J.D., Rambaldi, A., Vellenga, E., Young, D.C., Ostapovicz, D., and Cannistra, S.A.,** Secretion of interleukin-1 by acute myeloblastic leukemia cells in vitro induces endothelial cells to secrete colony stimulating factors, *Blood,* 70, 1218, 1987.
83. **Wetzler, M., Kurzrock, R., Taylor, K., Spitzer, G., Kantarjian, H., Baiocchi, G., Ku, S., Gutterman, J.U., and Talpaz, M.,** Constitutive and induced expression of growth factors in normal and chronic phase myelogenous leukemia Ph_1 bone marrow stroma, *Cancer Res.,* 50, 5801, 1990.
84. **Brizzi, M.F., Avanzi, G.C., and Pegoraro, L.,** Hematopoietic growth factor receptors, *Int. J. Cell Cloning,* 9, 274, 1991.
85. **Olsson, I., Gullberg, U., Lantz, M., and Richter, J.,** The receptors for regulatory molecules of hematopoiesis, *Eur. J. Haematol.,* 48, 1, 1992.

86. **Walker, F., Nicola, N.A., Metcalf, D., and Burgess, A.W.,** Hierarchical down-modulation of hemopoietic growth factor receptors, *Cell,* 43, 269, 1985.
87. **Gordon, M.Y.,** Hemopoietic growth factors and receptors: bound and free, *Cancer Cells,* 3, 127, 1991.
88. **Lotem, J. and Sachs, L.,** Regulation of cell surface receptors for different hematopoietic growth factors on myeloid leukemic cells, *EMBO J.,* 5, 2163, 1986.
89. **Iscove, N.N., Roitsch, C.A., Williams, N., and Guilbert, L.J.,** Molecules stimulating early red cell, granulocyte, macrophage, and megakaryocyte precursor in culture: similarity in size, hydrophobicity, and charge, *J. Cell. Physiol.,* Suppl. 1, 65, 1982.
90. **Abkowitz, J.L., Holly, R.D., Segal, G.M., and Adamson, J.W.,** Multilineage, non-species specific hematopoietic growth factor(s) elaborated by a feline fibroblast cell line: enhancement by virus infection, *J. Cell. Physiol.,* 127, 189, 1986.
91. **Bartelmez, S.H., Sacca, R., and Stanley, E.R.,** Lineage specific receptors used to identify a growth factor for developmentally early hemopoietic cells: assay of hemopoietin-2, *J. Cell. Physiol.,* 122, 362, 1985.
92. **Bartelmez, S.H. and Stanley, E.R.,** Synergism between hemopoietic growth factors (HGFs) detected by their effects on cells bearing receptors for a lineage specific HGF: assay of hemopoietin-1, *J. Cell. Physiol.,* 122, 370, 1985.
93. **Jubinsky, P.T. and Stanley, E.R.,** Purification of hemopoietin 1: a multilineage hemopoietic growth factor, *Proc. Natl. Acad. Sci. U.S.A.,* 82, 2764, 1985.
94. **Stanley, E.R., Bartocci, A., Patinkin, D., Rosendaal, M., and Bradley, T.R.,** Regulation of very primitive, multipotent hemopoietic cells by hemopoietin-1, *Cell,* 45, 667, 1986.
95. **Platzer, E., Welte, K., Grabrilove, J.L., Lu, L., Harris, P., Mertelsmann, R., and Moore, M.A.S.,** Biological activities of a human pluripotent hemopoietic colony stimulating factor on normal and leukemic cells, *J. Exp. Med.,* 162, 1788, 1985.
96. **Gabrilove, J.L., Welte, K., Harris, P., Platzer, E., Lu, L., Levi, E., Mertelmann, R., and Moore, M.A.S.,** Pluripoietin α: a second human hematopoietic colony-stimulating factor produced by the human bladder carcinoma cell line 5637, *Proc. Natl. Acad. Sci. U.S.A.,* 83, 5478, 1986.
97. **Platzer, E., Oez, S., Welte, K., Sendler, A., Gabrilove, J.L., Mertelsmann, R., Moore, M.A.S., and Kalden, J.R.,** Human pluripotent hemopoietic colony stimulating factor: activities on human and murine cells, *Immunobiology,* 172, 185, 1986.
98. **Miglioratti, G., Cannarile, L., Herberman, R.B., Bartocci, A., Stanley, E.R., and Riccardi, C.,** Role of interleukin 2 (IL 2) and hemopoietin-1 (H-1) in the generation of mouse natural killer (NK) cells from primitive bone marrow precursors, *J. Immunol.,* 138, 3618, 1987.
99. **Mochizuki, D.Y., Eisenman, J.R., Conlon, P.J., Larsen, A.D., and Tushinski, R.J.,** Interleukin 1 regulates hematopoietic activity, a role previously ascribed to hemopoietin 1, *Proc. Natl. Acad. Sci. U.S.A.,* 84, 5267, 1987.
100. **Zsebo, K.M., Wypych, J., Yuschenkoff, V.N., Lu, H., Hunt, P., Dukes, P.P., and Langley, K.E.,** Effects of hematopoietin-1 activities on early hematopoietic cells of bone marrow, *Blood,* 71, 962, 1988.
101. **Metcalf, D.,** Multi-CSF-dependent colony formation by cells of a murine hemopoietic cell line: specificity and action of multi-CSF, *Blood,* 65, 357, 1985.
102. **Broxmeyer, H.E., Maze, R., Miyazawa, K., Carow, C., Hendrie, P.C., Cooper, S., Hacgoc, G., Vadhanraj, S., and Lu, L.,** The *kit* receptor and its ligand, steel factor, as regulators of hemopoiesis, *Cancer Cells,* 3, 480, 1991.
103. **Williams, D.E., Devries, P., Namen, A.E., Widmer, M.B., and Lyman, S.D.,** The steel factor, *Develop. Biol.,* 151, 368, 1992.
104. **Williams, D.E., Eisenman, J., Baird, A., Rauch, C., Van Ness, K., March, C.J., Park, L.S., Martin, U., Mochizuki, D.Y., Boswell, H.S., Burgess, G.S., Cosman, D., and Lyman, S.D.,** Identification of a ligand for the c-*kit* proto-oncogene, *Cell,* 63, 167, 1990.
105. **Flanagan, J.G. and Leder, P.,** The *kit* ligand: a cell surface molecule altered in steel mutant fibroblasts, *Cell,* 63, 185, 1990.
106. **Zsebo, K.M., Wypych, J., McNiece, I.K., Lu, H.S., Smith, K.A., Karkare, S.B., Sachdev, R.K., Yuschenkoff, V.N., Birkett, N.C., Williams, L.R., Satyagal, V.N., Tung, W., Bosselman, R.A., Mendiaz, E.A., and Langley, K.E.,** Identification, purification, and biological characterization of hematopoietic stem cell factor from Buffalo rat liver-conditioned medium, *Cell,* 63, 195, 1990.
107. **Martin, F.H., Suggs, S.V., Langley, K.E., et al.,** Primary structure and functional expression of rat and human stem cell factor DNAs, *Cell,* 63, 203, 1990.

108. Zsebo, K.M., Williams, D.A., Geissler, E.N., Broudy, V.C., Martin, F.H., Atkins, H.L., Hsu, R.Y., Birkett, N.C., Okino, K.H., Murdock, D.C., Jacobsen, F.W., Langley, K.E., Smith, K.A., Takeishi, T., Cattanach, B.M., Galli, S.J., and Suggs, S.V., Stem cell factor is encoded at the *Sl* locus of the mouse and is the ligand for the c-*kit* tyrosine kinase receptor, *Cell,* 63, 213, 1990.
109. Huang, E., Nocka, K., Beier, D.R., Chu, T.-Y., Buck, J., Lahm, H.-W., Wellner, D., Leder, P., and Besmer, P., The hematopoietic growth factor KL is encoded at the *Sl* locus and is the ligand of the c-*kit* receptor, the gene product of the W locus, *Cell,* 63, 225, 1990.
110. Anderson, D.M., Lyman, S.D., Baird, A., Wignall, J.M., Eisenman, J., Rauch, C., March, C.J., Boswell, H.S., Rauch, C., March, C.J., Boswell, H.S., Gimpel, S.D., Cosman, D., and Williams, D.E., Molecular cloning of mast cell growth factor, a hematopoietin that is active in both membrane bound and soluble forms, *Cell,* 63, 235, 1990.
111. Mathew, S., Murty, V.V.V.S., Hunziker, W., and Chaganti, R.S.K., Subregional mapping of 13 single-copy genes on the long arm of chromosome 12 by fluorescence *in situ* hybridization, *Genomics,* 14, 775, 1992.
112. Nishikawa, M., Tojo, A., Ikebuchi, K., Katayama, K., Fujii, N., Ozawa, K., and Asano, S., Deletion mutagenesis of stem cell factor defines the C-terminal sequences essential for its biological activity, *Biochem. Biophys. Res. Commun.,* 188, 292, 1992.
113. de Vries, P., Brasel, K.A., Eisenman, J.R., Alpert, A.R., and Williams, D.E., The effect of recombinant mast cell growth factor on purified murine hematopoietic stem cells, *J. Exp. Med.,* 173, 1205, 1991.
114. Ulich, T.R., del Castillo, J., Yi, E.S., Yin, S., McNiece, I., Yung, Y.P., and Zsebo, K.M., Hematologic effects of stem cell factor in vivo and in vitro in rodents, *Blood,* 78, 645, 1991.
115. Tsai, M., Takeishi, T., Thompson, H., Langley, K.E., Zsebo, K.M., Metcalfe, D.D., Geissler, E.N., and Galli, S.J., Induction of mast cell proliferation, maturation, and heparin synthesis by rat c-*kit* ligand, stem cell factor, *Proc. Natl. Acad. Sci. U.S.A.,* 88, 6382, 1991.
116. Meininger, C.J., Yano, H., Rottapel, R., Bernstein, A., Zsebo, K.M., and Zetter, B.R., The c-*kit* receptor ligand functions as a mast cell chemoattractant, *Blood,* 79, 958, 1992.
117. Tsai, M., Shih, L-S., Newlands, G.F.J., Takeishi, T., Langley, K.E., Zsebo, K.M., Miller, H.R.P., Geissler, E.N., and Galli, S.J., The rat c-*kit* ligand, stem cell factor, induces the development of connective tissue-type and mucosal mast cells in vivo. Analysis by anatomical distribution, histochemistry, and protease phenotype, *J. Exp. Med.,* 174, 125, 1991.
118. Avraham, H., Vannier, E., Cowley, S., Jiang, S., Chi, S., Dinarello, C.A., Zsebo, K.M., and Groopman, J.E., Effects of the stem cell factor c-*kit* ligand on human megakaryocytic cells, *Blood,* 79, 365, 1992.
119. Ikuta, K., Ingolia, D.E., Friedman, J., Heimfeld, S., and Weissman, I.L., Mouse hematopoietic stem cells and the interaction of c-*kit* receptor and steel factor, *Int. J. Cell Cloning,* 9, 451, 1991.
120. Ratajzak, M.Z., Luger, S.M., and Gewirtz, A.M., The c-*kit* proto-oncogene in normal and malignant human hematopoieisis, *Int. J. Cell Cloning,* 10, 205, 1992.
121. Kuriu, A., Ikeda, H., Kanakura, Y., Griffin, J.D., Druker, B., Yagura, H., Kitayama, H., Ishikawa, J., Nishiura, T., Kanayama, Y., Yonezawa, T., and Tarui, S., Proliferation of human myeloid leukemia cell line associated with the tyrosine phosphorylation and activation of the proto-oncogene c-*kit* product, *Blood,* 78, 2834, 1991.
122. Blume-Jensen, P., Claesson-Welsh, L., Siegbahn, A., Zsebo, K., Westermark, B., Heldin, C.-H., Activation of the human c-*kit* product by ligand-induced dimerization mediates circular actin reorganization and chemotaxis, *EMBO J.,* 10, 4121, 1991.
123. Herbst, R., Lammers, R., Schlessinger, J., and Ullrich, A., Substrate phosphorylation specificity of the human c-*kit* receptor tyrosine kinase, *J. Biol. Chem.,* 266, 19908, 1991.
124. Alai, M., Mui, A.L.-F., Cutler, M.L., Bustelo, X.R., Barbacid, M., and Krystal, G., Steel factor stimulates the tyrosine phosphorylation of the proto-oncogene product, p95^{vav}, in human hemopoietic cells, *J. Biol. Chem.,* 267, 18021, 1992.
125. Kodama, H., Nose, M., Yamaguchi, Y., Tsunoda, J., Suda, T., Nishikawa, S., and Nishikawa, S., In vitro proliferation of primitive hemopoietic stem cells supported by stromal cells: evidence for the presence of a mechanism(s) other than that involving c-*kit* receptor and its ligand, *J. Exp. Med.,* 176, 351, 1992.
126. Ashman, L.K., Cambareri, A.C., To, L.B., Levinsky, R.J., and Juttner, C.A., Expression of the YB5.B8 antigen (c-*kit* proto-oncogene product) in normal human bone marrow, *Blood,* 78, 30, 1991.

127. **Wershil, B.K., Tsai, M., Geissler, E.N., Zsebo, K.M., and Galli, S.J.,** The rat c-*kit* ligand, stem cell factor, induces c-*kit* receptor-dependent mouse mast cell activation in vivo. Evidence that signaling through the c-*kit* receptor can induce expression of cellular function, *J. Exp. Med.,* 175, 245, 1992.
128. **Yasuda, H., Galli, S.J., and Geissler, E.N.,** Cloning and functional analysis of the mouse c-*kit* promoter, *Biochem. Biophys. Res. Commun.,* 191, 893, 1993.
129. **André, C., d'Auriol, L., Lacombe, C., Gisselbrecht, S., and Galibert, F.,** c-*kit* mRNA expression in human and murine hematopoietic cell lines, *Oncogene,* 4, 1047, 1989.
130. **Rolink, A., Streb, M., Nishikawa, S.I., and Melchers, F.,** The c-*kit*-encoded tyrosine kinase regulates the proliferation of early pre-B-cells, *Eur. J. Immunol.,* 21, 2609, 1991.
131. **Welham, M.J. and Schrader, J.W.,** Modulation of c-*kit* mRNA and protein by hemopoietic growth factors, *Mol. Cell. Biol.,* 11, 2901, 1991.
132. **Alexander, W.S., Lyman, S.D., and Wagner, E.F.,** Expression of functional c-*kit* receptors rescues the genetic defect of *W* mutant mast cells, *EMBO J.,* 10, 3683, 1991.
133. **Tsujimura, T., Hirota, S., Nomura, S., Niwa, Y., Yamazaki, M., Tono, T., Morii, E., Kim, H.-M., Kondo, K., Nishimune, Y., and Kitamura, Y.,** Characterization of *Ws* mutant allele of rats: a 12-base deletion in tyrosine kinase domain of c-*kit* gene, *Blood,* 78, 1942, 1991.
134. **Giebel, L.B. and Spritz, R.A.,** Mutation of the *KIT* (mast/stem cell growth factor receptor) protooncogene in human piebaldism, *Proc. Natl. Acad. Sci. U.S.A.,* 88, 8696, 1991.
135. **Steel, K.P., Davidson, D.R., and Jackson, I.J.,** TRP-2/DT, a new early melanoblast marker, shows that steel growth factor (c-kit ligand) is a survival factor, *Development,* 115, 1111, 1992.
136. **Rossi, P., Albanesi, C., Grimaldi, P., and Geremia, R.,** Expression of the messenger RNA for the ligand of c-*kit* in mouse Sertoli cells, *Biochem. Biophys. Res. Commun.,* 176, 910, 1991.
137. **Manova, K., Huang, E.J., Angeles, M., De Leon, V., Sanchez, S., Pronovost, S.M., Besmer, P., and Bachvarova, R.F.,** The expression pattern of the c-*kit* ligand in gonads of mice supports a role for the c-*kit* receptor in oocyte growth and proliferation of spermatogonia, *Develop. Biol.,* 157, 85, 1993.
138. **Brannan, C.I., Lyman, S.D., Williams, D.E., Eisenman, J., Anderson, D.M., Cosman, D., Bedell, M.A., Jenkins, N.A., and Copeland, N.G.,** Steel-Dickie mutation encodes a c-*kit* ligand lacking transmembrane and cytoplasmic domains, *Proc. Natl. Acad. Sci. U.S.A.,* 88, 4671, 1991.
139. **Godin, I., Deed, R., Cooke, J., Zsebo, K., Dexter, M., and Wylie, C.C.,** Effects of the *steel* gene product on mouse primordial germ cells in culture, *Nature,* 352, 807, 1991.
140. **Dolci, S., Williams, D.E., Ernst, M.K., Resnick, J.L., Brannan, C.I., Lock, L.F., Lyman, S.D., Boswell, H.S., and Donovan, P.J.,** Requirement for mast cell growth factor for primordial germ cell survival in culture, *Nature,* 352, 809, 1991.
141. **Tohda, S., Yang, G.S., Ashman, L.K., McCulloch, E.A., and Minden, M.D.,** Relationship between c-KIT expression and proliferation in acute myeloblastic leukemia cell lines, *J. Cell. Physiol.,* 154, 410, 1993.
142. **Bühring, H.-J., Ullrich, A., Schaudt, K., Müller, C.A., and Busch, F.W.,** The product of the proto-oncogene c-kit (P145$^{c\text{-}kit}$) is a human bone marrow surface antigen of hemopoietic precursor cells which is expressed on a subset of acute non-lymphoblastic leukemic cells, *Leukemia,* 5, 854, 1991.
143. **Wang, C., Curtis, J.E., Geissler, E.N., McCulloch, E.A., and Minden, M.D.,** The expression of the proto-oncogene c-kit in the blast cells of acute myeloblastic leukemia, *Leukemia,* 3, 699, 1989.
144. **Wang, C., Koistinen, P., Yang, G.S., Williams, D.E., Lyman, M.D., and McCulloch, E.A.,** Mast cell growth factor, a ligand for the receptor encoded by c-kit, affects the growth in culture of the blast cells of acute myeloblastic leukemia, *Leukemia,* 5, 493, 1991.
145. **Ikeda, H., Kanakura, Y., Tamaki, T., Kuriu, A., Kitayama, H., Ishikawa, J., Kanayama, Y., Tonezawa, T., Tarui, S., and Griffin, J.D.,** Expression and functional role of the proto-oncogene c-*kit* in acute myeloblastic leukemia cells, *Blood,* 78, 2962, 1991.
146. **Berdel, W.E., de Vos, S., Maurer, J., Oberberg, D., von Marschall, Z., Schroeder, J.K., Li, J., Ludwig, W.-D., Kreuser, E.D., Thiel, E., and Herrmann, F.,** Recombinant human stem cell factor stimulates growth of a human glioblastoma cell line expressing c-*kit* protooncogene, *Cancer Res.,* 52, 3498, 1992.
147. **Hibi, K., Takahashi, T., Sekido, Y., Ueda, R., Hida, T., Ariyoshi, Y., Takagi, H., and Takahashi, T.,** Coexpression of the stem cell factor and the c-*kit* genes in small-cell lung cancer, *Oncogene,* 6, 2291, 1991.
148. **Rygaard, K., Nakamura, T., and Spang-Thomsen, M.,** Expression of the proto-oncogenes c-*met* and c-*kit* and their ligands, hepatocyte growth factor/scatter factor and stem cell factor, in SCLC cell lines and xenografts, *Br. J. Cancer,* 67, 37, 1993.

149. **Natali, P.G., NIcotra, M.R., Sures, I., Mottolese, M., Botti, C., and Ullrich, A.,** Breast cancer is associated with loss of the c-*kit* oncogene product, *Int. J. Cancer,* 52, 713, 1992.
150. **Cutler, R.L., Metcalf, D., Nicola, N.A., and Johnson, G.R.,** Purification of a multipotential colony-stimulating factor from pokeweed mitogen-stimulated mouse spleen cell conditioned medium, *J. Biol. Chem.,* 260, 6579, 1985.
151. **Hiraoka, A., Ohkubo, T., and Fukuda, M.,** Production of human hematopoietic survival and growth factor by a myeloid leukemia cell line (KPB-M15) and placenta as detected by a monoclonal antibody, *Cancer Res.,* 47, 5025, 1987.
152. **Metcalf, D.,** The granulocyte-macrophage colony-stimulating factors, *Science,* 229, 16, 1985.
153. **Metcalf, D.,** The molecular biology and functions of the granulocyte-macrophage colony-stimulating factors, *Blood,* 67, 257, 1986.
154. **Clark, S.C. and Kamen, R.,** The human hematopoietic colony-stimulating factors, *Science,* 236, 1229, 1987.
155. **Kaushansky, K.,** The molecular biology of the colony-stimulating factors, *Blood Cells,* 13, 3, 1987.
156. **Groopman, J.E.,** Colony-stimulating factors: present status and future applications, *Semin. Hematol.,* 25, 30, 1988.
157. **Weisbart, R.H., Gasson, J.C., and Golde, D.W.,** Colony-stimulating factors and host defense, *Ann. Int. Med.,* 110, 297, 1989.
158. **Andreeff, M. and Welte, K.,** Hematopoietic colony-stimulating factors, *Semin. Oncol.,* 16, 211, 1989.
159. **Pimentel, E.,** Colony-stimulating factors, *Ann. Clin. Lab. Sci.,* 20, 36, 1990.
160. **Metcalf, D.,** The colony-stimulating factors: discovery, development, and clinical applications, *Cancer,* 65, 2185, 1990.
161. **Golde, D.W.,** Overview of myeloid growth factors, *Semin. Hematol.,* 27(Suppl. 3), 1, 1990.
162. **Heyworth, C.M., Vallance, S.J., Whetton, A.D., and Dexter, T.M.,** The biochemistry and biology of the myeloid haemopoietic cell growth factors, *J. Cell Sci.,* Suppl. 13, 57, 1990.
163. **Gregory, S.H., Magee, D.M., and Wing, E.J.,** The role of colony-stimulating-factors in host defenses, *Proc. Soc. Exp. Biol. Med.,* 197, 349, 1991.
164. **Metcalf, D.,** Control of granulocytes and macrophages: molecular, cellular, and clinical aspects, *Science,* 254, 529, 1991.
165. **Bazer, F.W., Worthington-White, D., Fliss, M.F.V., and Gross, S.,** Uteroferrin: a progesterone-induced hematopoietic growth factor of uterine origin, *Exp. Hematol.,* 19, 910, 1991.
166. **Malipiero, U.V., Frei, K., and Fontana, A.,** Production of hemopoietic colony-stimulating factors by astrocytes, *J. Immunol.,* 144, 3816, 1990.
167. **Oster, W., Lindemann, A., Mertelsmann, R., and Herrmann, F.,** Regulation of gene expression of M-, G-, GM-, and multi-CSF in normal and malignant hematopoietic cells, *Blood Cells,* 14, 443, 1988.
168. **Sakai, N.N., Kubota, M., Shikita, M., Yokota, M., and Ando, K.,** Intraclonal diversity of fibrosarcoma cells for the production of macrophage colony-stimulating factor and granulocyte colony-stimulating factor, *J. Cell. Physiol.,* 133, 400, 1987.
169. **Ernst, T.J., Ritchie, A.R., O'Rourke, R., and Griffin, J.D.,** Colony-stimulating factor gene expression in human acute myeloblastic leukemia cells is posttranscriptionally regulated, *Leukemia,* 3, 620, 1989.
170. **Eliason, J.F. and Odartchenko, N.,** Colony formation by primitive hemopoietic progenitor cells in serum-free medium, *Proc. Natl. Acad. Sci. U.S.A.,* 82, 775, 1985.
171. **Eliason, J.F.,** Granulocyte-macrophage colony formation in serum-free culture: effects of purified colony-stimulating factors and modulation by hydrocortisone, *J. Cell. Physiol.,* 128, 231, 1986.
172. **Burgess, A.W., Metcalf, D., Kozka, I.J., Simpson, R.J., Vairo, G., Hamilton, J.A., and Nice, E.C.,** Purification of two forms of colony-stimulating factor from mouse L-cell-conditioned medium, *J. Biol. Chem.,* 260, 16004, 1985.
173. **Begley, C.G., Nicola, N.A., and Metcalf, D.,** Proliferation of normal human promyelocytes and myelocytes after a single pulse stimulation by purified GM-CSF or G-CSF, *Blood,* 71, 640, 1988.
174. **Lazar, G.S., Quon, D.H., and Lusis, A.J.,** A gene-controlling response of bone marrow progenitor cells to granulocyte-macrophage colony stimulating factors, *J. Cell. Physiol.,* 124, 293, 1985.
175. **Falk, L.A. and Vogel, S.N.,** Comparison of bone marrow progenitors responsive to granulocyte-macrophage colony stimulating factor and macrophage colony stimulating factor-1, *J. Leukocyte Biol.,* 43, 148, 1988.
176. **Akagawa, K.S., Kamoshita, R., and Tokunaga, T.,** Effects of granulocyte-macrophage colony-stimulating factor and colony-stimulating factor-1 on the proliferation and differentiation of murine alveolar macrophages, *J. Immunol.,* 141, 3383, 1988.

177. **McNiece, I., Andrews, R., Stewart, M., Clark, S., Boone, T., and Quesenberry, P.,** Action of interleukin-3, G-CSF, and GM-CSF on highly enriched human hematopoietic progenitor cells: synergistic interaction of GM-CSF plus G-CSF, *Blood,* 74, 110, 1989.
178. **Williams, N., Sparrow, R., Gill, K., Yasmeen, D., and McNiece, I.,** Murine megakaryocyte colony-stimulating factor: its relationship to interleukin 3, *Leukemia Res.,* 9, 1487, 1985.
179. **Morla, A.O., Schereurs, J., Miyajima, A., and Wang, J.Y.J.,** Hematopoietic growth factors activate the tyrosine phosphorylation of distinct sets of proteins in interleukin-3-dependent murine cell lines, *Mol. Cell. Biol.,* 8, 2214, 1988.
180. **Ulich, T.R., del Castillo, J., McNiece, I.K., Yin, S., Irwin, B., Busser, K., and Guo, K.,** Acute and subacute hematologic effects of multi-colony stimulating factor in combination with granulocyte colony-stimulating factor in vivo, *Blood,* 75, 48, 1990.
181. **Vellenga, E., Rambaldi, A., Ernst, T.J., Ostapovicz, D., and Griffin, J.D.,** Independent regulation of M-CSF and G-CSF gene expression in human monocytes, *Blood,* 71, 1529, 1988.
182. **Wieser, M., Bonifer, R., Oster, W., Lindemann, A., Mertelsmann, R., and Herrmann, F.,** Interleukin-4 induces secretion of CSF for granulocytes and CSF for macrophages by peripheral blood monocytes, *Blood,* 73, 1105, 1989.
183. **Broxmeyer, H.E., Williams, D.E., Cooper, S., Shadduck, R.K., Gillis, S., Waheed, A., Urdal, D.L., and Bicknell, D.C.,** Comparative effects in vivo of recombinant murine interleukin 3, natural murine colony-stimulating factor-1, and recombinant murine granulocyte-macrophage colony-stimulating factor on myelopoiesis in mice, *J. Clin. Invest.,* 79, 721, 1987.
184. **Broxmeyer, H.E., Williams, D.E., Hangoc, G., Cooper, S., Gillis, S., Shadduck, R.K., and Bicknell, D.C.,** Synergistic myelopoietic actions *in vivo* after administration to mice of combinations of purified natural murine colony-stimulating factor 1, recombinant murine interleukin 3, and recombinant murine granulocyte/macrophage colony-stimulating factor, *Proc. Natl. Acad. Sci. U.S.A.,* 84, 3871, 1987.
185. **Seelentag, W.K., Mermod, J.-J., Montesano, R., and Vassalli, P.,** Additive effects of interleukin 1 and tumour necrosis factor-α on the accumulation of the three granulocyte and macrophage colony-stimulating factor mRNAs in human endothelial cells, *EMBO J.,* 6, 2261, 1987.
186. **Vogel, S.N., Douches, S.D., Kaufman, E.N., and Neta, R.,** Induction of colony stimulating factor in vivo by recombinant interleukin 1α and recombinant tumor necrosis factor α, *J. Immunol.,* 138, 2143, 1987.
187. **Ohta, M., Greenberger, J.S., Anklesaria, P., Bassols, A., and Massagué, J.,** Two forms of transforming growth factor-β distinguished by multipotential haematopoietic progenitor cells, *Nature,* 329, 539, 1987.
188. **Sing, G.K., Keller, J.R., Ellingsworth, L.R., and Ruscetti, F.W.,** Transforming growth factor β selectively inhibits normal and leukemic human bone marrow cell growth in vitro, *Blood,* 72, 1504, 1988.
189. **Ottmann, O.G. and Pelus, L.M.,** Differential proliferative effects of transforming growth factor-β on human hematopoietic progenitor cells, *J. Immunol.,* 140, 2661, 1988.
190. **Kishi, K., Ellingsworth, L.R., and Ogawa, M.,** The suppressive effects of type β transforming growth factor (TGFβ) on primitive hemopoietic progenitors are abrogated by interleukin-6 and granulocyte colony-stimulating factor, *Leukemia,* 3, 687, 1989.
191. **Cheng, G.Y.M., Kelleher, C.A., Miyauchi, J., Wang, C., Wong, G., Clark, S.C., McCulloch, E.A., and Minden, M.D.,** Structure and expression of genes of GM-CSF and G-CSF in blast cells from patients with acute myeloblastic leukemia, *Blood,* 71, 204, 1988.
192. **Griffin, J.D. and Young, D.C.,** The role of colony stimulating factors in leukaemogenesis, *Clin. Haematol.,* 15, 995, 1986.
193. **Vellenga, E., Young, D.C., Wagner, K., Wiper, D., Ostapovicz, D., and Griffin, J.D.,** The effects of GM-CSF in promoting growth of clonogenic cells in acute myeloblastic leukemia, *Blood,* 69, 1771, 1987.
194. **Lotem, J., Shabo, Y., and Sachs, L.,** Role of different normal hematopoietic regulatory proteins in the differentiation of myeloid leukemic cells, *Int. J. Cancer,* 41, 101, 1988.
195. **Begley, C.G., Metcalf, D., and Nicola, N.A.,** Purified colony-stimulating factors (G-CSF and GM-CSF) induce differentiation in human HL60 leukemic cells with suppression of clonogenicity, *Int. J. Cancer,* 39, 99, 1987.
196. **Schlick, E. and Ruscetti, F.W.,** In vivo induction of terminal differentiation of malignant myelopoietic progenitor cells by CSF-inducing biological response modifiers, *Blood,* 67, 980, 1986.

197. Groopman, J.E., Clinical applications of colony-stimulating factors, *Semin. Oncol.*, 15, 27, 1988.
198. Talmadge, J.E., Tribble, H., Pennington, R., Bowersox, O., Schneider, M.A., Castelli, P., Black, P.L., and Abe, F., Protective, restorative, and therapeutic properties of recombinant colony-stimulating factors, *Blood*, 73, 2093, 1989.
199. Kelleher, C., Miyauchi, J., Wong, G., Clark, S., Minden, M.D., and McCulloch, E.A., Synergism between recombinant growth factors, GM-CSF and G-CSF, acting on the blast cells of acute myeloblastic leukemia, *Blood*, 69, 1498, 1987.
200. Rein, A., Keller, J., Schultz, A.M., Holmes, K.L., Medicus, R., and Ihle, J.N., Infection of immune mast cells by Harvey sarcoma virus: immortalization without loss of requirement for interleukin-3, *Mol. Cell. Biol.*, 5, 2257, 1985.
201. Oppenheim, J.J., Antigen nonspecific lymphokines: an overview, *Methods Enzymol.*, 116, 357, 1985.
202. Gearing, A.J.H., Johnstone, A.P., and Thorpe, R., Production and assay of the interleukins, *J. Immunol. Methods*, 83, 1, 1985.
203. Horohov, D.W. and Siegel, J.P., Lymphokines: progress and promise, *Drugs*, 33, 289, 1987.
204. Billingham, M.E.J., Cytokines as inflammatory mediators, *Br. Med. Bull.*, 43, 350, 1987.
205. Dinarello, C.A. and Mier, J.W., Lymphokines, *N. Engl. J. Med.*, 317, 940, 1987.
206. Oppenheim, J.J., Matsushima, K., Yoshimura, T., and Leonard, E.J., The activities of cytokines are pleiotropic and interdependent, *Immunol. Lett.*, 16, 179, 1987.
207. Harrison, L.C. and Campbell, I.L., Cytokines: an expanding network of immuno-inflammatory hormones, *Mol. Endocrinol.*, 2, 1151, 1988.
208. Arai, K., Lee, F., Miyajima, A., Miyatake, S., Arai, N., and Yokota, T., Cytokines: coordinators of immune and inflammatory responses, *Annu. Rev. Biochem.*, 59, 783, 1990.
209. Kennedy, R.L. and Jones, T.H., Cytokines in endocrinology — their roles in health and disease, *J. Endocrinol.*, 129, 167, 1991.
210. Aggarwal, B.B. and Pocsik, E., Cytokines: from clone to clinic, *Arch. Biochem. Biophys.*, 292, 335, 1992.
211. Smith, E.M., Hormonal activities of cytokines, *Chem. Immunol.*, 52, 154, 1992.
212. Andus, T., Palitzsch, K.-D., Gross, V., and Schölmerich, J., Metabolische und endokrine Funktionen der Zytokine, *Dtsch. Med. Wochenschr.*, 118, 306, 1993.
213. Beck, G., O'Brien, R.F., and Habicht, G.S., Invertebrate cytokines: the phylogenetic emergence of interleukin-1, *Bioessays*, 11, 62, 1989.
214. Mosmann, T.R. and Fong, T.A.T., Specific assays for cytokine production by T cells, *J. Immunol. Methods*, 116, 151, 1989.
215. Thompson, C.B., Lindsten, T., Ledbetter, J.A., Kunkel, S.L., Young, H.A., Emerson, S.G., Leiden, J.M., and June, C.H., CD28 activation pathway regulates the production of multiple T-cell-derived lymphokines/cytokines, *Proc. Natl. Acad. Sci. U.S.A.*, 86, 1333, 1989.
216. Tovey, M.G., Coantent, J., Gresser, I., Gugenheim, J., Blanchard, B., Guymarho, J., Poupart, P., Gigou, M., Shaw, A., and Fiers, W., Genes for IFN-β-2 (IL-6), tumor necrosis factor, and IL-1 are expressed at high levels in the organs of normal individuals, *J. Immunol.*, 141, 3106, 1988.
217. Pober, J.S., Cytokine-mediated activation of vascular endothelium — physiology and pathology, *Am. J. Pathol.*, 133, 426, 1988.
218. Otten, U., Ehrhard, P., and Peck, R., Nerve growth factor induces growth and differentiation of human B lymphocytes, *Proc. Natl. Acad. Sci. U.S.A.*, 86, 10059, 1989.
219. Adashi, E.Y., The potential relevance of cytokines to ovarian physiology: the emerging role of resident ovarian cells of the white blood cell series, *Endocrine Rev.*, 11, 454, 1990.
220. Beresini, M.H., Lempert, M.J., and Epstein, L.B., Overlapping polypeptide induction in human fibroblasts in response to treatment with interferon-α, interferon-β, interleukin 1α, interleukin 1β, and tumor necrosis factor, *J. Immunol.*, 140, 485, 1988.
221. Kasakura, S. and Lowenstein, L., A factor stimulating DNA synthesis derived from the medium of leukocyte cultures, *Nature*, 208, 794, 1965.
222. Gordon, J. and Maclean, L.D., A lymphocyte-stimulating factor produced in vitro, *Nature*, 208, 795, 1965.
223. Dinarello, C.A. and Mier, J.W., Interleukins, *Annu. Rev. Med.*, 37, 173, 1986.
224. Malkovsky, M., Sondel, P.M., Strober, W., and Dalgleish, A.G., The interleukins in acquired disease, *Clin. Exp. Immunol.*, 74, 151, 1988.
225. Strober, W. and James, S.P., The interleukins, *Pediatr. Res.*, 24, 549, 1988.
226. Mizel, S.B., The interleukins, *FASEB J.*, 3, 2379, 1989.

227. **Paul, W.E.,** Lymphokine nomenclature, *Immunol. Today,* 9, 366, 1988.
228. **Larsson, E.L., Iscove, N.N., and Coutinho, A.,** Two distinct factors are required for induction of T-cell growth, *Nature,* 283, 664, 1980.
229. **Smith, K.A., Lachman, L.B., Oppenheim, J.J., and Favata, M.F.,** The functional relationship of the interleukins, *J. Exp. Med.,* 151, 1551, 1980.
230. **Maizel, A.L. and Mehta, S.R.,** Effect of interleukin 1 on human thymocytes and purified human T cells, *J. Exp. Med.,* 153, 470, 1980.
231. **Houssiau, F.A., Coulie, P.G., and Van Snick, J.,** Distinct roles of IL-1 and IL-6 in human T-cell activation, *J. Immunol.,* 143, 2520, 1989.
232. **Cardell, S. and Sander, B.,** Interleukin-2, interleukin-4 and interleukin-5 are sequentially produced in mitogen-stimulated murine spleen cell cultures, *Eur. J. Immunol.,* 20, 389, 1990.
233. **Yamamura, Y., Hattori, T., Obaru, K., Sakai, K., Asou, N., Takatsuki, K., Ohmoto, Y., Nomiyama, H., and Shimada, K.,** Synthesis of a novel cytokine and its gene (LD78) expressions in hematopoietic fresh tumor cells and cell lines, *J. Exp. Med.,* 84, 1707, 1989.
234. **Vigon, I., Mornon, J.-P., Cocault, L., Mitjavila, M.-T., Tambourin, P., Gisselbrecht, S., and Souyri, M.,** Molecular cloning and characterization of *MPL,* the human homolog of the v-*mpl* oncogene: identification of a member of the hematopoietic growth factor receptor superfamily, *Proc. Natl. Acad. Sci. U.S.A.,* 89, 5640, 1992.
235. **Skoda, R.C., Seldin, D.C., Chiang, M.K., Peichel, C.L., Vogt, T.F., and Leder, P.,** Murine c-*mpl* — a member of the hematopoietic growth factor receptor superfamily that transduces a proliferative signal, *EMBO J.,* 12, 2545, 1993.
236. **Wendling, F. and Tambourin, P.,** La superfamille des récepteurs de cytokines et l'oncogène v-*mpl, MS Méd. Sci.,* 7, 569, 1991.
237. **Meydani, S.N.,** Dietary modulation of cytokine production and biological functions, *Nutr. Rev.,* 48, 361, 1990.
238. **Mosmann, T., Cherwinski, H., Bond, M.W., Geidlen, M., and Coffman, R.L.,** Two types of murine T helper cell. I. Definition according to profile of lymphocyte activities and secreted proteins, *J. Immunol.,* 136, 2348, 1986.
239. **Kelso, A. and Owens, T.,** Production of two hemopoietic growth factors is differentially regulated in single T lymphocytes activated with an anti-T cell receptor antibody, *J. Immunol.,* 140, 1159, 1988.
240. **Kelso, A. and Gough, N.M.,** Coexpression of granulocyte-macrophage colony-stimulating factor, γ interferon, and interleukins 3 and 4 is random in murine alloreactive T-lymphocyte clones, *Proc. Natl. Acad. Sci. U.S.A.,* 85, 9189, 1988.
241. **Akiyama, Y., Stevenson, G.W., Schlick, E., Matsushima, K., Miller, P.J., and Stevenson, H.C.,** Differential ability of human blood monocyte subsets to release various cytokines, *J. Leukocyte Biol.,* 37, 519, 1985.
242. **Bollon, A.P., Berent, S.L., Torczynski, R.M., Hill, N.O., Lemeshev, Y., Hill, J.M., Jia, F.L., Joher, A., Pichyangkul, S., and Khan, A.,** Human cytokines, tumor necrosis factor, and interferons: gene cloning, animal studies, and clinical trials, *J. Cell. Biochem.,* 36, 353, 1988.
243. **Zucali, J.R., Elfenbein, G.J., Barth, K.C., and Dinarello, C.A.,** Effects of human interleukin 1 and human tumor necrosis factor on human T lymphocyte colony formation, *J. Clin. Invest.,* 80, 772, 1987.
244. **Potter, J.W. and Van Epps, D.E.,** Separation and purification of lymphocyte chemotactic factor (LCF) and interleukin 2 produced by human peripheral blood mononuclear cells, *Cell. Immunol.,* 105, 9, 1987.
245. **Van Damme, J., Van Beeumen, J., Opdenakker, G., and Billiau, A.,** A novel, NH_2-terminal sequence-characterized human monokine possessing neutrophil chemotactic, skin-reactive, and granulocytosis-promoting activity, *J. Exp. Med.,* 167, 1364, 1988.
246. **Smith, C.A. and Rennick, D.M.,** Characterization of a murine lymphokine distinct from interleukin 2 and interleukin 3 (IL-3) possessing a T-cell growth factor activity and a mast-cell growth factor activity that synergizes with IL-3, *Proc. Natl. Acad. Sci. U.S.A.,* 83, 1857, 1986.
247. **Symington, F.W.,** Lymphotoxin, tumor necrosis factor, and γ interferon are cytostatic for normal human keratinocytes, *J. Invest. Dermatol.,* 92, 798, 1989.
248. **Herrmann, F., Cannistra, S.A., Lindemann, A., Blohm, D., Rambaldi, A., Mertelsmann, R.H., and Griffin, J.D.,** Functional consequences of monocyte IL-2 receptor expression. Induction of IL-1β secretion by IFNγ and IL-2, *J. Immunol.,* 142, 139, 1989.

249. **Pukel, C., Baquerizo, H., and Rabinovich, A.,** Destruction of rat islet cell monolayers by cytokines. Synergistic interactions of interferon-γ, tumor necrosis factor, lymphotoxin, and interleukin 1, *Diabetes,* 37, 133, 1988.
250. **Saegusa, Y., Ziff, M., Welkovich, L., and Cavender, D.,** Effect of inflammatory cytokines on human endothelial cell proliferation, *J. Cell. Physiol.,* 142, 488, 1990.
251. **Cosman, D.,** The hematopoietin receptor superfamily, *Cytokine,* 5, 95, 1993.
252. **Black, R.J. and Friedman, R.M.,** Cytokines and oncogene activity, *Cancer Surv.,* 8, 725, 1989.
253. **Kawano, M., Kuramoto, A., Hirano, T., and Kishimoto, T.,** Cytokines as autocrine growth factors in malignancies, *Cancer Surv.,* 8, 905, 1989.
254. **Lange, W., Brugger, W., Rosenthal, F.M., Kanz, L., and Lindemann, A.,** The role of cytokines in oncology, *Int. J. Cell Cloning,* 9, 252, 1991.
255. **Chong, A.S.-F., Scuderi, P., Grimes, W.J., and Hersh, E.M.,** Tumor targets stimulate IL-2 activated killer cells to produce interferon-γ and tumor necrosis factor, *J. Immunol.,* 142, 2133, 1989.
256. **Shimizu, H., Wyatt, D., Knowles, R.D., Bucana, C.D., Stanbridge, E.J., and Kleinerman, E.S.,** Human monocytes selectively bind to cells expressing the tumorigenic phenotype, *Cancer Immunol. Immunother.,* 28, 185, 1989.
257. **Stötter, H., Wiebke, E.A., Tomita, S., Belldegrun, A., Topalian, S., Rosenberg, S.A., and Lotze, M.T.,** Cytokines alter target cell susceptibility to lysis. II. Evaluation of tumor infiltrating lymphocytes, *J. Immunol.,* 142, 1767, 1989.
258. **Axelrad, A.A.,** Some hemopoietic negative regulators, *Exp. Hematol.,* 18, 143, 1990.
259. **Raghavachar, A., Frickhofen, N., Digel, W., Porzsolt, F., and Heimpel, H.,** Lymphokines as inhibitors of hematopoietic cell proliferation, *Blood Cells,* 14, 471, 1988.
260. **Zipori, D.,** Regulation of hemopoiesis by cytokines that restrict options for growth and differentiation, *Cancer Cells,* 2, 205, 1990.
261. **Barlozzari, T., Herberman, R.B., and Reynolds, C.W.,** Inhibition of pluripotent hematopoietic stem cells of bone marrow by large granular lymphocytes, *Proc. Natl. Acad. Sci. U.S.A.,* 84, 7691, 1987.
262. **Keller, J.R., Mantel, C., Sing, G.K., Ellingsworth, L.R., Ruscetti, S.K., and Ruscetti, F.W.,** Transforming growth factor β1 selectively regulates early murine hematopoietic progenitors and inhibits the growth of IL-3-dependent myeloid leukemia cell lines, *J. Exp. Med.,* 168, 737, 1988.
263. **Strassmann, G., Cole, M.D., and Newman, W.,** Regulation of colony-stimulating factor 1-dependent macrophage precursor proliferation by type β transforming growth factor, *J. Immunol.,* 140, 2645, 1988.
264. **Lee, G., Ellingsworth, L.R., Gillis, S., Wall, R., and Kincade, P.W.,** β Transforming growth factors are potential regulators of B lymphocytes, *J. Exp. Med.,* 166, 1290, 1987.
265. **Mitjavila, M.T., Vinci, G., Villeval, J.L., Kieffer, N., Henri, A., Testa, U., Breton-Gorius, J., and Vainchenker, W.,** Human platelet α granules contain a nonspecific inhibitor of megakaryocyte colony formation: its relationship to type β transforming growth factor (TGF-β), *J. Cell. Physiol.,* 134, 83, 1988.
266. **Trucco, M., Rovera, G., and Ferrero, D.,** A novel human lymphokine that inhibits haematopoietic progenitor cell proliferation, *Nature,* 309, 166, 1984.
267. **Santoli, D., Tweardy, D.J., Ferrero, D., Kreider, B.L., and Rovera, G.,** A suppressor lymphokine produced by human T leukemia cell lines: partial characterization and spectrum of activity against normal and malignant hemopoietic cells, *J. Exp. Med.,* 163, 18, 1986.
268. **Montaldo, P.G., Lanciotti, M., Castagnola, E., Parodi, M.T., Cirillo, C., Cornaglia-Ferraris, P., and Ponzoni, M.,** A human leukemia-derived T-cell line produces two inhibitor factors which suppress lymphocyte proliferation: characterization and purification of the molecules, *Lymphokine Res.,* 7, 413, 1988.
269. **Douer, D., Ben-Bassat, I., Froom, P., Shaked, N., and Ramot, B.,** T-cell acute lymphoblastic leukemia with severe leukopenia: evidence for suppression of myeloid progenitor cells by leukemic blasts, *Acta Haematol.,* 80, 185, 1988.
270. **Zarling, J.M., Shoyab, M., Marquardt, H., Hanson, M.B., Lioubin, M.N., and Todaro, G.J.,** Oncostatin M: a growth regulator produced by differentiated histiocytic lymphoma cells, *Proc. Natl. Acad. Sci. U.S.A.,* 83, 9739, 1986.
271. **Brown, T.J., Lioubin, M.N., and Marquardt, H.,** Purification and characterization of cytostatic lymphokines produced by activated human T lymphocytes. Synergistic antiproliferative activity of transforming growth factor β1, interferon-γ, and oncostatin M for human melanoma cells, *J. Immunol.,* 139, 2977, 1987.

272. **Malik, N., Kallestad, J.C., Gunderson, N.L., Austin, S.D., Neubauer, M.G., Ochs, V., Marquardt, H., Zarling, J.M., Shoyab, M., Wei, C.-M., Linsley, P.S., and Rose, T.M.,** Molecular cloning, sequence analysis, and functional expression of a novel growth regulator, oncostatin M, *Mol. Cell. Biol.,* 9, 2847, 1989.
273. **Linsley, P.S., Bolton-Hanson, M., Horn, D., Malik, N., Kallestad, J.C., Ochs, V., Zarling, J.M., and Shoyab, M.,** Identification and characterization of cellular receptors for the growth regulator, oncostatin M, *J. Biol. Chem.,* 264, 4282, 1989.
274. **Grove, R.I., Eberhardt, C., Abid, S., Mazzucco, C., Liu, J., Kiener, P., Todaro, G., and Shoyab, M.,** Oncostatin M is a mitogen for rabbit vascular smooth muscle cells, *Proc. Natl. Acad. Sci. U.S.A.,* 90, 823, 1993.
275. **Nair, B.C., DeVico, A.L., Nakamura, S., Copeland, T.D., Chen, Y., Patel, A., O'Neil, T., Oroszlan, S., Gallo, R.C., and Sarngadharan, M.G.,** Identification of a major growth factor for AIDS-Kaposi's sarcoma cells as oncostatin M, *Science,* 255, 1430, 1992.
276. **Miles, S.A., Martínez-Maza, O., Rezai, A., Magpantay, L., Kishimoto, T., Nakamura, S., Radka, S.F., and Lindsley, P.S.,** Oncostatin M as a potent mitogen for AIDS-Kaposi's sarcoma-derived cells, *Science,* 255, 1432, 1992.
277. **Gearing, D.P., Comeau, M.R., Friend, D.J., Gimpel, S.D., Thut, C.J., McGourty, J., Brasher, K.K., King, J.A., Gillis, S., Mosley, B., Ziegler, S.F., and Cosman, D.,** The IL-6 signal transducer, gp130: an oncostatin M receptor and affinity converter for the LIF receptor, *Science,* 255, 1434, 1992.
278. **Liu, J., Modrell, B., Aruffo, A., Marken, J.S., Taga, T., Yasukawa, K., Murakami, M., Kishimoto, T., and Shoyab, M.,** Interleukin-6 signal transducer gp130 mediates oncostatin M signaling, *J. Biol. Chem.,* 267, 16763, 1992.
279. **Liu, J.W., Clegg, C.H., and Shoyab, M.,** Regulation of EGR-1, c-*jun*, and c-*myc* gene expression by oncostatin-M, *Cell Growth Differ.,* 3, 307, 1992.
280. **Kasukabe, T., Okabe-Kado, J., Honma, Y., and Hozumi, M.,** Production by undifferentiated leukemia cells of a novel growth-inhibitory factor(s) for partially differentiated myeloid leukemic cells, *Jpn. J. Cancer Res.,* 78, 921, 1987.
281. **Borish, L. and Rocklin, R.E.,** Effects of leukocyte inhibitory factor (LIF) on neutrophil phagocytosis and bactericidal activity, *J. Immunol.,* 138, 1475, 1987.
282. **Borish, L. and Rocklin, R.,** Effects of leukocyte inhibitory factor (LIF) on neutrophil mediated antibody-dependent cellular cytotoxicity, *J. Immunol.,* 138, 1480, 1987.
283. **Borish, L., Rosenbaum, R., and Rocklin, R.,** Role of calcium in the activation of neutrophils by leukocyte inhibitory factor (LIF), *Lymphokine Res.,* 6, 341, 1987.
284. **Pojda, Z., Dexter, T.M., and Lord, B.I.,** Production of a multipotential cell (CFU-S) proliferation inhibitor by various populations of mouse and human macrophages, *Br. J. Haematol.,* 68, 153, 1988.
285. **Graham, G.J., Wright, E.G., Hewick, R., Wolpe, S.D., Wilkie, N.M., Donaldson, D., Lorimore, S., and Pragnell, I.B.,** Identification and characterization of an inhibitor of haemopoietic stem cell proliferation, *Nature,* 344, 442, 1990.
286. **Hardy, C.L. and Balducci, L.,** Hemopoietic alterations of cancer, *Am. J. Med. Sci.,* 290, 196, 1985.
287. **Cohen, M.C. and Cohen, S.,** The role of lymphokines in neoplastic disease, *Hum. Pathol.,* 17, 264, 1986.
288. **Löwenberg, B. and Touw, I.P.,** Hematopoietic growth factors and their receptors in acute leukemia, *Blood,* 81, 281, 1993.
289. **Lu, C., Vickers, M.F., and Kerbel, R.S.,** Interleukin 6: a fibroblast-derived growth inhibitor of human melanoma cells from early but not advanced stages of tumor progression, *Proc. Natl. Acad. Sci. U.S.A.,* 89, 9215, 1992.
290. **Bernstein, S.H.,** Growth factors in the management of adult acute leukemia, *Hematol. Oncol. Clin. N. Am.,* 7, 255, 1993.
291. **Russell, N.H.,** Autocrine growth factors and leukaemic haemopoiesis, *Blood Rev.,* 6, 149, 1992.
292. **Metcalf, D. and Nicola, N.A.,** Role of the colony stimulating factors in the emergence and suppression of myeloid leukemia populations, in *Molecular Biology of Tumor Cells,* Wahren, B., Ed., Raven Press, New York, 1985, 215.
293. **Lange, B., Valtieri, M., Santoli, D., Caracciolo, D., Mavilio, F., Gemperlein, I., Griffin, C., Emanuel, B., Finan, J., Nowell, P., and Rovera, G.,** Growth factor requirements of childhood acute leukemia: establishment of GF-CSF-dependent cell lines, *Blood,* 70, 192, 1987.

294. Motoji, T., Takanashi, M., Fuchinoue, M., Masuda, M., Oshimi, K., and Mizoguchi, H., Effect of recombinant GM-CSF and recombinant G-CSF on colony formation of blast progenitors in acute myeloblastic leukemia, *Exp. Hematol.,* 17, 56, 1989.
295. Kitamura, T., Tange, T., Terasawa, T., Chiba, S., Kuwaki, T., Miyagawa, K., Piao, Y.-F., Miyazono, K., Urabe, A., and Takaku, F., Establishment and characterization of a unique human cell line that proliferates dependently on GM-CSF, IL-3, and erythropoietin, *J. Cell. Physiol.,* 140, 323, 1989.
296. Miyauchi, J., Kelleher, C.A., Wong, G.G., Yang, Y.-C., Clark, S.C., Minkin, S., Minden, M.D., and McCulloch, E.A., The effects of combinations of the recombinant growth factors GM-CSF, G-CSF, IL-3, and CSF-1 on leukemic blast cells in suspension culture, *Leukemia,* 2, 382, 1988.
297. Delwel, R., Salem, M., Pellens, C., Dorssers, L., Wagemaker, G., Clark, S., and Löwenberg, B., Growth regulation of human acute myeloid leukemia: effects of five recombinant hematopoietic factors in a serum-free culture system, *Blood,* 72, 1944, 1988.
298. Santoli, D., Yang, Y.-C., Clark, S.C., Kreider, B.L., Caracciolo, D., and Rovera, G., Synergistic and antagonistic effects of recombinant human interleukin (IL) 3, IL-1α, granulocyte and macrophage colony-stimulating factors (G-CSF and M-CSF) on the growth of GM-CSF-dependent leukemic cell lines, *J. Immunol.,* 139, 3348, 1987.
299. O'Garra, A., Barbis, D., Wu, J., Hodgkin, P.D., Abrams, J., and Howard, M., The BCL_1 B lymphoma responds to IL-4, IL-5, and GM-CSF, *Cell. Immunol.,* 123, 189, 1989.
300. Touw, I., Groot-Loonen, J., Broeders, L., van Agthoven, T., Hählen, K., Hagemeijer, A., and Löwenberg, B., Recombinant hematopoietic growth factors fail to induce a proliferative response in precursor B acute lymphoblastic leukemia, *Leukemia,* 3, 356, 1989.
301. Leslie, K.B. and Schrader, J.W., Growth factor gene activation and clonal heterogeneity in an autostimulatory myeloid leukemia, *Mol. Cell. Biol.,* 9, 2414, 1989.
302. Delmer, A. and Zittoun, R., Utilisation des facteurs de croissance hématopoïétiques en cancérologie, *Bull. Cancer,* 68, 115, 1991.
303. Metcalf, D., Clonal analysis of the response of HL60 human myeloid leukemia cells to biological regulators, *Leukemia Res.,* 7, 117, 1983.
304. Metcalf, D., The induction and inhibition of differentiation in normal and leukaemic cells, *Philos. Trans. R. Soc. London,* B327, 99, 1990.
305. Appelbaum, F.R., The clinical use of hematopoietic growth factors, *Semin. Hematol.,* 26(Suppl. 3), 7, 1989.
306. Irvine, A.E., Berney, J.J., and Francis, G.E., Dissociation of the proliferation and differentiation stimuli of granulocyte colony-stimulating factor (G-CSF), *Leukemia,* 4, 203, 1990.
307. Lang, R.A., Metcalf, D., Gough, N.M., Dunn, A.R., and Gonda, T.J., Expression of a hemopoietic growth factor cDNA in a factor-dependent cell line results in autonomous growth and tumorigenicity, *Cell,* 43, 531, 1985.
308. Vellenga, E., Ostapovicz, D., O'Rourke, B., and Griffin, J.D., Effects of recombinant IL-3, GM-CSF, and G-CSF on proliferation of leukemic clonogenic cells in short-term and long-term cultures, *Leukemia,* 1, 584, 1987.
309. Inoue, C., Murate, T., Hotta, T., and Saito, H., Response of leukemic cells to the sequential combination of GM-CSF and G-CSF, *Int. J. Cell Cloning,* 8, 54, 1990.
310. Karray, S., Merle-Béral, H., Vazquez, A., Gerard, J.-P., Debre, P., and Galanaud, P., Functional heterogeneity of B-CLL lymphocytes: dissociated responsiveness to growth factors and distinct requirements for a first activation signal, *Blood,* 70, 1105, 1987.
311. Löwenberg, B., Salem, M., and Delwel, R., Effects of recombinant multi-CSF, GM-CSF, G-CSF, and M-CSF on the proliferation and maturation of human AML in vitro, *Blood Cells,* 14, 539, 1988.
312. Jinnai, I., *In vitro* growth response to G-CSF and GM-CSF by bone marrow cells of patients with acute myeloid leukemia, *Leukemia Res.,* 14, 227, 1990.
313. Humphries, R.K., Abraham, S., Krystal, G., Lansdorp, P., Lemoine, F., and Eaves, C.J., Activation of multiple hemopoietic growth factor genes in Abelson virus-transformed myeloid cells, *Exp. Hematol.,* 16, 774, 1988.
314. Spooncer, E., Boettiger, D., and Dexter, T.M., Continuous *in vitro* generation of multipotential stem cell clones from src-infected cultures, *Nature,* 310, 228, 1984.
315. Lichtman, A.H., Williams, M.E., Ohara, J., Paul, W.E., Faller, D.V., and Abbas, A.K., Retrovirus infection alters growth factor responses of T lymphocytes, *J. Immunol.,* 138, 3276, 1987.

316. Eiseman, E. and Bolen, J.B., src-Related tyrosine protein kinases as signaling components in hematopoietic cells, *Cancer Cells,* 2, 303, 1990.
317. Harrison, M.L., Low, P.S., and Geahlen, R.L., T and B lymphocytes express distinct tyrosine protein kinases, *J. Biol. Chem.,* 259, 9348, 1984.
318. Kastan, M.B., Stone, K.D., and Civin, C.I., Nuclear oncoprotein expression as a function of lineage, differentiation stage, and proliferative status of normal human hematopoietic cells, *Blood,* 74, 1517, 1989.
319. Kastan, M.B., Radin, A.I., Kuerbitz, S.J., Onyekwere, O., Wolkow, C.A., Civin, C.I., Stone, K.D., Woo, T., Ravindranath, Y., and Craig, R.W., Levels of p53 protein increase with maturation in human hematopoietic cells, *Cancer Res.,* 51, 4279, 1991.
320. Reed, J.C., Alpers, J.D., Nowell, P.C., and Hoover, R.G., Sequential expression of protooncogenes during lectin-stimulate mitogenesis of normal human lymphocytes, *Proc. Natl. Acad. Sci. U.S.A.,* 83, 3982, 1986.
321. Reed, J.C., Tsujimoto, Y., Alpers, J.D., Croce, C.M., and Nowell, P.C., Regulation of *bcl*-2 protooncogene expression during normal human lymphocyte proliferation, *Science,* 236, 1295, 1987.
322. Kelly, K., Cochran, B.H., Stiles, C.D., and Leder, P., Cell-specific regulation of the c-*myc* gene by lymphocyte mitogens and platelet-derived growth factor, *Cell,* 35, 603, 1983.
323. Persson, H., Hennighausen, L., Taub, R., DeGrado, W., and Leder, P., Antibodies to human c-*myc* oncogene product: evidence of an evolutionary conserved protein induced during cell proliferation, *Science,* 225, 687, 1984.
324. Ferrari, S., Torelli, U., Selleri, L., Donelli, A., Venturelli, D., Narni, F., Moretti, L., and Torelli, G., Study of the levels of expression of two oncogenes, c-*myc* and c-*myb*, in acute and chronic leukemias of both lymphoid and myeloid lineage, *Leukemia Res.,* 9, 833, 1985.
325. Smeland, E., Godal, T., Ruud, E., Beiske, K., Funderud, S., Clark, E.A., Pfeifer-Ohlsson, S., and Ohlsson, R., The specific induction of *myc* protooncogene expression in normal human B cells is not a sufficient event for acquisition of competence to proliferate, *Proc. Natl. Acad. Sci. U.S.A.,* 82, 6255, 1985.
326. Krönke, M., Leonard, W.J., Depper, J.M., and Greene, W.C., Sequential expression of genes involved in human T lymphocyte growth and differentiation, *J. Exp. Med.,* 161, 1593, 1985.
327. Reed, J.C., Nowell, P.C., and Hoover, R.G., Regulation of c-*myc* mRNA levels in normal human lymphocytes by modulators of cell proliferation, *Proc. Natl. Acad. Sci. U.S.A.,* 82, 4221, 1985.
328. Depper, J.M., Leonard, W.J., Drogula, C., Krönke, M., Waldmann, T.A., and Greene, W.C., Interleukin 2 (IL-2) augments transcription of the IL-2 receptor gene, *Proc. Natl. Acad. Sci. U.S.A.,* 82, 4230, 1985.
329. Farrar, W.L. and Anderson, W.B., Interleukin-2 stimulates association of protein kinase C with plasma membrane, *Nature,* 315, 233, 1985.
330. Farrar, W.L. and Taguchi, M., Interleukin 2 stimulation of protein kinase C membrane association: evidence for IL-2 receptor phosphorylation, *Lymphokine Res.,* 4, 87, 1985.
331. Rapp, U.R., Cleveland, J.L., Brightman, K., Scott, A., and Ihle, J.N., Abrogation of IL-3 and IL-2 dependence by recombinant murine retroviruses expressing v-*myc* oncogenes, *Nature,* 317, 434, 1985.
332. Caubet, J.-F., Mitjavila, M.-T., Dubart, A., Roten, D., Weil, S.C., and Vanchenker, W., Expression of the c-*fos* protooncogene by human and murine erythroblasts, *Blood,* 74, 947, 1989.
333. Müller, R., Müller, D., and Guilbert, L., Differential expression of c-*fos* in hematopoietic cells: correlation with differentiation of monomyelocytic cells in vitro, *EMBO J.,* 3, 1887, 1984.
334. Kelly, K. and Siebenlist, U., The role of c-myc in the proliferation of normal and neoplastic cells, *J. Clin. Immunol.,* 5, 65, 1985.
335. Mitchell, R.L., Zokas, L., Schreiber, R.D., and Verma, I.M., Rapid induction of the expression of proto-oncogene *fos* during human monocytic differentiation, *Cell,* 40, 209, 1985.
336. Sariban, E., Mitchell, T., and Kufe, D., Expression of the c-*fms* proto-oncogene during human monocytic differentiation, *Nature,* 316, 64, 1985.
337. Gewirtz, A.M., Anfossi, G., Venturelli, D., Valpreda, S., Sims, R., and Calabretta, B., G_1/S transition in normal human T-lymphocytes requires the nuclear protein encoded by c-*myb*, *Science,* 245, 180, 1989.
338. Todokoro, K., Watson, R.J., Higo, H., Amanuma, H., Kuramochi, S., Yanagisawa, H., and Ikawa, Y., Down-regulation of c-*myb* gene expression is a prerequisite for erythropoietin-induced erythroid differentiation, *Proc. Natl. Acad. Sci. U.S.A.,* 85, 8900, 1988.

339. **Weinstein, Y., Ihle, J.N., Lavu, S., and Reddy, E.P.,** Truncation of the c-*myb* gene by a retroviral integration in an interleukin 3-dependent myeloid leukemia cell line, *Proc. Natl. Acad. Sci. U.S.A.,* 83, 5010, 1986.
340. **Katzav, S.,** *vav:* A molecule for all haemopoiesis, *Br. J. Haematol.,* 81, 141, 1992.
341. **Hu, P., Margolis, B., and Schlessinger, J.,** *vav:* A potential link between tyrosine kinases and *ras*-like GTPases in hematopoietic cell signaling, *Bioessays,* 15, 179, 1993.
342. **Bustelo, X.R., Rubin, S.D., Suen, K.-L., Carrasco, D., and Barbacid, M.,** Developmental expression of the *vav* protooncogene, *Cell Growth Differ.,* 4, 297, 1993.
343. **Coppola, J., Bryant, S., Koda, T., Conway, D., and Barbacid, M.,** Mechanism of activation of the *vav* protooncogene, *Cell Growth Differ.,* 2, 95, 1991.
344. **Bustelo, X.R., Ledbetter, J.A., and Barbacid, M.,** Product of *vav* proto-oncogene defines a new class of tyrosine protein kinase substrates, *Nature,* 356, 68, 1992.
345. **Margolis, B., Hu, P., Katzav, S., Li, W., Oliver, J.M., Ullrich, A., Weiss, A., and Schlessinger, J.,** Tyrosine phosphorylation of *vav* proto-oncogene product containing SH2 domain and transcription factor motifs, *Nature,* 356, 71, 1992.
346. **Bustelo, X.R. and Barbacid, M.,** Tyrosine phosphorylation of the *vav* proto-oncogene product in activated B cells, *Science,* 256, 1196, 1992.
347. **Westin, E.H., Wong-Staal, F., Gelmann, E.P., Dalla Favera, R., Papas, T.S., Lautenberger, J.A., Eva, A., Reddy, E.P., Tronick, S.R., Aaronson, S.A., and Gallo, R.C.,** Expression of cellular homologues of retroviral *onc* genes in human hematopoietic cells, *Proc. Natl. Acad. Sci. U.S.A.,* 79, 2490, 1982.
348. **Reitsma, P.H., Rothberg, P.G., Astrinb, S.M., Trial, J., Bar-Shavit, Z., Hall, A., Teitelbaum, S.L., and Kahn, A.J.,** Regulation of *myc* gene expression in HL-60 leukaemia cells by a vitamin D metabolite, *Nature,* 306, 492, 1983.
349. **Craig, R.W. and Bloch, A.,** Early decline in c-*myb* oncogene expression in the differentiation of human myeloblastic leukemia (ML-1) cells induced with 12-*O*-tetradecanoylphorbol 13-acetate, *Cancer Res.,* 44, 442, 1984.
350. **Grosso, L.E. and Pitot, H.C.,** The expression of the *myc* proto-oncogene in a dimethylsulfoxide resistant HL-60 cell line, *Cancer Lett.,* 22, 55, 1984.
351. **Grosso, L.E. and Pitot, H.C.,** Modulation of c-*myc* expression in the HL-60 cell line, *Biochem. Biophys. Res. Commun.,* 119, 473, 1984.
352. **Filmus, J. and Buick, R.N.,** Relationship of c-*myc* expression to differentiation and proliferation of HL-60 cells, *Cancer Res.,* 45, 822, 1985.
353. **Grosso, L.E. and Pitot, H.C.,** Transcriptional regulation of c-*myc* during chemically induced differentiation of HL-60 cultures, *Cancer Res.,* 45, 847, 1985.
354. **Watanabe, T., Sariban, E., Mitchell, T., and Kufe, D.,** Human c-myc and N-ras expression during induction of HL-60 cellular differentiation, *Biochem. Biophys. Res. Commun.,* 126, 999, 1985.
355. **Simpson, R.U., Hsu, T., Begley, D.A., Mitchell, B.S., and Alizadeh, B.N.,** Transcriptional regulation of c-myc protooncogene by 1,25-dihydroxyvitamin D_3 in HL-60 promyelocytic leukemia cells, *J. Biol. Chem.,* 262, 4104, 1987.
356. **Koeffler, H.P.,** Induction of differentiation of human acute myelogenous leukemia cells: therapeutic implications, *Blood,* 62, 709, 1983.
357. **Lachman, H.M. and Skoultchi, A.I.,** Expression of c-*myc* changes during differentiation of mouse erythroleukaemia cells, *Nature,* 310, 592, 1984.
358. **Lachman, H.M., Hatton, K.S., Skoultchi, A.I., and Schildkraut, C.L.,** c-*myc* mRNA levels in the cell cycle change in mouse erythroleukemia cells following inducer treatment, *Proc. Natl. Acad. Sci. U.S.A.,* 82, 5323, 1985.
359. **Jonak, G.J. and Knight, E., Jr.,** Selective reduction of c-*myc* mRNA in Daudi cells by human β interferon, *Proc. Natl. Acad. Sci. U.S.A.,* 81, 1747, 1984.
360. **Einat, M., Resnitzky, D., and Kimchi, A.,** Close link between reduction of c-*myc* expression by interferon and G_0/G_1 arrest, *Nature,* 313, 597, 1985.
361. **Gambari, R., del Senno, L., Piva, R., Barbieri, R., Amelotti, F., Bernardi, F., Marchetti, G., Citarella, F., Tripodi, M., and Fantoni, A.,** Human leukemia K562 cells: relationship between hemin-mediated erythroid induction, cell proliferation, and expression of c-*abl* and c-*myc* oncogenes, *Biochem. Biophys. Res. Commun.,* 125, 90, 1984.
362. **Gonda, T.J. and Metcalf, D.,** Expression of *myb, myc* and *fos* proto-oncogenes during the differentiation of a murine myeloid leukaemia, *Nature,* 310, 249, 1984.

363. **Müller, R., Curran, T., Müller, D., and Guilbert, L.,** Induction of c-*fos* during myelomonocytic differentiation and macrophage proliferation, *Nature,* 314, 546, 1985.
364. **Mitchell, R.L., Henning-Chubb, C., Huberman, E., and Verma, I.M.,** c-*fos* Expression is neither sufficient nor obligatory for differentiation of monomyelocytes to macrophages, *Cell,* 45, 497, 1986.
365. **Oliff, A., Oliff, I., Schmidt, B., and Famulari, N.,** Isolation of immortal cell lines from the first stage of murine leukemia virus-induced leukemia, *Proc. Natl. Acad. Sci. U.S.A.,* 81, 5464, 1984.
366. **Oliff, A., Agranovsky, O., McKinney, M.D., Murty, V.V.V.S., and Bauchwitz, R.,** Friend murine leukemia virus-immortalized myeloid cells are converted into tumorigenic cell lines by Abelson leukemia virus, *Proc. Natl. Acad. Sci. U.S.A.,* 82, 3306, 1985.
367. **Pimentel, E.,** *Oncogenes,* Vols. I and II, 2nd ed., CRC Press, Boca Raton, FL, 1989.

Chapter 2

Interleukins and Cytokines

I. INTRODUCTION

In general, for stem cells, renewal and differentiation are incompatible alternatives, and differentiation is usually associated with progressive limitation in the proliferative capacity of the cell lineage. A terminally differentiated cell is usually a "dead cell", in relation to its inability to reproduce. However, this general concept does not appear to hold for lymphopoiesis.[1] Cells phenotypically recognized as differentiated T lymphocytes can be maintained in long-term culture provided the specific growth factor, IL-2, is included in the medium. A clone of differentiated B cells, capable of synthesizing a particular Ig species, may be expanded by cell proliferation *in vivo* under the appropriate antigenic stimulus. Thus, T and B lymphocytes are differentiated cells that maintain their capacity for proliferation after specific stimulation.

Lymphocyte mitogenic and activating factors, including the lymphokines, monokines, and interleukins, were originally identified in the supernatants of human lymphocyte cultures.[2,3] Since it later becomes apparent that the action of these mediators is not limited to lymphocytes and monocytes, but may affect a wide diversity of cell types including endothelial cells and fibroblasts, they are currently known generically as cytokines. A number of factors have been classified in this category.[4-9] In addition to their roles in hematopoietic, inflammatory, and immunologic processes the cytokines are importantly involved in metabolic and endocrine functions.[10] A functional cytokine network exists in the placenta.[11]

Due to their origin and functions, as well as to the assay systems used for their identification, the cytokines have been designated and classified in confusing terms.[12] Soluble mediators required for optimal stimulation of T-cell mitogenesis are IL-1 and IL-2.[13,14] IL-6 may also be an essential factor in T-cell activation, but activation of human T lymphocytes by IL-1 and IL-6 could be due to their effects on the production of and response to IL-2. Thus, IL-2 is a second messenger in the cascade of events triggered by the interaction of human T lymphocytes by IL-1 and IL-6.[15,16] Other interleukins may be produced thereafter in an orderly fashion, according to the cellular system and the physiologic conditions. The interleukins IL-2, IL-4, and IL-5 are sequentially produced in mitogen-stimulated murine spleen cell cultures.[17] Recently, other interleukins have been added to this growing list. Different combinations of interleukins may act selectively on target cells such as thymocytes at different developmental stages.[18] Since it is clear that these substances have important physiological roles in cells and tissues outside the hematopoietic system, such as the neuroendocrine and immune systems, the name cytokines is a more appropriate designation for these agents. The human endometrium is an active site of cytokine production and action.[19] The cytokines act as modulators of the growth and function of the pituitary gland.[20] In general, the cytokines can act as paracrine, autocrine, and endocrine factors capable of modulating an array of cellular functions, including cell proliferation and differentiation.

Certain hormones may display cytokine-like activity. Human lymphocytes express the prolactin gene and produce prolactin with a predicted amino acid sequence that is identical to that of pituitary prolactin.[21,22] Lymphoid cells such as thymocytes and splenocytes express both prolactin and its cell surface receptor, suggesting that prolactin may function as an autocrine growth factor for these cells. Prolactin may be a T-cell-derived cytokine involved in immune responses as well as in T-cell development.

The cell surface receptors for several interleukins (IL-2, IL-3, IL-4, IL-5, IL-6, and IL-7), as well as the receptors for CSF-2, erythropoietin, prolactin, and growth hormone, are members of a superfamily of transmembrane glycoproteins — the hematopoietin receptor superfamily. The members of this family are closely related in the structure of their extracellular, ligand-binding domains.[23] The biological significance of these homologies is unknown. The human cell surface receptors for IL-3, IL-5, and CSF-2 are composed of cytokine-specific α subunits but share a common β subunit.[24] In contrast, the murine receptors for these three factors have two distinct β subunits. The reason for this difference between the two species is not understood. After receptor binding, the transductional mechanisms of cytokines are associated with the action of second messengers, alteration of protein phosphorylation, and changes in gene expression.[25] Although cytokine receptors do not possess intrinsic tyrosine kinase activity, binding of the physiologic ligand to these receptors may result in the phosphorylation of distinct cellular proteins on tyrosine residues. The mechanism of this effect is not understood, but may implicate the secondary activation of specific tyrosine kinases. Interestingly, cytokines transmit signals for activation of cellular tyrosine kinases through the extracellular rather than cytoplasmic domains of the receptors.[26]

The interleukins and cytokines may play important roles in many tumorigenic processes.[27] Tumor cells are able to induce the expression of various cytokines *in vitro*,[28] and the cytokines may be involved in the regulation of tumor growth *in vivo*. Certain cytokines have an inhibitory activity on the proliferation of tumor cells, whereas other cytokines may stimulate tumor cell growth. The actions of cytokines on tumorigenesis may depend, at least in part, on the expression of specific proto-oncogenes.[29] Transfer of cytokine genes into tumor cells may represent a valuable approach for the analysis of cytokine-mediated effects on tumor cells. In some cases, the expression of cytokine genes may result in tumor rejection or eradication, which requires the action of CD8+ T lymphocytes.[30] However, the effectivity of the vaccination of mice with tumor cells genetically engineered to produce different types of cytokines may not be superior to that of parental cells admixed with a classical bacterial adjuvant.[31] Further experimental and clinical studies are required for a proper evaluation of the possible application of preventive or therapeutic strategies based on tumor cells manipulated to produce cytokines.

II. INTERLEUKIN 1

Interleukin 1 (IL-1), initially called lymphocyte-activating factor, was defined as a soluble factor produced by activated monocytes that is required for T-cell immune response. However, IL-1 is produced by a diversity of cell types and elicits a wide variety of physiological effects in hematic and nonhematic cells.[32-36] Protein with IL-1 activity has been characterized from several sources, including a human acute monocytic leukemia cell line.[37] IL-1 is constitutively produced by the human hepatic adenocarcinoma cell line SK-hep-1, in which addition of LPS or calcium ionophore results in a 30-fold enhancement in the release of IL-1 activity.[38] Two distinct proteins, IL-1α and IL-1β, are responsible for the manifold physiological activities attributed to IL-1.[39] Although IL-1α and IL-1β have only limited amino acid identity, they are recognized by the same receptor on the cell surface and express very similar biological activities. However, the two forms of IL-1 are differentially presented by the cells in which they are produced. Whereas IL-1β is a soluble protein, IL-1α is expressed as a membrane-associated protein in macrophages, monocytes, and B lymphocytes as well as in human endothelial cells and dermal fibroblasts.[40,41] The membrane-associated form of IL-1 may have distinct functions *in vivo* and may be crucial in the cognate interactions required for induction of immune responses. The tumor-inhibitory factor TIF-2, isolated from the conditioned medium of the A673 human rhabdomyosarcoma cell line, was recently identified with IL-1.[42]

A. BIOLOGICAL EFFECTS OF IL-1

IL-1 has important effects, not only in blood cells but also in tissue injury, immunologic reactions, and inflammatory processes, as well as in the pathogenesis of the acute phase response to noxious factors including microbial infection.[43,44] The acute-phase response is characterized by an acute shift from energy storage to energy utilization. The symptoms of this response include fever and leukocytosis, as well as changes in the concentrations of plasma protein and divalent cations, breakdown of muscle protein, alterations of intravascular coagulation, and lymphocyte activation. Important alterations in the plasma concentrations of a set of plasma proteins, collectively known as the acute-phase reactants, occur during the acute-phase response associated with inflammation, irrespective of its cause.[45] IL-1 may be an endogenous mediator of fever and appears to be identical with the endogenous pyrogen which acts on the hypothalamus.[46]

IL-1 and TNF-α share important activities in physiological processes such as fever and acute phase changes, in spite of their different structures and their action through binding to different receptors.[47-49] Both IL-1 and TNF-α possess the ability to induce hemodynamic and hematological changes typical of septic shock in the rabbit.[50]

1. Effects of IL-1 on Hematopoietic Cells

IL-1 has an important role in modulating the proliferation, maturation, and functional activation of hematopoietic cells, including lymphoid and nonlymphoid cells. These effects may be exerted through the stimulation of marrow stromal cells, which are able to produce and secrete factors that contribute to the regulation of hematopoiesis within the marrow microenvironment. IL-1α induces the production of CSF-2 in immature marrow cells.[51] Human marrow stromal cell layers in culture are stimulated by IL-1 to produce both CSF-1 and CSF-3.[52] CSF-1 production by human term placenta is stimulated by IL-1β.[53]

The human stromal fibroblastoid cell line, ST-1, is stimulated by IL-1 to produce CSF-2, CSF-3, and IL-6.[54] The factors produced by IL-1-stimulated stromal cells may contribute to support hematopoiesis both *in vitro* and *in vivo*. Administration of IL-1 to intact mice may lead within 20 h to an enhanced proportion of marrow cells entering the cell cycle.[55] IL-1 is involved in regulating the production of humoral stimulators of early human hematopoietic progenitors.[56]

IL-1 is a cofactor required by concanavalin A to stimulate growth of T lymphocytes and is capable of inducing the differentiation of B lymphocytes into antibody-producing cells.[57-59] Both IL-1 and TNF-α can stimulate T-cell colony formation by human peripheral blood lymphocytes.[60] IL-1 may, in association with antigen, be a signal capable of activating the generation of cytolytic T lymphocytes through an activation of the helper T-cell pathway, which may result in the generation of helper differentiation factors and activation and differentiation of precursor cytolytic T cells. An antiserum that inhibits IL-1-mediated functions is immunosuppressive of T-cell functions both *in vivo* and *in vitro*.[61] IL-1 appears to have little direct effect on peripheral T lymphocytes, but it may enhance T-cell-dependent immune responses by amplifying the accessory function of dendritic cells.[62]

IL-1 is a second mediator in the cascade of events triggered by the binding of IL-2 to human T lymphocytes.[63] IL-1 costimulates IL-2 gene expression by enhancing the activity of the IL-2 gene promoter, which is associated with increases in the levels of transcriptional factors that bind to IL-2 gene regulatory sequences.[64] The secretion of IL-2 and the expression of IL-2 receptors in lymphoid cells are IL-1-dependent processes.[65] An exceptional murine T-cell line, MD10, responds directly to the IL-1 stimulus without requiring the induction of intermediary growth factors.[66] An autocrine factor (BLAST-2), detected in lymphocytes immortalized by EBV, has properties similar to those of IL-1.[67]

The effects of IL-1 on B lymphocytes are controversial. IL-1 may act on resting B cells as a differentiation-inducing factor in the presence of antigen.[68] In particular, IL-1 would primarily control the maturation of proliferating B cells into antibody-forming cells.[69] IL-1 also induces or increases the expression of IL-5 receptors on B cells. BSF-1-stimulated proliferation of B cells can be enhanced by IL-1.[70] However, IL-1 alone has no stimulating activity in the colony-formation assay of B cells in soft agar and would only provide a synergistic effect with the specific B-cell-stimulating factor, BSF-1/IL-4, on already activated B cells, resulting in an increased size of B-cell clones stimulated by BSF-1/IL-4. Purified recombinant IL-1 has no effect on the proliferation of human splenic B cells *in vitro* when added simultaneously with or after B-cell activation with anti-Ig, but incubation of the B cells with IL-1 for 24 h before stimulation with anti-Ig results in an amplified mitogenic response.[71] It may be concluded that IL-1 does not activate B cells, but primes them to respond to subsequent activation.

The production and functional properties of nonlymphoid blood cells are also affected by IL-1. Granulocytopoiesis is regulated by IL-1 *in vitro* and probably also *in vivo*.[72-74] Injection of IL-1 in rabbits causes immediate granulocytosis at a low dose, while a profound granulopenia followed by hypergranulocytosis is observed at a high dose.[75] The effects of IL-1 on granulocytopoiesis are indirect, probably being mediated by CSF-3, and are exerted in synergy with CSF-1. IL-1 is a complete secretagogue for neutrophils, stimulating the release of granule constituents from these cells.[76] Human and murine polymorphonuclear neutrophils have IL-1 receptors, suggesting a role for this interleukin in the mediation of inflammatory responses.[77] The transendothelial passage of neutrophils from the vascular bed to the interstitial tissue is stimulated by IL-1 in the absence of an externally applied chemotactic gradient.[78] Highly purified preparations of IL-1 antagonize the capacity of erythropoietin to stimulate the proliferation of mouse spleen and bone marrow erythroid precursor cells in culture.[79] This antagonizing effect apparently is not mediated by inhibition of erythropoietin binding to its receptor, but would occur by interference with some late postreceptor event(s) of erythropoietin action. These results suggest that IL-1 may have a role in the pathogenesis of hypoplastic anemias associated with infections, rheumatoid arthritis, systemic lupus erythematosus, and other diseases.

IL-1 may have a selective effect on primitive hematopoietic precursors. Recombinant IL-1α acts synergistically with CSF-2 or CSF-3 in the stimulation of clonogenic cells from AML patients, and can promote the growth of multipotential progenitors from normal human marrow cells in the presence of CSF-2.[80] IL-1 can induce *in vitro* the differentiation of certain murine myeloid leukemia cell clones.[81] This effect is indirect, however, and is associated with the production of CSF-2 and a differentiation-inducing activity (MGI-2). IL-1-induced differentiation of normal myeloid precursor cells is associated with the production of CSF-2 and MGI-2.

The pluripotential effects of IL-1 on hematopoiesis have been confirmed *in vivo*. A single injection of recombinant human IL-1α into normal mice resulted in a generalized stimulation of hematopoiesis with a marked stimulation in the numbers of spleen and marrow immature erythroid, macrophage, granulocyte, granulocyte-macrophage, and megakaryocyte progenitor cells.[82] A suppressive effect of IL-1α was found in late-stage erythropoiesis, which can be prevented by administration of erythropoietin. The multiple effects of IL-1 on hematopoietic cells could be exploited for therapeutic purposes, especially for the mitigation of marrow toxicity that occurs during treatment of malignant diseases.

In addition to its effects on hematopoietic cells, IL-1 may have important effects on mature blood cells. IL-1 may be involved in the initiation and amplification of immune and inflammatory responses, and may play a role in host defense against tumor cells through activation of monocytes.[83,84] Human dermal fibroblasts stimulated by IL-1 or TNF-α produce a basic heparin-binding monocyte chemotactic and cell activating factor (MCAF).[85] This factor is a potent chemoattractant for monocytes *in vitro* and also augments the cytostatic activity of monocytes on several types of tumor cell lines. MCAF is a member of the superfamily of genes which includes the gene encoding IL-8.

2. Effects of IL-1 on the Digestive Tract

IL-1 may have an important function in the regulation of liver metabolism and be responsible for some of the marked changes in hepatic protein synthesis that occur in the acute phase response to inflammation or tissue injury.[86,87] IL-1 decreases the number of glucocorticoid receptors in the liver and may play a role in glucocorticoid-regulated hepatic metabolism.[88] The synthesis of serum amyloid A in the liver and other tissues is stimulated by IL-1 and, to a lesser extent, also by TNF-α.[89,90] Serum amyloid A is a sensitive indicator of inflammation and may have a role as an effector of nonspecific host resistance.

IL-1 induces changes in the expression of some of the genes encoding liver-derived plasma proteins that are affected during the acute phase response to inflammation or tissue injury, including albumin and the complement protein factors B and C3.[91] IL-1 and TNF-α stimulate the production of a third component of the complement, but do not elevate any other member of the acute phase response group in the human hepatoma cell line HEP 3B2.[92] In rat hepatocyte primary cultures, IL-1 stimulates $α_2$-macroglobulin synthesis, whereas albumin synthesis is decreased.[93] However, IL-1 may not be able to stimulate hepatocyte metabolism *in vitro*, suggesting that the presence of hormones may be important for IL-1 action in the liver.[94] It is clear that IL-1 is not able to elicit a full acute phase response, and should instead be considered as a modulator of certain aspects of this response.[45] Other hormones and growth factors, including glucocorticoids, TNF-α, IL-5, and IL-6 are also involved in the acute phase response.[95-97]

IL-1β is a potent inhibitor of the growth of rat hepatocytes maintained in primary culture.[98] Addition of IL-1β to the hepatocytes stimulated by insulin and EGF results in a growth-inhibitory effect. IL-1β acts at two stages in the G_1 phase of the cell cycle and its actions at both of these stages are necessary for the inhibition of hepatocyte growth. Kupffer cells and hepatic macrophages are known to produce IL-1 during hepatitis and liver injury, and these cells may be involved in the regulation of liver regeneration by synthesis and secretion of IL-1. In addition to the production of IL-1, stimulated human monocytes can produce an activity, termed hepatocyte-stimulating factor (HSF), which induces specific metabolic changes in cultured hepatocytes.[99,100] IL-1 and HSF are produced by LPS-stimulated monocytes, but they are regulated by different mechanisms and may have distinct biological activities. The functions of organs of the digestive tract other than the liver may be regulated by IL-1. However, some of these effects may be indirect. Gastric pepsin secretion is inhibited by peripherally or centrally injected IL-1 in rats.[101]

3. Effects of IL-1 on Bone, Cartilage and Connective Tissue

IL-1 is involved in the regulation of bone remodulation. IL-1β is identical with an activity, the osteoclast-activating factor (OAF), that was described as a bone-resorptive cytokine present in the culture supernatant of antigen- or mitogen-stimulated human peripheral blood mononuclear cells.[102] Infusions of IL-1α or IL-1β into mice cause effects similar to those of PTH, with a dose-dependent increase in the plasma calcium level associated with increased numbers of osteoclasts and bone resorption surfaces.[103] High doses of IL-1 cause many of the animals to die, and these animals are hypocalcemic and hyperphosphatemic immediately prior to death. Since IL-1β mRNA and protein are expressed by ATL cells, the interleukin may be responsible, at least in part, for the hypercalcemia that is frequently associated with ATL.[104] IL-1α may be involved in the hypercalcemia and leukocytosis observed in some cancer patients, in particular in patients with squamous cell carcinoma.[105] Other cytokines involved in bone resorption are IL-1α, TNF-α, and TNF-β. However, IL-1β is 13-fold more potent than IL-1α and 1000-fold more potent than TNF-α and TNF-β in stimulating bone resorption.[106] However, there are synergistic actions between these factors in relation to bone resorption. The bone-resorptive effects of IL-1, as well as those of TGF-α, are associated with increased prostaglandin synthesis and can be blocked by inhibitors of prostaglandin synthesis such as indomethacin and flufenamic acid.[107]

Osteoblasts mediate IL-1 stimulation of bone resorption by rat osteoclasts.[108] The osteoblastic cell line MC3T3-E1, derived from newborn mouse calvaria, spontaneously produces IL-1 or an IL-1-like cytokine.[109] IL-1 has independent effects on DNA and collagen synthesis in rat calvaria.[110] IL-1 stimulates calvarial DNA synthesis as well as collagen and noncollagen calvarial protein synthesis, however, while the IL-1 effect on DNA synthesis is observed in the presence of indomethacin the stimulatory effect of IL-1 on collagen and noncollagen protein synthesis is blocked by indomethacin. Stimulation of bone resorption in fetal mouse bones by human IL-1α is associated with increased production of PGE_2.[111]

Specific interactions between cells and extracellular matrix components including fibronectin, collagen, vitronectin, laminin, and proteoglycans are fundamental in cell differentiation, cell division, and cell migration. These interactions are mediated by the integrins, which are integral membrane glycoproteins which act as receptors for extracellular matrix components and serve to connect them to cytoplasmic cytoskeletal components. IL-1β, acting as a mediator of osteoblastic cell function, can regulate the expression of integrins in human osteosarcoma cells.[112] In addition, IL-1β is an inhibitor of osteosarcoma cell proliferation and is able to increase alkaline phosphatase activity in these cells and to alter their morphological characteristics.

The synthesis of extracellular matrix molecules depends on a complex interplay between different types of hormones and growth factors. TGF-β is a potent regulator of connective tissue metabolism and is capable of increasing the synthesis and decreasing the degradation of collagen and other matrix molecules. IL-1β is a potent antagonist of the action of TGF-β on connective tissue and can inhibit TGF-β-stimulated collagen synthesis in human skin fibroblasts, whereas it does not change or may even stimulate collagen gene expression in nonactivated cells.[113]

IL-1 could be involved in the pathogenesis of chronic inflammatory joint diseases such as rheumatoid arthritis as well as in osteoarthritis, and may also play a role in the mechanisms of articular cartilage destruction that occurs in degradative arthropathies.[114,115] IL-1 is spontaneously produced in long-term culture by cloned adherent synovial cells from rheumatoid synovitis, which include dendritic cells as well as macrophage-and fibroblast-like cells. These synovial cells may be important for bone destruction in rheumatoid joints. IL-1, or a related substance called mononuclear cell factor, induces stimulation of proteoglycan synthesis in human neonatal articular chondrocytes, and the addition of indomethacin reduces the stimulation effect by 60 to 70%.[116] The effects of IL-1 on chondrocytes may, at least in part, be indirect. IL-1β induces synthesis and secretion of IL-6 in human chondrocytes.[117] Stimulation of osteoblasts stimulated with IL-1 results in increased production of IL-6.[118] This effect is mediated by the type-1 IL-1 receptor and is increased by calcitriol. PGE_2 may act as a mediator of IL-1-induced bone resorption, and macrophage colony-stimulating activity (M-CSA) produced by osteoblasts may synergistically potentiate this process by recruiting osteoclast precursors.[119] TNF-α has effects similar to those of IL-1α on PGE_2 and M-CSA production and osteoblast-mediated osteoclastic bone resorption.[120] In addition, both IL-1α and TNF-α inhibit alkaline phosphatase activity, which may lead to a decrease in bone formation.

Human IL-1 is capable of increasing collagen protein and mRNA levels in cultured normal human dermal fibroblasts.[121] Dermal fibroblasts from scleroderma patients are characterized by exhibiting increased collagen production, but the cells grown from both affected and unaffected skin areas are unresponsive to the effects of IL-1. IL-1 may have a role in the earlier stages of scleroderma and other fibrotic diseases.

IL-1 produced by monocyte/macrophage cells is capable of inducing a proliferative response in fibroblasts, although other factors produced by blood cells, possibly including TNF-α and PDGF, may also be important for the growth of fibroblasts.[122] In a study of the effect of human IL-1 on the growth of mouse fibroblasts, it was concluded that IL-1 alone is not a potent mitogen for fibroblasts and does not bring the cells out of the growth-arrest phase, G_0, but treatment with PDGF renders the cells more responsive to IL-1.[123] Part of the IL-1 action on replication competent fibroblasts may be characterized as progression-inducing activity. Available evidence suggests that the mitogenic activity of IL-1 for fibroblasts and smooth-muscle cells is indirect and mediated by induction of the PDGF A-chain (PDGF-AA) gene and the subsequent synthesis and secretion of PDGF-AA polypeptide.[124]

IL-1 stimulates human marrow fibroblasts to produce multilineage HGFs and CSFs.[125,126] It also acts as an inducer of IFN-β production by human fibroblasts.[127] Complex interactions between stromal cells, including endothelial cells and fibroblasts, and hematopoietic cells may occur in the bone marrow hematopoietic microenvironment. Such interactions are of utmost importance for the regulation of normal hematopoiesis by IL-1 and other factors.

4. Effects of IL-1 on Vascular Cells

IL-1 may have important effects on vascular cells. Both IL-1 and IFN-γ induce modifications in the morphological and physiological properties of endothelial cells.[128] IL-1 alone has little effect on the proliferation of endothelial cells, but it inhibits the mitogenic effect of ECGF on these cells.[129] IL-1 stimulates the expression of mRNAs for several CSFs in cultured human umbilical vein endothelial cells.[130,131] The release of CSFs from endothelial cells in response to IL-1 may be a mechanism for stimulating the production of neutrophils and mononuclear phagocytes, and for attracting and activating these cells at sites of inflammation. In addition to its effects on endothelial cells, IL-1 may also have some important effects on vascular smooth muscle cells by regulating HBGF-2 gene expression in these cells.[132]

5. Effects of IL-1 on the Skin

IL-1 and IL-1-like proteins are present in the normal human epidermis,[133,134] and they probably play an important role in dermal morphology and physiology. Human peripheral blood monocytes can stimulate G_1-arrested mouse skin keratinocytes to enter the cell cycle and synthesize DNA, and this growth-promoting activity depends on IL-1 released by monocytes.[135] Highly purified human IL-1 and recombinant human monocyte IL-1 are highly active in stimulating DNA synthesis in keratinocyte cultures. These results suggest that IL-1, or a similar protein released by monocytes-macrophages may be involved in the pathogenesis of certain skin diseases, including chronic diseases such as psoriasis and epithelial fungus infections.

6. Effects of IL-1 on the Endocrine System and the Gonads

The effects of IL-1 on metabolic processes occurring in the liver and other organs and tissues may be mediated, at least in part, by modifications of the hormonal environment of the body. IL-1 may have important effects on the function of the hypothalamus-pituitary axis. Administration of subpyrogenic doses of either natural or recombinant IL-1 to mice and rats induces increased blood levels of ACTH and glucocorticoids.[136] IL-1-induced stimulation of ACTH secretion is due to PGE_2-stimulated secretion of CRH.[137,138] Expression of the CRH gene in the rat hypothalamus is stimulated by IL-1.[139] Both IL-1 and IL-2 exert an effect similar to that of CRF, stimulating the transcriptional expression of the POMC gene, which encodes the precursor for ACTH, MSH, and endorphins.[140] IL-1 potentiates agonist-induced secretion of β-endorphin by anterior pituitary cells.[141] IL-1 also acts directly on pituitary cells to stimulate the release of ACTH, LH, TSH, growth hormone, and prolactin.[142,143] These effects have been observed in rat pituitary cells maintained in monolayer culture as well as in a perifusion system at concentrations of IL-1 that are similar to those observed *in vivo*. In cultured AtT-20 mouse pituitary cells, IL-1 stimulation of ACTH secretion is tightly associated with production of cAMP and activation of protein kinase A.[144] In general, the results from these studies support the existence of important dynamic regulatory interactions between the immune system and the neuroendocrine system. Since IL-1 is present at relatively high concentrations in the median eminence of the hypothalamus, it seems likely that IL-1 secretion into the hypophyseal portal vessels directly affects pituitary hormone release. IL-1 may also exert a regulatory action on the secretion of hormones by the placenta. IL-1β rapidly stimulates hCG secretion from perifused first-trimester trophoblasts.[145]

The thyroid gland may also be a target for the regulatory actions of IL-1. Recombinant IL-1 produces, in the presence of serum or IGF-I, a marked stimulation of DNA synthesis in the rat thyroid follicular cell line FRTL5.[146] This effect is associated with increased expression of *c-myc* gene transcripts. IL-1 stimulates the growth of thyrocytes derived from normal human thyroid gland tissue as well as from the glands of patients with Graves' disease.[147] Local production of IL-1 by infiltrating monocytes may contribute to the development of thyroid enlargement in patients with autoimmune thyroid disease. Thyrocytes stimulated with LPS *in vitro* produce a substance with IL-1-like activity.

IL-1 has an important role in the regulation of insulin secretion by β cells in the pancreatic islets of Langerhans.[148-151] The insulin-secreting β cells possess receptors for IL-1β.[152] The stimulatory effects of IL-1 on insulin secretion are reversible and glucose-dependent and may be mediated, at least in part, by phosphoinositide-derived second-messenger molecules.[153,154] However, there is evidence that human IL-1β can stimulate insulin secretion by a mechanism which is not dependent on changes in phospholipase C and protein kinase C activities or Ca^{2+} handling of the β cells.[155] Glucose-induced insulin secretion by isolated rat pancreatic islets can be either inhibited or stimulated by IL-1, depending on its concentration and the exposure time. High concentrations of IL-1 reduce insulin release by rat islets maintained in tissue culture and abolish glucose-stimulated insulin release in short-term incubations. Moreover, the pancreatic islets incubated with IL-1 exhibit decreased content of DNA, and marked signs of degeneration as well as cell death are observed in these islets by light microscopy.[156] Since insulitis with infiltration of mononuclear cells in the islets of Langerhans is commonly observed in type 1 diabetes mellitus (insulin-dependent diabetes), these results suggest that monocyte-derived IL-1 may contribute to islet cell damage and β-cell destruction associated with type 1 diabetes mellitus in genetically susceptible individuals. However, IL-1 is probably not directly responsible for the destruction of β cells associated with type 1 diabetes. IL-1 reversibly inhibits the release of insulin by rat islet cell monolayer cultures in a dose- and time-dependent manner without producing cell destruction. The effects of IL-1 are incompatible with the specific and irreversible destruction of islet β cells characteristic of the insulitis lesion in type I diabetes.[157] Consequently, factors other than IL-1, produced by macrophage/monocyte and NK cells, must be responsible for the damage of β cells that occur in type 1 diabetes.

IL-1 has important effects on the gonads. IL-1β functions as a potent stimulator of DNA synthesis in immature rat Leydig cells and may interact with LH, the steroidogenesis-inducing protein (SIP), IGF-I, TGF-α, and other growth-promoting factors to cause an increase in the number of Leydig cells during prepubertal development.[158] However, IL-1 is a potent inhibitor of Leydig cell-associated steroidogenesis, and this effect is enhanced by TNF-α.[159,160] IL-1β inhibits the expression in Leydig cells of mRNA coding for IGF-I, a factor that functions as an autocrine modulator of Leydig cell function.[161] In the ovary, IL-1 inhibits FSH-induced differentiation of granulosa cells, as assessed by LH receptor formation and progesterone secretion.[162] Proliferation of cultured porcine granulosa cells obtained from immature or developing follicles is stimulated by IL-1, but the cells lose response to IL-1 in terms of growth and progesterone secretion as they mature and become luteal cells.[163] In rat granulosa cells, IL-1β is more potent than IL-1α in suppressing FSH-induced LH receptor formation and secretion of progesterone.[164] Since the major form of circulating IL-1 is IL-1β, it seems likely that the β form of IL-1, acting as a humoral factor, may have a greater affinity for the receptors in the ovary. Some of the effects of IL-1 on ovarian function may be exerted at the hypothalamus-hypophysis level. IL-1 inhibits ovarian steroid-induced LH surge and LHRH release in rats.[165]

7. Effects of IL-1 on Neural Tissues

IL-1 may have an important role in the physiology of neural tissues. Although IL-1 may enter the central nervous system from the circulation, the study of glial cell lines suggests that IL-1 may be locally produced by ameboid microglia.[166] IL-1 is contained in neural elements within the human hypothalamus, where it may serve as a neuromodulator in the central component of the acute phase reaction.[167] At least some of the actions of IL-1 on neural tissues may be indirect and may be mediated by stimulation of the secretion of other growth factors, including NGF. In primary cultures of fibroblasts isolated from adult rat sciatic nerves, IL-1 not only enhances NGF gene transcription but also increases the stability of NGF mRNA.[168] Macrophages invading a site of nerve injury may contribute to the repair of the lesion through secretion of IL-1, which stimulates the production of NGF.[169]

B. IL-1 STRUCTURE AND THE IL-1 GENE

cDNAs corresponding to the human, mouse, and rat IL-1 genes have been produced and the cloned genes were expressed in *Escherichia coli* as well as in mammalian cells.[170-173] The murine IL-1 cDNA codes for a IL-1 polypeptide precursor of 270 amino acids, and biologically active IL-1 was produced by expressing the carboxy-terminal 156 amino acids of the IL-1 precursor. The 37-kDa IL-1 precursor is processed by proteolysis and generates a diversity of IL-1-related substances with molecular weights of between 13 and 19 kDa, which would explain the microheterogeneity previously detected in IL-1 by physicochemical procedures. mRNA isolated by hybridization to a human IL-2 cDNA clone has been translated in a reticulocyte cell-free system, yielding immunoprecipitable IL-1.[171] Microinjection of this hybrid-selected mRNA into *Xenopus laevis* oocytes resulted in the production of biologically active IL-1.

1. IL-1α and IL-1β

Sequence analysis of human IL-1 yielded evidence for the existence of biochemically distinct forms of IL-1.[174] The purification to homogeneity and the amino acid sequence analysis of two anionic species of human IL-1 has been reported.[175] There are two distinct genes for human IL-1, and two distinct IL-1 molecules are responsible for the manifold physiological activities attributed to IL-1.[176] Two distantly related cDNAs encoding proteins sharing human IL-1 activity were isolated from a macrophage cDNA library and were designated IL-1α and IL-1β.[39] The human genome contains a single gene coding for IL-1β, and it is located on the long arm of chromosome 2, at region 2q13-q21.[177] Evidence obtained with serologic analysis using a monoclonal antibody to recombinant IL-1α showed that the activity detected in serum-free supernatants of the human bladder tumor cell line HBT 5637 is due to IL-1α.[178] Since the activity detected in HBT 5636 cells was previously designated hemopoietin 1, this hemopoietin 1 and IL-1α are identical molecules. Two types of natural IL-1 protein molecules were also identified in porcine and murine cells.[179,180]

2. Human IL-1α and IL-1β Genes and Their Products

The IL-1α gene is located on human chromosome region 2q13.[181] The complete nucleotide sequence and structural organization of the human gene coding for IL-1α has been determined.[182] The human IL-1α gene contains 10,206 bp and is composed of 7 exons and 6 introns. The human IL-1β gene was expressed in *Escherichia coli* and the nucleotide sequence of the human IL-1 gene was determined.[183-186] The gene is composed of 7 exons and the primary transcription product is 7008 nucleotides in length. The exon sequence, exon boundaries, and general genomic organization of the pro-IL-1β gene are similar to those of the human pro-IL-1α gene. The human pro-IL-1β gene may have arisen by a reverse transcriptase-mediated duplication of the related pro-IL-1α gene, i.e., it may represent a functional retroposon.

Biologically active IL-1 proteins are expressed by transfected simian COS cells.[187] The primary translation products of the two human IL-1 genes expressed in *E. coli* are 271 (IL-1α) and 269 (IL-1β) amino acids long. Both molecules are synthesized as large precursors that are processed to smaller forms. The mature IL-1β is a polypeptide of 153 amino acid residues that is generated from the IL-1β precursor by the action of a converting enzyme whose gene has been cloned and localized to human chromosome band 11q23.[188] The IL-1β precursor (pro-IL-1β) is biologically active, as demonstrated by its binding to specific cellular receptors and its capability for the stimulation of helper T cells.[189] Treatment of pro-IL-1β with trypsin or chemotrypsin generate 22- and 17-kDa polypeptide fragments, respectively, that are up to 600-fold more active than pro-IL-1β.[190] Removal of the first 114 amino acids from pro-IL-1β generate a fully active molecule. Pro-IL-1β appears to be biologically inactive because it is incapable of binding to the IL-1 receptor. The biological activity attributed to pro-IL-1β in earlier studies could be due to the formation of proteolytic fragments of the precursor in the assay system. The recombinant human IL-1β protein has been purified and characterized.[191] The purified recombinant IL-1β protein has a molecular weight of 18 kDa and an isoelectric point of 6.9, the same as natural human IL-1β.[186] The carboxy-terminal 153 amino acids of human IL-1β expressed in *E. coli* exhibits the same biological, biochemical, and immunological properties as the native protein.[192] A synthetic peptide corresponding to the sequence of the extreme carboxy-terminal region of IL-1β can function as a ligand for the IL-1 receptor on murine cell lines and competes with intact radiolabeled IL-1β.[193] The peptide antagonizes native IL-1β in a thymocyte bioassay.

3. Rodent IL-1 Genes and Their Products

Mouse IL-1 is synthesized as a 270-amino acid precursor protein. Studies with recombinant constructs and site-directed mutagenesis technology indicated that biologically active murine IL-1 polypeptides must be at least 127 amino acids long and are derived from the carboxyl terminus of the precursor.[194] The genes coding for the two forms of IL-1, α and β, were identified in the mouse genome and their products were characterized.[180] The two genes are closely linked on mouse chromosome 2.[195] Both murine IL-1 forms appear to be recognized by the same receptor. Comparison of the cloned murine IL-1β gene with the human IL-1α gene showed that the organization of the intron-exon structure is highly conserved between the two species, suggesting that both genes derive from a common ancestor.[196] Sequence homologies existing upstream of the 5' end of the coding regions may represent regulatory sequences common to both genes. A cDNA encoding the rat IL-1α gene was isolated and the biologically active IL-1α protein was expressed in monkey COS-1 cells.[173] The rat IL-1α cDNA encodes a 270-amino acid protein which is 65% homologous to human IL-1α.

4. Secretion of IL-1α and IL-1β and Binding to the IL-1 Receptor

IL-1α and IL-1β proteins have limited homology at the amino acid level (23% homology). However, both proteins compete for binding to the same plasma membrane receptor. According to site-directed mutagenesis studies, a unique histidine residue at position 30 may contribute directly or indirectly to the molecular architecture of the receptor binding site on the IL-1β polypeptide.[197] Using an *in vitro* expression system to generate truncated forms of IL-1α and IL-1β, it was shown that core sequences of 147 amino acids for

IL-1β (residues 120–266) and 140 amino acids for IL-1α (residues 128–267) must be left intact to retain full biological activity.[198] Studies with site-directed mutagenesis showed that conversion of Arg-127 to Gly-127 in the mature human IL-1β protein reduces bioactivity by 100-fold, while the receptor binding affinity decreases by only 25%.[199] These results suggest that the IL-1β mutein is defective in activating signal transduction events and indicate that binding of IL-1β protein to its receptor is necessary but insufficient for biological activity.

IL-1 precursors do not possess a signal peptide and are apparently not associated with the Golgi or the endoplasmic reticulum. The human histiocytic leukemia cell line, U-937, secretes IL-1 into the medium upon activation by treatment with PMA and LPS, and the IL-1β precursor in these cells was found to be associated with microtubules of the cytoskeleton.[200] The 30-kDa precursor forms of IL-1α and IL-1β differ in their affinities toward the IL-1 receptor. The initial translation product from IL-1β mRNA must be processed in order to bind to the IL-1 receptor, whereas the similar product of the IL-1α mRNA can bind to the IL-1 receptor without further processing.[201] The biological significance of this difference is unknown, but IL-1α is the form associated with the monocyte membrane, whereas IL-1β is not.[202] Thus, IL-1α may be preferentially associated with the surface of cells, particularly those involved in antigen presentation, while IL-1β would be present in the cytoplasm and secreted upon stimulation. In a first step, IL-1β is secreted by activated macrophages as an unprocessed precursor. This precursor is then cleaved in a second, postsecretory step by a LPS-inducible protease to generate the 20-kDa IL-1β protein which is the biologically active interleukin.[203] Phosphorylation of serine close to the dibasic/tetrabasic amino acid sequence of the human IL-1α precursor may facilitate the release of a more mature extracellular form of IL-1α.[204]

5. Biological Activities of IL-1α and IL-1β

Some biological activities of IL-1α are not shared by IL-1β. IL-1α, but not IL-1β, induces S phase entry of TPA-stimulated B cells of human B-cell CLL.[205] IL-1β, but not IL-1α, stimulates glucose transport in rat adipose cells.[206] Injection of IL-1β in rats induces an increase in the plasma levels of ACTH in a dose-dependent manner, whereas the injection of IL-1α does not induce this increase.[207]

IL-1 produced by stimulated human peripheral blood monocytes, as well as recombinant IL-1β purified to homogeneity, is directly cytotoxic for the A375 human melanoma cell line.[208] TNF-α, also released by activated monocytes, is not cytotoxic for the same melanoma cell line. The mechanism of action of IL-1 for killing tumor cells is unknown.

The amino-terminal portion of the IL-1 molecule is essential for its biological activity and deletion of this portion results in a total loss of biological activity. A series of amino-terminal variants (muteins) of human IL-1 have been constructed by using recombinant DNA techniques.[209] Two of these muteins exhibited a four- to sevenfold increase in bioactivity as compared to that of native IL-1. The enhanced biological potency coincided with an increase in both receptor binding affinity and *in vivo* tumor inhibitory activity. By site-directed mutagenesis procedures, it was shown that the arginine at the fourth position of the IL-1 molecule is one of the key residues in the function of IL-1.

A monoclonal antibody directed to the biologically active site of human IL-1 is able to block IL-1-mediated thymocyte and fibroblast proliferation, and may help to determine whether both of the described subspecies of human IL-1 (IL-1α and IL-1β), which are different in their amino acid sequences, share a common sequence responsible for their biological functions.[210] This antibody could be used to determine whether the multiplicity of the biological effects of IL-1 are due to the same moiety of the molecule.

6. IL-1-Related Proteins

There is evidence of the existence of a family of IL-1-like proteins, but the precise relationship between these proteins and IL-1 produced by activated macrophages is not clear. At least some of these proteins may be produced by proteolysis of the IL-1 precursor molecule. Both EBV-positive and EBV-negative human lymphoblastoid B-cell lines can constitutively produce an IL-1-like activity of low molecular weight that may be serologically distinct from IL-1 produced by macrophages.[211] IL-1 may be processed to peptides of only 2- to 4-kDa, which have been detected in human urine and which are still biologically active.[212]

C. IL-1 PRODUCTION AND SECRETION

IL-1 was first characterized as a cytokine produced by activated leukocytes including macrophages, monocytes, and dendritic cells. The macrophage (mononuclear phagocyte) is the principal leukocyte that synthesizes IL-1.[213] Freshly isolated human monocytes stimulated with LPS produce large amounts of

IL-1, with IL-1β exceeding IL-1α, and this production is controlled at the levels of IL-1β mRNA concentration and IL-1β protein secretion.[214] Release of IL-1α, IL-1β, and a non-IL-1 activity (25K thymocyte mitogenic factor) by human mononuclear cells is regulated in a differential manner, suggesting that these factors may play different roles in immune or inflammatory response.[215]

In addition to monocytes, IL-1 and IL-1-like factors are produced by other types of cells under the stimulus of a wide diversity of agents. Production of IL-1 is a common property of murine T-cell clones, where IL-2 appears to serve an autocrine role in the activation of these cells inasmuch as anti-IL-1α antiserum blocks the proliferation of these cells when they are the only source of IL-1.[216] Both T and B lymphocytes produce IL-1 or substances with IL-1-like activities.[217] Other cells capable of producing IL-1 include keratinocytes, kidney mesangial cells, corneal epithelium, fibroblasts, smooth muscle cells, astrocytes, glioma cells, and endothelial cells, as well as some types of transformed cells. Sertoli cells are the site of IL-1α secretion in rat testis.[218] Studies with normal mice using *in situ* hybridization in tissue sections indicate that many organs contain IL-1 mRNA, but the highest frequency is found in lymphoid organs.[219] Both IL-1α and IL-1β are normally present in the human amniotic fluid.[220] A unique high molecular weight form of IL-1β exists in the human amniotic fluid due to the aggregation of IL-1β with an unknown molecule.

IL-1 genes are expressed in human chondrocytes and it has been suggested that this expression may represent a mechanism for autocrine control of cartilage matrix degradation.[221] Normal keratinocytes produce a factor, termed epidermal cell-derived thymocyte activating factor, which is identical to IL-1.[222] The keratinocyte factor is mainly IL-1α, while LPS-stimulated human peripheral blood monocytes produces mainly IL-1β. Production of IL-1α varies according to the state of keratinocyte differentiation — being more abundant in undifferentiated keratinocytes and ceasing in the terminally differentiated cells.[223] Chondrocytes also synthesize IL-1α.[224] Production of human IL-1 *in vitro* may be enhanced by sodium acetate.[225] Transcription of the IL-1β gene in lymphoid cells is inhibited by glucocorticoids.[226]

1. Production of IL-1 by Malignant Cells

IL-1 is produced by cells of some hematopoietic neoplasms. Human leukemic cells may constitutively produce and secrete IL-1. An unregulated secretion of IL-1 by AML cells may induce stromal cells to overproduce CSFs, thus contributing to the unrestricted growth of AML cells.[227] Bone marrow and peripheral blood cells from children with juvenile chronic granulocytic leukemia, but not with the adult form of the disease, show spontaneous granulocyte-macrophage colony growth. The unusual pattern of colony growth observed in juvenile chronic granulocytic leukemia depends on the production by mononuclear phagocytes of IL-1 which, in turn, by a paracrine mechanism, stimulates the release of high levels of colony-stimulating activity by auxiliary cells.[228] IL-1-dependent production of granulopoietic CSFs may represent a mechanism by which granulopoietic hyperplasia develops in children with this juvenile chronic granulocytic leukemia. In about half of the cases of Hodgkin's disease, IL-1 can be identified by immunohistological methods in Reed-Sternberg cells, granulocytes, and small to medium cells of undetermined origin.[229] Demonstration of IL-1-positive cells in Hodgkin's disease does not correlate with the presence of constitutional symptoms of the disease such as fever, weight loss, and night sweats. In addition to Hodgkin's disease, IL-1 has been detected in neoplastic cells from patients with histiocytic lymphoma and malignant histiocytosis.[230] No IL-1 expression was detected in other lymphomas, including T- and B-cell lymphomas. No IL-1 is apparently present in normal human B or T lymphocytes as well as in normal endothelial cells or fibroblasts.

HL-60 human promyelocytic leukemia cells do not secrete IL-1, but monocytic differentiation induced in these cells by a combined treatment with IFN-γ and calcitriol results in the induction of IL-1 secretion.[231] Production of both IL-1α and IL-1β occurs when the human histiocytic lymphoma cell line, U-937, is induced to differentiate into macrophages and these cells are stimulated with LPS.[232] The production of IL-1 by transformed cells such as the U-937 tumor cell line has been used for the purification and characterization of the IL-1.[233] Dexamethasone selectively inhibits transcription of the IL-1α and IL-1β genes and decreases the stability of IL-1β mRNA in U-937 cells.[234] EBV-transformed human B lymphocytes as well as ATL cells associated with HTLV-I infection express IL-1β mRNA and protein.[104,235,236] Since IL-1β is identical with the osteoclast-activating factor (OAF) expressed in ATL,[102] IL-1β could contribute to the pathogenesis of the ATL-associated hypercalcemia. IL-1 is produced by certain transformed cells of nonhematopoietic cell origin. The PAM-12 cell line, a spontaneously transformed BALB/c-derived keratinocyte cell line, constitutively express IL-1α mRNA, and this expression is markedly augmented in PAM-12 cells by exposure to LPS.[222]

In addition to hematopoietic neoplasms, production of IL-1 is also observed in some human solid tumors. Nasopharyngeal carcinoma cells, which usually harbor the EBV genome, may constitutively produce IL-1α.[237] Significant levels of IL-1α can be detected in conditioned medium from fresh nasopharyngeal carcinoma biopsies. A feature of this tumor is the presence of a T-cell infiltrate which accounts for a major part of the tumor mass. IL-1 released from the malignant epithelial cells of the tumor may contribute to the presence of this infiltrate through stimulation of T-cell migration and activation of the cells within the tumor. Human melanoma cells in culture frequently produce and secrete IL-1.[238] Constitutive production of IL-1-like activity was detected in the conditioned media of 4 of 7 primary melanomas and 5 of 20 metastatic melanoma cell lines.[239] The possible role of IL-1 in the biology of melanomas is unknown, but interleukin could be important in the immune responses occurring in patients bearing these tumors.

2. Regulation of IL-1 Production and Secretion

Numerous physiologic and nonphysiologic factors may be involved in the regulation of IL-1 production and secretion. IL-1 itself stimulates IL-1 gene expression in different systems, including smooth muscle cells, endothelial cells, and monocytes.[240] Stimulation of human polymorphonuclear leukocytes with either LPS or IL-1α induces expression of the IL-1α and IL-1β genes at both the transcriptional and translational levels.[241] IL-1β can induce IL-1α mRNA expression in primary cultures of Leydig cells.[242] Both IL-1α and IL-1β increase the levels of IL-1β gene transcripts in cultured human fibroblasts.[243] Blockage of PGE_2 production reduces the stimulatory effect exerted by IL-1, suggesting that IL-1 and PGE_2 may act in synergism to enhance IL-1 gene expression in the cultured cells.

Human peripheral blood mononuclear cells, freshly isolated from normal donors, do not express either IL-1α or IL-1β gene transcripts.[244] Stimulation of the mononuclear cells with lectin (PHA/concanavalin A) induces expression of both IL-1α and IL-1β, but at different levels. IL-1β mRNA exhibits a much higher level of induction than IL-1α mRNA at all time points after lectin induction. IL-2 also stimulates human peripheral blood mononuclear cells to produce IL-1α and IL-1β.[245,246] Protein kinase C, but not calcium/calmodulin kinase, is involved in the transduction of signals initiated by IL-2 for the expression of IL-1β mRNA in human monocytes. Tyrosine kinase activity is involved in the protein kinase C-induced IL-1β gene expression in monocytic cells.[247] IL-4 regulates IL-1 expression in human monocytes through transcriptional and posttranscriptional mechanisms.[248]

A membrane-associated form of IL-1 may be structurally and functionally different from the usually detected soluble form of the interleukin. T cells may induce macrophages to express the membrane associated form of IL-1 both by direct cell-cell contact and through the release of an unidentified lymphokine after activation.[249] A membrane-associated form of IL-1 is induced on the human macrophage tumor cell line U-937 by pretreatment with phorbol ester.[250] IL-1 production by human monocyte cell lines can be enhanced by treatment with the DNA-demethylating agent, azacytidine.[251]

The production and secretion of IL-1 may be altered in a diversity of nonmalignant human diseases. Bacterial endotoxin and TNF-α may cause accumulation of IL-1β mRNA in human vascular endothelial cells.[252,253] The induction of IL-1 production by IL-1 in human vessel wall cells represents a positive feedback loop which may have an important role in the pathogenesis of vascular disease, including vasculitis and atherosclerosis. Hyaluronic acid, which coexists with macrophages and other leukocytes in synovial fluid from patients with rheumatoid arthritis, induces IL-1 production in macrophages and may contribute to the pathological and physiological changes in connective tissues.[254] IL-1 secreted by activated monocyte-macrophages induce synovial cells and chondrocytes to secrete increased levels of PGE_2 and proteases, leading to the breakdown of cartilage matrix. This effect of IL-1 may be enhanced by other factors, especially by FGF.[255] Production of IL-1 is increased in HIV-positive patients with AIDS-related complex.[256] However, IL-1 production by LPS-activated monocytes-macrophages is decreased in patients with fully developed AIDS.

3. Mechanisms of Regulation of IL-1 Production and Secretion

The mechanisms involved in the control of IL-1 production and secretion are little understood. IL-1 is apparently not preformed, and increased levels of IL-1 mRNA are detected when cells such as monocytes-macrophages are stimulated. The IL-1 precursor molecule (pro-IL-1) lacks a typical leader sequence, suggesting that IL-1 secretion does not involve the endoplasmic reticulum, the Golgi apparatus, or secretory vesicles. The results of an immunoelectron microscopic study suggest that IL-1β is not anchored on the plasma membrane but is localized to the cytosolic ground substance after LPS stimulation of human monocytes.[257] The precise mechanism of IL-1 secretion remains to be characterized.

Complex interactions involving arachidonic acid metabolites, cyclic nucleotides, and IFNs may participate in the regulation of IL-1 production and secretion by cells such as mouse peritoneal macrophages.[258,259] Calcium does not appear to play a central role in the induction and secretion of IL-1 by activated monocytes.[260] Other cytokines may contribute to regulate the generation of IL-1 in different types of cells. IFN-α, but not IFN-γ, directly induces production and secretion of IL-1 by human monocytes.[261] On the other hand, IFN-γ, but not IFN-α, renders the monocytes more sensitive to certain other IL-1-inducing stimuli. TNF-α induces the production of both IL-1α and IL-1β mRNA and protein in human fibroblasts.[262] The production of IL-1 by mouse macrophages may depend on the concentration of TNF-α. Whereas at low levels TNF-α induces the production of IL-1 as well as that of a factor that synergizes with IL-1, at higher concentrations TNF-α blocks the production of IL-1.[263] TNF-α-induced production of IL-1 by murine resident peritoneal macrophages is augmented by indomethacin (an inhibitor of the cyclooxygenase pathway of arachidonic acid metabolism and PGE_2 synthesis).[264] Indomethacin also increases bacteriotoxin-stimulated IL-1 expression by human peripheral blood monocytes and the promyelocytic tumor cell line U-937.[265] These data indicate that prostaglandins participate in an autoregulatory pathway that posttranscriptionally reduces the expression of IL-1 activity. Protein kinase C and other unknown signal pathways may also be involved in the control of IL-1 production by stimulated macrophages.[266] Phorbol ester-induced differentiation of U-937 cells is associated with IL-1 gene expression, and this effect is mediated by the activation of protein kinase C.[267]

Tumor cells may stimulate IL-1 production from enriched large granular lymphocytes.[268] Moreover, a relationship may exist between the ability of tumor cells to stimulate IL-1 release from large granular lymphocytes and their susceptibility to lysis by these cells. Adoptive tumor immunotherapy, and possibly primary antitumor immune response, results in an increased production of IL-1.[269] Systemic activation of the IL-1 pathway in tumor-bearing animals may be reflected by the increased levels of IL-1 in the peritoneal cavity, which is probably due to the secretory activity of peritoneal macrophages.

D. IL-1 INHIBITORS

A number of heterogeneous molecules that inhibit one or more of the activities of IL-1 have been identified and partially characterized.[270] These inhibitors might act at several levels, including the binding of IL-1 to its receptor, the receptor function after IL-1 binding, and postreceptor events of IL-1 cellular actions. IL-1 inhibitors have been detected in body fluids (blood and urine) as well as in solid tissues. Human neutrophils are the source of a specific IL-1 inhibitor.[271] This inhibitor is heat-labile, heterogeneous in size, and appears to be constitutively present in polymorphonuclear neutrophils. UV irradiation of normal and transformed murine epidermal cells *in vitro* results in the release of a 40-kDa IL-1 inhibitor.[272] The biological significance of IL-1 inhibitors is unknown.

1. Urine-Derived Inhibitors of IL-1

Human urine is a rich source of IL-1 inhibitors. IL-1 inhibitors of 20 to 40 and 29 to 67 kDa have been detected in the urine of febrile patients.[273,274] A 18- to 25-kDa IL-1 inhibitor partially purified from the urine of leukemic and other febrile patients affected the various biological activities of both IL-1α and IL-1β, but not TNF-α.[275] This inhibitor apparently acts by interfering with the interaction of IL-1 and its receptor.

An IL-1 inhibitor isolated from human urine is uromodulin, an 85-kDa glycoprotein rich in sialic acid and with immunosuppressive properties.[276-279] Uromodulin regulates the biological activity IL-1 and its activity depends on intact N-linked glycosylation. It is distinct from the IL-1 inhibitor derived from the urine of febrile individuals, although both proteins are potent inhibitors of antigen-induced human lymphocyte proliferation and may prove to be physiologically significant immunoregulators of IL-1. The mechanism of action of IL-1 inhibitors is unknown.

2. α-Melanocyte-Stimulating Hormone

The pituitary hormone, α-melanocyte-stimulating hormone (α-MSH), may act as an inhibitor of the ability of IL-1 to augment the proliferation of murine thymocytes and the production of prostaglandin by human fibroblasts *in vitro*.[280] These inhibitory effects of α-MSH occur in a dose-dependent manner and show a biphasic type of response. Both native α-MSH and an analog of α-MSH are capable of inhibiting the capacity of IL-1β to elicit a number of its reported *in vivo* activities in mice, including fever, neutropenia, hepatocyte production of serum amyloid P, and stimulation of increased plasma levels of corticosterone.[281] However, α-MSH is not a universal inhibitor of the physiological activities of IL-1 since some of these activities, either *in vivo* or *in vitro*, are not inhibited by α-MSH.

3. Protein p15E

The retroviral transmembrane envelope protein p15E, contained in the human retroviruses HTLV-I and HTLV-II, as well as a putative envelope protein encoded by an endogenous type C human retroviral DNA, exhibits immunosuppressive activity on human lymphocytes, monocytes, and macrophages.[282] A synthetic peptide, termed CKS-17, corresponding to the p15E region, inhibits the proliferation of an IL-2-dependent murine cytotoxic T-cell line as well as that of alloantigen-stimulated murine and human lymphocytes. The CKS-17 peptide neither binds directly to IL-1 nor interferes with the ability of the receptor to bind or internalize IL-1, but it is capable of inhibiting the secretion of IL-2 by murine thymocytes stimulated with IL-1 or by phorbol esters.[283] CKS-17 inhibits the effector phase of monocyte-mediated cytotoxicity and may exert an immunosuppressive effect by blocking the production of IL-1, which would eliminate the stimulus necessary for IL-2 production.[284] Apparently, CKS-17 inhibits IL-1-mediated responses by interfering with signal transduction through a protein kinase C pathway.

4. IL-1 Receptor Antagonist

An IL-1 inhibitory activity purified from the medium conditioned by monocytes grown on adherent immune complexes or IgG has been shown to be represented by one nonglycosylated and two glycosylated forms of a polypeptide that can block the action of IL-1 by binding to IL-1 receptors with the same activity as IL-1.[285,286] A similar or identical IL-1 inhibitor was purified and characterized from the culture medium conditioned by the PMA-differentiated human monocyte cell line THP-1.[287] These inhibitors do not have IL-1-like actions and may act through a mechanism corresponding to the action of a pure IL-1 receptor antagonist protein (IRAP or IL-1ra).[288] Analysis of cDNAs coding for human IRAP indicated that its structure is partially similar to that of IL-1β.[289,290] Comparison of the sequences of genomic clones for IRAP from human, mouse, and rat with sequences for IL-1α and IL-1β from the same sources suggests that the three proteins have a common ancestor, and that the gene leading to IRAP diverged early in the evolution of the IL-1 family.[291] The human gene encoding the IL-1 receptor antagonist has been mapped to chromosome region 2q14, near the IL-1α and IL-1β loci.[292,293] Analysis of monocyte RNA showed that IRAP expression is regulated at the transcriptional level. Both TNF-α and IL-1 markedly increase the synthesis of IRAP by synovial fibroblasts.[294] IRAP inhibits IL-1 bioactivity on T lymphocytes and endothelial cells *in vitro* and is a potent inhibitor of IL-1-induced corticosterone production *in vivo*.

E. IL-1 RECEPTORS

The effects of IL-1 at the cellular level are initiated by the binding of IL-1 to a specific, high-affinity cellular receptor located at the level of the plasma membrane.[295] Analysis of cDNA clones encoding the murine and human IL-1 receptor indicate that the receptor molecule contains a large cytoplasmic region, a single transmembrane domain, and an extracellular, IL-1-binding portion composed of three Ig-like domains.[296] The cytoplasmic portion of the receptor is composed of 215 amino acids and does not resemble other sequenced molecules of known function.

IL-1 receptors are expressed in both hematic and nonhematic cells, but among T-lymphocyte populations this expression is restricted to the L3T4+ subset of mature T cells.[297] Rat hepatocytes express abundant IL-1 receptors.[298] The IL-1 protein and its receptor are evolutionarily conserved. Human IL-1 potentiates the proliferative response of catfish lymphocytes to concanavalin A,[299] suggesting that fish IL-1 receptors can recognize IL-1 protein of mammalian origin.

1. Classes of Surface IL-1 Receptors

IL-1 receptors with high and low affinity for the ligand have been detected in a variety of cell types. Whereas cells such as the EL4-6.1 mutant subline of EL4 mouse thymoma express large amounts of both classes of IL-1 receptors, other cells, including normal T cells, also express both classes of receptors, but the absolute number of receptors per cell is considerably less.[300] The effects of IL-1, however, are mediated exclusively via interaction with the minor class of high-affinity IL-1 receptors. The receptors for IL-1α and IL-1β are identical in human, murine, and porcine cells.[179,301,302] The biological significance of two different IL-1 molecules sharing a common receptor is not understood.

IL-1 receptors present on murine T-cell lymphoma and fibroblast cell lines are very similar despite the fact that the biological response of the two cell types to IL-1 differ by several orders of magnitude.[303] However, due to the wide diversity of cell types responding to IL-1 and the wide variety of physiological effects caused by IL-1, it seems likely that IL-1 may be recognized by different receptors in different types of cells. Human and murine B-cell and T-cell lines express different IL-1 receptors.[304,305] In the EL4-6.1 murine thymoma cell line, the IL-1 receptor is represented by a membrane-associated glycoprotein of about 80 kDa containing N-linked glycan units.[306,307] In EBV-transformed human B cells the IL-1 receptor is a protein of 60 kDa.[308] Studies on human B-cell lines indicate marked heterogeneity in IL-1 receptor binding, suggesting that the effects of IL-1 on B-lymphocyte proliferation and differentiation may not be mediated via binding to the 80-kDa receptor only.[309] An IL-1 receptor of 60 kDa expressed in many types of human and murine cells, including B and T lymphocytes, has been characterized. The 60-kDa IL-1 receptor consists of a ligand-binding portion comprised of three Ig-like domains, a single transmembrane region, and a short cytoplasmic domain of 29 amino acids — in contrast to the 215 amino acids of the 80-kDa IL-1 receptor.[310] Thus, there are two distinct classes of high-affinity IL-1 receptors: an 80-kDa receptor (type I IL-1 receptor) and a 60-kDa receptor (type II IL-1 receptor). The two classes of murine high-affinity IL-1 receptors are encoded by distinct genes.[311] The possible functional significance of IL-1 receptor heterogeneity is not understood, but IL-1α and IL-1β may bind independently to the type I and type II receptors.[312] The two types of IL-1 receptors may interact with different intracellular transduction pathways. IL-1 induces in lymphocytes expression of the transcription factor NF-kappa B (NF-κB) through its type I, but not its type II receptor.[313]

2. Expression of IL-1 Receptors on the Cell Surface

Expression of IL-1 receptors depends on both homologous and heterologous regulatory factors. The levels of IL-1 receptor expression on the cell surface are partially controlled by IL-1 itself. Exposure of cultured human fibroblasts to IL-1 results in a marked reduction in the expression of IL-1 receptors on the cell surface, but this initial phase is followed by upregulation of the receptor expression through production of prostaglandins.[314] Exogenously added PGE_2 and glucocorticoid enhance IL-1 receptor expression by the cultured human fibroblasts and peripheral blood mononuclear cells in an additive manner. In the YT human large granular lymphocyte cell line, IL-1 induces downregulation of its own receptor, caused by internalization of the IL-1-receptor complex after ligand binding.[315] After internalization, IL-1 is transferred to membranous intracellular organelles, and finally to lysosomes. As with other growth factors, the IL-1 receptor may be released in a soluble form from the cell surface into the extracellular fluids.[316] Soluble IL-1 receptors may contribute to the regulation of the physiological action of IL-1 on the cell surface.

Heterologous regulation of the IL-1 receptor occurs in many different types of cells under different conditions. Several hormones and growth factors are involved in the regulation of IL-1 receptor expression. Glucocorticoid hormones induce an increase in the expression of the IL-1 receptor on human peripheral blood mononuclear cells without any significant alteration in the receptor binding affinity.[317] CSF-3 can also stimulate IL-1 receptor expression in these cells, and this effect is synergistically enhanced by glucocorticoids.[318] TGF-β-induced inhibition of IL-1 activity in cultured chondrocytes involves downregulation of IL-1 receptors.[319] In contrast, FGF enhances IL-1 receptor expression in the chondrocytes.[320] PDGF induces an increase in the expression of IL-1 receptors in mouse fibroblasts and enhances the response of the cells to IL-1.[321,322] The effect of PDGF on IL-1 receptor expression occurs at the transcriptional level and requires the products of immediate early genes. The intracellular signal transductional mechanisms involved in the regulation of IL-1 receptor expression are unknown, but studies on BALB/c 3T3 mouse fibroblasts indicate that stimulation of either the protein kinase C pathway or the cAMP-dependent pathway may lead to the induction of IL-1 binding and IL-1 receptor mRNA accumulation.[323] These two pathways appear to mediate IL-1 receptor expression in a manner independent of each other.

3. Nuclear IL-1 Receptors

Receptor-mediated endocytosis of IL-1 is associated in different types of cells with its transportation into the nucleus.[324] Accumulation of IL-1α in the nucleus of EL4-6.1 cells has been attributed to the presence of specific nuclear receptors which could mediate some of the cellular actions of the interleukin.[325] However, the structure and possible physiologic role of the IL-1 nuclear receptors remain to be established. Internalization and nuclear localization of IL-1 may not be sufficient to elicit IL-1 activation of gene expression in T cells.[326]

4. Bacterial IL-1 Receptors

IL-1 may enhance bacterial growth through its interaction with receptor-like structures localized on the surface of the microorganism. Human IL-1β, but not TNF-α or IL-4, can enhance the growth of virulent, but not avirulent, strains of *Escherichia coli* through its interaction with a receptor-like protein on the bacterial surface.[327] This enhancement is blocked by the action of the IL-1 receptor antagonist (IRAP). Radiolabeled IL-1 binds to the virulent, but not the avirulent, *E. coli* in a specific and saturable fashion, and IRAP inhibits this binding. These findings suggest that IL-1, produced in the intact animal as a result of inflammation or in the course of bacterial infection, could serve as a growth factor for some types of virulent bacteria, thereby worsening the course of the infection. The precise nature and biological role of the putative bacterial IL-1 receptor(s) remains to be elucidated.

F. POSTRECEPTOR MECHANISMS OF ACTION OF IL-1

The postreceptor mechanisms of action of IL-1 are very complex and are understood only in part. After binding to its surface receptor in responsive cells, IL-1 and its receptor are slowly internalized and translocated to the nucleus.[324] The possible role of this translocation is unknown. Cellular changes occurring in IL-1-responsible cells may include the adenylate cyclase system, ion fluxes, production of prostaglandins, protein phosphorylation, phosphoinositide turnover, protein synthesis, and proto-oncogene expression. IL-1-induced changes at the level of the plasma membrane may include stimulation of hexose transport by increasing the expression of glucose transporters.[328]

1. Production of Cyclic Nucleotides

The adenylate cyclase system may mediate at least some of the cellular actions of IL-1. cAMP mediates IL-1-induced lymphocyte penetration through endothelial monolayers and cytostasis of K-562 human leukemia cells.[329,330] Exposure of mouse Swiss 3T3 or human FS-4 fibroblasts to IL-1 causes a rapid accumulation of cAMP and an increase in the level of cAMP-dependent protein kinase activity.[331,332] This kinase can phosphorylate histone HII-B protein *in vitro*, but the endogenous substrates of the IL-1-activated kinase have not been identified. At least in certain cells, cAMP is not directly involved in mediating IL-1 action but may have a modulatory effect on this action.[333]

cGMP may have a role in the mechanism of IL-1 action. Both IL-1 and TNF-α stimulate cGMP formation in rat renal mesangial cells.[334] IL-1 induces increased GTP binding and hydrolysis in membranes of the murine thymoma cell line EL4.[335]

2. Changes in Ion Fluxes

The cellular actions of IL-1 may be mediated, at least in part, by changes in ion fluxes across the plasma membrane. IL-1 enhances the exchange of Na^+/H^+ across the membrane of lymphoid cells, thus increasing the total concentration of intracellular sodium and causing sustained cytoplasmic alkalinization and a transient decrease in the intracellular concentration of calcium.[336,337] In a murine T-cell line (MD10 cells), IL-1 activates the Na^+/H^+ antiporter by a mechanism that is unrelated to changes in $[Ca^{2+}]_i$, but may involve protein kinase C activation.[338] The precise role of IL-1-induced alterations in the influx of monovalent ions is not understood. An increase in Na^+ influx may not be required for the expression of differentiated functions induced by IL-1 in target cells. For example, IL-1 induces an increase in pH_i and in total sodium concentration in the 70Z/3 murine pre-B-like lymphoid cell line, but as demonstrated by using an amiloride analog which inhibits the Na^+/H^+ antiporter, these increases are not required for the IL-1-induced synthesis of IgM and the expression of IgM on the surface of 70Z/3 cells.[339] Moreover, in contrast to previous experiments, purified recombinant human IL-1 has no effect on $[Ca^{2+}]_i$ in human polymorphonucleated neutrophils.[340] In cultured rat mesangial cells, the effects of IL-1 are not associated with pH_i alterations.[341] In cultured rabbit osteoclasts, IL-1α induces a sustained increase in $[Ca^{2+}]_i$.[342] In general, the physiological significance of changes in monovalent and divalent ions in the postreceptor cellular mechanisms of IL-1 action is unknown.

3. Production of Polyamines

The activity of ODC, the rate-limiting enzyme in polyamine biosynthesis, is stimulated by IL-1 in human and murine cells that are stimulated to proliferate by the cytokine — including a mouse helper T-cell line, a NK cell-like line, and a human glioblastoma cell line.[343] IL-1 also induces ODC activity in normal T lymphocytes.[344] The effect of IL-1 on ODC activity precedes, and directly correlates in a dose-dependent manner, with its effect on DNA synthesis. Furthermore, putrescine, a product of the ODC reaction and a precursor of polyamines, is able to overcome most, but not all of the antiproliferative action of IL-1 in the A375 human melanoma cell line, which is very sensitive to suppression by IL-1. However, putrescine is not able to reverse the cytostatic effect of IL-1 on MCF-7 and T-47D human breast carcinoma cells.

4. Production of Prostaglandins

Prostaglandins may mediate some of the cellular actions of IL-1. Addition of IL-1 to mouse Swiss 3T3 cells results in stimulated synthesis of PGE_2 which, in turn, stimulates the synthesis of cAMP.[334] The activity of phospholipase A_2 and the metabolism of arachidonic acid with production of PGE_2 is increased in human lung fibroblasts, rat mesangial cells, and rabbit chondrocytes exposed to IL-1α or IL-1β.[345,346] Synergistic effects are observed when IL-1α or IL-1β and TNF-α are added together. The effects of IL-1 on PGE_2 and phospholipase A_2 are inhibited by pretreatment of the cells with either actinomycin D or cycloheximide, suggesting that they are mediated, at least in part, by transcriptional and translational processes. The gene coding for cyclooxygenase, an enzyme involved in the synthesis of prostaglandins, is rapidly and markedly induced in endothelial cells by the action of IL-1.[347] IL-1α may be more potent than IL-1β in stimulating fibroblasts to synthesize PGE_2.[348] However, IL-1 alone is not sufficient to induce PGE_2 synthesis in fibroblasts, which requires the presence of other growth factors such as PDGF or FGF.[349]

IL-1 stimulates the resorption of bone in cultured mouse calvaria and this effect is associated with the production of PGE_2, PGI_2, and $PGF_2α$.[350] The effects are abrogated or reduced by treatment with either indomethacin (an inhibitor of cyclooxygenase activity) or IFN-γ (which inhibits prostaglandin production in bone). A membrane-associated form of IL-1 markedly enhances PGE_2 production from the human chondrosarcoma cell line SW-1353.[250]

IL-1-induced production of PGE by cultured human fibroblasts is not due to a direct mobilization of arachidonic acid but involves the synthesis of new protein(s), different from phospholipase A_2, in the stimulated cells.[351] Synthesis of this protein may be required for the conversion of free arachidonic acid to PGE_2. The protein may correspond to cyclooxygenase, an enzyme involved in the conversion of arachidonate into prostaglandin. IL-1 also stimulates the production of prostacyclin (PGI_2) by vascular endothelial cells *in vitro*.[352] IL-1 stimulates the synthesis of cyclooxygenase by fibroblasts in a time- and dose-dependent fashion.[353]

5. Protein Phosphorylation

Phosphorylation of cellular proteins may play an important role in the mechanism of IL-1 action, but the kinases involved in IL-1-induced protein phosphorylation remain to be identified. Studies on the human leukemia cell line K562 had suggested that the IL-1 receptor has an ATP-binding site and possesses tyrosine kinase activity.[354,355] However, no evidence has been obtained that the IL-1 receptor has an intrinsic kinase activity, and the phosphorylations occurring in the IL-1 receptor and other cellular proteins after IL-1 binding to their receptors are probably due to the secondary activation of protein kinases. Binding of IL-1 to its receptor induces a rapid phosphorylation of the receptor on serine/threonine residues due to activation of an extrinsic protein kinase.[356] IL-1 stimulates serine phosphorylation of an acidic cytosolic protein of 65 kDa in glucocorticoid-pretreated normal human peripheral blood mononuclear leukocytes.[317] This phosphorylation may not be due to protein kinase C activity. However, phorbol esters, which induce phosphorylation of cellular proteins through activation of protein kinase C, can display IL-1-like activity. A PMA-protein complex mimics IL-1 activity in some cellular systems.[357] PMA, but not IL-1, can induce phosphorylation of the murine IL-1 receptor on a single threonine residue (Thr-537), near the carboxy-terminus of the receptor molecule.[358] The possible functional significance of this modification is unknown.

The effects of IL-1 *in vivo* may partially depend on the stimulated phosphorylation of specific cellular proteins. However, most studies on this subject have been performed *in vitro*. In a mouse anterior pituitary tumor cell line, IL-1 induces phosphorylation of proteins of 19, 20, and 60 kDa and stimulates secretion of β-endorphin.[359] In human fibroblast monolayers, IL-1β causes a transient increase in the phosphorylation of the cytoskeletal protein talin, and this effect is followed by changes in the attachment and shape of the cells.[360] The phosphorylation of talin would occur via activation of a serine/threonine-specific protein kinase and may lead to changes in transmembrane linkage proteins and the cytoskeleton. Alterations at focal adhesions provides a mechanism by which IL-1 may modulate cell-matrix interactions during inflammation and wound healing.

6. Phosphoinositide Metabolism

The possible role of phosphoinositide metabolism in the mechanisms of IL-1 action is a subject of controversy, with different results being obtained in different cell types and different experimental systems. Enhanced phosphoinositide turnover, associated with an increase in $[Ca^{2+}]_i$ and protein kinase C activation, may not be required for mediating actions of IL-1 such as the induction of IL-2 production by some human leukemia cells.[361] Studies using a plasmid construct also indicate that the IL-1 signal required for the induction of IL-2 gene expression is not mediated by protein kinase C.[362] Protein kinase C is probably not a mediator of IL-1 action in rabbit articular chondrocytes.[363] However, IL-1 may stimulate phospholipid metabolism and arachidonic acid release by human synovial cells.[364] Treatment of rat chondrocytes with either IL-1 or TNF-β results in a dose-dependent activation of membrane-bound phospholipase.[365] IL-1 can stimulate phosphatidylinositol kinase activity in human fibroblasts.[366]

IL-1 is able to generate 1,2-diacylglycerol in certain types of cells (peripheral blood T cells, murine T-cell lines, and Jurkat cells) directly from phosphatidylcholine, in the absence of increased phosphatidylinositol turnover.[367] In Jurkat cells, IL-1 modulates protein kinase C activity through stimulation of the synthesis of phosphatidylserine.[368] In the murine pre-B-like cell line 70Z/3, IL-1α enhances Na^+/H^+ exchange across the membrane and induces translocation of protein kinase C to the plasma membrane, but protein kinase C activation is not required in these cells for IL-1α to stimulate Na^+/H^+ exchange across the membrane.[337] In rat mesangial cells, IL-1 activates a phospholipase C which is predominantly linked to phosphatidylethanolamine.[341] These results suggest that IL-1-induced cellular activation may be mediated, at least in part, by phospholipid-derived second messengers generated through some novel metabolic pathways.

7. Protein Synthesis

Cytokines such as IL-1α, IL-1β, IFN-α, IFN-β, and TNF-α induce or enhance, in a partially overlapping form, the synthesis of various proteins in target cells such as human fibroblasts.[369] The greater numbers of proteins are induced in common between IFN-α and IFN-γ and between IL-1α and TNF-α. The two forms of IL-1 and TNF-α each induced several polypeptides in the human fibroblasts, but little is known of the structure and function of these polypeptides. Recent evidence indicates that one of the polypeptides induced by IL-1 in fibroblasts and smooth muscle cells is a homodimer of the PDGF A-chain (PDGF-AA).[124] Most probably, the mitogenic effects of IL-1 in fibroblasts and smooth muscle cells are indirect and mediated by the production of PDGF-AA.

8. Gene Expression

Some of the effects of IL-1 on its target cells may be exerted through modification of gene expression. IL-1 activates the expression of several genes in lymphoid cells, including the genes for TGF-β and the IL-2 receptor, the proto-oncogene c-*myc*, and the tumor suppressor gene p53.[370] Expression of the genes encoding the neutrophil-activating protein, IL-8, and the monocyte chemotactic peptide are stimulated by IL-1 in human synovial cells.[371]

The mechanisms by which IL-1 can induce specific alterations in gene expression are not known, but one of them may consist in the activation of the nuclear factor kappa B (NF-κB), an ubiquitous transcription factor that is capable of affecting the expression of many genes.[372] In contrast to phorbol ester-induced NF-κB activation, IL-1-induced activation of NF-κB occurs through pathways independent of protein kinase C, whereas this enzyme may be involved in IL-1β induction of TNF-α gene expression.[373] Complexes of IL-1β and its receptor may be internalized into the nucleus, and may form a complex with DNA, suggesting a direct regulation of gene expression by this mechanism.[374]

9. Proto-Oncogene Expression

IL-1α alters the level of expression of c-*fos* and c-*myc* in both human peripheral blood T lymphocytes and the IL-1-dependent mouse helper T-cell line D10.G4.1.[375] Untreated human T cells produce minimal amounts of c-*fos* and c-*myc* mRNA and are induced to produce high levels of these mRNAs after stimulation with IL-1. Other cell types stimulated with IL-1 may express the c-*fos* and c-*myc* genes. Secretion of β-endorphin by the mouse anterior pituitary cell line AtT-20 depends on c-*fos* and c-*myc* gene expression by the cells.[376] Exposure of quiescent diploid human FS-4 fibroblasts to IL-1 and/or TNF-α results in a rapid induction of c-*fos* and c-*myc* gene expression.[377] IL-1 induced of c-*myc* expression in fibroblasts is mediated by NF-κB-like transcription factors.[378] IL-1β increases the concentration of c-*myc* mRNA and stimulates the growth of the rat thyroid follicular cell line FRTL5.[146] This effect is synergistically enhanced by the presence of serum or IGF-I. Expression of the c-*fos* gene is rapidly and transiently increased when human vascular smooth-muscle cells maintained in culture are exposed to IL-1.[379] IL-1 is involved in the local regulation of insulin secretion and induces rapid and transient expression of c-*fos* gene expression in isolated pancreatic islets and in purified pancreatic β cells, as well as in the clonal insulin secretory cell line HIT-T15.[380,381] Accumulation of c-*fos* mRNA and protein may represent an early signal transduction event in the β cell and a component of the mechanisms by which IL-1 influences β-cell function.

G. EFFECTS OF IL-1 ON THE PROLIFERATION AND DIFFERENTIATION OF NORMAL AND NEOPLASTIC CELLS

Depending on the cell type and the physiological conditions, IL-1 may either inhibit or stimulate, or may have no effect on cellular proliferation.[382] IL-1 inhibits the proliferation of normal human endometrial stromal cells.[383] Different types of mechanisms may be responsible for the effects of IL-1 on cell proliferation. The antiproliferative effect of IL-1 on the human melanoma cell line A375 are due to arrest of the cells in the $G_0 + G_1$ phases of the cycle.[384] The growth of human vascular smooth muscle cells is not stimulated by IL-1 under usual conditions, but inhibition of prostaglandin synthesis with cyclooxygenase inhibitors such as indomethacin or aspirin in the tissue incubated in the presence of IL-1 results in a marked increase in cell growth.[379] Prolonged exposure of the cells to IL-1 may cause growth in the absence of cyclooxygenase inhibitors.

A variety of solid human tumors produce and secrete IL-1 *in vitro* and probably also *in vivo*. Human ovarian epithelial cancer cells cultured *in vitro* express both IL-1α and IL-1β genes.[385] However, the biological significance of this expression is not understood. IL-1 exerts variable effects on the growth of tumor cells *in vitro*. Whereas some human mammary carcinoma cell lines (MCF-7, T47D, and MDA-MB-415) are growth inhibited in the presence of either native or recombinant forms of human IL-1, other normal and malignant cell lines, including the lung carcinoma (CALU-1) and colon carcinoma (SW-48) lines, are not inhibited by IL-1.[386,387] IL-1 has no effect on the growth of the milk mammary line HBL-100. The reasons for these differences, as well as the mechanisms of IL-1-induced inhibition of cell growth, are unknown, but both inhibition and stimulation of malignant cell growth by IL-1 are related to the presence of receptor sites. However, the differential effect of IL-1 on the growth of different human breast cancer cell lines may be due to differences in the expression of IL-1 receptors in these cells.[388] The cell line MCF-7, whose growth is inhibited by IL-1, possesses IL-1 receptors, whereas growth of the cell line MDA-231 is not inhibited by IL-1 and these cells do not possess IL-1 receptors. In any case, the inhibitory effect of IL-1 on the growth of human breast cancer cell lines corresponds to that of a hormone acting on nonimmune target organs or tissues.

Human AML cells frequently produce IL-1, and IL-1 may act as an autocrine growth factor for these cells.[389] However, the activity of IL-1 to potentiate blast progenitor growth in AML may be indirect — via production of CSFs by the leukemic cells.[390] The endogenous production of IL-1 by AML cells may stimulate autocrine secretion of CSF-2, thus inducing autonomous growth of the blast cell population.[391,392] In contrast, IL-1 can inhibit in a reversible fashion the growth of the K562 human myelogenous leukemia cell line.[355,393] The effect of IL-1 on K562 cells is accompanied by signs of differentiation, including increased expression of HLA antigens. A similar growth-inhibitory and differentiation-inducing effect is exerted by IL-1 on the mouse myeloid leukemia cell line M1.[394]

Complex interactions occurring between IL-1 and other factors may explain, at least in part, the variable effects of IL-1 on the proliferation and differentiation of tumor cells. IL-1 and IL-6 exhibit additive or synergistic effects on the differentiation of human and murine myeloid leukemic cell lines, including M1 and U-937 cells.[395] IL-1 and TNF-α have cooperative effects on the differentiation of M1 cells.[396] IL-1α inhibits the proliferation of human melanoma cells A375 *in vitro*,[397] and this inhibition is synergized by TNF-α.[398] The antiproliferative effect of IL-1 on human melanoma cells involves at least two pathways, one IL-6-dependent and another IL-6-independent.[399] The growth-inhibitory effects of IL-1 and IFN-γ are additive in the mammary carcinoma cell lines MCF-7 and MDA-MB-415, but other cell lines (cervical carcinoma HeLa and myelogenous leukemia K562) are refractory to IL-1, although they respond to IFN-γ alone.[400] In other cell lines (lung carcinoma CALU-1 and colon carcinoma SW-48), IL-1 stimulates cell growth and abrogates the growth inhibitory effect of IFN-γ. Autocrine secretion of IL-1β can be involved in proliferation of the M7 AML cell line.[401] IL-1 enhances the anchorage-independent growth of the adrenal-derived human adenocarcinoma cell line SW-13.[402] The mechanisms involved in the altered proliferation and differentiation of cells exposed *in vitro* to IL-1 are unknown. The cytostatic effects of IL-1 on tumor cells may also occur *in vivo*. Tumor-bearing hosts may be capable of producing compounds that induce a high secretion of IL-1, which may enable macrophages to mount an antiproliferative effect against tumor cells.[403]

IL-1 released by the endothelium may have important effects on tumorigenesis. The conditioned media of human endothelial monolayers contains a chemoattractant activity for tumor cells which appears to be identical with IL-1.[404] The chemoattractant present in endothelial-derived conditioned media is blocked after preincubation with antibodies against IL-1α and IL-1β. These results suggest that the behavior of intravascular tumor cells and their egress from the microvasculature may be affected by endothelial-derived IL-1. In addition to locally produced IL-1, animals bearing tumors may exhibit a systemic increase in the level of IL-1 activity, which may be due to the release of growth factors such as CSF-1 by the tumor cells.[405] In general, complex interactions between growth factors produced by tumor cells and blood cells, or cells from the local stroma and endothelial cells, may be of great importance for the evolution of tumors *in vivo*.

III. INTERLEUKIN 2

Interleukin-2 (IL-2), originally called T-cell growth factor (TCGF),[406] is produced in T lymphocytes stimulated by the binding of antigen to the T-cell receptor/CD3 complex. IL-2 is also produced by T lymphocytes stimulated with specific mitogens such as plant lectins. IL-2 is present in PHA-stimulated lymphocyte-conditioned media and is capable of maintaining normal lectin-activated T cells in continuous proliferative culture.[407-413] The stimulation of T-cell proliferation by IL-2 occurs by an autocrine type of mechanism which involves IL-2-induced expression of its own receptor. In addition to its growth-stimulating activity on T cells, IL-2 has other important influences on the immune response and the development of natural cytotoxic activity.[414] IL-2 has remarkable antitumor effects both *in vivo* and *in vitro*, which is probably related to its ability to induce the generation of NK cells and other cytotoxic T cells that can counteract tumor growth. The activation of lymphocyte-mediated cytotoxicity by IL-2 may occur, at least in part, through induction of TNF-α receptor expression in the lymphocytes.[415] However, IL-2 is not an exclusively lymphocytotropic factor since it can directly augment the cytotoxicity of human monocytes.[416]

In addition to IL-2, other factors may have a role in T-cell activation. A keratinocyte-derived TCGF, which is functionally distinct from IL-2,[417,418] is probably identical to IL-1a.[222] Another lymphokine, IL-4/BSF-1, may also be considered as a TCGF since it is capable of activating a subpopulation of T cells (type II T helper cells) in the absence of IL-2.[419] IL-4/BSF-1 is produced by stimulated immature thymocytes and is a potent costimulator for some populations of both mature and immature thymocytes.[420] CSF-2 can also function as a growth factor for certain T cells.[421] Cloned T cells (HT-2 cells) can grow for up to 2 months in the presence of CSF-2 as the sole TCGF. Human T cells are capable of proliferating, although to a limited extent, in the absence of both IL-2 and IL-4.[422] The results from several studies strongly suggest that in addition to IL-2, IL-4, and CSF-2, there are other TCGFs and other mechanisms involved in the stimulation of proliferation of T-cell subsets. A thymic stroma-derived T-cell growth factor is capable of inducing the proliferation of various helper T-cell clones, but not of cytotoxic T-cell clones.[423] This growth factor is distinct from IL-2 and IL-4, as well as from the keratinocyte-derived TCGF, according to several functional criteria. The identification of a TCGF derived from the thymic stroma indicates that cellular components of this stroma produce growth factors with activity directed to particular subsets and/or natural stages of lymphocytic cells from the T-cell lineage.

A. BIOLOGICAL EFFECTS OF IL-2
IL-2 exerts important physiological effects on hematic cells including both T and B lymphocytes as well as natural killer cells (NK cells) and cells from the myelopoietic system.

1. Effects of IL-2 on T Lymphocytes
IL-2 is an essential element in the control of T-cell growth and in T-cell mediated immune responses. Activation of T cells requires at least two signals.[424] The first signal consists of processed antigen presented in the context of MCG (Ia) by antigen-presenting cells. This signal can be substituted for by mitogens such as PHA or concanavalin A. A second signal is provided by IL-1 produced by macrophages or other types of cells. Activation of T cells induces the transition from a resting G_0 state into the G_1 phase of the cycle and the subsequent induction of IL-2 secretion and the expression of IL-2 receptors on the surface. Progression of the activated cells from G_1 through the S, G_2, and M phases of the cycle is initiated and regulated by IL-2 binding to high-affinity IL-2 receptors and leads to an expansion of the T-cell population. IL-2 is capable of inducing the proliferation of certain T-cell populations in the absence of any other known external stimulation. IL-2-directed T-cell mitosis is a quantal response determined by a critical threshold of signals generated by the interaction between IL-2 and the IL-2 receptor.[425] Three factors are involved in T-cell cycle progression: IL-2 concentration, IL-2 receptor density, and the duration of the interaction of IL-2 with its receptor.

IL-2 alone may be sufficient to induce the majority of resting NK cells to enter the cell cycle and proliferate, but T cells require antigen or other mitogenic stimuli to respond to IL-2.[426] However, there is clear evidence that a subpopulation of resting T cells is able to proliferate in response to IL-2, in the presence of IL-1, without any antigenic of mitogenic triggering.[427] Most helper T cells expressing the T4 surface glycoprotein antigen (OKT4+ cells) are capable of proliferating in an autocrine fashion in response to the IL-2 that they themselves produce, but an indefinite clonal expansion of these cells (which may result in uncontrolled neoplastic cell growth) does not occur because T4+ cells become refractory to IL-2 at some point after the interaction of IL-2 with its receptor.[428] The mechanisms of acquisition of IL-2 refractoriness by T4+ cells are not understood but are not related to changes in the number, affinity, or functional capacity of the IL-2 receptors expressed in the stimulated cells. Autocrine growth and tumorigenicity may be observed in IL-2-dependent helper T cells transfected with an IL-2 gene.[429] Thus the IL-2 gene, as genes encoding other growth factors, may display oncogene-like properties under specific experimental conditions.

The activation signal requirements for the induction of IL-2 responsiveness are different in the two major subsets of human T lymphocytes, CD4/T4+ (helper/inducer T cells) and CD8/T8+ (cytotoxic/suppressor T cells).[430] Under total monocyte-depleted conditions, T8+ resting small lymphocytes can be activated by concanavalin A, anti-T3 monoclonal antibody, calcium ionophore, and phorbol ester, either alone or in various combinations, to become responsive to IL-2. In contrast, none of these stimuli could, by themselves, induce IL-2 responsiveness in T4+ resting small lymphocytes; this activation requires combinations of PMA plus concanavalin A, anti-T3 monoclonal antibody, or ionomycin. Under optimal conditions *in vitro*, growth of both resting T4+ and T8+ lymphocyte subsets may be independent of monocytes.

IL-2 stimulates the progression of T cells from the G_1 to S phase of the cycle, inducing their "blastic transformation".[431] In the constant presence of IL-2, mature T lymphocytes can be grown indefinitely *in vitro*, and this is valid for both normal and neoplastic human T cells. Whereas normal T cells show an absolute requirement for prior antigenic stimulation for response to IL-2, some malignant cells from leukemias and lymphomas of mature T-cell origin respond directly to lectin-free, partially purified IL-2.

Not all T cells respond to IL-2. T helper cells can be classified into two groups (I and II) based on the profile of lymphokines they produce.[419] Type I T helper cells produce IL-2 and proliferate in response to this factor. In contrast, type II T helper cells produce a distinct factor, IL-4/BSF-1, and this molecule may represent an autocrine growth factor for type II T helper cells.[432] However, the presence of another lymphokine, IL-1, is required for the transduction of the signal generated by IL-4 in type II T helper cells.

2. Effects of IL-2 on NK and Large Granular Lymphocytes

Normal splenic or peripheral human lymphocytes can be activated to become potent NK cells by prolonged exposure to IL-2. Such lymphokine-activated cells (LAK cells) have been described in mouse and human systems and are defined as being able to kill a wide range of tumor cell targets while leaving normal cells undamaged. IL-3 and IL-4 can strongly inhibit *in vitro* human LAK cell function and are also able to reduce the ability of IL-2 to generate LAK cells.[433] LAK cells that proliferate in response to IL-2 in the absence of antigenic of mitogenic stimulation are contained exclusively within the CD11+ lymphocyte subpopulation, which is recognized by anti-CD11 monoclonal antibodies that react with receptors for the iC3b component of complement.[434] IL-2 can act directly upon NK cells to increase their cytotoxicity.[435,436] Human large granular lymphocytes, the morphologic homologues of NK activity, can proliferate in direct response to IL-2 without needing previous activation.[437] Although PHA induces the expression of IL-2 receptors on large granular lymphocytes and T cells, IL-2 alone is able to induce IL-2 receptor mRNA, IL-2 receptor expression, and proliferation of large granular cells with an associated enhancement of their cytotoxicity.[438] In addition to IL-2, IL-3 may have a role in the regulation of growth and differentiation of a subset of large granular lymphocytes committed to T-cell lineage.[439]

Large granular lymphocytes play a central role in natural immunity against tumors. Tumor-infiltrating lymphocytes from metastatic melanoma are primarily cytotoxic cells that can recognize and kill autologous tumor cells after *in vitro* culture. IL-2 induces these cells to proliferate and enhances their cytotoxic activity such that they can eliminate the autologous tumor cells during short-term culture.[440] IL-2 has a crucial role in the generation of LAK cells which display cytotoxic activity against a diversity of tumor cells. This action is synergized by TNF-α and antagonized by TGF-β.[441]

3. Interaction of IL-2 with Other Lymphokines

IL-2 regulates the expression of other lymphokines. The production of IL-1α and IL-1β by human peripheral blood mononuclear cells is stimulated by IL-2.[245] Activation of cytotoxic T cells and NK cells is partially determined by IL-2-independent pathways that may include the action of other lymphokines.[442,443] IL-1α may cooperate with IL-2 in increasing the development of NK cells, which may be due to induction of IL-2 receptors.[444] A combination of TNF-α with IL-2 induces a much more marked increase in NK cell activity than that induced by TNF-α alone.[445] IL-3 and CSF-2 markedly potentiate the IL-2 responsiveness of both freshly isolated human lymphocytes and *in vitro* stimulated T cells.[446]

IL-2 induces IFN-γ expression at both the transcriptional and translational levels.[447] Arachidonic acid plays a pivotal role as mediator of the signal initiated by IL-2 for the stimulation of IFN-γ production.[448] Both IFN-α and IFN-γ would act as modulators of cytotoxic cell responses to IL-2.[449] Release of IL-3 activity by T4+ human T-cell clones may also depend on IL-2.[450]

4. Abrogation of IL-2 Requirement by Oncoproteins

Viral oncoproteins may abrogate the requirement of T cells for the exogenous supply of IL-2. Infection of IL-2-dependent T cells with the acute retrovirus A-MuLV, which carries the v-*abl* oncogene, may result in abrogation of the requirement for IL-2.[451] The precise mechanism of this abrogation is unknown, but does not involve an autocrine phenomenon with endogenous production of IL-2 and expression of IL-2 receptors.

5. Effects of IL-2 on B Lymphocytes

IL-2 could have modulatory actions not only on T lymphocytes but also on B lymphocytes. Both IL-1 and IL-2 may contribute to controlling the maturation of proliferating B cells into antibody-forming cells.[69] IL-2 and IFN-γ may act synergistically at different steps of terminal maturation of human B cells.[452] IL-2 appears to stimulate the growth of large but not small B cells, and this stimulatory effect is not mediated through T cells.[453] Direct induction of human B-cell differentiation has been obtained by treatment with recombinant IL-2.[454] Administration of IL-2 *in vivo* may induce a polyclonal IgM response capable of protecting mice against septic death.[455,456] Glucocorticoids may act as potentiators of the effects of IL-2 on B-cell differentiation.[457] IL-2 regulates the activity of the Lyn tyrosine kinase in a B-cell line.[458] However, it is not totally clear as to whether IL-2 exerts direct effects on B lymphocytes. Studies with an *in vivo* system indicate that murine B cells, but not T cells, proliferate and differentiate polyclonally into Ig-secreting cells without expressing substantial amounts of IL-2 receptors.[459] In other studies, it was found that human IL-2 does not perturb the physiology of purified B cells in any state of activation, suggesting that the previously described effects of IL-2 on B cells are mediated through additional cell types.[460] Similar negative findings were obtained with IFN-γ. These results cast doubt on the necessity for IL-2 or IFN-γ for T-cell-dependent B-cell proliferation and differentiation. However, in a recent critical study it was concluded that "IL-2 induces both B-cell proliferation and differentiation which are independent of any other cells" and that "IL-2 directly affects the function of activated B cells."[461] Further studies are required in order to clarify the possible direct effects of IL-2 on B cells.

6. Effects of IL-2 on Monocytes

Human monocytes exposed *in vitro* to IFN-γ express IL-2 receptor mRNA and protein, and addition of IL-2 to monocytes pretreated with IFN-γ results in release of IL-1β induced by endotoxin (LPS).[462] IFN-γ and IL-2 would act in a sequential fashion on monocytes to amplify the immune response by establishing a positive feedback circuit.

7. Effects of IL-2 on Myelopoiesis

In addition to its important physiological effects on T and B lymphocytes, IL-2 may have a regulatory effect on myelopoiesis. Recombinant human IL-2 increases bone marrow cellularity and proliferation of stem cells in normal mice as well as in mice receiving lethal or sublethal doses of cyclophosphamide or lethal doses of γ-irradiation.[463] These effects are probably secondary to stimulation of CSF activities. In other experimental conditions, IL-2 may exert an inhibitory effect on myelopoiesis.[464] This effect depends on T cells and is mediated by the T-cell IL-2 receptor, but other humoral mechanisms, involving IFN-γ and other IL-2-induced T-cell lymphokines, are also implicated in mediating the effects of IL-2 on myelopoiesis. The results suggest that IL-2 can function as a potent growth regulator of a nonlymphoid compartment of the human immune system, and that IL-2 may play a role in the negative feedback regulation occurring between T lymphocytes and granulocyte/macrophage progenitor proliferation.

8. Effects of IL-2 on Endocrine Cells

IL-2 may exert physiological effects in endocrine cells. IL-2 is locally produced in the gonads and may play a paracrine function in modulating Leydig cell function. IL-2 is a potent inhibitor of steroidogenesis in primary cultures of rat Leydig cells, inhibiting the hCG-stimulated production of testosterone and cAMP, but has no effects on the binding of hCG to Leydig cells.[465]

B. THE HUMAN T-CELL ANTIGEN RECEPTOR COMPLEX

The differentiation of T lymphocytes occurs mainly within the thymus and includes the formation and expression of surface receptors (T-cell antigen receptors or T-cell receptors) which are capable of recognizing foreign antigens.[466] Specific interaction between T-cell receptors on immature thymocytes and MHC antigens expressed in the thymus determines the differentiation of the thymocytes into mature T cell.[467] Induction of an immune response to a foreign antigen requires the activation of T lymphocytes expressing antigen-specific receptors.[468] Unlike immunoglobulins, which recognize free antigens, T lymphocytes can recognize cell-bound antigens, but these antigens must be presented in the context of antigen molecules encoded by MHC genes. However, it is still unknown how T-cell receptors recognize target cell MHC and antigen. Collection of antigens in lymphoid organs, processing of these antigens in accessory cells such as macrophages and dendritic cells, and presentation of the processed antigen to antigen-specific lymphocytes promote the proliferation, interaction, and differentiation to effector cells for the development of the immune response. Migration of recirculating lymphocytes from the bloodstream to particular lymphoid organs or sites by a process called homing, which is mediated by lymphocyte homing receptors, would facilitate the recognition of the cells involved in the specific immune response.[469]

1. T Lymphocyte Subsets

The differentiation of two functionally distinct classes of T lymphocytes is associated with the acquisition of the CD4 and CD8 antigens represented by glycoproteins expressed on the cell surface.[470] These markers divide T cells into two major subsets: CD4$^+$ (OKT4 or T4$^+$) with helper/inducer activity, and CD8$^+$ (OKT8 or T8$^+$) with cytotoxic/suppressor properties. Mature T cells expressing one or the other of the CD antigens arise in the thymus from "double negative" (CD4$^-$/CD8$^-$) precursors, with "double positive" (CD4$^+$/CD8$^+$) thymocytes postulated to be intermediate in lymphocyte ontogeny.[471] Helper/inducer T cells tend to recognize cognate antigens presented in the context of a class II MHC molecule, whereas cytotoxic/suppressor T cells recognize antigens presented in conjunction with a class I MHC molecule.[472] The molecular basis for this correlation is unknown.

Tyrosine phosphorylation is required for T-cell receptor-mediated signal transduction.[473] The CD4/CD8 antigens are complexed on the surface of human T lymphocytes to the protein p56^{lck}, which is the product of the putative proto-oncogene *lck*.[474] The *lck* gene is a member of the *src* gene family and its product possesses tyrosine kinase activity. There is genetic evidence for the involvement of the Lck tyrosine kinase in signal transduction through the T-cell antigen receptor.[475] The Lck protein interacts with the membrane-proximal cytoplasmic domain of CD4 and CD8 through its unique amino-terminal region.[476-478] T-cell receptor complexes CD4-Lck and CD8-Lck include a 32-kDa phosphoprotein that is recognized by an antiserum to a consensus GTP-binding region in G proteins.[479] Activated Lck tyrosine kinase can stimulate antigen-independent IL-2 production in T cells.[480] However, the precise role of Lck in the intracellular transductional mechanism of T cells is not clear. Another member of the Src protein family, the Fyn tyrosine kinase, is an important component of the T-cell receptor transduction apparatus.[481] In HPB-ALL T cells, the CD45 tyrosine phosphatase regulates Fyn, but not Lck, and tyrosine kinase activity. Activation of Fyn results in Ca^{2+} influx, diacylglycerol production, and protein kinase C activation.[482] Phospholipase Cγ_1 may be a substrate for Fyn- and Lck-induced phosphorylation in T cells. In addition to Fyn and Lck, other members of the Src family or protein kinases, including Src and Fgr, are expressed during the process of activation of murine T lymphocytes.[483] The precise role of each tyrosine kinase in T-cell activation is unknown, but it is known that there are important functional interactions between tyrosine kinases and Ras proteins, and Ras activity is essentially required for T-cell receptor signal transduction.[484] The precise functions of tyrosine kinases and Ras proteins in T-cell antigen receptor function are not totally clear as yet, but there is evidence that Ras proteins mediate IL-2 synthesis through activation of the IL-2 gene promoter and stimulate T-cell antigen receptor function through protein kinase C activation.[485]

Lymphocytes of the helper/inducer (CD4$^+$) subset recognize antigen in the context of class II MHC molecules. Cytochemical and ultrastructural analyses have demonstrated the existence of at least two distinct cell types within the CD4$^+$ subset — one with typical lymphocyte morphology and the other with large granular lymphocyte morphology. Large granular lymphocytes are mature T cells expressing the CD11 differentiation marker and have T-cell receptor activity. The CD11$^+$/CD4$^+$ large granular lymphocytes have a minimal response to IL-2 alone and can proliferate in response to soluble antigen even in the absence of exogenous IL-2. The human retrovirus HIV, which is associated with the etiology of AIDS, interacts largely with CD4+ cells, and the virus infection can be specifically inhibited by using monoclonal antibodies against the CD4 molecule.[486] The CD4 gene is located on the short arm of human chromosome 12, at region 12p12-pter.[487]

2. Structure of the T-Cell Antigen Receptor

The general structure of the human and murine T-cell antigen receptor has been characterized.[472,488-491] The human T-cell receptor is a polymorphic heterodimer of 75 to 90 kDa composed of an acidic α chain of 39 to 46 kDa and a basic β chain of 40 to 44 kDa, which are extensively glycosylated. The single α chain of the antigen receptor molecule is linked via a disulfide bond to the single β chain of the same molecule. In addition to the interchain disulfide bond, the molecule has intrachain bonds within both the α and β chains. Both subunits of the receptor molecule exhibit charge and size microheterogeneity which depends on variable levels of glycosylation. Each chain of the receptor contains at least three sites for N-linked glycosylation.

The α and β chains of the T-cell antigen receptor are encoded by different genes. The organization of the T-cell antigen receptor genes has been determined and the genes have been mapped on human chromosomes 7 (chain β) and 14 (chain α).[492,493] The protein product of the c-ets-1 proto-oncogene binds in a sequence-specific fashion to the transcriptional enhancer of the human T-cell receptor α gene and regulates the expression of the gene.[494] The T-cell antigen receptor genes encode transmembrane proteins that exhibit an organization which is reminiscent of that of the immunoglobulins. In a manner similar to the Ig light and heavy chains, both the antigen receptor α and β chains are composed of variable (V) and constant (C) regions. Both Ig genes and T-cell receptor genes consist of separated germline segments that encode the V and C regions of the polypeptide chains, and which become rearranged during differentiation of the somatic cells to form functionally active proteins by similar mechanisms.[495-498] Both classes of genes are members of an evolutionarily related superfamily of genes characterized by acquisition of the ability to rearrange DNA. The germline configuration for the β chain of the T-cell receptor consists, in addition to the V and C regions, of separate diversity (D) and joining (J) region segments which participate in the molecular rearrangements occurring in lymphoid cells.

The αβ heterodimer of the T-cell antigen receptor is intimately associated with the antigen CD3 on the surface of T cells in order to form a functionally active structure: the T-cell antigen receptor/CD3 complex. Class I or class II MHC molecules participate in the formation of the active antigen receptor complex on the surface of T cells. CD3 is a 25-kDa glycoprotein with a 16-kDa peptide backbone and is composed of three distinct polypeptide subunits designated as CD3-gamma, CD3-delta, and CD3-epsilon. The T-cell receptor/CD3 complex undergoes phosphorylation on serine and tyrosine residues and is probably involved in signal transduction within T cells. However, in addition to the CD3 complex, several accessory molecules on the T-cell surface may participate in different ways in the formation of a conjugate between T cells and the presented antigen as well as in the subsequent activation of the T cell.

The αβ T-cell receptor is expressed in about 95% of mature T cells, especially in functional helper and cytotoxic T cells. The remaining 5% of T cells express a second type of T-cell receptor which is a dimer composed of a single γ chain and a δ chain. These chains undergo rearrangement early in T-cell differentiation.[499] Cells expressing the γδ T-cell receptor may also be involved in cytotoxicity but, while αβ dimers are necessary and sufficient for T-cell recognition of antigen in association with MHC molecules, cells bearing the γδ receptor show MHC-unrestricted cytotoxicity.

Mature functional T lymphocytes can undergo rearrangement of T cell receptor genes, which may result in the appearance of new specificities.[500] The results of a study on the T-cell receptor in cloned murine large granular lymphocyte lines, which are the morphological counterparts of NK cells, revealed that NK cells represent a population of lymphocytes genetically committed to the T-cell lineage.[501] The results also suggested that the cytotoxic activity in NK cells is not directly mediated by their T-cell antigen receptors. Truncated mRNA transcripts of the genes coding for the α and β chains of the T-cell receptor may be present at low levels in some human B-cell lines as well as in some freshly purified human tonsillar B-cell specimens, but these transcripts arise from unrearranged genes and do not encode T-cell receptor proteins.[397]

Isolation of a cDNA clone encoding the T-cell receptor β-chain from a beef insulin-specific hybridoma has been reported.[503] A total of 15 independent cDNA clones containing genes encoding for the V region of the T-cell receptor β chain were derived from a human tonsil cDNA library screened with a murine T-cell receptor probe.[504] The 15 genes were grouped into 10 distinct subfamilies. Minimal polymorphism was observed between individuals, except in multimember families.

3. The T3 Molecule

The antigen receptor α and β chains are associated with three nonpolymorphic peptide chains of 20 to 28 kDa, identified by the T-3 monoclonal antibody.[505] cDNA clones encoding the 20-kDa nonglycosylated polypeptide chain of the human T cell receptor complex have been generated.[506] The antigen receptor molecule and the T3 molecule are spatially associated on the lymphocyte surface, forming the so-called T3/T-cell receptor complex. The predominant association of this complex occurs between the 28-kDa T3 heavy subunit and the receptor β subunit.[507] Two of the three subunits of T3 proteins are glycoproteins. The complete amino acid sequence of one of the human T3 components, the T3 δ chain, was deduced from a cDNA clone.[508]

4. The T-Cell Activating Protein

An additional protein involved in T-cell activation, but not forming part of the T-cell receptor/T3 molecule complex, is the T-cell-activating protein (TAP).[509] TAP is a glycoprotein of 10 to 12 kDa under nonreducing conditions and 15 to 18 kDa under reducing conditions. It is not a transmembrane protein, but is anchored to the membrane by a phosphatidylinositol lipid linkage. Antibody cross-linking of TAP activates T lymphocytes to produce lymphokines and to enter the cell cycle. It can also positively or negatively modulate T-cell activation through the T-cell antigen receptor complex.

5. Activation of the T-Cell Receptor Complex

Ligand binding to the T-cell receptor complex initiates signaling events which activate effector cell functions including lymphokine secretion and cytolytic activity, followed by cell proliferation.

Intracellular second messengers produced after T-cell receptor-antigen interaction include inositol 1,4,5-trisphosphate and 1,2-diacylglycerol, which are generated by activation of phospholipase C. T-cell receptor functional activation induces phosphorylation on tyrosine of phospholipase $C\gamma_1$.[510,511] The second messengers generated by activation of phosphoinositide metabolism induce an increase in $[Ca^{2+}]_i$ by mobilizing intracellular Ca^{2+} and activating membrane Ca^{2+} channels. Diacylglycerol activates protein kinase C, which may result in the phosphorylation of the T3/T-cell receptor complex on the lymphocyte surface.[512] This phosphorylation occurs on serine residues in the γ and δ chains of the T3 molecule and may lead to the downregulation of the T3/T-cell receptor complex. The γ subunit of T3 is phosphorylated on a specific residue (Ser-126) when protein kinase C is activated by treatment of T cells with phorbol ester.[513] In addition, a 21-kDa protein (p21) associated with the T-cell antigen receptor complex is phosphorylated on tyrosine upon antigenic activation of T cells.[514] Constitutive phosphorylation of p21 on tyrosine residues may occur in lymphoproliferative disorders.[515] Stimulation of T cells or the Jurkat T-cell line with PMA or soluble antibodies to the T-cell receptor complex causes activation of protein kinase C, which is associated with phosphorylation of the c-Src protein at an amino-terminal residue (Ser-12).[516] Although the physiological significance of these phosphorylations of the T-cell antigen receptor complex on serine and tyrosine is unknown, they occur within minutes after addition of the antigen. Killing of certain target cells by cytotoxic T lymphocytes depends not only on the activation of the phosphoinositide pathway, but may also occur in the absence of stimulation of phosphatidylinositol hydrolysis.[517]

6. T-Cell Receptor Gene Rearrangements

Rearrangement of T-cell receptor genes can occur in human T-cell malignancies.[496,499,518,519] These neoplasms encompass a spectrum of intrathymic T-cell developmental stages, ranging from primitive cells whose antigen receptor genes were retained in the germline configuration, to cells with rearranged and transcribed antigen receptor genes and a nearly mature T-cell phenotype.[520]

T-cell leukemias and non-Hodgkin lymphomas can be regarded as representing the malignant counterparts of normal hematopoietic cells, and expression of the T-cell receptor-CD3 antigen complex can be used to analyze the different stages of differentiation arrest of lymphocytic leukemias.[521] The results of these studies indicate the following aspects:

1. CD3 gene transcription is one of the earliest events during T-cell differentiation and already occurs in prothymocytes.
2. The T-cell receptor γ and β genes rearrange early during thymocytic differentiation and can be subsequently transcribed.
3. High levels of T-cell receptor γ gene transcription may only occur in part of the T cells during thymic differentiation, while T-cell receptor β gene transcription continues during further differentiation.

4. T-cell receptor a gene transcription may be the final step in the production of the complete set of T-cell receptor and CD3 antigen proteins, resulting in the expression of T-cell receptor-CD3 complex at the cell surface of mature T cells.

The data also indicate a predetermined rearrangement and expression of the T-cell receptor and CD3 antigen genes during early stages of human T-cell differentiation.[521]

The monoclonal rearrangements of the T-cell antigen receptor complex can be used as markers of lineage and clonality in human lymphoid neoplasms.[522-524] Most frequently, tumor samples from T-cell ALL exhibit rearrangement of the T-cell receptor γ and β chains.[525] The majority of human leukemias corresponding to the earliest stages of T-cell differentiation lack cell surface expression of the antigen receptor and do not produce mRNA coding for the α chain of the receptor, but transcribe mRNA coding for the β chain of the receptor.[526] Approximately 10% of human malignant lymphoproliferative disorders, representing the majority of the significant clinical and histopathological subtypes of lymphoid neoplasias, are bigenotypic in having rearrangements of both Ig and T-cell antigen receptor β-chain genes.[527] These dual genotypes are probably not characteristic of neoplastic lymphoid cells, but may also occur in normal lymphoid cells. When Ig and T-cell receptor probes are utilized, the more mature leukemia cells show an unambiguous pattern of Ig or T-cell antigen receptor gene rearrangements.[528]

Fusion of an Ig variable gene and a T-cell receptor constant gene was detected in the chromosome 14 inversion associated with human T-cell tumors.[529] There is evidence for a mechanism involving chromosomal inversion during T-cell receptor β-chain gene rearrangements.[530] An established cell line (SKW-3), derived from the malignant cells of a patient with T-cell CLL, contains a t(8;14) chromosome translocation in which the constant region of the T-cell receptor α-chain gene, which is normally located on human chromosome bands 14q11-q12, was translocated to the 8q+ chromosome, distal to the c-*myc* proto-oncogene.[531] Moreover, translocation of the α-chain locus of the T cell receptor 3' to the c-*myc* gene in human T-cell leukemias associated with t(8;14)(q24;q11) chromosome translocation may result in transcriptional deregulation of c-*myc* gene expression.[532] The possible role of c-*myc* alteration in the origin or development of T-cell leukemias is unknown, but only some of these leukemias are associated with the above-mentioned type of translocation.

Rearrangements of T-cell receptor genes can occur in nonlymphoid malignancies. Rearrangements of these genes were detected in the blast cells of 3 out of 24 AML patients, but the rearranged gene configurations differed in these 3 positive patients, which is consistent with the concept of lineage infidelity in hematologic malignant diseases.[533] In an independent series, illegitimate clonal rearrangements at Ig heavy-chain and/or T-cell receptor β-chain genes were detected in 5 of 17 AML patients.[534] The biological significance of T-cell receptor gene rearrangements in AML and other nonlymphoid neoplasms remains to be determined.

7. Role of the T-Cell Antigen Receptor Complex and IL-2 in Activation of T Cells

Activation of T cells is initiated following the interaction of antigen with the T-cell receptor which, upon interaction with macrophage-derived IL-1, induces T cells to synthesize and secrete IL-2. In order to exert its biological effects, IL-2 must interact with high-affinity specific membrane receptors, and these receptors are rapidly expressed on T cells following activation with antigen or mitogen. Thus, both IL-2 and its receptor are absent in resting T cells, but following activation the genes for both proteins become expressed.[505] It is thus clear that both the production of IL-2 and the expression of IL-2 receptors are pivotal events in the development of the immune response.

Previous activation of T lymphocytes may not be necessary for IL-2 response. IL-2 can support the proliferation of human peripheral blood lymphocytes in the absence of exogenous stimulation. A subpopulation of large granular lymphocytes, which are morphologic homologues of natural killer activity and are TAC-positive, are initially the predominant cell population responding directly to IL-2.[437] The activity induced clinically with high doses of IL-2, as monitored in peripheral blood lymphocytes, may be a result of IL-2-induced stimulation of large granular lymphocytes.

Separate pathways may be involved in the induction of cytotoxicity and IL-2 synthesis by T lymphocytes.[535] Interleukins and other HGFs may participate in the different stages of the chain of events leading to the specific immune response. IFN-α is able to induce rearrangement of T-cell antigen receptor α-chain genes and maturation to cytotoxicity in T cell clones *in vitro*.[536] Moreover, there is definite evidence that activation of particular types of T cells may depend solely on the action of BSF-1 as an autocrine growth factor, and that the lymphokine secreted by a particular T-cell (IL-2 or BSF-1) is also the lymphokine that mediates the proliferative response of that T cell to antigen receptor-specific signals.[537]

C. STRUCTURE OF IL-2

Human IL-2 purified to homogeneity has been characterized as a protein of 15,400 Da released by a subset of mature T cells upon lectin-antigen activation.[538] Its amino acid sequence and posttranslational modification have been determined.[539,540] Nucleotide sequence analysis of the human IL-2 gene cloned from the Jurkat cell line showed that the IL-2-encoded protein contains three cysteines located at residues 58, 105, and 125 of the mature protein. Studies with site-directed mutagenesis indicated that substitution of serine for cysteine at either position 58 or 105 of the IL-2 protein substantially reduced biological activity. These two cysteine residues are thus necessary for maintenance of the biologically active conformation and may therefore be linked by a disulfide bridge. In contrast, the modified IL-2 protein containing a substitution at position 125 retained full biological activity, suggesting that the cysteine at this position is not involved in a disulfide bond and that a free sulfhydryl group at that position is not necessary for receptor binding.[541] The use of antibodies prepared against IL-2 and IL-2 fragments indicates that two nonoverlapping epitopes in the region defined by amino acid residues 8-54 of the IL-2 molecule are involved in establishing contact with the IL-2 receptor.[542] Computer-assisted predictive methods for the assignment of secondary protein structure, together with a method to predict the tertiary structure of a protein from data on its primary sequence and secondary structure, were applied to the construction of IL-2 structural models.[543] The IL-2 protein may be folded such that the amino terminus, the carboxyl terminus, and the internal amino acid residues 30 to 60 are juxtaposed to form the binding site recognized by the IL-2 receptor.[544]

Human IL-2, secreted by stimulated peripheral blood lymphocytes, consists of a mixture of glycosylated and nonglycosylated forms.[545] During the first 30 h of incubation the cells secrete only the nonglycosylated form of IL-2, the glycosylated form being detected only after prolonged culture times. IL-2 glycosylation is paralleled by an increase in glycosyltransferase activities involved in the formation of sialylated oligosaccharides O-linked to proteins. The biological significance of IL-2 glycosylation is not clear.

D. THE IL-2 GENE

The structural gene of IL-2 is located on human chromosome region 4q26-28, and on the feline chromosome B1.[546,547] The gene coding for human IL-2 was cloned from normal and leukemic cells and was expressed in *Escherichia coli* as well as in mammalian cells, and the amino acid sequence of the protein was deduced from the cDNA nucleotide sequence.[548-554] A procedure for the solubilization, refolding, and purification of recombinant human IL-2 expressed in *E. coli* was reported.[555] The purity and homogeneity of the recombinant human IL-2 protein was confirmed by X-ray structure analysis.[556] The human IL-2 gene was also cloned and expressed in *Streptomyces lividans* using the *E. coli* consensus promoter.[557] The IL-2 cDNA encodes a protein of 153 amino acids, the first 20 of which constitute a signal peptide and are not present in the secreted protein. There is only a single copy of the human IL-2 gene and its organization in a variety of human malignant lymphoid cell types is apparently identical to that of normal human cells, the gene not being rearranged in the malignant cells.[546,548]

The cloning, expression, and sequence analysis of murine and bovine IL-2 cDNA have also been reported.[558,559] The murine IL-2 cDNA sequence contains an ORF which encodes 169 amino acids and its most peculiar feature is the presence of tandem repeats of a CAG sequence (nucleotides 150 to 185) which produces 12 consecutive glutamine residues in the IL-2 polypeptide. As for human IL-2, there is no potential N-glycosylation site in murine IL-2. Three cysteine residues, two of which seem to have a critical role in maintaining the human IL-2 molecule in the active conformation, are present in the murine IL-2 sequence. There is only one gene for IL-2 in the mouse genome, and the molecular heterogeneity of the native IL-2 protein may be due to the different extent of posttranslational modifications of a single product.[558] Mature bovine IL-2 is composed of 135 amino acids and has a molecular weight of 14,450 Da.[559] The bovine IL-2 is more homologous to the human (65%) than to the murine (50%) protein sequence and murine cells are totally refractory to stimulation with recombinant bovine IL-2. Bovine IL-2 is unique among the characterized IL-2 protein homologs in that it has a single N-linked glycosylation site.

1. Transcriptional Expression of the IL-2 Gene

IL-2 mRNA is not synthesized constitutively in T cells, but is produced only after stimulation with activators of these cells. Both ubiquitous and lymphocyte-specific *trans*-acting factors are involved in the induction and regulation of IL-2 expression in human lymphocytes through their binding to specific IL-2 gene sequences.[560] DNA-binding proteins that may participate in intrathymic changes involving developmental regulation of IL-2 gene expression are either inducible or constitutively expressed, and include transcription factors such as NF-κB, NF-AT, and AP-1.[561] The transcription factor Oct-1, which contains a homeodomain sequence, and a 40-kDa auxiliary protein, OAP[40], participate in activating the transcriptional expression of the IL-2 gene in stimulated T lymphocytes.[562] The IL-2 gene promoter is activated by Ras proteins in T lymphocytes by a mechanism involving protein kinase C.[563] IL-2 gene transcripts have a half-life of 1 to 2 h in T-cell lines and human peripheral blood lymphocytes.[564] Degradation of IL-2 mRNA is sensitive to inhibitors of protein and RNA synthesis such as cycloheximide and actinomycin D. After removal of the inducing agents, IL-2 mRNA levels decline rapidly in the lymphoid cells, indicating that transcription of the IL-2 gene continues only as long as the activating signal is present. The transience of IL-2 mRNA may be important in relation to immunoregulation.

2. Homologies of the Flanking Regions of the IL-2 Gene

DNA sequences located in the 5' flanking region of the human IL-2 gene are involved in regulating the expression of the IL-2 gene in activated T lymphocytes.[565] A DNA sequence located in the 5' regulatory region of the human IL-2 gene, approximately 300 bp upstream from the IL-2 promoter, shows 83% homology to a sequence which is directly in the intronic DNase-I hypersensitive area of the human IFN-γ gene.[566] The 5' flanking region of the human IL-2 gene also shows sequence homology with HTLV-I,[567] a human virus that may be associated with adult T-cell leukemia/lymphoma.[568-573] Regions contained within the 5' flanking region of the human IL-2 gene also show homology to LTR sequences contained in the human retrovirus HIV, which may be associated with AIDS.[565] A viral LTR was detected in the IL-2 gene of a gibbon leukemia cell line (MLA 144) that constitutively produces IL-2.[574] This viral LTR is integrated at the 3' end of the IL-2 gene, but sequences related to gibbon leukemia virus (GLV) were also detected at the 5' end of the rearranged IL-2 gene. The integration event results in transcription of a composite mRNA made up of the protein coding sequences of the IL-2 gene transcript but incorporating the viral LTR in the 3' nontranslated region of the mRNA. The MLA 144 cell line responds to mitogen stimulation by increasing about 30-fold the synthesis and secretion of IL-2 over the constitutive level.

Structural homology has been detected between the flanking regions of the c-*myc* and c-*fos* protooncogenes and the region located immediately 5' to the IL-2 gene, where the transcriptional control on the level of IL-2 expression is probably exerted.[575] Moreover, the region of homology, represented by the consensus sequence TGGANNGNANCCAA, is also shared with sequences of viruses with oncogenic potential, including the LTRs of the human T-cell leukemia viruses HTLV-I and HTLV-II, and the E1a region of human adenovirus 5 (Ad5). The presence of a consensus sequence in cellular and viral genomes suggests the existence of common mechanisms related to the control of cell proliferation.

E. PRODUCTION OF IL-2

Stimulation of T lymphocytes by antigen, anti-CD3 antibody, or mitogenic lectins results in the production of IL-2 and expression of high-affinity IL-2 receptors on the lymphocyte surface. Binding of the secreted IL-2 to its high-affinity receptor on the cell surface leads to proliferation of the activated cells.

Expression of the IL-2 gene is cell-specific, being restricted to T lymphocytes, and strictly depends on activation of the producing T cell.[576] Control of IL-2 synthesis immediately after lymphocyte stimulation occurs exclusively at the level of transcription. Biosynthesis of IL-2 does not require DNA synthesis and can occur in terminally differentiated T cells, but it requires binding of a stimulatory agent and protein synthesis. Secretion of IL-2 by activated T lymphocytes requires phosphorylation of tyrosine residues in a variety of protein substrates as an obligatory event in transmembrane signaling processes.[577] Production of the IL-2 protein can be quantitated by a sensitive radioimmunoassay.[578]

The synthesis of IL-2 in stimulated human T cells depends on the expression of early genes and the synthesis of proteins which are necessary for IL-2 gene transcription.[579] The IL-2 and IFN-γ genes may be coordinately expressed, and activation of transcription of these genes may represent a primary event of T cell activation.[580] Human peripheral T lymphocytes treated with PHA or IL-2 exhibit an accumulation of mRNAs for IL-2, IL-2 receptor, and IFN-γ, which is paralleled by the expression of the respective proteins.[581] The wave of IL-2 mRNA synthesis corresponding to the initial phase of the response to stimulation is followed by an active shutoff phase which depends on protein synthesis, most probably representing synthesis of a short half-life repressor protein.[582]

IL-2 has been classically considered to be synthesized only by T cells, but there is evidence that some subsets of stimulated B cells are able to produce IL-2. Stimulation of the A20.2J B-cell lymphoma cell line and normal murine splenic B cells with PMA or the calcium ionophore A23187 may result in the production of IL-2 by these cells.[583] Since B lymphocytes express IL-2 receptors, it is possible that antigenic stimulation of these cells can promote their proliferation and differentiation through activation of the IL-2 system. However, the precise role of IL-2 in B-cell function has not been defined. In addition to lymphocytes, the IL-2 gene is expressed in the human placental syncytiotrophoblast.[584] The placental expression of the IL-2 gene is apparently constitutive and occurs at all stages of gestation. The possible functional role of IL-2 synthesis in the placenta is unknown, but may be related to the control of local immune function at the interface between the host mother and the developing fetal allograft.

1. Role of Calcium Ions and Phosphoinositide Turnover

Autocrine production of IL-2 by activated T cells requires an increased $[Ca^{2+}]_i$ and phosphoinositide hydrolysis with protein kinase C activation. Both the production and secretion of IL-2 are regulated by protein kinase C.[585] Early precursor thymocytes produce IL-2 upon stimulation with calcium ionophore and phorbol ester, which induces a direct activation of protein kinase C.[586] Developing T cells acquire the ability to produce IL-2 upon induction with calcium ionophore and phorbol ester before they are capable of responding to concanavalin stimulation. Cultures of human peripheral blood mononuclear cells incubated with the calcium ionophore A23187 in the presence of PMA produce five to ten times more IL-2 and IFN-γ than cultures stimulated with other combinations of inducing agents and PMA.[587]

2. IL-1 and Phorbol Esters

In certain systems, such as EL4-6.1 murine thymoma cells, IL-1 is involved in the induction of both the secretion of IL-2 and the expression of the IL-2 receptor.[65] Transcription of the IL-2 gene is modulated by IL-1 and phorbol esters.[588] IL-1 has limited effect on IL-2 receptor expression and IL-2 secretion by T lymphocytes or thymocytes when added either alone or in combination with the antibiotic calcium ionophore, ionomycin. However, it synergizes with TPA plus ionomycin to cause an increase in IL-2 receptor expression and IL-2 secretion.[589] IL-1 may not cause these effects on T cells via the same mechanism of TPA-induced protein kinase C activation. Whereas in the Jurkat E6.1 T-cell lymphoma line PMA-induced IL-2 secretion depends on the translocation and activation of protein kinase C, in the HUT-78 T-cell lymphoma cell line the production of IL-2 is independent of translocation of the enzyme to the plasma membrane.[590] A variant of the phorbol ester-sensitive cell line EL4 is resistant to the effects of phorbol esters. These cells show no differences in phorbol ester-binding or protein kinase C activity, but lack a 45-kDa protein substrate present in sensitive cells and do not synthesize IL-2 mRNA in response to treatment with phorbol esters.[591] Transcription of the IL-2 gene is stimulated by phorbol ester in sensitive EL4 cells. This stimulation can be blocked by cycloheximide or puromycin, which indicates that it depends on an intact protein synthesis.

3. Steroid Hormones

Steroid hormones such as glucocorticoids and calcitriol can exert inhibitory effects on IL-2 production by T cells. Glucocorticoids inhibit T-cell proliferation by suppressing IL-2 production through inhibition of arachidonic acid metabolism at the step of endogenous leukotriene B_4 production.[592] Dexamethasone inhibits both IL-2 mRNA and IL-2 secretion induced by PHA. Accumulation of mRNAs for IL-2, IFN-γ, and cMyc induced *in vitro* by the mitogen PHA, the phorbol ester TPA, or the calcium ionophore A23187 in human T cells can be suppressed by treatment with calcitriol.[593] Accumulation of IL-2 receptor mRNA is inhibited by calcitriol.

4. Platelet-Activating Factor

The platelet-activating factor (1-*O*-alkyl-2(R)-acetyl-*sn*-glycero-3-phosphate), abbreviated to PAF-acether or PAF, is a potent phospholipid mediator affecting several biological functions. PAF acts through binding to a specific G protein-coupled receptor on the cell surface.[594,595] The actions of PAF are mediated by increases in phospholipid turnover, calcium fluxes, arachidonic acid liberation, eicosanoid generation, tyrosine phosphorylation, and proto-oncogene expression[596-599] PAF is released from various inflammatory cells and may play a role in inflammatory responses. Nanomolar concentrations of PAF are able to markedly decrease both lymphocyte proliferation and IL-2 production.[600] These inhibitory effects can be reversed by a specific PAF antagonist, BN 52021.

5. Age-Related Changes in IL-2 Secretion and Action

Immune reactivity is reduced in elderly humans and animals. The proliferative response of human T lymphocytes to a specific antigen, the tuberculin-active peptide, is reduced with aging, and this reduction is associated with a decrease in both IL-2 production and IL-2 receptor expression in the aged-derived cells.[601] The age-associated decline in T cell proliferation is not entirely due to the decreased production of IL-2, since the magnitude of increment of tritiated thymidine incorporation after the addition of recombinant IL-2 to tuberculin active peptide-stimulated T cells is lower than that of the young controls. PHA-stimulated peripheral blood lymphocytes from older individuals (>60-year-old blood donors) exhibit the following defects: decreased IL-2 secretion, decreased percentage of IL-2 receptor-positive cells, diminished IL-2 receptor density per cell, and a decrease in both IL-2 and IL-2 receptor mRNA expression.[602] The results of these studies suggest that decreased expression of both IL-2 and IL-2 receptor mRNA contribute to the low level of synthesis of IL-2 and membrane IL-2 receptors, respectively, and that these alterations are partially responsible for the diminished proliferative capacity observed in lymphocytes from the elderly.

Similar results in relation to age-associated alterations in IL-2 and IL-2 receptor expression have been obtained in mice and rats. The functions of murine T lymphocytes are impaired with increasing age, which may be due, at least in part, to deficient IL-2 production by helper T cells.[603] In aging mice, the significant population of T cells is unable to express sufficient high-affinity IL-2 receptors to support concanavalin A-induced proliferative response mediated by IL-2.[604] The transcriptional expression of the IL-2 gene is reduced with increasing age in rats.[605] However, in an independent study, it was found that lymphocytes of aged rats responded similarly to those of young rats in the expression of both IL-2 and IL-2 receptors following mitogenic stimulation.[606] Thus, the defect responsible for decreased proliferative capacity of mitogen-induced aged lymphocytes may be related to other aspects of T-cell activation.

6. Constitutive Production of IL-2
Constitutive production of IL-2 occurs in the T-cell line MLA-144, which was established from a gibbon ape lymphosarcoma and is infected with a chronic retrovirus, the gibbon ape leukemia virus (GALV).[607] MLA-144 cells contain two GALV insertions in the IL-2 gene, one in the 3′-untranslated region and the other 1200 bp 5′ to the gene. It is thus likely that one or both of these viral insertions is involved in activation of IL-2 gene expression.

Expression of the v-Src oncoprotein in a murine T-cell hybridoma resulted in constitutive phosphorylation of the T-cell receptor and IL-2 production — two events associated with activation of T cells.[608] Protein kinase C activation is apparently not necessary for IL-2 production in cells constitutively expressing the v-Src oncoprotein.

7. Serum Inhibitors of IL-2
A number of specific serum inhibitors of IL-2 have been described and partially characterized.[609] The distinction between inhibitors of IL-2 production and inhibitors of IL-2 action is not clear. An IL-2 inhibitor present in normal serum is a T-cell-derived protein which may act in a homeostatic mechanism to restrict IL-2 action to the vicinity of activated T cells. Changes in the inhibitory activity have been detected in various normal and abnormal states, including infectious and malignant diseases. Low levels of plasma IL-2 inhibitory activity were detected in patients with systemic lupus erythematosus (SLE) compared to normal individuals.[610] SLE is a disease characterized by a complex of disturbed immune processes. The possible role of serum IL-2 inhibitors in AIDS and other immunodeficiency states is unknown.

F. THE IL-2 RECEPTOR
The effects of IL-2 on its target cells are initiated by its binding to a specific receptor located on the cell surface.[611-617] Activation of T lymphocytes by antigens or mitogens stimulates the production of IL-2 and the expression of high-affinity IL-2 receptors, which allows the cell to receive an IL-2-dependent proliferation signal in either an autocrine of paracrine fashion. Interaction between IL-2 and its receptor induces a rapid clonal expansion of the lymphocyte population originally activated. Termination of the T-cell immune response involves both the decline of IL-2 production and the decreased expression of IL-2 receptors.

The IL-2 receptor, first named Tac antigen, was purified by using monoclonal antibodies and was chemically characterized from normal human T cells and lymphoma cell lines.[618] The receptor isolated from normal PHA-activated T cells has a molecular weight of 60 kDa, whereas the receptor isolated from a human T-cell lymphoma cell line exhibits a molecular weight of 55 kDa. The difference between normal and malignant T cells is probably not caused by structural differences in the polypeptide chains of the receptor molecule, but by differences in posttranslational processes of the receptor. In addition to T lymphocytes, B lymphocytes express IL-2 receptors, and IL-2 is capable of promoting the growth of B cells and their differentiation into Ig-secreting cells. Functional IL-2 receptors are also expressed by human eosinophils.[619]

The IL-2 receptor (IL-2R) comprises two distinct polypeptide chains: one of 55 kDa, termed p55, Tac antigen, or IL-2Rα, and the other of 70 to 75 kDa, termed p70/p75 or IL-2Rβ. IL-2 binding to IL-2Rα occurs with low affinity and to IL-2Rβ with intermediate affinity, but together IL-2Rα and IL-2Rβ form a noncovalently linked heterodimer which binds IL-2 with high affinity. In addition to the α and β chains, the high-affinity IL-2 receptor may require for its normal function the interaction with the β chain of a distinct 56-kDa protein (p56).[620] This protein may be a component of the IL-2 receptor complex and has been termed IL-2Rγ, but its precise function is not understood. The gene encoding IL-2Rγ has been characterized recently.[621] The high-affinity, functional IL-2 receptor complex includes the α, β, and γ chains.

1. The IL-2 Receptor α-Chain

The gene for IL-2Rα is located on human chromosome 10, at region 10p14-15.6[22] The gene consists of 8 exons spanning over 25 kb.[623] The gene for the intermediate-filament protein, vimentin, is located on human chromosome region 10p13, not far from the IL-2Rα gene.[624] The vimentin gene is growth-regulated and the steady-state levels of vimentin mRNA increase rapidly after peripheral blood mononuclear cells are stimulated by mitogens, preceding the appearance of c-*myc* mRNA. In purified T lymphocytes, the induction of both vimentin and IL-2Rα mRNAs requires the addition of IL-2, and it is conceivable that the IL-2Rα and vimentin genes are coordinately regulated in human lymphocytes.[625] The human IL-2Rα gene contains on its 5′ flanking region a 130-bp portion located between 220 and 90 bp upstream of the major transcription initiation site, which exerts a positive regulatory enhancing effect and is responsible for the cell-specific expression of the receptor and its induction by a lymphokine.[626] Cloning, sequence, and expression of the human IL-2Rα gene has been reported.[627-633] The bacterially produced human IL-2R protein binds IL-2 in spite of the fact that it is not glycosylated, which indicates that carbohydrate components and other modifications of the natural receptor are not essential for IL-2 binding.

The IL-2Rα protein is composed of 251 amino acids and is separated into two domains by a 19-residue transmembrane region.[622,627,628] An IL-2 binding site is located in the amino-terminal portion of the IL-2Rα molecule.[634] Limited proteolytic cleavage of the human receptor provides evidence that the extracellular region of the receptor is organized into two domains and that the amino-terminal domain, which includes the segment coded by exon 2, forms part of the IL-2 binding site.[635] The region coded by exon 4, homologous to exon 2, is in the carboxy-terminal domain which is disulfide bonded to the amino-terminal domain. Limited proteolysis and structural analysis of the human receptor showed that a highly symmetrical core of the molecule, consisting of two homologous domains encoded by exons 2 and 4, with a total of 135 amino acids, is the smallest protein moiety so far known to be capable of binding IL-2.[636] Expression in COS cells of artificially mutated forms of Tac cDNA, as well as analysis of a naturally occurring alternatively spliced form of Tac, suggest that the 72 amino acids encoded by exon 4 of the Tac gene may interact with residues in exon 2 to produce the IL-2 binding site.[637] A structural model of the IL-2 receptor has been proposed on the basis of the determined disulfide bonds of the receptor molecule.[638]

The intracytoplasmic region of human IL-2Rα is composed of 13 amino acids and is too small for an enzymatic function. A serine residue of this region (Ser-247) is phosphorylated by protein kinase C in response to PMA and other stimuli.[639] The possible functional role of this phosphorylation is unknown. The amino acid sequence of the IL-2 receptor does not show significant homology with any known proto-oncogene protein.

Studies with the products of chimeric genes may contribute to elucidate the transductional mechanisms of IL-2 action. Chimeric genes consisting of sequences encoding the extracellular domain of the IL-2Rα protein, joined to the transmembrane domain and either full-length or truncated cytoplasmic domain of the human insulin receptor, were constructed.[640] Studies using the mouse T-cell line EL-4 showed that the chimeric receptor molecules are capable of transmitting the IL-2-specific signal and exhibit properties indistinguishable from those of the authentic IL-2 receptor. The kinase activity of the chimeric receptor was not modulated by IL-2 binding and the precise nature of the IL-2-specific signal transmitted to the cell machinery remains unknown.

2. The IL-2 Receptor β-Chain

The high-affinity IL-2 receptor in human and monkey T cells is composed, in addition to the 55-kDa α-chain (p55 or Tac antigen), of a polypeptide chain of 70 to 78 kDa, termed p70, p75, p78, or β-chain.[641-646] It was proposed that the human IL-2 receptor on activated T cells results from the noncovalent interaction of the α- and β-chain molecules, and that the low-affinity IL-2 receptor is represented by the α-chain component, while the high-affinity IL-2 receptor is formed by the interaction of the α- and β-chain components.[647] The human T-cell line MT-1, which was derived by HTLV-I infection and manifests only low-affinity IL-2 receptors, expresses the IL-2Rα, but not the IL-2Rβ polypeptide. The MT-1 line can be converted to another expressing high-affinity IL-2 receptors by fusion of its cell membranes with membranes from MLA 144 cells bearing the β-chain alone.[648]

The IL-2Rβ gene is located on human chromosome region 22q12-q13. The human IL-2Rβ gene has been isolated and characterized.[649,650] Analysis of a cDNA clone coding for human IL-2Rβ showed that it contains an ORF encoding a receptor polypeptide of 551 amino acids which contains an extracellular region of 214 amino acids, and a hydrophobic transmembrane stretch of 25 amino acids. A cytoplasmic region of IL-2Rβ consists of 286 amino acids in which a functional domain (or domains) mediating an intracellular transduction pathway may be embodied. The molecular mechanism of this transduction is not apparent, as could be deduced from the structure of the polypeptide. A cysteine-rich extracellular region of the IL-2Rβ sequence which exhibits homology to other cytokine receptors, as well as to growth hormone and prolactin receptors, is encoded primarily by exons 3 and 4 of the IL-2Rβ gene. The proximal membrane is a cysteine-poor domain exhibiting homology to type III modules of fibronectin, and is encoded by exon 7. Sequence analysis of the 5′-flanking region of the gene demonstrated the presence of potential binding sites for transcription factors.

IL-2Rβ alone is able to mediate endocytosis of surface-bound IL-2 and can also mediate IL-2 signal transduction.[645,646,651-655] IL-2Rβ, and not the α chain of the receptor, participates in the initial binding of IL-2 and in the transmission of activating signals to T and B cells as well as to large granular lymphocytes. The signaling capacity for the IL-2-induced phosphorylation of tyrosine residues in specific cellular proteins resides in IL-2Rβ.[656] A unique region contained within the cytoplasmic domain of the human IL-2Rβ is essential for signal transduction, but not for ligand binding and internalization.[657] The study of structurally altered IL-2 proteins, produced by site-directed mutagenesis, indicates that binding of these proteins to the β chain, rather than to other components of the IL-2 receptor, is essential for the initiation of IL-2-specific biological activities including NK cell activation, T-cell proliferation, and IFN-γ production.[658] IL-2Rβ is responsible for signaling cell growth, and the α-chain component of the receptor would only facilitate IL-2 binding by serving as a helper of binding sites, having no discernible signaling role by itself.[659] Interaction of IL-2 with IL-2Rβ alone is sufficient to stimulate the Na^+/H^+ antiport, thus transducing a signal to the T cells.[660]

Normal and leukemic human large granular lymphocytes express IL-2Rβ, but do not express the α-chain/Tac peptide.[525] Normal human monocytes constitutively express IL-2Rβ, and this expression is involved in the activation of monocytes by IL-2.[661] Antibody to IL-2Rβ, but not to the α chain of the IL-2 receptor (IL-2Rα), inhibits the activation of monocytes to a cytotoxic stage induced by IL-2 but does not block IFN-γ-induced cytotoxicity. A model of IL-2 signaling, well supported by the available evidence, proposes that IL-2Rα represents the low-affinity form of the receptor, IL-2Rβ the intermediate-affinity form, and the complex formed by IL-2Rα and IL-2Rβ the high-affinity form of the receptor. IL-2-dependent proliferation of T cells requires expression of both the IL-2Rα and IL-2Rβ subunits of the IL-2 receptor.[662]

3. Phosphorylation of the IL-2 Receptor

IL-2Rβ is phosphorylated *in vitro* in the presence of IL-2.[663] The IL-2R complex could contain an IL-2-responsive protein kinase activity and would signal the T lymphocyte upon ligand binding through a phosphorylation event. Binding of IL-2 to its receptor on the surface of T cells results in rapid stimulation of the phosphorylation of several cellular proteins on tyrosine residues, and this effect is mediated by the IL-2Rβ chain.[664] IL-2Rβ itself is the substrate for a tyrosine kinase which is activated by IL-2 binding to the receptor.[665] Since the IL-2 receptor does not possess the structural features that characterize tyrosine kinases, the phosphorylation of the receptor on tyrosine must depend on the activity of cellular proteins possessing this type of activity. The β-chain of the IL-2 receptor forms a complex with the lymphocyte-specific tyrosine kinase, $p56^{lck}$ (Lck), which is a member of the Src family of proteins.[666] As a result of this interaction, IL-2Rβ becomes phosphorylated. The Lck tyrosine kinase may be a critical signaling molecule downstream of IL-2Rβ. Association of Lck with the IL-2 receptor is crucial for the IL-2-induced activation of Lck.[667]

In addition to Lck, other protein kinases may be involved in IL-2R-mediated signal transduction. Stimulation of the IL-2R in human peripheral blood mononuclear cells results in phosphorylation and activation of the serine/threonine kinase Raf-1, encoded by the c-*raf*-1 proto-oncogene. The Raf-1 kinase is physically associated with the β chain of IL-2R, and is translocated from the IL-2 receptor complex into the cytosol after lymphocyte stimulation, which depends on Lck activation.[668] The Raf-1 kinase mediates signal transduction by several receptors with a tyrosine kinase-associated activity, including the receptors for insulin, PDGF, CSF-1, and erythropoietin.

G. EXPRESSION OF THE IL-2 RECEPTOR

Quiescent, unstimulated T lymphocytes neither produce IL-2 nor usually express high-affinity IL-2 receptors. However, it has been suggested that there is a small population of IL-2 receptor-bearing T lymphocytes in fresh, unstimulated spleen cells from unimmunized mice; these cells would exclusively correspond to L3T4+Lyt-2− population of lymphocytes.[669] After stimulation of resting (G_0) peripheral mononuclear cells with mitogens, T cells enter the G_1 phase of the cycle and express IL-2 receptors on the surface. This expression, which is critical to the development of an immune response, is regulated in an uncommon way because the receptor is not expressed in the absence of activation determined by immunostimulatory ligands such as antigens, T-cell-specific monoclonal antibodies, mitogenic lectins, or phorbol esters, and the levels of expression of IL-2 receptors decline progressively upon removal of the immunostimulatory signal.[670]

Exposure of a T-cell population to immunostimulatory ligands results in the expression of IL-2 receptors at different rates by individual cells, giving rise to the asynchronous entry of cells into the S phase of the cell cycle. If IL-2 is excluded from an antigen-activated cell population, IL-2 receptor expression still occurs, but DNA synthesis does not take place. In the thymus, IL-2 receptors are preferentially expressed by a small subpopulation of T cells characterized by the absence of two differentiation antigens, Lyt-2 and L3T4.[671,672] Such cells may be considered as intrathymic stem cells, and it is likely that IL-2 plays a role in thymus cell ontogeny. Thymic hormones may be involved in the modulation and maintenance of IL-2 receptor expression in normal human lymphocytes.[673] The agent responsible for the enhancement of IL-2 receptor expression was identified as thymosin fraction 5 (TF5), and was partially purified from the calf thymus. TF5 increases *in vitro* production of IL-2 by PHA-activated human lymphocytes. Cyclosporin A, a potent immunosuppressive cyclic peptide of fungal origin, prevents induction of IL-2 receptors in rat thymocytes.[674]

IL-2-induced regulation of IL-2 receptors on the surface of a human tumor T-cell line (IARC 301), which constitutively expresses the receptor, is a biphasic phenomenon with a rapid downregulation of the receptor after exposure to IL-2, followed by upregulation which reaches a maximum after 24 h.[675] An acceleration of the rate of internalization of the receptor is responsible for the early downregulation of the IL-2 receptor and the upregulation involves new synthesis of the IL-2 receptor protein.

1. Factors Involved in the Induction of IL-2 Receptors

The cellular mechanisms involved in the induction of IL-2 receptor expression are not understood. In particular, the intracellular mediators involved in the induction of IL-2 receptors are unknown. Forskolin (a direct activator of adenylyl cyclase) and cAMP analogues are capable of inducing activation of the IL-2 gene, suggesting that the adenylyl cyclase system plays a role in the regulation of IL-2 receptor expression.[676] Other mediators may exist, however. An intracellular protein of 41 kDa, termed rpt-1, selectively produced by activated CD4+ helper/inducer T cells, may be involved in regulating IL-2 receptor expression by affecting the promoter region of the gene encoding the α chain of the IL-2 receptor.[677] An IL-2 receptor-inducing factor, secreted by the macrophage cell line P388-D1, is required for IL-2 receptor expression in murine Lyt-2+ T cells exposed *in vitro* to concanavalin A.[678] The factor is a heat-labile protein of 44 kDa which does not need glycosylation to exert its physiological action. Monocyte-derived receptor-inducing factor is required, in conjunction with antigen, for the expression of IL-2 receptors by CD8+ cytotoxic T cells as well as for the expression of the c-*myc* gene by these cells.[679] Accessory cells, IL-2 receptor-inducing factor, or phorbol ester can substitute for each other and are equally active for the induction of IL-2 responsiveness in high-density Lyt-2+ T cells exposed to concanavalin A.

Regulation of IL-2 receptor expression *in vivo* depends on complex interactions between multiple factors, and the sole expression of IL-2 receptors may not be sufficient to elicit a response to IL-2. Stimulation of responsive cells with IL-2, despite causing an increase in the number of high-affinity IL-2 receptors, can actually decrease the sensitivity of T lymphocytes to IL-2.[680] Activation with antigen, on the other hand, results in a marked increase in the number of IL-2 receptors, and the T lymphocytes are more sensitive to IL-2. Even though 50 to 70% of immature thymocytes from fetal or adult mice have receptors for IL-2, they need to be stimulated *in vitro* to be able to respond to IL-2.[681] The best inducer for T-cell activation consists of a combination of phorbol ester (PMA) and ionomycin, which generate an appropriate Ca^{2+}- and protein kinase C-associated signal required for the IL-2-induced cellular response. In summary, IL-2 receptor number and affinity are not the only parameters that can affect the proliferative response of lymphocytes to IL-2, and the operation of some uncharacterized postreceptor mechanism should be taken into account in relation to the magnitude of this response.

2. Low-Affinity IL-2 Receptors

In addition to high-affinity IL-2 receptors, there are low-affinity receptors on activated T cells.[682] However, all known biological actions of IL-2 have been correlated with occupancy of high-affinity receptors, and internalization of IL-2 occurs only when bound to these high-affinity sites.[683] The functions and biological significance of the low-affinity sites are unknown. The presence of high- and low-affinity IL-2 receptors could be explained by the presence of some component (converter protein) on the lymphocyte membrane which modulates the affinity and functionality of the IL-2 receptor protein.[684,685] The nature of such a hypothetical membrane component(s) is unknown. β-Adrenergic receptor agonists downregulate IL-2 receptors primarily by affecting low-affinity IL-2 receptor sites.[686]

3. Expression of IL-2 Receptors in Non-T Cells

IL-2 receptors are expressed not only in T lymphocytes but also in B lymphocytes. Interaction of IL-2 with its receptor on the surface of B cells induces a proliferative B-cell response, which is sharply inhibited by anti-Tac antibodies.[687] IL-2 induces T-cell-dependent IgM production in human B cells.[688] However, although there is evidence in favor of a role for IL-2 in B-cell growth and differentiation in *in vitro* culture systems, little evidence is available to support the view that IL-2 has a similar role *in vivo*, and B cells can be induced to express IL-2 receptors much more easily *in vitro* than *in vivo*.[459]

Human peripheral blood monocytes, as well as the monocytic cell line U-937, can be induced to express IL-2 receptors by exposure to IFN-γ.[462,689] This expression is due to induction of IL-2 receptor gene transcription and not to translocation of a cryptic pool of receptors to the cell surface. The addition of IL-2 to human monocytes pretreated with IFN-γ results in increased secretion of IL-1β. However, in contrast to T and B lymphocytes, there is no evidence that IL-2 induces monocyte DNA synthesis and cell proliferation. Since an interaction between monocytes and T cells is critical in the generation of an immune response, these results suggest that a humoral circuit involving IFN-γ and IL-2 may serve to amplify the immune response.

4. Internalization and Degradation of the IL-2 Receptor

After IL-2 binding, high-affinity IL-2 receptors in human cells contribute to the internalization and degradation of the ligand in a temperature-dependent process which terminates IL-2 action.[690] Internalization of IL-2 receptor complexes occurs in a manner similar to that of other peptide hormones, i.e., by endocytosis via coated pits, passage through endosomes, and final accumulation and degradation in multivesicular bodies and lysosome-like structures.[691] The half-life for surface high-affinity IL-2 receptors in the human tumor T-cell line IARC 301 was calculated to be about 1 h. The turnover rate of surface IL-2 receptors suggests that the receptor molecules are constantly internalized even in the absence of IL-2, and that they do not recycle to the membrane after receptor-mediated endocytosis.[692] Both chains, α and β, of the receptor are internalized and remain associated inside the cell after IL-2 endocytosis.[693]

5. Soluble IL-2 Receptors

Activated normal peripheral blood mononuclear cells (T and B cells and monocytes), as well as T- and B-cell lines and cells from a variety of lymphoproliferative and hematologic malignancies, may release a soluble form of the IL-2 receptor.[694-696] The soluble form of the IL-2 receptor is smaller (40 to 45 kDa) than its cell-associated counterpart, but retains the ability to bind IL-2. Soluble IL-2 receptors are present in the sera from normal and tumor-bearing mice. The levels of cell-free, soluble IL-2 receptors were found to be elevated in the serum of mice bearing a T-cell lymphoma, especially in those with a highly metastatic variant of the tumor.[697] Activated normal human lymphocytes, as well as HTLV-I-positive lymphoid-cell lines, produce both cell-associated and cell-free soluble IL-2 receptors.[698,699] High concentrations of IL-2 receptors have been detected in the sera of patients with leukemias and lymphomas, including children with newly diagnosed ALL.[700] Serum levels of soluble IL-2 receptors are markedly increased in patients with hairy-cell leukemia and have been considered as a tumor marker for following up this disease.[701] Soluble IL-2 receptors could have an immunoregulatory role in patients with AIDS or lymphoid malignancies. The levels of soluble IL-2 receptors in serum have been found to be elevated in HIV-seropositive asymptomatic intravenous drug abusers and in patients with HIV-associated lymphadenopathy or AIDS.[702-704] Increased levels of soluble IL-2 receptors have been detected in the serum from patients with nonmalignant diseases including infectious mononucleosis, cytomegalovirus infection, viral hepatitis, bacterial infections, chronic renal failure, and sarcoidosis.[694] The levels in nonmalignant diseases are generally lower than those found in cancer patients.

H. REGULATION OF IL-2 RECEPTOR EXPRESSION

High-affinity IL-2 receptors are not expressed in quiescent, unstimulated T lymphocytes. Antigenic stimulation via the T-cell antigen receptor/CD3 complex on the T-cell surface results in the transcriptional activation of both the IL-2 gene and the gene encoding IL-2 receptor subunits. A number of endogenous and exogenous factors may have a role in the regulation of IL-2 receptor expression.

1. Inducers of IL-2 Receptors

In addition to antigenic stimulation, other factors may have a role in increasing the expression of IL-2 receptors of the T-cell surface. IL-2 itself augments the expression of its own receptor as well as the synthesis of IFN-γ by human T cells.[670,705-707] IL-2 stimulation of human peripheral blood mononuclear cells results in increased accumulation of IL-2 receptor mRNA within 4 h, while an increase in IL-2 receptor transcription is observed within 30 min in isolated nuclei.[708] However, IL-2 alone is insufficient to maintain a continuous state of maximal transcriptional activity of the IL-2 receptor gene. PHA lymphocyte stimulation induces larger nuclear precursor forms of IL-2 receptor mRNA within 1 h after stimulation.[709] IL-2 is a sufficient signal to induce the expression of its own receptor on PHA-stimulated T cells, with subsequent cell proliferation, but it is not sufficient to cause endogenous IL-2 synthesis and secretion.[710] The intracellular pathway involved in regulation of IL-2 receptor expression, but not necessarily that of IL-2 synthesis and secretion, may include the phosphorylation of a 70-kDa protein located in the cytosol.[711]

Cytokines other than IL-2 may be involved in regulating the expression of IL-2 receptors. In certain systems, such as EL4-6.1 murine thymoma cells, IL-1 is involved in inducing the expression of the IL-2 receptor as well as the secretion of IL-2.[65] Expression of IL-2 receptors in $CD16^+$ LGl cells is only slightly stimulated by IL-2 alone, but is greatly enhanced by preincubation of the cells with a combination of IL-2 and TNF-α.[445] TNF-α may directly induce IL-2 receptor expression and does not appear to act via an indirect mechanism.[712] Phorbol esters such as PMA stimulate IL-2 receptor mRNA and protein expression on activated T cells, and IL-3 contributes to the regulation of IL-2 receptor expression on hematopoietic cells.[713] Phorbol ester-stimulated IL-2 receptor expression in human T leukemia cell lines correlates with an induction of the 3.5- and 1.5-kb IL-2 receptor mRNAs.[714]

2. Inhibitors of IL-2 Receptor Expression

Cyclosporin A and dexamethasone diminish the expression of IL-2 receptors in human peripheral blood mononuclear cells and block the PHA-mediated induction of signals necessary for T cells to become capable of proliferating in response to IL-2.[715] This inhibition involves a reduction of both high- and low-affinity forms of the IL-6 receptor. The glucocorticoid receptor can exert a negative regulation of IL-2 gene transcription.[716]

Human serum may inhibit the IL-2-dependent proliferation of mouse cells in IL-2 bioassays.[717] A soluble factor interferes with the mechanism of T-cell activation induced by IL-2.[718] The suppressive activity was detected in suppressor T cells obtained from mice treated with antilymphocyte antiserum. However, the inhibitory activity detected in human serum may be due to antibody-complement-mediated lysis of the IL-2-dependent mouse cells used in the bioassay, and would not be biologically relevant.[719]

3. Regulatory Mechanisms of IL-2 Receptor Expression

The transmembrane signaling mechanisms involved in the regulation of IL-2 receptor expression after activation of the T-cell antigen receptor/CD3 complex are little known. However, there is evidence that triggering of the receptor can induce phosphatidylinositol breakdown with generation of second messengers such as inositol 1,4,5-trisphosphate and 1,2-diacylglycerol.[720] The inositol trisphosphate induces intracellular mobilization of Ca^{2+}, whereas diacylglycerol activates protein kinase C. The role of these molecules in the autocrine mechanisms related to T lymphocyte proliferation is not clear, however. The dual signals of Ca^{2+} mobilization and protein kinase C activation may be necessary for IL-2 production, whereas IL-2 receptor expression can be induced by the stimulus of protein kinase C only.[721] Thus, IL-2 production and the expression of IL-2 receptors are not coordinate events and can be dissociated in experimental systems.

The product of the c-*rel* proto-oncogene, the c-Rel protein, is involved in the positive regulation of IL-2Rα gene expression through its binding to the kappa-B site which is present in the promoter of the IL-2Rα gene.[722] c-Rel shares extensive homology with the p50 and p65 subunits of the NF-κB complex, which has an important role in the regulation of RNA transcription.

I. IL-2 RECEPTOR IN LEUKEMIA AND LYMPHOMA CELLS

The IL-2 receptor is expressed in a variety of hematopoietic malignancies. However, the two subunits of the IL-2 receptor may be differentially expressed in the different types of these diseases. Cells from most T-cell malignancies, common ALL and ANLL, express only the p70-75/β-subunit of the IL-2 receptor, while the mature B-cell neoplasms including CLL and well-differentiated lymphocytic lymphoma, predominantly express the complexed αβ form of the IL-2 receptor.[723] In contrast, most cell lines established from human hematopoietic malignancies do not express either subunit of the IL-2 receptor. In the mouse lymphoma cell line EL-4, the gene for the β subunit of the IL-2 receptor is rearranged due to the insertion of an intracisternal A particle LTR sequence, which gives rise to constitutive expression of IL-2 receptor β-chain mRNA.[724]

The role of IL-2 receptor expression in human hematopoietic malignancies is not clear. In contrast to normal T cells, neoplastically transformed T cells may grow independently from the presence of IL-2. Acute T-cell leukemic populations and lines derived from them, as well as most populations of Sézary's leukemic T cells, do not express IL-2 receptors.[505] IL-2-independent cell lines with tumorigenic potential may arise during prolonged cultivation of IL-2-dependent cell lines, probably as a result of exposure to chemicals or viruses.[725] However, not all transformed lymphoid cells become IL-2 independent.

1. Adult T-Cell Leukemia and HTLV-I-Infected Cells

Adult T-cell leukemia (ATL) is almost always associated with infection by the human chronic retrovirus HTLV-I.[569-573] The mechanisms of HTLV-I transforming potential would be associated with the Tax protein encoded by the retroviral genome. Tax would behave analogous to a secreted cytokine.[726] Leukemic cell populations of ATL patients may spontaneously and continuously express high amounts of the Tac antigen without requiring prior activation.[505,727] When ATL cells are cultured in a low-calcium medium there is little expression of IL-2 receptors, but addition of $CaCl_2$ to the medium results in expression of the IL-2 receptors in a dose-dependent manner.[728] Furthermore, addition of a calcium antagonist or a calmodulin inhibitor to the medium inhibits the expression of IL-2 receptors on ATL cells, suggesting that this expression is regulated by the calcium/calmodulin system.

HTLV-I-infected T-cell lines may display aberrantly sized IL-2 receptors which are not downregulated by anti-Tac antibody and are spontaneously phosphorylated. The constant presence of high numbers of IL-2 receptors on the ATL cells and/or the aberrancy of these receptors could play a role in the growth of these malignant cells. The observation that ATL cells constitutively express IL-2 receptors, whereas normal resting cells and their precursors do not, may provide a basis for therapeutic trials with agents to eliminate the IL-2 receptor-expressing cells.[729] Clinical remission of the disease can be obtained in patients with ATL upon treatment with i.v.-administered anti-Tac monoclonal antibody.[505]

2. T-Cell Chronic Lymphocytic Leukemia

Examination of leukemic cells with monoclonal antibodies specific for particular types of cell surface antigens may contribute to a better definition of their biological characteristics.[730] Tumor cells of patients with HTLV-1-negative T-cell CLL and with an OKT3+/T4+/T8– phenotype express IL-2 receptors which are inducible and upregulatable when the cells are cultured with IL-2 for two days.[731] In contrast, leukemic T cells with an OKT3+/T4–/T8+ phenotype neither express the IL-2 receptor nor respond to IL-2.

3. B-Cell Leukemias and Other Leukemias

Increased production of IL-2 may occur in B-cell CLL,[732] but IL-2 is rapidly removed and absorbed by the neoplastic B cells in CLL.[733] IL-2 can act on CLL B-cell progenitors which express IL-2 membrane receptors upon activation with PHA or TPA.[734] Expression of IL-2 receptors by leukemic B cells is confined to a defined maturation stage and is lost after the prolymphocyte stage that precedes plasma cell transformation.[735] Hairy cell leukemia cells express IL-2 receptors and rearrange Ig genes.[736] Non-T ALL cells can also respond to IL-2 and proliferate in culture.[737]

4. Hodgkin's and Non-Hodgkin's Lymphoma

Determination of IL-2 receptor expression may be useful for risk assignment in children with non-Hodgkin's lymphomas.[738] Highly soluble IL-2 receptor levels in these lymphomas are associated with more advanced disease and greater tumor burden and may predict a poor treatment outcome. In adult patients with malignant T- or B-cell lymphomas, serum IL-2 receptor levels correlate with disease activity and size of the tumor, but not with grade or stage of the tumor.[739] Patients with Hodgkin's disease in active phase have increased values of soluble IL-2 receptors in their serum, which correlate with the severity of the disease.[740]

5. Chronic Myelogenous Leukemia

CML cells do not express IL-2 receptors during the chronic phase of the disease, but large proportions of these cells can be induced to express IL-2 receptors by incubation in suspension for 18 h at 37°C.[741] In contrast, IL-2 receptors are not inducible by the same procedures in the normal marrow progenitors, which are usually IL-2 receptor-negative. The possible pathophysiological significance of this difference is not understood.

6. Role of IL-2 in the Proliferation of Leukemic Cells

In a detailed study on the role of IL-2 in the proliferation of human neoplastic lymphoid cells it was found that IL-2 is capable of stimulating the *in vitro* colony formation of a broad spectrum of these cells, including malignancies of both B and T maturation lineages.[742] Variations between different lymphoid neoplasms from this series were related to the inducibility of IL-2 receptors and the proliferative response to IL-2, and included the following aspects:

1. B-CLL cells spontaneously express IL-2 receptors.
2. Fresh non-T ALL cells do not express receptors for IL-2 as assessed with a monoclonal anti-Tac antibody, but IL-2 receptors appear on the membrane of 25 to 100% of these cells within 18 h following incubation with either PHA or TPA
3. Different types of leukemic cells may have different requirements for activation with PHA or TPA: in general, the mature T immunological phenotype of lymphoid neoplasias is stimulatable with either PHA or TPA, whereas cells with more immature features respond to TPA only
4. Usually, induction of IL-2 receptors in ALL cells directly correlates to their proliferation, but in a minority of patients the ALL cells, though displaying IL-2 receptors, do not respond to IL-2 in colony culture even when very high concentrations of the factor are supplied
5. Some leukocyte factor(s) additional to IL-2 may be required for stimulation in non-T ALL cells
6. Certain leukemia/lymphoma cells are capable of an autocrine production of IL-2.[742]

7. Mechanisms of IL-2 Receptor Expression in Leukemic Cells

The mechanisms responsible for the production of IL-2 and the expression of IL-2 receptors by human leukemic cells are unknown. However, there is evidence that immature leukemic T cells release a T-cell colony-promoting activity which can induce both the expression of IL-2 receptors and the production of IL-2 by normal resting peripheral blood T cells.[743] The same activity, or a similar one, could act in an autocrine fashion to stimulate the expression of IL-2 receptors and the production of IL-2 by leukemic cells, thus favoring their proliferation.

8. Significance of Altered IL-2 Receptor Expression

The precise biological significance of altered expression of IL-2 receptors in neoplastic and nonneoplastic cells, as well as the function of IL-2 receptors in non-T cells, are unknown. It has been suggested that a mechanism for lymphomagenesis could consist in the transformation of IL-2-dependent T lymphoblasts into IL-2-independent T-lymphoma cells.[744,745] This change could be due to an endogenous production of IL-2 or an IL-2-like growth factor by the transformed cells, consistent with the autocrine hypothesis of neoplasia. However, a simple autostimulation model is probably not realistic for human T-cell leukemia associated with infection by HTLV-I because extremely low levels of IL-2 mRNA transcripts are detected in HTLV-I-infected human cell lines, and IL-2 is not expressed in fresh leukemic cells from patients with T-cell leukemia.[746,747] The leukemic cells from patients with T-cell ALL and T-cell non-Hodgkin's lymphoma remain dependent on IL-2, either added to the cultures or endogenously produced, for proliferation.[748] Besides IL-2, these cells require activation by TPA for colony growth. Both IL-1 and phorbol esters may induce the expression and phosphorylation of the human IL-2 receptor.[588,749]

Leukemic human T cells may release factors capable of activating normal resting lymphocytes. Media conditioned by human leukemic T cells induce the expression of IL-2 receptors on normal T lymphocytes.[750] At least a part of the IL-2 receptor-inducing activity in ATL cells and ATL cell lines seems to be due to the production of IL-1α by the tumor cells.[104,229]

J. POSTRECEPTOR MECHANISMS OF ACTION OF IL-2
The postreceptor mechanisms of action of IL-2 are complex and include the following aspects:

1. Activation of phosphoinositide turnover
2. Stimulation of protein kinase C activity
3. Alteration in the intracellular distribution of Ca^{2+}
4. Changes in the Na^+/H^+ antiport activity and cytoplasmic alkalinization
5. Modulation of adenylyl cyclase activity
6. Stimulation of GTP hydrolysis
7. Phosphorylation of the ribosomal protein S6, and
8. Induction of gene transcription.[751]

The precise sequence and categorization of these complex changes in relation to IL-2-regulated cellular processes is unknown. Moreover, the role of known intracellular second messengers in the IL-2 stimulus-response coupling remains controversial. In a study using the IL-2-dependent murine T-lymphocyte clone CTLL-2, no evidence was obtained to suggest that Ca^{2+} mobilization, protein kinase C activation, cytoplasmic alkalinization, alterations in membrane potential, or the action of G proteins are involved in IL-2 signal transduction.[752] Recent evidence clearly indicates that increases in the phosphorylation of cellular proteins on tyrosine residues is an early event in the stimulation of both IL-2-dependent cell lines and normal human T lymphocytes.[753,754] Since the IL-2 receptor does not possess tyrosine kinase activity, the IL-2-stimulated phosphorylation of cellular proteins on tyrosine would depend on the coupling of the IL-2 receptor to some intracellular tyrosine kinases, which may include members of the Src family.

1. Production of cAMP
IL-2 exerts an inhibitory effect on both the basal and the stimulated cAMP production in human T lymphocytes.[755] The inhibitory effect of IL-2 on the adenylyl cyclase system in human T cells is apparently mediated by protein kinase C. Elevation of the intracellular levels of cAMP antagonizes IL-2-stimulated T-cell progression through the G_1 phase of the cell cycle, leading to accumulation of asynchronous proliferating T cells at a very early stage of G_1.[756] Both the differentiation and proliferation-inducing effects of IL-2 on human lymphocytes can be inhibited by PGE_2, a potent stimulator of adenylyl cyclase.[757] Agents which inhibit adenylyl cyclase directly or indirectly can stimulate the differentiation and proliferation of lymphocytes, but to a lesser extent than IL-2. These results strongly suggest that decreased intracellular levels of cAMP are an important signal for IL-2-induced proliferation and differentiation of lymphocytes.

2. GTP Binding and Hydrolysis
Transductional mechanisms represented by receptor-coupled G proteins may have some role in IL-2-elicited transmembrane signaling. GTP binding and hydrolysis activities are stimulated in the lymphocyte membrane by the action of IL-2.[758]

3. Phosphoinositide Metabolism, Calcium Influx, and Protein Kinase C Activity
IL-2 stimulates the translocation of protein kinase C to the plasma membrane,[759] which may result in activation of the enzyme and phosphorylation on serine and threonine of some cellular proteins,[760-762] probably including the IL-2 receptor.[763] Tumor promoters such as phorbol esters, which directly activate protein kinase C, may induce the expression of IL-2 receptor in IL-2 receptor-negative human T leukemic cell lines as well as in EBV-immortalized human B lymphocytes, and may also induce the rapid phosphorylation of the receptor on serine and threonine residues.[749,764] The hypothesis that protein kinase C plays an essential role in the activation of T lymphocytes is reinforced by the observation that a synthetic inhibitor of protein kinase C inhibits the proliferation of T-cell lines induced by antigen and IL-2.[765] However, protein kinase C inhibitors may have significant toxic effects on a number of metabolic pathways, which makes the interpretation of results obtained with them difficult. The study of a murine

T-cell clone (mutant P1 cells), which lacks protein kinase C, shows that activation of protein kinase C is not required for IL-2-induced cell proliferation.[766]

Protein kinase C may be involved in the regulation of IL-2 receptor expression and T-cell proliferation.[767] There is evidence for a direct phosphorylation of the IL-2 receptor by protein kinase C.[768] The enzyme is activated by diacylglycerol, which functions as a second messenger to induce an increase in the affinity for calcium ions.[769] Activation of protein kinase C may be associated with the control of cell proliferation and differentiation.[770]

IL-2 triggers in both human and murine lymphocytes a direct association of PI 3-kinase with the IL-2 receptor.[771] Moreover, the activated IL-2 receptor may induce phosphorylation of the enzyme on tyrosine, suggesting a role for PI 3-kinase in the mechanism of IL-2 signal transduction.[772] The enzyme is involved in the phosphorylation at the D3 position of the inositol ring, thereby creating a novel family of phosphoinositides. The possible role of these metabolites in the mechanism of IL-2 action is not understood, but PI 3-kinase has been found to be associated with receptors possessing tyrosine kinase activity, suggesting that it may be a component of the signaling mechanism of these receptors.

Calcium may play an important role in the events occurring at the membrane level in activated T cells.[773] Activation of NK cells by interaction with ligands such as immune complexes is associated with phosphoinositide hydrolysis and a rapid rise in $[Ca^{2+}]_i$.[774] Part of the initial rise of $[Ca^{2+}]_i$ that occurs in activated NK cells is due to intracellular mobilization of Ca^{2+}, but maintenance of these levels depends on an increased influx of extracellular Ca^{2+} into the cell. IL-2 is capable of inducing a rapid influx of extracellular calcium into quiescent cells bearing specific receptors for the ligand, which may result in increased $[Ca^{2+}]_i$.[775] There is clear evidence, however, that Ca^{2+} cannot be considered, in the strict sense, as an intracellular messenger involved in the IL-2-induced DNA synthesis and mitogenic response of the activated T cells.[771,776] The calcium ionophores A23187 and ionomycin do not activate mouse T lymphocytes, but either one in combination with phorbol ester can induce in lymphoid cell populations the expression of receptors for IL-2 and the secretion of IL-2.[777] While IL-2 production and IL-2 receptor expression depend on increased phosphoinositide turnover, activation of protein kinase C, and intracellular mobilization of Ca^{2+}, IL-2-induced lymphocyte proliferation appears to be independent of these processes.[778-780] In addition to an increase in $[Ca^{2+}]_i$ and protein kinase C activation, stimulation of T-cell proliferation requires the activation of a different costimulatory signaling pathway whose nature remains to be determined.[781]

Diacylglycerol mimics phorbol ester induction of leukemic cell differentiation *in vitro*.[782] Treatment of cloned cytotoxic T lymphocytes with PMA results in inactivation of their cytolytic function, and IL-2 may provide a sufficient signal to restore cytolytic activity to the inactivated T lymphocytes by a process that is independent of cell proliferation and IFN-γ production.[783]

4. Monovalent Ion Transport

IL-2 induces a rapid increase in pH_i through activation of a Na^+/H^+ antiport, but cytoplasmic alkalinization may not be required for lymphocyte proliferation.[784] However, IL-2-induced activation of the Na^+/K^+-ATPase at the membrane of cytotoxic T lymphocytes may be required for the growth of these cells.[785] Activation of this enzyme is associated with pumping of Na^+ out of the cells against a chemical gradient, which represents an early mitogenic signal in certain cellular systems. Interaction of IL-2 with the β-chain (p70/p75) component of the IL-2 receptor alone is sufficient to stimulate the Na^+/H^+ antiport and transduce an activation signal across the cell membrane of T lymphocytes.[786] The study of mutant murine T cells which lack functional protein kinase C indicates that activation of protein kinase C is not required for IL-2-induced Na^+/H^+ exchange.[766]

5. Polyamine Synthesis

IL-2 induces increased ODC activity and polyamine synthesis in IL-2-sensitive lymphocytes, and intracellular polyamine synthesis is required for IL-2 responsiveness in mitogen-stimulated lymphocytes.[787] Polyamines may have a role as second messengers required following binding of IL-2 to its receptor, prior to DNA synthesis, during induced lymphocyte mitogenesis.

6. Pteridine Synthesis

The biosynthetic pathway of pteridines starts from guanosine and GTP. Accumulation of pteridines (neopterin, biopterin, and 6-hydroxymethylpterin) is triggered by the interaction of IL-2 with its specific membrane receptor on T cells.[788] The biological significance of this accumulation is unknown, but the period of accumulation clearly precedes the main period of DNA synthesis in the IL-2-stimulated T cells.

7. Protein Phosphorylation

Protein phosphorylation has a key role in lymphocyte activation and mitogenesis associated with IL-2 action. Interaction of IL-2 with its receptor on the surface of T lymphocytes is followed by the increased phosphorylation of various cellular protein on tyrosine or serine/threonine residues through activation of specific kinases. However, the cytoplasmic domain of the IL-2 receptor is structurally insufficient to include a sequence with receptor-associated tyrosine kinase activity. Neither the α nor the β subunit of the IL-2 receptor exhibit significant homology with the intracellular domains of growth factor receptors or other molecules involved in signal transduction. The IL-2 receptor subunits lack homology with both the serine/threonine and tyrosine kinase families. Phosphorylation of proteins in cells exposed to IL-2 would thus result from the secondary activation of kinases with specificity for tyrosine or serine/threonine residues. In addition, IL-2 action could be associated with the secondary activation of some protein phosphatases.

IL-2 transiently stimulates the activity of Lck, a tyrosine kinase which is expressed at high levels in T lymphocytes.[789] T-cell proliferation induced by IL-2 correlates with a transient increase in Lck kinase activity and the tyrosine phosphorylation of a 97-kDa protein.[790] Lck, as well as serine/threonine kinases, may participate in IL-2-mediated signal transduction in T lymphocytes. However, the mechanism of activation of these kinases and their precise role in IL-2 signal transduction are not clear. The level of expression of Lck may not correlate with the amount of IL-2-stimulated protein tyrosine phosphorylation, suggesting that other kinases are probably involved.[791] A T-cell-specific tyrosine kinase of 72 kDa, Itk, is inducible by IL-2.[792] On addition of IL-2 to responsive T cells, Itk mRNA may increase in parallel with that of IL-2Rα, implicating Itk in the activation of T cells.

The β chain of the IL-2 receptor itself is phosphorylated *in vitro* in the presence of exogenously added IL-2,[663,665] suggesting that the IL-2 receptor complex is tightly associated with an IL-2-responsive protein kinase activity, and may signal the cell through a phosphorylation event. The β chain of the IL-2 receptor would be sufficient to induce tyrosine phosphorylation of cellular substrates involved in IL-2 signal transduction.[664] The IL-2 receptor does not possess intrinsic tyrosine kinase activity, but it may form a noncovalent association with a tyrosine kinase.[793] Thus, in addition to the α and β subunits, a protein with tyrosine kinase activity appears to be a component of the high-affinity IL-2 receptor complex. Two phosphotyrosyl-containing proteins of 58 and 97 kDa have been found to be associated with the high-affinity IL-2 receptor complex in extracts of membrane glycoproteins from activated normal human T cells. The 97-kDa protein possesses tyrosine kinase activity, suggesting that it may be involved in the IL-2 signaling pathway.[794]

IL-2-induced activation of human and murine T lymphocytes is tightly associated with the phosphorylation of cellular proteins on tyrosine. Among multiple substrates with molecular weights ranging from 180 to 32 kDa, IL-2 rapidly increases in human T cells the phosphorylation on tyrosine of a 92-kDa protein, and this effect requires only the action of the β chain of the receptor.[795]

Treatment of either the IL-2-dependent, cytotoxic murine T-cell line CTLL-2, or short-term cultures of human T lymphocytes with IL-2, results in an increase in tyrosine phosphorylation of several proteins ranging from 38 to 120 kDa.[754] Tyrosine phosphorylation of proteins in the activated T cells reaches a maximum level within 15 min, and the concentration of IL-2 required for induction of this phosphorylation correlates with the ability of IL-2 to stimulate the proliferation of lymphoid cells, suggesting that the physiological effects of IL-2 are partially mediated by the secondary activation of protein kinases with specificity for tyrosine residues. Studies using the human leukemia T-cell line Hut 78, which expresses both the IL-2 receptor and the T-cell antigen receptor complex, showed that these receptors are coupled to different signal transduction pathways responsible for an independent activation of distinct tyrosine kinases.[796]

IL-2-induced activation of protein kinase C may result in the phosphorylation on serine of substrates that include proteins of 80 and 60 kDa.[797] These proteins are also phosphorylated in T cells by a synthetic diacylglycerol derivative, suggesting that IL-2 and phorbol ester may share some common pathways in lymphocyte activation. A 65-kDa protein whose phosphorylation on serine is stimulated by IL-2 in human T cells has two calcium-binding sites and belongs to actin-binding proteins.[798,799] It may be identical with L-plastin, a protein which was first identified in chemically transformed human fibroblasts.

The c-Raf serine/threonine-specific protein kinase, which is the product of the *c-raf* proto-oncogene, is an endogenous substrate for IL-2-stimulated phosphorylation.[800] In the IL-2-dependent murine T-cell line CTLL-2, IL-2 induces c-Raf phosphorylation, and this modification is associated with increased kinase activity of the protein. These results suggest that c-Raf participates in IL-2-mediated signal transduction events leading to cell proliferation.

Phosphorylation of some cellular proteins may be shared by IL-2 and other hormones or growth factors. Both IL-2 and growth hormone stimulate the proliferation of the rat T-cell line Nb2, and this stimulation is associated with increased phosphorylation of two cellular proteins, one of 18,600 Da and the other of 15,600 Da.[801] The mitogenic action of both IL-2 and growth hormone on Nb2 cells is potentiated by PMA, which is able, by itself, to inhibit the phosphorylation of the 15,600-Da protein, but is not able to stimulate the phosphorylation of the 18,600-Da protein. IL-2 and growth hormone may act on Nb2 cells through separate receptors and their mitogenic action is mediated, at least in part, by phosphorylation/dephosphorylation processes affecting some specific cellular proteins.

8. Induction of Gene Expression

IL-2 induces the expression of specific genes in sensitive cells such as lymphocytes. The majority of genes induced by IL-2 in a T helper lymphocyte cell line were represented by "housekeeping" genes which include six glycolytic enzymes, vimentin, α-tubulin, β-actin, γ-actin, ERp99, elongation factor 2, and the ribosomal phosphoprotein P1.[802] An IL-2-induced gene, *dbpB*/YB-1, encodes a DNA-binding protein that may be involved in regulation of gene expression, and some genes regulated by IL-2 do not correspond to previously identified sequences. In murine T cells, IL-2 can induce the transcription and translation of the IFN-γ gene by a mechanism which involves protein kinase C activation and intracellular mobilization of Ca^{2+}.[803] In the cloned murine B lymphoma cell line BCL_1, IL-2 induces J-chain gene transcription, which is the limiting factor in pentamer IgM synthesis.[804] The mechanism of this induction is unknown, but the effect is associated with altered sensitivity to nuclease at a site within the 5′ flanking sequence of the J-chain gene, suggesting that the IL-2 signal produces an alteration of the chromatin structure at this site, thus favoring transcription. Regulation of the activity of DNA-binding transcription factors such as NF-κB may be part of the mechanism of IL-2 signal transduction.[805] Activation of human T cells via the CD28 cell surface molecule involves members of the NF-κB family of nuclear proteins: c-Rel, p50, and p65.[806] CD28 is an accessory component of the T-cell receptor complex, and is required for the induction of T-cell proliferation and the production of cytokines such as IL-2 and IFN-γ by the activated cells. IL-2-induced immediate-early genes have been identified and isolated recently.[807]

9. IL-2-Induced Proto-Oncogene Expression

The levels of expression of several proto-oncogenes are altered by IL-2 stimulation in T cells. Treatment with IL-2 of G_1-arrested cultures of the cloned murine cytotoxic T-cell line CT6, which solely requires IL-2 for viability and cell cycle progression, results in sequential expression of proto-oncogenes encoding nuclear products such as Fos, Myc, and Myb, but does not affect the expression of proto-oncogenes whose products are localized in the cytosol or are associated with the membrane.[808]

The level of c-*myc* gene expression is altered in mitogen-stimulated lymphoid cells. Stimulation of murine splenocytes with either concanavalin A (a T-cell-specific mitogen) or LPS (a B-cell-specific mitogen) results in a rapid and marked increase in the levels of c-*myc* mRNA.[809,810] The level of c-Myc protein is increased in PHA-stimulated human peripheral blood mononuclear cells.[811] A role for IL-2 in c-*myc* expression in lymphoid cells stimulated by mitogens is suggested by the observation that accumulation of c-*myc* mRNA can be induced in murine T cells by IL-2 during the G_1 phase of the cell cycle.[812] It is known that T cells stimulated with specific T-cell mitogens produce and express receptors for IL-2.[813] Transient induction of the expression of c-*myc* mRNA and IL-2 receptors occurs in human peripheral blood lymphocytes after activation with PHA.[814] IL-2 has little effect on c-*myc* expression in lymphoid cells, but in combination with PHA it augments levels of c-*myc* mRNA measured at 24 h, but not at 3 h after stimulation.[812,813] Anti-Tac antibody, which interferes with IL-2-mediated events by binding to the IL-2 receptor, inhibits the increase of c-*myc* mRNA levels at 24 h, but not at 3 h, after PHA stimulation. Cloned T cells stimulated with either IL-2 or concanavalin A exhibit increased expression of c-*myc* mRNA.[815] The biological significance of c-*myc* expression in IL-2-stimulated lymphocytes is not understood. The kinetics of c-*myc* expression may exhibit large differences in different subpopulations of stimulated T cells, in spite of similar or identical proliferative responses of the cells.[810] A strong correlation between the onset and strength of c-*myc* gene expression or the steady-state level of c-*myc* transcripts and commitment of the cells to grow is not apparent in many cases. Expression of the c-*myc* gene induced by IL-2 in human thymocytes is not dependent on the rate of cell proliferation.[816] Expression of c-*myc* is inducible by IL-2, even in quiescent T cells, and is not sufficient for IL-2-dependent proliferation.[817] It seems that IL-2-induced expression of c-*myc* is elicited by the binding of the growth factor to its receptor, rather than by the proliferative response. The precise relationship between this response and the expression of c-*myc* remains to be determined.

In addition to c-*myc*, human lymphocytes stimulated with IL-2 show an accumulation of c-*myb*, N-*ras*, p53, and transferrin receptor mRNAs.[818] Expression of the c-*myb* gene was found to be rapidly induced by IL-2 in T lymphocytes and it was suggested that this expression may be associated with T-cell progression through the G_1 phase of the cell cycle.[819] However, in another study, no alteration of c-*myb* expression was detected in cloned lymphocytes stimulated by IL-2, which argues against a role for the c-Myb protein in the proliferation of T cells.[815] Expression of c-*fos* is not upregulated in IL-2-stimulated T lymphocytes, suggesting that c-*fos* gene expression is not directly associated with cell cycle progression in T cells. Stimulation of human T cells may result in transient accumulation of c-*fos* gene transcripts, but the precise role of this accumulation is unknown.

Exposure of human monocytes to IL-2 results in enhanced expression of c-*fms*/CSF-1 receptor mRNA and protein.[820] Treatment of the cells with CSF-1 sustains cytotoxicity induced by IL-2, but not by IFN-γ. Through increased expression of macrophage CSF-1 receptors, IL-2 may lead to prolongation of monocyte-mediated tumoricidal activity.

Expression of the c-Raf-1 serine/threonine kinase is barely detectable in T lymphocytes freshly isolated from human peripheral blood, but activation of the T-cell receptor in these cells results in a severalfold increase in c-*raf* mRNA, and stimulation of the IL-2 receptor leads to a further induction of c-*raf* mRNA, resulting in an accumulation of c-Raf protein through the G_1 phase of the cycle.[821] Expression of c-*raf* remains elevated through DNA synthesis, implicating the c-*raf* gene product as functioning in later stages of the cycle. The c-Raf protein is an endogenous substrate for IL-2-stimulated phosphorylation.[799] IL-2 regulates Raf-1 kinase activity through a tyrosine phosphorylation-dependent mechanism in a T-cell line.[822]

Other proto-oncogenes may have a role in the mechanism of IL-2 action. As mentioned, the tyrosine kinase encoded by the putative proto-oncogene *lck* is activated by the binding of Il-2 to its receptor. The Ras protein is activated by IL-2 in murine lymphoid cells, and this activation is required for IL-2-induced tyrosine phosphorylation of an 85-kDa protein and for the expression of the c-*fos* and c-*myc* genes in these cells.[823] In contrast, the c-*fgr* proto-oncogene is constitutively expressed in resting lymphocytes, and its level of expression is unaffected by lymphocyte mitogens, including IL-2. Expression of the putative proto-oncogene *bcl*-2, which is frequently involved in human follicular B-cell lymphomas associated with the chromosome translocation t(14q32;18q21), is induced in B and T lymphocytes by IL-2 and other mitogens.[824] Regulation of *bcl*-2 expression occurs at the transcriptional level and is subjected to both positive and negative control mechanisms. Expression of the product of the p53 tumor suppressor gene may be increased by the action of IL-2 on human peripheral blood lymphocytes.[825] In the IL-2-stimulated cells, expression of p53 protein is inhibited by a monoclonal antibody to the IL-2 receptor. In general, the biological significance of IL-2-induced proto-oncogene and tumor suppressor gene expression remains an enigma.

10. Induction of DNA Synthesis

The mechanisms involved in IL-2-induced DNA synthesis are unknown, but there is evidence that activation of lymphocyte proliferation is associated with the appearance of an intracellular factor that can induce DNA synthesis in isolated quiescent nuclei.[826] This factor, referred to as activator of DNA replication (ADR), may play a role in the sequence of intracellular events leading to activation for IL-2-mediated lymphocyte proliferation. Although lymphocytes from aged individuals respond poorly to proliferative stimuli, they appear to produce normal to above-normal levels of ADR; however, their nuclei would be only poorly responsive to ADR. Preparations rich in ADR activity have proteolytic activity, and protease inhibitors suppress ADR-induced DNA synthesis in a dose-dependent manner, suggesting that ADR is an endogenous protease whose endogenous substrate has not been identified.

ADR may be present in an inactive form through the early part of the cell cycle, rather than being rapidly synthesized immediately prior to the onset of DNA replication. An inhibitor of ADR would thus be present in quiescent cells. The ADR inhibitor was characterized as a protein of around 60 kDa. In addition to suppressing the interaction of ADR with quiescent nuclei, the ADR inhibitor is able to suppress DNA synthetic activity of nuclei isolated from mitogen-activated lymphocytes. Nuclei from neoplastic cells are relatively insensitive to the suppressive effects of the ADR inhibitor, which suggests that the continuous DNA replication of neoplastic cells may be associated with their insusceptibility to respond to the inhibitory signal.[826] The possible general significance of ADR and the ADR inhibitor, as well as their relation to the physiological effects of hormones, growth factors, and proto-oncogene products remains to be elucidated.

K. IL-2 AND THE IL-2 RECEPTOR FUNCTIONS IN NEOPLASTIC CELLS

Deficient production of IL-2 and/or deficient response of T cells to IL-2 is observed in some cancer patients. For example, patients with primary malignant brain tumors manifest a variety of abnormalities in cell-mediated and humoral immunity which are linked to deficiencies in IL-2 production as well as to diminished IL-2 responses.[827] The number of lymphocytes that can be induced to express IL-2 receptors may be reduced in these patients when compared to normal values.

1. Adult T-Cell Leukemia

The role of IL-2 and the IL-2 receptor in human leukemogenic processes has been addressed in several studies. Particular interest has been focused on the subject of dysfunction of the IL-2 receptor in adult T-cell leukemia/lymphoma (ATL).[828] ATL is very frequently associated with infection by the chronic human retrovirus HTLV-I, and HTLV-I may be one of the etiologic agents of ATL.[568-573] However, HTLV-I-negative cases of ATL have been observed, suggesting that factors other than HTLV-I are involved in some cases of ATL leukemogenesis.[829]

The pathogenetic mechanisms of ATL are complex,[830] and the precise relationships between HTLV-I infection, IL-2 secretion and response, and ATL development are not clear. ATL cells associated with clinically high-grade HTLV-I-positive leukemia and large-cell morphology (immunoblastic lymphomas) may have higher levels of expression of IL-2 and TGF-β genes than low-grade T-cell neoplasms such as mycosis fungoides and Sézary's syndrome.[831] LAK cells, but not resting NK cells, are able to lyse HTLV-infected T- and B-cell lines.[832] HTLV-I-infected human umbilical cord blood T lymphocytes can be propagated in culture indefinitely and exhibit a diminished requirement for IL-2, may have an increased density of IL-2 receptors, and often become completely independent of the exogenous supply of IL-2.[833] Leukemic cells from ATL patients may constitutively express IL-2 receptors, but paradoxically, they do not respond to IL-2 simulation and do not grow as cell lines in the presence of IL-2.[726,834] Only in a few cases do the leukemic cells from ATL patients proliferate in the presence of IL-2.[835]

A short region of homology exists between the envelope protein of HTLV-I (amino acids 20 to 27) and the sequences of the IL-2 protein.[836] This homology raises the possibility of a direct interaction between HTLV-I and the IL-2 receptor on the lymphocyte surface. Such an interaction could result in the generation of an IL-2-like signal in the infected lymphocytes. Several IL-2-independent cell lines infected with HTLV-I do not contain IL-2 mRNA, suggesting that the immortalization of mature T cells by HTLV-I may sometimes occur by mechanisms that bypass the IL-2/IL-2-receptor system.[837] It has been suggested that HTLV-I-infected T cells and HTLV-I virions are both able to induce the proliferation of T colony-forming cells in the absence of exogenous IL-2.[838] Thus, loss of the exogenous requirement for IL-2 may define an early event in HTLV-I infection. However, ATL cells exhibit striking heterogeneity in both the production of IL-2 and the response to this cytokine.[839]

IL-2 does not stimulate growth of T cells unless they are first activated by lectin-antigen. In contrast, T-cells from patients with T-cell malignancies can be grown in long-term culture directly with IL-2.[840] These cells may express IL-2 receptors on the cell surface constitutively, in the absence of known activators that induce IL-2 receptor on normal resting T cells. Exogenous IL-2 may augment IL-2 receptor expression in leukemic cells from ATL patients, although IL-2 does not induce proliferation of these cells.[841] A subset of T-cell colony-forming cells from patients with T-cell ALL may display functional IL-2 receptors, which suggests that the IL-2/IL-2-receptor system could be involved in the spontaneous proliferation of some immature T-cell colony-forming cells in these patients.[842]

Constitutive expression of the IL-2 receptor has been detected in rat lymphoid cell lines producing HTLV-I,[843] and there is evidence for IL-2 receptor induction by HTLV-I in EBV-transformed human B-cell lines.[746] Deregulation of IL-2 receptor gene expression may occur in ATL.[844] One of the *trans*-activator products of HTLV-I, the p40^x or Tax protein, can induce expression of IL-2 and IL-2 receptor in some human T-cell lines (Jurkat and HSB-2), but not in other human T-cell lines (CEM, Molt 3, and RPMI 8402).[845,846] HTLV-I infection of T cells that have differentiated to a certain stage would induce expression of IL-2 receptors. Extracellular Tax protein can activate IL-2Rα expression, suggesting a role for Tax in HTLV-I-associated pathogenesis.[847]

In one case of ATL, the operation of an autocrine mechanism involving IL-2 and IL-2R was documented.[848] However, the possible role of IL-2 and the IL-2 receptor in HTLV-I-associated leukemogenesis remains unclear.[849] The *trans*-activator gene of another member of the HTLV family of human retroviruses, the HTLV-II virus, may induce both IL-2 and IL-2 receptor expression,[850] but HTLV-II may not have an etiologic role in human leukemia. HTLV-I can infect normal mature human B lymphocytes *in vitro* and can induce in these cells the expression of IL-2 receptors.[851] HTLV-I induces the differentiation of human B cells into Ig-secreting cells, without affecting their proliferation. In conclusion, the role of IL-2 and the IL-2 receptor in HTLV-I-associated leukemogenesis is unclear. ATL cells show a marked heterogeneity in the production of IL-2 and the response to this cytokine.[839] Thus, the development of ATL is probably mediated by heterogeneous mechanisms and HTLV-I is neither necessary nor sufficient for the origin of ATL.

2. Other Hematologic Diseases

IL-2 receptors are present in a wide spectrum of human hematologic malignancies, though always with lower density than on the surface of activated T lymphocytes.[852] IL-2 may have important effects, not only on leukemic T cells but also leukemias of B-cell origin, which may express IL-2 receptors with structural characteristics similar to those of the receptor expressed on normal activated T cells.[853] Purified leukemic cells from B-cell CLL show an increased rate of DNA synthesis upon exposure to IL-2 without preactivation *in vitro*, and in some patients with CLL IL-2 stimulates the secretion of IgM and IgG.[854] Peripheral blood leukemic T cells in ATL associated with HTLV-I infection express IL-2 receptors (Tac antigen) of similar weight to that of normal activated T cells and can bind IL-2, but paradoxically, these cells respond very poorly to exogenous IL-2.[726] Both normal and leukemic human large granular lymphocytes express p75/IL-2Rβ, but do not express Tac/IL-2Rα.[651] Large granular lymphocyte leukemia cells show proliferative response to IL-2, but require much higher concentration than that required for the growth of normal PHA-stimulated T cells that express high-affinity IL-2 receptors. ALL cells may express IL-2 receptors after stimulation with phorbol ester, but addition of IL-2 to these cells has no effect on cell proliferation.[855]

In a detailed immunohistochemical study on the expression of IL-2 receptors in 166 cases of lymphoid lesions it was found that IL-2 receptors are present in a variety of human lymphoid proliferative disorders, including not only T-cell lymphomas but also neoplastic and nonneoplastic histiocytic proliferations, Hodgkin's disease, and some intermediate and high-grade B-cell lymphomas.[856] The data support the view that IL-2 receptors are expressed on a variety of cell types and indicate that the use of anti-IL-2-receptor antibodies as a diagnostic tool in immunopathology is of limited value. In most circumstances, the pattern of IL-2 receptor staining does not definitely distinguish reactive from neoplastic proliferations.

3. Solid Tumors

The possible role of IL-2 in the growth of solid human tumors remains poorly defined. Patients with advanced head and neck cancer are frequently immunosuppressed, but no evidence of defective IL-2 production was obtained in 67 of these patients after stimulation of peripheral blood lymphocytes with PHA.[857] IL-2 receptors may be expressed by human melanoma cells, suggesting a direct role of the cytokine in the growth or these tumors.[858]

L. IL-2 AND THE ACQUIRED IMMUNE DEFICIENCY SYNDROME

The acquired immune deficiency syndrome (AIDS) has been observed at a worldwide level with increased frequency since 1981, when unprecedented occurrences of Kaposi's sarcoma, malignant lymphomas, and opportunistic infections, including *Pneumocystis carinii* pneumonia were observed among homosexual men, intravenous drug abusers, hemophiliacs and other persons receiving blood transfusions, immunosuppressed patients, and other groups of persons.[859-864] The AIDS epidemic increasingly includes heterosexual contacts and children.[865-868] Most AIDS patients die from pulmonary infections or infections of the central nervous system, but the pathologic lesions found in these patients include the alimentary canal, the liver, the lymph nodes, and the skin.[869] The central nervous system is frequently involved in AIDS.[870] The patients may have encephalitis accompanied by neuropsychiatric symptoms, and the cells most commonly involved in the infection are from the monocyte-macrophage lineage. Cancer may be one of the manifestations of the AIDS syndrome. In addition to Kaposi's sarcoma,[871] patients with AIDS have an increased propensity to develop non-Hodgkin's lymphomas, including brain lymphomas.[872] The association of HIV infection with tumors other than Kaposi's sarcoma and non-Hodgkin's lymphomas may not be significant.

An etiologic agent of AIDS may be a chronic retrovirus, the human immunodeficiency virus (HIV), previously designated as HTLV-III or LAV.[873-877] Two distinct types of HIV have been detected in AIDS patients, HIV-1 and HIV-2, but AIDS is etiologically associated mainly with HIV-1 infection.[878] The pathogenic mechanisms of AIDS are complex and the precise role of HIV in these processes is not totally clear, but there may be little doubt that HIV is the major cause of the disease. The genetic, biochemical, and pathogenetic properties of HIV are well characterized.[879-885] HIV infects and destroys CD4+/OKTK+/T4+ helper/inducer T cells after its initial interaction with the CD4 receptor on the surface of T cells.

Immunosuppression induced by HIV, due to selective depletion of T4+ cells, plays a central role in the mechanisms of HIV-associated pathogenicity. HIV does not transduce oncogenes and cannot be considered as an oncogenic virus. IL-2, as well as other cytokines and growth factors, may have an important role in the pathogenesis of AIDS and other HIV-associated diseases, including HIV infection of the brain.

AIDS patients usually have a severe deficiency of the immune system with a reduction in the number of helper/inducer T cells (CD4+/T4+ lymphocytes). The prodromes of AIDS (pre-AIDS syndrome) include unexplained chronic lymphadenopathy and leukopenia with diminished number of circulating helper T lymphocytes. In general, patients with fully developed AIDS have reduced T-helper:T-suppressor (T4+/T8+) ratios in peripheral blood. However, most persons infected with the HIV-1 virus are asymptomatic carriers, and in these individuals HIV-1 is harbored predominantly as full-length, unintegrated cDNA.[886] Such extrachromosomal DNA forms of HIV-1 retain the ability to integrate upon T-cell activation *in vitro*. In AIDS patients, there may be an increase in integrated relative to extrachromosomal DNA forms of HIV-1. Quiescent T cells may act as an inducible virus reservoir in HIV-1 infection.

The nature of the T-cell defect in AIDS is unknown. HIV infection does not affect the normal regulation of IL-2 and IFN-γ gene expression.[887] Spontaneous production of IL-2 by unstimulated T cells is decreased in AIDS, and IL-2 produced by PHA-activated T cells may also be decreased in patients with AIDS and AIDS-related complex.[256] T-helper lymphocytes from AIDS may be able to produce adequate amounts of IL-2 upon mitogenic stimulation, but the ability of these cells to produce IL-2 or to proliferate as a response to a soluble antigenic stimulus is diminished.[888] T cells from these patients produce adequate amounts of IL-2 following stimulation with lectins, but their T-cell blasts have a diminished response to exogenously supplied IL-2.[889] This defect may be related to the failure of IL-2 receptor expression on the cell surface following lectin stimulation, which is recognized by the anti-Tac (T-cell activation) antibody in AIDS patients.

Expression of the IL-2 receptor from retrovirus vectors containing HIV-1 *trans*-acting elements results in autonomous growth of lymphoid cells.[890] However, IL-2 receptor expression is diminished on lectin-stimulated T cells from AIDS patients.[891] The serum from AIDS patients would contain an inhibitor that interferes with normal T-cell growth in response to external stimuli. The immunosuppressive effect of this inhibitor is mediated by the IL-2-responsive target lymphocyte and culminates in a reduction of the normal levels of IL-2 receptor expression.[892]

Elevated levels of soluble IL-2 receptors have been detected in the serum of the majority of patients with AIDS, AIDS-related complex, HIV-positive lymphadenopathy syndromes, HIV-positive hemophiliacs, and HIV-positive asymptomatic homosexual males, drug abusers, and heterosexual contacts.[702] Increased levels of soluble IL-2 receptors were also found in a study of blood donors seropositive for HIV.[703] While the release of an excess of soluble IL-2 receptors is not unique to HIV infection (it is also found in patients with leukemia, including HTLV-I-positive ATL), it is possible that it may contribute to the immune deficiency seen in AIDS by blocking the binding of IL-2 to its surface receptors, thus producing a downregulation of the immune system.

A region of the human IL-2 sequence which was predicted to be a contact point with its receptor contains an amino acid sequence that is homologous to a hexapeptide from the carboxyl terminus of the HIV envelope (env) protein.[893,894] This hexapeptide was found to inhibit the biological activity of human IL-2 in a murine spleen cell proliferation assay and, when conjugated to a carrier protein, the hexapeptide inhibited the binding of radiolabeled IL-2 to its receptor. Unique DNA sequences spanning about 200 bp in the 5' region of the human IL-2 gene exhibit sequence homology to HIV LTR sequences.[565] These sequences are involved in the control of T-cell-specific gene expression induced by different agents.

In many respects, activation of the HIV-1 LTR resembles that of the IL-2Rα promoter. An inducible 86-kDa nuclear protein specifically binds to both the HIV-1 LTR enhancer element and a closely related 12-bp sequence (positions −267 to −256) present in the 5' regulatory region of the IL-2 receptor α-subunit gene.[895] The amino acid sequence of a stretch of 25 residues (positions 91 to 116) of the middle portion of the 27-kDa 3'-ORF protein of HIV shares homology with both an intracytoplasmic phosphorylation domain of the IL-2 receptor and the ATP-binding site of the catalytic subunit of cAMP-dependent protein kinase, as well as with the protein-tyrosine kinases of the *src* gene family.[896] These homologies suggest possible mechanisms by which HIV might cause cellular alterations leading to the development of AIDS.

Complex interactions between IL-2 and other cytokines and HGFs may be of great importance for the development of AIDS. HIV-infected human monocytic cells produce increased amounts of cytokines, such as TNF-α and IL-1β, in response to stimuli that could be present *in vivo*.[897] The level of HIV-1 expression may depend, in part, on the presence of TNF-α and IL-1, which are capable of activating the HIV-1 enhancer.[898] This effect may be mediated by specific nuclear factors.

Endogenous production of IFNs, especially IFN-γ, may have an important role in HIV-1 infection. It was suggested that IL-2 treatment may enhance NK cell activity in AIDS patients through an IFN-independent mechanism.[899] However, IL-2 addition is necessary to detect HIV-1-specific induction of IFN-γ in cultures of mononuclear leukocytes from HIV-1 seropositive homosexual men.[900] The requirement of exogenous IL-2 may be necessary to compensate for the direct inhibition of IL-2 gene expression by HIV-1. Treatment with IL-2 alone is apparently inefficient in patients with established AIDS and not a regression, but a progression of AIDS-associated Kaposi's sarcomas was found in a clinical trial involving IL-2 administration.[901]

Growth of AIDS-associated Kaposi's sarcoma requires the endogenous stimulation by a diversity of interleukins and growth factors. IL-1 and TNF-α stimulate the growth of cultured cells derived from Kaposi's sarcoma lesions.[902] Kaposi's sarcoma cells synthesize and release relatively large amounts of biologically active basic FGF-like molecules and IL-1, which can induce self proliferation of the cells by an autocrine mechanism as well as proliferation of normal endothelial cells by a paracrine mechanism.[903]

Infection of susceptible mice with F-MuLV results in a dysfunction of immune responsiveness that resembles human AIDS. IL-2 production and response are strongly suppressed in F-MuLV-infected mice.[904] In contrast, IL-1 production and response are intact in the same animals. The suppression of humoral and cell-mediated immune responses that occur in F-MuLV-infected mice are probably related to the observed alterations in IL-2 production and action.

M. IL-2 AS AN AGENT FOR CANCER TREATMENT

The possibility of using IL-2 for cancer treatment has been explored in a number of clinical and experimental studies.[905-912] Human cancer may be associated with immunological abnormalities and relative deficiency of IL-2, and treatment with recombinant human IL-2, lymphokine (IL-2)-activated killer (LAK) cells, or a combination of both may be beneficial in selected cases of malignant diseases. In particular, renal cell carcinomas, melanomas, and AMLs may be benefited by treatments including IL-2 administration. Even some patients with metastatic cancer may be ameliorated by this adoptive immunotherapy. High doses of IL-2 are usually required for a therapeutic response. Local or regional administration of IL-2 may provide a strategy for immunotherapy of tumors.[913] Unfortunately, the majority of patients either do not respond to IL-2 or exhibit only a partial response of short duration. The reasons for the nonresponse are unclear. However, application of recombinant human IL-2 as a modality for cancer treatment is still promising. The mechanisms possibly involved in IL-2-induced tumor regression remain uncharacterized.

N. ALTERATIONS OF IL-2 IN NONMALIGNANT DISEASES

Changes in the production and secretion of IL-2 and/or in the expression of IL-2 receptors may occur in a diversity of nonmalignant diseases, including diabetes mellitus, multiple sclerosis, and systemic lupus erythematosus. An acquired defect in the production of IL-2 is observed in patients with type 1 (insulin-dependent) diabetes mellitus.[914] This type of diabetes is associated with an autoimmune disorder including destruction of pancreatic β cells, and this alteration can be delayed by prolonged treatment with immunosuppressive drugs such as cyclosporine.[915,916]

IL-2 may act in the central nervous system by inhibiting the proliferation of oligodendrocyte progenitor cells through an IL-2 receptor-mediated mechanism.[917] IL-2 and other interleukins, including IL-1 and IFN-γ, may have important effects on the development of certain lesions occurring in particular diseases of the central nervous system. Antigen- and mitogen-induced T-cell lines and clones obtained from peripheral blood and cerebrospinal fluid of patients with multiple sclerosis show differences in the expression of IL-2 receptors and responsiveness to IL-2 when compared to those obtained from normal individuals.[918]

Systemic lupus erythematosus (SLE) is a severe human disease attributed to an autoimmune mechanism. Autoimmune MRL-*lpr/lpr* mice have clinical features similar to those of human SLE, including autoantibody production, arthritis, vasculitis, and glomerulonephritis.[919] Rapidly growing T-cell lines and clones developed from these mice exhibit a defect in IL-2 receptor expression and unusually high levels of expression of the proto-oncogenes c-*myb* and c-*raf*.[920] Long-term lines and clones derived from MRL-*lpr/lpr* T cells bear large numbers of IL-2 receptors continuously and without stimulation and, paradoxically, they are poorly inhibited by anti-IL-2 receptor antibody, which suggests that the rapidly growing abnormal T cells may be stimulated by some kind of autocrine mechanism. The phorbol ester TPA and the calcium ionophore A23187 synergistically induce both IL-2 receptor and c-*myc* mRNA expression by *lpr* Lyt-2⁻ L3T4⁻ cells, as well as by normal T cells.[921] However, the response on *lpr* T cells was attenuated in comparison to that of normal T cells. BXSB male mice can also spontaneously develop a progressive autoimmune disorder that closely resembles human SLE, and which is associated with intrinsic defects in the capacity of their T lymphocytes to produce and respond to IL-2.[922] Treatment with IL-2 could restore the depressed allogeneic cell-mediated lympholysis and NK cell activity in human patients with SLE.[923]

The mechanisms of altered responses to IL-2 in autoimmune humans and mice are unknown. However, there is evidence that normal mouse serum contains a factor capable of inhibiting IL-2-dependent proliferation of cytotoxic T lymphocytes, and decreased activity of this inhibitor has been detected in serum from autoimmune-prone mice.[924] The IL-2 inhibitor is adsorbed by IL-2-dependent cells but not by IL-2 molecules.

The IL-2 receptor provide a basis for specific immune intervention strategies directed against neoplastic and autoimmune disorders. Since the receptor is not expressed by normal resting lymphocytes, but is selectively expressed by abnormal T cells in patients with certain lymphoid malignancies or autoimmune disorders and in subjects rejecting allografts, monoclonal antibodies and toxin-lymphokine conjugates directed toward IL-2 receptors may represent therapeutic agents for these clinical conditions.[925,926]

IV. INTERLEUKIN 3

Interleukin 3 (IL-3) is one of the soluble factors produced by activated T lymphocytes.[927-930] It can stimulate the growth and differentiation of progenitor cells for most of the hematopoietic cell lineages.[931] IL-3 is identical to hemopoietin 2, multicolony-stimulating factor (multi-CSF), multilineage colony-stimulating activity, and CSF-2α. IL-3 is probably also identical to a factor with erythroid burst-promoting activity,[932] as well as to the mast-cell growth factor (MCGF).[933]

Activated T cells are an important source of IL-3. Both of the major T-cell subsets, OKT4$^+$ cells (helper/inducer cells) and OKT8^1 cells (suppressor/cytotoxic cells), produce IL-3 or a similar factor.[934] Recently, it was found that IL-3 gene induction in T cells is under strict control, and occurs only after T-cell receptor/CD3 complex activation in the CD28$^+$ subset of lymphocytes and has an obligate requirement for increased $[Ca^{2+}]_i$.[935] In a manner similar to IL-2, the production of IL-3 by murine T cells declines with age.[936] It has been suggested that IL-3 may not act directly on lymphocytes or their precursors, but may potentiate the humoral immune response to T-cell-dependent antigens, presumably by acting on accessory cells.[937] Normal and neoplastic B lymphocytes do not produce IL-3.[938]

Cells other than T lymphocytes may synthesize and secrete IL-3. IL-1 stimulates endothelial cells to release IL-3.[939] IL-3 is produced by human placental cells as well as by several cell lines of human origin, including the squamous cell carcinoma cell line Colo-16, and the osteosarcoma cell line R97KL4.[940] The murine myelomonocytic leukemia cell line WEHI-3B produces IL-3 constitutively.[941] The alteration occurring in WEHI-3B cells is due to the insertion of an intracisternal A particle (IAP) close to the promoter region of the IL-3 gene.[942] The constitutive expression of IL-3 in WEHI-3B cells may contribute to the maintenance of their transformed phenotype by an autostimulatory mechanism. WEHI-3B cells can be induced to differentiate by treatment with calcitriol and this induction is accompanied by suppression of IL-3 production in a time- and dose-dependent manner.[943] The relationship between the suppression by calcitriol of WEHI-3B cell growth and the suppression of IL-3 production remains to be elucidated. The kidney appears to be an active site of degradation of IL-3.[944]

A. BIOLOGICAL EFFECTS OF IL-3
IL-3 is a multilineage HGF, capable of stimulating primitive multipotent hematopoietic cells that generate more than one fully differentiated cell type.[945] Human IL-3 can stimulate *in vitro,* and probably also *in vivo,* the proliferation and differentiation of erythroid, granulocyte, macrophage, eosinophil, and mixed colonies of hematopoietic cells, as well as megakaryocytes, from human bone marrow cells. Moreover, IL-3 can act on IL-3-sensitive cells, not only as a competence factor capable of stimulating cells to undergo the transition from G_0 to G_1 phases of the cycle, but if exposure persists it can also act as a progression factor, allowing cells to traverse from G_1 into S, G_2, and M.[946] The effect of IL-3 depends on the state of differentiation.

Induction of differentiation of murine bone marrow cells by IL-3 is associated with transient expression of the Thy-1 antigen.[947] This antigen is specifically expressed on immature myeloid cells that are undergoing lineage restrictions to granulocytes, macrophages, and mast cells. Cells of the neutrophilic myeloid series lose their responsiveness to IL-3 as they differentiate.[948] IL-3 is a differentiation factor for human basophils.[949] It is also capable of inducing the differentiation of cultured murine bone marrow cells into cells resembling osteoclasts.[950] The cells resulting from treatment with IL-3 are multinucleated and show tartrate resistant acid phosphatase activity, as do resident osteoclasts found in bone. Osteoclasts, the cells involved in bone resorption, are normally derived from hematopoietic precursors in the bone marrow.

Administration of recombinant IL-3 to intact animals results in the production of profound effects on the hematopoietic system. IL-3 is active *in vivo* at a concentration as low as 1 ng per mouse, i.e., 4×10^{10} molecules of IL-3, which means that it is an effective stimulator even at only a few molecules per cell.[951] Bacterial endotoxin (LPS) given at high doses can mimic the *in vivo* effects of recombinant IL-3. So far, IL-3 has not been detected *in vivo* in normal animals. Concurrent administration of IL-3 and CSF-3 to intact rats results in additive effects for the production of peripheral neutrophilia.[952]

IL-3 acts directly on multipotential hematopoietic progenitors in culture, exerting a permissive role in their proliferation and differentiation. IL-3 does not trigger hematopoietic progenitors into active proliferation, but is necessary for cell cycle progression and for the continued proliferation of sensitive cells.[953,954] Both IL-3 and CSF-1 can support the formation of macrophage and neutrophil-macrophage colonies from marrow cells of normal mice, but there is evidence that the macrophage-forming cells that respond to IL-3 are more primitive than those that are sensitive to CSF-1.[955] IL-3 contributes to the regulation of IL-2 receptor expression on the surface of hematopoietic cells.[713]

IL-3 does not appear to act directly on lymphopoiesis, nor on mature lymphocytes, but may enhance the immune response by exerting specific effects on accessory cells.[937] Both IL-3 and CSF-2 potentiate the growth of IL-2-responsive cells, suggesting a role for these factors in T-cell-mediated immune responses.[446] Bone marrow-derived IL-3-dependent T cells display natural cytotoxicity (NC) but do not contain rearranged T cell receptor β-chain genes.[956] These cells with NC activity are different from NK cells and may be of a mast cell/basophil origin. These IL-3-dependent cells may mediate their NC activity through the release of TNF contained in intracellular granules. IL-3 enhances the antibody-independent cytotoxicity of monocytes against tumor cells, and this effect is mediated by an increased release of TNF-α.[957] IL-3 is a major negative regulator of the generation of NK cells from bone marrow precursors.[958]

Human IL-3 may be a growth factor for normal B cells.[959] IL-3 supports the growth of B-cell precursors, favoring the development of pre-B-cell clones that can be induced to mature into antibody-secreting cells *in vitro*.[960] Other growth factors, including IL-1, IL-2, IFN-γ, and BCGF are unable to induce differentiation of B-cell precursors into antibody-producing cells.[961] IL-3 can also promote the maturation of murine megakaryocytes *in vitro*.[962] IL-3 directly stimulates both megakaryocyte progenitor cells and immature megakaryocytes.[963] Although IL-3 alone does not stimulate colony formation by mature blood monocytes and tissue-derived macrophages, it can enhance the capacity of both types of cells to proliferate in response to suboptimal concentrations of CSF-1.[964] This effect is mediated by an IL-3-stimulated increased expression of CSF-1 receptors.

Recombinant IL-3 of nonhuman primate (gibbon) origin is an effective stimulator of blast stem cells from AML patients in cell culture.[965] Both renewal and determination of blast cells are stimulated by IL-3, but marked variation may be observed from patient to patient. Human IL-3 has direct stimulative effects on human hematopoietic progenitor cells *in vitro*.[966] However, addition of IL-3 without other growth factors results in a plating efficiency much lower than that achieved with a combination of other HGFs.[967] When combined with the lineage-restricted factor CSF-3 or erythropoietin, IL-3 augments the formation of neutrophil colonies or erythroid bursts, respectively. These results are compatible with a model in which IL-3 supports the proliferation of human hematopoietic progenitor cells in the early stages of development, but not the later stages of maturation. IL-3 can stimulate the development of many erythroid BFUs even in the absence of serum and detectable erythropoietin.[968] However, IL-3 alone is unable to support the terminal differentiation of the erythroid cell lineage, and both IL-3 and erythropoietin are required for supporting the terminal differentiation of hematopoietic progenitors in serum-free culture.[969]

The multiple biological effects of IL-3 obtained with the murine factor were confirmed in human bone marrow cells with IL-3 cloned from a gibbon cell line.[970] The factor can stimulate human cells to produce granulocyte, macrophage, granulocyte-macrophage, and eosinophil colonies. IL-3 is a powerful stimulator of mature human eosinophil function but has no effect on any neutrophil function. The overlapping activities of IL-3 and CSF-2 on eosinophil function may be due to their interaction at the level of the cell surface, where they partially inhibit the binding of each other to its specific receptor.[971] The precise mechanism of this reciprocal inhibition is not understood. In the presence of human plasma, IL-3 stimulates megakaryocytopoiesis. The stimulatory activity of IL-3 is limited primarily to the early, mitotic component of megakaryocyte colony development, with no effect on later events such as megakaryocyte nuclear endoreduplication.[972] IL-3 alone is not able to induce burst formation of human early erythroid progenitors, but in collaboration with erythropoietin it stimulates the growth of these erythroid progenitors.[973]

B. IL-3 STRUCTURE AND THE IL-3 GENE

The genes for IL-3, IL-5, and CSF-2 are closely linked on mouse chromosome 11.[974,975] Repeated DNA sequences present in the mouse IL-3 gene share extensive homology with similar sequences from the human genome which was shown to have enhancer activity. These repeated sequences may play a role in the expression of the IL-3 gene in concanavalin A- or antigen-stimulated T lymphocytes.[933] IL-3 purified to homogeneity from murine WEHI-3 cells is a glycoprotein of 28 kDa.[976] The mature IL-3 protein consists of 140 amino acids.[977] The murine IL-3 gene cloned from inducer T cells, WEHI-3B cells, and a mouse sperm DNA library has been sequenced and expressed in *Escherichia coli* and COS monkey cells.[933,978,979] The IL-3 precursor, as deduced from its cDNA, is composed of 166 amino acids and shows no significant homology to either human IL-2 or human immune interferon (IFN-γ).[978] A cell line producing high levels of IL-3 was produced by superinfection with a constructed retroviral vector carrying multiple cloning sites for the murine IL-3 gene.[980] Cloning and expression of the rat IL-3 gene has also been reported.[981]

A cDNA clone encoding IL-3 has been derived from a gibbon T cell line (UCD-144-MLA), which allowed the identification of the human IL-3 gene.[982] The deduced protein sequences of the gibbon and human IL-3 molecules differ by only 11 amino acids. Recently, a cDNA clone which expresses biologically active IL-3 was isolated from activated human T cells.[983] This clone, 922 bp in length, encodes a polypeptide of 152 amino acids. The human IL-3 gene has been localized to human chromosome region 5q23, a region that is frequently deleted in patients with myeloid disorders.[984-986] The chromosome region 5q23-33 is deleted in the 5q- syndrome which is associated with refractory anemia and other symptoms.[987] This segment of human chromosome 5 contains the genes coding for IL-3, IL-4, IL-5, CSF-1, CSF-2, the PDGF receptor, and the c-*fms* proto-oncogene which encodes the CSF-1 receptor. Loss of some of these genes may play an important role in the pathogenesis of hematologic disorders associated with the 5q-syndrome.

The biological activity of bacterial recombinant human IL-3 is identical to that of mature glycosylated IL-3 in terms of target cell specificity, spectrum of effects, and specific activity, indicating that the carbohydrate moiety of the IL-3 molecule is not required for its activity.[988] Continuous injection of recombinant IL-3 into normal mice results in at least a doubling of the total hematopoietic activity. Moreover, the decreased hematopoietic activity resulting from sublethal irradiation of animals can be compensated for by exogenously administered recombinant IL-3, with hematopoiesis being enhanced by about tenfold. The IL-3-induced increase in hematopoiesis occurs in the spleen and is accompanied by a marked decrease in progenitor cells in the marrow, suggesting that IL-3-stimulated progenitor cells are mobilized to leave the bone marrow and colonize the spleen.[988] Erythropoiesis is as strongly stimulated as myelopoiesis in the IL-3-treated animals.

IL-3 was also synthesized by means of an automated peptide synthesizer and the synthetic 140-amino acid product was found to have the spectrum of biological activity attributed to the native molecule.[989] The results indicated that glycosylation or other posttranslational modifications are not essential for IL-3 functional capacity. Experiments with fragments of the synthetic protein showed that while the complete IL-3 molecule is required for maximal activity, an amino-terminal fragment (residues 1 to 79) was sufficient to stimulate cell lines. It was shown that a disulfide bond incorporating the cysteine at position 17 is essential for IL-3 activity and that residues 7 to 16 are required for maximal biological activity. Antibodies generated in rabbits against synthetic peptides corresponding to specific sequences of the IL-3 molecule (sequences 1–29, 91–112, and 123–140) inhibit, although with different dose-response characteristics, the biological activities of IL-3.[990] These antibodies may be useful tools in determining the structure of native IL-3, as well as for experiments designed to analyze the role of IL-3 in normal conditions and neoplastic processes.

1. Regulation of IL-3 Gene Expression

Regulation of IL-3 gene expression can occur at both the transcriptional and posttranscriptional levels. In mast cells, regulation of IL-3 mRNA expression occurs mainly at the posttranscriptional level and is mediated by Ca^{2+}.[991]

2. IL-3-Like Proteins

A pluripotent CSF is constitutively produced by the 5637 human carcinoma cell line.[992] The purified 18-kDa protein can support the growth of human mixed hematopoietic cell colonies, granulocyte/macrophage colonies, and early erythroid colonies. In addition, it can induce the differentiation of the human promyelocytic cell line HL-60 and the murine myelomonocytic leukemia cell line WEHI-3B(D+).

Astrocytes and glioma cells of the brain produce and secrete an IL-3-like protein factor which can promote the growth of macrophages and microglia cells.[993,994] Since infiltration of lymphocytes, activation of astrocytes, and accumulation of macrophages are constant features of multiple sclerosis, and are considered to be of primary significance for the development of demyelinization, it can be hypothesized that the IL-3-like factor produced in the brain may contribute to the brain lesions occurring in patients with multiple sclerosis. The accumulation of macrophages observed in this disease is probably due to invasion and proliferation of blood-derived monocytes as well as to an expansion of the macrophages normally resident in the brain, which are usually called microglia cells.

An unidentified factor with IL-3 activity may be produced by adherent cell lines.[995] The precise relationship of IL-3-like proteins to other pluripotent hematopoietic growth factors remains to be established.

3. Homology Between IL-3 and HTLV Sequences

The tat-I/x-lor/pX gene region of the human retroviruses HTLV-I and HTLV-II contains a region coding for a 38-amino acid sequence in the p40^x protein which shows highly significant homology with murine IL-3.[996] This homology suggests that the biological functions of the retroviral p40^x protein may be related to those exerted by IL-3 in leukemogenic processes.

C. IL-3 RECEPTORS

High-affinity receptors for IL-3 are present in the membrane of cells sensitive to IL-3 action, such as freshly isolated cells from fetal liver and bone marrow which proliferate in response to IL-3, as well as in cell lines established from long-term bone marrow cell cultures.[997,998] Receptors for IL-3 exist in all neutrophilic granulocyte, eosinophilic granulocyte, and monocytic cells, but are not present in nucleated erythroid and lymphoid cells.[999] In each of the IL-3 receptor-positive cell lineages, the receptor numbers per cell decrease with increased cell maturation, but a small subpopulation of bone marrow cells including blast cells, monocytes, promyelocytes, and myelocytes exhibits very high numbers of IL-3 receptors. The biological role of marrow cells possessing very high numbers of IL-3 receptors is not understood.

Proteins of different size may exhibit IL-3 binding activity in different types of hematopoietic cells. At least some of these proteins may be the products of proteolytic cleavage of the authentic receptor expressed on the cell surface.[1000,1001] The high-affinity human IL-3 receptor is composed of an IL-3-specific α-subunit (IL-3Rα) of 60 to 80 kDa and a β-subunit (IL-3Rβ) of 120 to 135 kDa that is shared by the IL-3, CSF-2, and IL-5 receptor proteins.[1002,1003] The receptor α subunits determine ligand specificity and are capable of binding with low affinity to their ligand in the absence of the β subunit. The shared β subunit is not capable of binding IL-3, CSF-2, or IL-5 by itself, but confers high-affinity specific binding to the α subunits. The IL-3, CSF-2, and IL-5 receptors can interact on the surface of human basophils.[1004]

The highly purified murine IL-3 receptor would be a 140-kDa protein phosphorylated on tyrosine and serine residues.[1005] However, analysis of specific cDNA clones shows that, as in the human IL-3 receptor, the murine receptor is composed of two subunits: an α subunit of 70 kDa and a β subunit of 135 to 150 kDa which is shared with the CSF-2 receptor. In contrast to the human, the mouse IL-3 receptor β chain is encoded by two genes, AIC2A and AIC2B.[1006] Whereas ACI2B is common between mouse IL-3, CSF-2, and IL-5 receptors, AIC2A is unique to the mouse. The two β-chain gene products of the mouse are capable of forming functional high-affinity IL-3 receptors, and the possible physiologic significance of the existence of two distinct IL-3 receptor β chains in the mouse is not understood.

The transductional mechanism of the IL-3 receptor is unknown, but phosphorylation of cellular proteins on tyrosine occurs after activation of the IL-3 receptor by ligand binding,[1007-1010] and one of the tyrosine phosphorylated proteins is the IL-3 receptor itself.[1011] However, no direct proof exists that the activated IL-3 receptor acts as a tyrosine kinase, and no consensus sequence for a tyrosine kinase is present in the cytoplasmic domain of the receptor molecule.[1012] Thus, additional components are probably required for the phosphorylation events associated with the high-affinity IL-3 receptor. Moreover, tyrosine phosphorylation mediated by the β chain shared by the IL-3, IL-5, and CSF-2 receptors may be separated from the transduction of growth-inducing signals.[1013] However, in a cell line that responds to IL-3 and CSF-2, both factors stimulate the phosphorylation on tyrosine of an almost identical set of proteins.[1014]

The physiologic factors implicated in the regulation of IL-3 receptor expression are little known. IL-3 may induce downregulation of its receptor on the surface of sensitive cells *in vitro* under both short- and long-term conditions of cell exposure to the interleukin.[1015] The surface-bound IL-3 is rapidly internalized and degraded in lysosomes, while its receptor may be recycled back to the cell surface.

D. POST-RECEPTOR MECHANISMS OF ACTION OF IL-3

The postreceptor mechanisms of action of IL-3 are very complex. Many different biochemical changes occur in IL-3-sensitive cells after binding of IL-3 to its high-affinity receptor on the cell surface. Proliferation of hematopoietic stem cells stimulated by IL-3 is independent of G protein mitogenic signaling events.[1016] Phosphoinositide turnover and protein phosphorylation may be the two main signaling pathways of IL-3 action.

1. Phosphoinositide Metabolism

The possible role of increased phosphoinositide turnover in the cellular mechanism of IL-3 action remains controversial, which may be attributed, at least in part, to the different systems used to study these changes. In K562 human myeloblast cells, IL-3 and CSF-2 induced the expression of inositol trisphosphate receptors.[1017]

Interaction of IL-3 with its receptor may result in a rapid and transient redistribution of protein kinase C from the cytosol to the plasma membrane.[1018,1019] Phorbol esters activate protein kinase C and glucose transport and can replace the requirement for IL-3 in IL-3-dependent stem cells.[1020] However, studies with a recombinant expression vector indicate that IL-3-mediated growth of IL-3-dependent cells, such as the FDC-P1 myeloid cell line, occurs through pathways other than those involving protein kinase C.[1021] Exposure of the IL-3-dependent leukemic cell line DA-1 to IL-3 results in redistribution of another phosphoinositide-stimulated enzyme, the protein kinase P, between cytosolic and particulate fractions of the cell.[1022] However, IL-3 can stimulate proliferation of murine bone marrow-derived macrophages without inducing inositol lipid breakdown.[1023]

Release and metabolism of membrane-associated arachidonic acid through the cyclooxygenase or lipooxygenase pathway, with the subsequent augmentation of eucosanoid metabolism, may not play a role in IL-3-induced cell proliferation.[1024] Another possibility for the IL-3 signal transduction is the stimulation of phosphatidylcholine hydrolysis, which may result in the generation of diacylglycerol.[1025] In addition, there is evidence that IL-3 induces a rapid influx of extracellular calcium into quiescent cells bearing specific receptors for the ligand, which may result in an increase in the $[Ca^{2+}]_i$.[776] Further studies are required for a proper evaluation of the possible role of these changes in the transductional mechanism of IL-3 action.

2. Protein Phosphorylation

Phosphorylation of proteins on serine/threonine and tyrosine residues may be an important transductional mechanism of IL-3 action. A protein of 33 kDa, which may be involved in signal transduction, is rapidly phosphorylated in IL-3-dependent murine cell lines stimulated to grow by the addition of IL-3.[1026] Treatment of the murine myeloid cell line FDC-P1 with either IL-3 or PMA results in protein kinase C activation and phosphorylation of cellular protein on serine/threonine residues.[1027,1028] However, the role of protein kinase C in the mediation of IL-3 action is unknown. Some of the proteins that are phosphorylated by IL-3 in hematopoietic cells are also phosphorylated by CSF-2, and most of these phosphorylations may not be mediated by protein kinase C.[1029] Phosphorylation of the Raf-1 kinase in human myeloid cells may have a role in the mechanism of action of both IL-3 and CSF-2.[1030]

Sodium orthovanadate, which is an inhibitor of protein-tyrosine phosphatase activity and is capable of increasing the content of phosphotyrosine in cellular proteins, can transiently replace IL-3 in the stimulation of DNA, RNA, and protein synthesis in IL-3-dependent murine cells.[1031] Stimulation of the murine cell line IC-2.9 with IL-3 causes an increase in tyrosine phosphorylation of proteins with molecular weights of 160, 95, 90, 70, and 55 kDa.[753] Treatment with IL-3 or CSF-2 of MO7E cells, derived from an infant with acute megakaryocytic leukemia, resulted in increased levels of phosphorylation of a similar or identical set of cellular proteins on tyrosine residues.[1032] Since IL-3 and CSF-2 receptors do not possess intrinsic tyrosine kinase activity, the receptor would be coupled to tyrosine kinases that could be represented, at least in part, by members of the Src family. IL-3 regulates the activity of the Lyn tyrosine kinase in myeloid-committed leukemic cell lines.[1033] Although the proteins phosphorylated on tyrosine by the action of IL-3 have not been characterized, they may have a role in the abrogation of the requirement for the exogenous supply of IL-3 in cells transformed by oncogenes whose products induce a similar phosphorylation.

In conclusion, a coactivation of serine/threonine-specific and tyrosine-specific protein kinases may be implicated in the transductional mechanisms of IL-3 action. However, further studies are required in order to clarify the cellular mechanisms involved in the transduction of signals elicited by IL-3 upon its binding to the IL-3 receptor on the cell surface.

E. IL-3 REQUIREMENT AND ONCOGENE EXPRESSION

IL-3-dependent cells may become independent of the growth factor by mechanisms involving stable genetic changes. The frequency of spontaneous mutations responsible for the acquisition of independency to IL-3 is similar to that of other known loci: for example, the hypoxanthine-guanine phosphoribosyltransferase (HGPRT) locus.[1034] At least two different mechanism for the acquisition of IL-3 independency may exist in IL-3-dependent myeloid cell lines — one of them implicating activation of the IL-3 gene by mutation, which results in constitutive expression of IL-3 and autocrine-regulated growth. The other mechanism does not involve constitutive tyrosine kinase activity, but c-*myc* gene transcription is constitutively activated.

The acute transforming retrovirus A-MuLV, which transduces the v-*abl* oncogene, potentiates long-term growth of mature B cells.[1035] A-MuLV induces transformation of nontumorigenic murine blood cells (lymphoid, myeloid, and mast cells) and the transformed cells become independent of the exogenous supply of IL-3.[1036-1042] The A-MuLV-derived mast cell transformants may not express or secrete IL-3 and their growth may not be inhibited by anti-IL-3 serum, which argues against an autocrine type of stimulation as a general mechanism of A-MuLV-induced transformation. A-MuLV-infected individual multilineage hematopoietic colonies express features characteristic of mast cells and produce not IL-3 but CSF-2.[1040]

Requirement of human hematopoietic cells for exogenous IL-3 supply is abrogated through a nonautocrine mechanism by transfection with a replication-defective murine retrovirus expressing an activated (translocated) human *trk* gene.[1043] In the *trk*-transformed cells many of the cellular proteins which are phosphorylated on tyrosine residues following IL-3 stimulation are constitutively phosphorylated, with the notable exception of a 140-kDa membrane protein which corresponds to the IL-3 receptor.

An autocrine mechanism not involving IL-3 may be activated in IL-3-dependent hematopoietic cell lines infected with acute retroviruses. Infection of the IL-3-dependent murine myeloid progenitor cell line 32D cl3 with retroviruses carrying a v-*src* oncogene resulted in the growth of IL-3-independent clones. This growth was directly associated with the production of a functional v-*src* gene product, as ascertained by using *ts* mutants of the v-Src oncoprotein.[1044] The cells expressing the v-*src* gene released into the medium a growth factor distinct from IL-3 and capable of stimulating the growth of intact 32D cl3 cells. The nature of this putative autocrine growth factor was not elucidated.

Oncogene-induced neoplastic transformation is not always associated with abrogation of the requirement for exogenous supply of a specific growth factor. Murine hematic cells infected with the acute retrovirus H-MuSV, which transduces the v-H-*ras* oncogene, although converted in immortal cell lines, do not loss their requirement for IL-3.[1036,1045] Moreover, in spite of high-level expression of the v-Ras oncoprotein, the H-MuSV-infected cells (immune mast cells) retain a differentiated phenotype. However, immortalized IL-3-dependent mouse mast cells (PB-3c cells), transfected with an activated c-H-*ras* gene under the glucocorticoid-dependent transcriptional control of MMTV LTR, exhibited progressive growth in the absence of exogenous IL-3, leading to complete abrogation of IL-3 requirement at high levels of c-H-Ras expression.[1046] The maintenance of the IL-3-independent state required a continuous expression of the c-H-*ras* gene, since dexamethasone removal from the medium was followed by rapid cell death. Expression of the activated c-H-*ras* gene induced PB-3c cells to produce IL-3 and CSF-2, suggesting that their IL-3-independent proliferation may be due to an autocrine mechanism. However, other mechanisms should also be considered in relation to these effects. Acquisition of IL-3 independence and tumorigenic conversion of murine bone marrow-derived FDC-P2 cells transfected with an a plasmid carrying an activated c-H-*ras* gene may not be associated with an autocrine mechanism.[1047] In a fastidious immortal myeloid cell line, IL-3 and the mutationally activated c-H-*ras* gene stimulate cell proliferation by acting through a common pathway involving protein kinase C activation.[1048]

Complex interactions may occur in different types of cells between the products of oncogenes or proto-oncogenes and the expression of IL-3 or other interleukins. Introduction of recombinant murine retroviruses expressing v-*myc* oncogenes may abrogate IL-3 and IL-2 dependence in cultured cells and may suppress endogenous c-myc proto-oncogene expression.[1049,1050] On the other hand, constitutive expression of a c-*myc* proto-oncogene driven by a recombinant retrovirus enhances the response of murine mast cells to IL-3, but is not sufficient to eliminate their requirement for growth factors.[1051] Expression of the endogenous c-*myc* gene is suppressed in clones expressing the exogenous c-*myc,* and the transfected cells exhibit constitutive ODC expression.[1052]

F. INFLUENCE OF IL-3 IN PROTO-ONCOGENE EXPRESSION

The physiological effects of IL-3 may be mediated, at least in part, by proto-oncogene induction. The effect of IL-3 on proto-oncogene expression has been evaluated in mast cells as well as in mast cell lines derived from murine bone marrow.[1053,1054] Expression of the c-*myc* proto-oncogene is required for the IL-3-induced proliferation of the normal IL-3-dependent murine mast cell line PB-3, in particular for traverse through the G_1 phase of the cycle. The c-*fos* proto-oncogene is also induced by IL-3 in PB-3 cells. In contrast, proliferation of the murine mast cell line PB-1, which is tumorigenic and shows a lack of IL-3 requirement, is associated with expression of the c-*fos* and c-*myc* genes independent of the presence of IL-3 in the medium. In both cell lines, PB-3 and PB-1, there is a strict correlation between c-*myc* gene expression and active cell proliferation. In normal human monocytes, IL-3 induces expression of the c-*jun* proto-oncogene.[1055] This effect is independent of tyrosine kinase activity and involves the action of protein kinase C. In the growth factor-dependent myeloid cell line FDC-P1, IL-3 strongly stimulates transcriptional expression of c-*myc* by a mechanism involving protein kinase C, but poorly stimulates c-*jun* gene expression.[1056] The precise role of proto-oncogene products in the cellular mechanisms of IL-3 action remains to be elucidated.

G. ROLE OF IL-3 IN NEOPLASTIC PROCESSES

The role or IL-3 in human neoplasias, including leukemias and lymphomas, is little understood. KG-1 AML cells possess high-affinity IL-3 receptors, and human CSF-2 compete with IL-3 for binding to these sites in KG-1 cells.[1057] Analysis of cell lines and samples obtained from patients with acute leukemias (ANLL and ALL) showed that IL-3 and CSF-2 can partially compete for specific binding sites.[1058] Constitutive expression of IL-3 receptors was observed in leukemic B-cell precursors from some ALL patients.[1059] IL-3 stimulates the proliferative activity of ALL cells in a dose-dependent manner without inducing differentiation. IL-3 is a growth factor for human follicular B-cell lymphoma cells.[1060]

Some solid tumors may express IL-3 receptors and may respond to IL-3. The proliferation of 1 of 11 human small-cell lung carcinoma cell lines tested was stimulated by IL-3 when measured with a proliferative as well as a clonogenic assay.[1061] In other types of tumor cells IL-3 may have growth inhibiting and/or tumor suppressing properties. IL-3 may be involved in autocrine loops operating in some tumor cells, and suppression of the transformed phenotype by somatic cell hybridization may involve altered IL-3 expression.[1062] The possible role of IL-3 in the mechanisms of action of tumor suppressor genes in unknown. It has been suggested that recombinant human IL-3 may be useful for the treatment of malignant diseases.[1063]

Oncogene expression may abrogate IL-3 requirement of certain neoplastic cell lines. For example, expression of the v-Abl oncoprotein encoded by the acute retrovirus A-MuLV abrogates the requirement for IL-3 of the murine myeloid leukemic cell line NSF-60 and promotes their partial differentiation.[1064] The mechanism by which v-*abl* oncogene expression can induce NSF-60 cell differentiation remains to be elucidated, but it may partially reflect a role of its normal cellular counterpart, the c-*abl* proto-oncogene, in hematopoietic cell differentiation. Overexpression of the *bcl*-2 gene, which is associated with the t(14;18) translocation that occurs in human follicular B-cell lymphomas, does not abolish long-term growth factor dependence of hematopoietic cell lines but can prolong the short-term survival of IL-3-dependent cell lines after IL-3 deprivation.[1065,1066]

H. IL-3-INDUCED NEOPLASTIC TRANSFORMATION

Expression of high amounts of IL-3 in an autocrine fashion may be capable of inducing the expression of a transformed phenotype. Expression in the FDC-P1 (FD) myeloid cell line of a retroviral vector carrying the IL-3 gene is capable of inducing the generation of an autocrine leukemia in mice inoculated with the genetically manipulated cells.[1067] The *in vitro* growth of these cells is inhibited by an antiserum to IL-3.

Transfection of a constructed plasmid bearing the murine IL-3 gene, ligated to the metallothionein I promoter element, into the factor-dependent myeloid cell line 32D c15 resulted in the production of biologically active IL-3 by the transfected cells.[1068] The transfected cells exhibited autonomous growth and secreted IL-3 into the medium. These cells consistently produced large tumors when injected subcutaneously into syngeneic mice. However, hematopoietic cells may require previous genetic changes for expressing an IL-3-induced transformed phenotype. Dysregulated CSF-3 expression by normal hematopoietic cells produces a fatal but nonneoplastic myeloproliferative syndrome.[1069]

V. B-CELL GROWTH FACTORS

The repertoire of antibodies or immunoglobulins (Igs) in the immune system is created by B lymphocytes.[1070] These cells derive from a pluripotent hematopoietic stem cell whose identity is unknown. Mature B cells are characterized by the synthesized Igs, which are molecules composed of light-chain and heavy-chain polypeptides. The genes coding for these two types of chains are separated from each other on different chromosomes in the most primitive B-cell precursors.[1071,1072] Specific rearrangements of the Ig genes occur during differentiation along the B-cell lineage, thus allowing an appropriate synthesis of the different molecular Ig species and subspecies. It is not known whether stochastic or deterministic phenomena are responsible for B-lymphocyte differentiation, but in recent years there has been much progress in the isolation and characterization of the factors specifically involved in B-cell differentiation.

A. REGULATION OF B-CELL DIFFERENTIATION AND PROLIFERATION

The differentiation of B-lymphoid cells comprises two distinct phases, the first one being antigen-independent and including a number of interdependent gene activation and rearrangement steps that assemble functional Ig heavy-and light-chain genes, and the second one being antigen-dependent and requiring external signals that trigger a differentiation cascade which produces the mature Ig-secreting plasma cell. The expression of Ig genes in B cells requires the interaction of transcriptional regulators with their cognate binding sites in the promoters and enhancers of the Ig loci. An important factor involved in these processes of B-cell development is Oct-2, a member of the POU family of transcription factors.[1073] Oct-2 binds to an octamer motif represented by the consensus sequence ATGCAAAT. The Oct-2 transcription factor plays an essential role in B-cell differentiation, when cells increase Ig expression in response to external stimuli.

Several growth factors related to the differentiation of the immediate precursors of mature peripheral B lymphocytes have been characterized, but little is known about those controlling the early stages of commitment and expansion of the B-cell lineage. Later stages of B-cell development are associated with the formation of lymphocytes capable of synthesizing Igs. Generation of primary antibody responses involves interactions between different cell types, including B lymphocytes, T lymphocytes, and macrophages. T cells are crucially involved in the activation of antibody-producing B cells.[1074] The interaction between resting B cells and helper T cells involves an MHC-restricted linked recognition of antigen-specific resting B lymphocytes by specific helper T cells, which leads to the stimulation of the B cells to enter exponential growth and develop into clones, some of which differentiate into Ig-secreting cells.[1075]

There exists a cascade of sequential steps from a resting B cell to an Ig-secreting mature B cell in the growth-factor-dependent differentiation of human B cells.[1076] This cascade comprises three phases: the activation step (G_0 to G_1), the proliferation step (G_1 to S, G_2/M), and the final maturation step to Ig-secreting cells. While some B cells may require direct interaction with T cells and macrophages in order to differentiate to antibody production, other B cells would require only antigen-nonspecific lymphokines to trigger antibody synthesis.[1077] Soluble factors produced by the B cells themselves may be involved in the regulation of their activation, proliferation, and differentiation.[1078] Multiple second messengers may modulate, both positively and negatively, the activation of quiescent B cells.[1079] Cross-linking of membrane Ig promotes the activation of mature B cells for clonal expansion and antibody production against foreign antigen. The mechanisms of this activation may include enhanced phosphoinositide turnover, increased $[Ca^{2+}]_i$, protein kinase C activation, and protein tyrosine phosphorylation.[1080,1081] The synthetic lymphokine-like molecules, 7,8-disubstituted guanine ribonucleosides, may drive B lymphocytes through the cell cycle by acting on second-messenger pathways to augment the responses of the cells without involvement of G protein interactions, $[Ca^{2+}]_i$ elevation, phosphoinositide hydrolysis, and protein kinase C translocation.[1082] Activation of human B lymphocytes is accompanied by phosphorylation of a tyrosine-specific protein kinase of 72 kDa.[1083]

Regulatory factors acting on B lymphocytes include B-cell growth factor (BCGF), B-cell differentiation factor (BCDF), IL-1, IL-2, IFN-γ, CSF-2, neuroleukin, and other factors whose respective activities reside in different molecules.[1077,1084] BCGF and BCDF activities are represented by a set of factors specifically involved in the growth and differentiation of B cells.[1085] Two main types of BCGFs were initially described, BCGF type I (BCGF-I) and BCGF type II (BCGF-II). It was later shown that these two BCGFs are partially or completely identical to factors described under other names, including T-cell-replacing factor and B-cell stimulatory factors (BSFs) as well as some interleukins. Three HGFs involved in the regulation of B cells are the interleukins IL-4, IL-5, and IL-6.[1086] The precise role of each of these factors in B cell activation and function is not totally clear, but expression of the genes encoding these factors is regulated in a differential fashion.[1087]

In addition to the known BCGFs and BSFs, other similar but distinct B-cell stimulatory factor(s) may exist.[1088] The cloning and expression in *Escherichia coli* of a cDNA sequence encoding a 12-kDa human BCGF was reported.[1089] Two molecular species of BCGF, termed BCGF-IIA and BCGF-IIB, would have similar but not identical biological activities.[1090,1091] A distinct molecular species of BCGF (high molecular weight BCGF, HMW-BCGF), is antigenically related to the complement component factor B. HMW-BCGF and factor B are mitogenic for B cells and compete for binding to the B-cell membrane, but they activate distinct sets of second messengers.[1092] Although both HMW-BCGF and factor B cause in human B cells a biphasic increase in diacylglycerol, HMW-BCGF, but not factor B, induces an increase in cytoplasmic cAMP concentrations and $[Ca^{2+}]_i$.

Both the activation stimulus and the origin of B cells (peripheral blood, spleen, or lymph node) contribute to determine the lymphokine requirements of human B cells to respond with proliferation and differentiation.[1093] The development of cell lines that respond only to one specific growth factor, but not to other factors, may contribute to a better characterization of these complex regulatory phenomena. The human lymphoblastoid cell line B-A3 responds to BCGF, but is not influenced by IL-2 or IFN-γ.[1094]

BCGFs produced by normal human B lymphocytes have been purified and partially characterized.[1095,1096] BCGFs may function as autocrine growth factors in both normal and transformed B lymphocytes.[1097] EBV has the specific property to infect and immortalize B lymphocytes, depending on its initial interaction with a receptor on the cell surface. Irradiated EBV has no effect on B-cell proliferation on its own, but can synergize with BCGF to stimulate cell division.[1098]

IL-2 may play a role in B-cell activation, which would result from a pathway including the ordered and sequential action of anti-μ antibody, a 50-kDa BCGF, and IL-2.[1099] Activated B cells express IL-2 receptors, and at least some of the effects of BCGFs on B cells would depend on IL-2 action.[687,1100] However, specific BCGFs and BCDFs interact with receptors distinct from the IL-2 receptor.[1101,1102] IFN-γ may act as a BCGF and may be one of several BCDF molecules with a direct role in driving the maturation of resting B cells to active Ig secretion.[1103] The stimulatory effects of BCGFs and other factors on B-cell differentiation may be counterbalanced by TGF-β, which exerts an inhibitory effect on the transition of pre-B cells to mature, functional B cells.[1104] The inhibitory effect of TGF-β on the differentiation of B cells is exerted at the transcriptional level and is associated with the blocking of kappa-light-chain expression.

The following general model is proposed for B-cell activation and differentiation:

1. The initial activation of B cells is associated with the expression of receptors for growth factors, including BCGF receptors.
2. Activated B cells, in turn, can respond by proliferation to BCGF, probably via binding of this factor to the cellular receptors.
3. These cells continue to proliferate without terminal differentiation if BCGF remains present and BCDF is absent.
4. This phenomenon may result in the clonal expansion of B cells of various specificities.
5. If BCDF is supplied to the proliferating B cells, they preferentially are driven to differentiate and secrete Ig.[1076] As little as 1 p*M* purified BCGF induces Ig secretion in activated B cells without inducing any cell growth.[1105]

Proliferation of B cells involves at least two signals. The first signal includes cross-linkage of surface membrane Ig with a given antigen (excitation phase) and the second signal is when antigen activated B cells acquire BCGF to proliferate (replication phase).[1106] TGF-β inhibits DNA synthesis in normal and neoplastic human B lymphocytes stimulated to proliferate with anti-Ig and BCGF.[1107] Both IFN-α$_2$ and IFN-β inhibit the BCGF-induced growth of hairy-cell leukemia cells, which are of B-cell origin.[1108] In general, the response of a neoplastic B cell to HGF is characterized by its heterogeneity. Different patients with B-cell chronic lymphocytic leukemia may exhibit different responses to a given HGF or to combinations of HGFs.[1109]

B. EFFECT OF BCGFs ON PROTO-ONCOGENE EXPRESSION

Treatment of purified human B cells with either BCGF or anti-Ig (anti-μ) results in induction of c-*myc* expression.[1110] These findings indicate that the induction of c-*myc* is not a mitogen-specific response. However, the role of c-*myc* expression in BCGF-stimulated lymphocytes is not clear. Expression of c-*myc* is not, by itself, sufficient for the cell cycle progression of BCGF-stimulated human peripheral blood B cells into the S phase.[1111] B cells from patients with SLE show either normal or depressed expression of the c-*myc* gene after stimulation with anti-IgM or BCGF.[1112]

C. PRODUCTION OF BCGFs BY NEOPLASTIC CELLS

Malignant cells may produce substances with BCGF activity. A spontaneous pre-B-cell transformant (H9 cells) and two independently derived A-MuLV-transformed pre-B-cell lines produce pre-B-cell stimulating factors which seem to act in an autocrine manner and are distinct from any known HGF.[1113] Human HTLV-I-negative malignant T-cell lines and B-lymphoblastoid cell lines constitutively produce a B-cell differentiating activity which is apparently represented by a protein of 40 to 60 kDa.[1114] Immortalized B-cell lines derived from Burkitt's lymphomas and EBV-induced B-cell transformation produce autostimulatory B-cell growth factors *in vitro*.[1115-1117] A BCGF produced by a human B-cell lymphoma cell line (Namalva) and a human T-cell line (T-ALL) is a 60-kDa protein that binds specifically to activated, but not to resting, B cells.[1118] The production of BCGFs with autostimulatory properties by neoplastic lymphoid cells reinforces the validity of the autocrine hypothesis of neoplastic cell transformation.

D. ACTIONS OF BCGFs ON NEOPLASTIC AND IMMORTALIZED CELLS

Functional BCGF receptors are present in B-cell precursor ALL, which suggests that BCGFs may play a role in regulating the growth of this neoplasm.[1119] In contrast, receptors for BCGF may be absent from the tumor cells of patients with B-cell CLL, and B-cell-derived lymphokines may influence the response of normal B cells, but not that of leukemic B cells.[1106,1120] However, in one study it was found that 60% of CLL cases constitutively expressed receptors for a 60-kDa BCGF and showed a marked proliferative response to BCGF.[1121] A monoclonal antibody to 60-kDa BCGF inhibited the BCGF-stimulated B-lineage CLL colony formation *in vitro*.

Although there has been a great deal of controversy over the origin of the malignant cell in hairy-cell leukemia, recent evidence indicates that leukemic hairy cells have Ig gene rearrangements characteristic of B cells.[736] Purified BCGF induces growth of hairy cells in short-term culture, and anti-Ig heavy-chain antibodies can further augment this response.[1122] Factors with BCGF activity are produced by neoplastic B cells from patients with hairy-cell leukemia.[1123]

Human B lymphocytes infected by EBV become immortalized and produce an autocrine growth factor, BLAST-2, which has properties similar to those of IL-1.[67] In addition, the growth of EBV-infected human B lymphocytes is promoted by paracrine factors, and one of these factors is identical to IL-6.[1124]

E. NEUROLEUKIN

Neuroleukin is a lymphokine produced by lectin-stimulated T cells that induces Ig secretion by cultured human peripheral blood mononuclear cells.[1125,1126] The neuroleukin target is the B cell but it does not have BCGF or BCDF activity. The neuroleukin-evoked induction of Ig secretion by B cells is both monocyte/macrophage- and T-cell-dependent. In addition to the effects on blood cells, neuroleukin promotes the survival in culture of a subpopulation of embryonic spinal neurons that probably includes skeletal motor neurons, and also supports the survival of cultured sensory neurons that are insensitive to NGF. Neuroleukin has no apparent effect on sympathetic or parasympathetic neurons.

Neuroleukin is a 56-kDa protein that was initially found in the mouse salivary gland. The mouse neuroleukin gene has been cloned and sequenced and has been expressed in monkey COS cells.[1125] The sequence contained in the cloned gene predicts a protein of 558 amino acids which shows no significant homology to other known growth factors, but a region of the neuroleukin molecule is partially homologous to a segment of the gp120 *env* gene product of the AIDS-associated HIV retrovirus. The significance of this homology is unknown, but it could enable the virus to mimic the biological activities of neuroleukin.

Neuroleukin is expressed in mouse tissues, the highest levels being present in skeletal muscle, brain, and bone marrow. The factor is not produced by mouse 3T3 cells, hamster CHO cells, or monkey COS-1 cells, but detectable amounts of neuroleukin have been found in human cell lines of lymphoma-leukemia origin.[1126] Moreover, infection of human B cells with EBV induces neuroleukin expression.

VI. INTERLEUKIN 4

The lymphokine BCGF-I/BSF-1/IL-4 was first described as a cofactor in the proliferation of resting B cells stimulated through the cross-linkage of their membrane Ig by anti-Ig antibody.[1127] IL-4 acts as a differentiation or activation factor for resting B cells and may not induce B-cell growth.[1128-1130] IL-4 is secreted by activated T cells during the course of *in vivo* T-cell-dependent immune responses.[1131] In addition to activated T cells, IL-4 mRNA is expressed by the majority of transformed murine mast-cell lines as well as by some IL-3-dependent nontransformed mast-cell lines, but IL-4 activity is not present in the culture supernatants of all the IL-4 mRNA-positive cell lines.[1132] By means of a specific monoclonal antibody it was shown that IL-4 is distinct from IL-1, IL-2, and IL-3.[1133] IL-4 is identical with a BCDF for IgG1.[1134] IL-4 has a broad spectrum of biological activities and its actions are not limited to B and T lymphocytes but include immature erythroid, myelomonocytic, and megakaryocytic precursors, as well as macrophages and mast cells.[1135,1136]

A. THE IL-4 GENE AND IL-4 STRUCTURE

Murine IL-4 is a 20-kDa glycoprotein which was purified to homogeneity.[1137-1139] The IL-4 molecule contains disulfide bonds whose reduction results in completely destroyed biological activity. The single IL-4 gene contained in the mouse genome was mapped to chromosome 11 by RFLP analysis.[1140] The IL-4 gene was cloned from a mouse liver cDNA library.[1141] The human IL-4 gene was also cloned and sequenced.[1142,1143] The mouse IL-4 and IL-5 genes are located on chromosome 11 and are closely linked, being 110 to 180 kb apart.[1144] Physical linkage studies indicate that the IL-4 and IL-5 genes are a minimum of 600 kb apart from the closely linked IL-4 and CSF-2 genes on mouse chromosome 11. The presence of this cluster of genes related to hematopoiesis suggests the possibility that they may have evolved by ancient gene duplication and may be important in the regulation of their expression.

The human IL-4 gene occurs as a single copy and is located on human chromosome region 5q23.3-q31.2, in a cluster that includes the genes encoding IL-3, IL-4, IL-5, CSF-1, CSF-2, the CSF-1 receptor/c-*fms* proto-oncogene, and the PDGF receptor.[986,1145,1146] This gene cluster is deleted in myeloid leukemias associated with a del(5q). The human IL-4 gene spans 10 kb and its 5'-flanking region is able to respond to stimulation with TPA and calcium ionophore A23187 in Jurkat cells. Human IL-4 is a protein of 133 residues and 15.4 kDa, and its three-dimensional structure is remarkably similar to that of growth hormone and CSF-2, despite the absence of any sequence homology.[1147] Human IL-4 is able to induce proliferation of preactivated B cells, and its activity is potentiated by another BCGF of low molecular weight as well as by IFN-γ.[1148] The biological actions of human and mouse IL-4 proteins, at least in part, are species-specific.[1149]

B. BIOLOGICAL EFFECTS OF IL-4

IL-4 plays a central role in the control and regulation of the immune and inflammatory systems. It is involved in the regulation of B-cell proliferation and differentiation. IL-4 stimulates the growth of B cells by acting during the G_1 phase of the cycle. It induces an increased B-cell volume and prepares resting B cells to enter S phase in response to stimuli such as anti-IgM and LPS.[1150] The number of B cells that proliferate under the influence of IL-4 in a colony-formation assay in soft agar can be significantly enhanced by costimulation with anti-IgM antibody.[76] However, IL-4 may have an inhibitory effect on the growth of selected B-cell populations, for example, in monoclonal lymphocytes from B-type CLL induced to proliferation by IL-2.[1151] IL-4 inhibits IL-2-induced activation of peripheral human blood lymphocytes.[1152] It blocks the upregulation of IL-2 receptors induced by IL-2 in normal human B cells.[1153] In human tonsillar B cells, IL-4 can antagonize the proliferative effect of IL-2 without altering IL-2-induced differentiation.[1154]

IL-4 does not induce the maturation of pre-B cells, but may be important in the process of B-lymphocyte generation by providing a signal for survival of these cells.[1155] IL-4 induces activated B lymphocytes to produce immunoglobulins such as IgG, IgM, and IgE.[1156-1158] IL-4 functions to cause differentiation of membrane IgM+ cells into membrane IgA+ cells and IL-5 then enhances the secretion of IgA by the newly differentiated B cells.[1159] IL-4 has an important role in the generation of IgE antibodies which are involved in allergic responses as well as in host reactions against parasites.[1160] IL-4 also induces the expression of low-affinity receptors for IgE on B cells.[1161,1162] Production of IL-6 is stimulated in human B lymphocytes by IL-4, but not by other interleukins of cytokines.[1163] However, IL-4 may downregulate the production of IL-6 in human peripheral blood mononuclear cells.[1164]

Expression of some antigens on the surface of B lymphocytes is stimulated by IL-4. The interleukin is responsible for the induction of increased levels of class II MHC molecules (Ia antigens) on resting lymphocytes. IL-4-induced increased selective expression of class II MHC antigens on the surface of B cells depends on both transcriptional and translational processes.[1165] Other lymphokines, including IL-1, IL-2, and IFN-γ, cannot duplicate this effect. IFN-γ inhibits the action of IL-4 on resting B cells, including the stimulated increase in expression of class II MHC and IgE receptor molecules, although it has little effect on B cells already stimulated by IL-4.[1150,1166] Expression of Thy-1, a cell-surface glycoprotein of undetermined function, is induced by IL-4 on mouse B cells.[1167] Recombinant IFN-γ inhibits Thy-1 induction by B cells stimulated with LPS and IL-4.

In addition to its action on B cells, IL-4 is involved in the stimulation or maintenance of a state of activation in T cells and promotes the proliferation of helper T cells.[1168-1172] IL-4 appears to be an important TCGF during the immune response to some antigens.[1173] IL-4 potentiates the IL-2-dependent proliferation of mouse cytotoxic T cells.[1174,1175] Generation of CD4+/CD8+ T cells in cultures of neonatal lymphocytes may be induced by IL-4.[1176] A subpopulation of CD4+/CD8– cells circulating in the human neonate can be induced to express both markers by short-term culture with IL-4, and these cells may further differentiate to express only the CD8 surface glycoprotein molecule.

IL-4 has profound effects on the generation of cytolytic T lymphocytes through mechanisms which may be independent of IL-2 induction.[1177] The autocrine growth of helper T cells after antigenic stimulation may be mediated by IL-4.[1178] It has been recognized recently that not all helper T cells proliferate in response to IL-2 and that these cells can be classified, according to their response, into two groups.[419] Type I helper T cells produce IL-2 and proliferate in response to this factor. In contrast, type II helper T cells produce IL-4, which may act as an autocrine factor for these cells in the presence of IL-1.[421] However, secretion of IL-4 is not necessarily associated with proliferation of helper T cells.[1179]

IL-4 is the sole autocrine growth factor for certain cloned lines of inducer T lymphocytes, and the lymphokine secreted by a particular T cell (IL-2 or IL-4) is also the lymphokine that mediates the proliferative response of that cell to antigen receptor-specific signals.[537] Thus, activation of particular types of T cells may be independent of the IL-2 activation system. IL-4, and not IL-2, may be an important growth factor for immature thymocytes, and as such it may play a crucial role in T-cell ontogeny.[420] Protein produced by a human cDNA clone with homology to mouse IL-4 displays stimulating activities for both B and T cells.[1142] IL-4-deficient mutant mice produced by gene targeting in murine embryonic stem cells exhibit normal T and B cell development, but the serum levels of IgG1 and IgE are not detectable after parasitic infection, indicating that IL-4 is critical for the physiology of the immune system.[1180] The potent immunologic effects of IL-4 may be put to use for the treatment of specific forms of human cancer.[1181]

IL-4 is a multifunctional cytokine that has important effects on blood cells other than B and T lymphocytes. IL-4 may contribute to the downregulation and resolution of an inflammatory response by selectively promoting expression of the IL-1 receptor antagonist (IRAP or IL-1ra).[1182] Administration of IL-4 to cancer patients results in a marked increase in the concentration of IRAP mRNA in monocytes, and a similar effect is observed in monocytes exposed to IL-4 *in vitro*. Expression of class II MHC antigens on human monocytes is increased by IL-4 in a dose-dependent manner *in vitro*.[1183] IL-4 inhibits expression of the IL-8 gene from human monocytes stimulated by LPS, TNF-α, or IL-1, but has no effect on the production of IL-8 by nonimmune cells such as fibroblasts and endothelial cells.[1184,1185] IL-4 can increase the proliferative rate of certain mast cell lines costimulated with IL-3.[419] The factor is required for *in vitro* clonal growth of connective tissue-type mast cells.[1186] IL-4 alone is not able to support colony formation by human hematopoietic progenitor cells, but it enhances pure neutrophil colony formation in the presence of CSF-3.[1187] The development of eosinophils and basophils is regulated by different sets of factors, and IL-4 has an enhancing effect on both cell lineages in association with the other factors.[1188] Mature human basophils express IL-4 receptors,[1189] and an eosinophil-dependent mechanism is implicated in the antitumor effect of IL-4.[1190]

IL-4 may be involved in macrophage activation and may play a role in the regulation of macrophage antigen-presenting function.[1191] Macrophages possess receptors for IL-4, and binding of IL-4 to these receptors results in development of potent tumoricidal activity of the activated macrophages against malignant cells such as fibrosarcoma target cells.[1192] IL-4 not only causes aggregation of macrophages and diminishes their migration, but also stimulates directly the formation of giant multinucleated cells via fusion of CSF-dependent bone marrow and alveolar macrophages.[1193] Giant multinucleated cells are associated with granulomatous lesions that occur in response to various infectious and noninfectious agents. However, the production of IL-1β, TNF-α, and PGE_2 is suppressed by the action IL-4 in human peritoneal macrophages.[1194] IL-4 may function as an autocrine factor secreted by Reed-Sternberg cells.[1195]

IL-4 is able to affect the proliferation of myeloid, erythroid, megakaryocyte, and multipotent hematopoietic progenitors.[1196,1197] IL-4 can inhibit the growth of megakaryocyte progenitor cells in culture.[1198] It may be considered as a multi-CSF similar to IL-3, with a direct action on the growth of primitive hematopoietic progenitor cells.[1199] Moreover, IL-4 may directly or indirectly regulate positive and negative aspects of progenitor cell growth and inhibits stromal cell-dependent growth of bone marrow-derived pre-B cells. The synthesis of a reversible inhibitory activity by adherent cells of normal bone marrow is regulated by IL-4.[1200] Induction of this activity, which may act as a negative regulator for both factor-dependent and factor-independent hematopoietic cell proliferation, is a unique property of IL-4. In addition to its actions on hematic cells, IL-4 may have important effects on other tissues. IL-4 is a mitogen for capillary endothelium.[1201] It may also function as a potent inhibitor of bone resorption.[1202] It is clear that IL-4 is a factor with multifunctional properties.

C. THE IL-4 RECEPTOR

The biological activities of IL-4 on human and murine cells are mediated by a single high-affinity receptor of 140 kDa.[1203-1206] Expression of the receptor on unstimulated B and T lymphocytes is low, but activation with mitogens such as LPS or concanavalin A produces a marked increase in IL-4 receptor numbers. Expression of IL-4 receptors on T and B cells is also enhanced by IL-4 stimulation of these cells.[1139] Low levels of IL-4 receptors are present in mast cell, macrophage, and myelomonocytic lineages. IL-4 receptors are present in human hematopoietic cells as well as on cells of epithelial and endothelial origin and primary human gingival fibroblasts.[1206,1207] Human monocytes and AML cells contain both high- and low-affinity binding sites for IL-4, and the expression of both types of sites is downmodulated by protein kinase C activation.[1208] IFN-γ induces and regulates IL-4 receptor expression on murine macrophage cell lines and marrow-derived macrophages.[1209] IL-4 receptors are expressed by nonhematopoietic murine cells, but the physiologic effects of IL-4 on these cells are little known.

A murine cell line expressing high levels of IL-4 receptors was used for the purification, protein sequencing, and cDNA cloning of the IL-4 receptor.[1210] The functional murine receptor has a molecular weight of 140 kDa.[1211] An IL-4 receptor-related polypeptide of 70 kDa (p70) represents a degradation product of the native receptor, and another IL-4-binding molecule of 40 kDa (p40), detected in IL-4-responsive murine cells, appears to be the product of an mRNA coding for a soluble form of the receptor. The soluble form blocks the ability of IL-4 to induce cell growth, and may represent a regulatory molecule specific for IL-4-dependent immune response.

The isolation and characterization of cDNAs encoding the murine and human IL-4 receptor indicate that the receptor is represented by a protein of 130 to 140 kDa that belongs to the cytokine receptor family. Little is known, however, about the mechanism of signal transduction induced by the ligand-activated IL-4 receptor, which lacks known consensus motifs for a signal-transducing molecule such as tyrosine kinase or nucleotide-binding sites. The critical region for signal transduction in the cytoplasmic domain of the human IL-4 receptor is located between amino acid residues 433 and 473, numbering from the carboxyl terminus.[1212] This region is highly conserved between mouse and human IL-4 receptors but lacks homology with other known cytokine receptors. The cytoplasmic domain of the IL-4 receptor is not essential for forming high-affinity sites nor for ligand internalization.

The IL-4 receptor is internalized after ligand binding. IL-4 is involved in the regulation of IL-4 receptor expression, being capable of inhibiting the expression of high-affinity IL-4 receptors in monoclonal human B cells.[1213] In the Burkitt's lymphoma cell line Jijoye, more than 90% of the internalized IL-4 receptor is released in a degraded form into the medium following first-order kinetics.[1214] Internalization of IL-4 receptor-ligand complexes can be inhibited by cytoskeletal disruption and lysosomotropic agents.

D. POSTRECEPTOR MECHANISMS OF ACTION OF IL-4

The postreceptor mechanisms of action of IL-4 are probably very complex and are little understood. IL-4 action on resting B cells may not require enhanced phosphoinositide turnover or increased influx of Ca^{2+}.[1215] Two distinct ion channels are activated by IL-4 in B lymphocytes: an inward rectifying K^+ channel and a large-conductance anion channel.[1216] Interaction of IL-4 with membrane receptors stimulates a membrane-associated protein kinase that phosphorylates an endogenous 44-kDa protein.[1217] The IL-4-stimulated kinase may be distinct from protein kinase C. However, IL-4 signal transduction in human monocytes is associated with translocation of protein kinase C.[1218] Stimulation of murine hematopoietic cell lines with IL-4 causes an increase in the phosphorylation of 170- and 140-kDa cellular proteins on tyrosine residues.[753] IL-4 induces tyrosine phosphorylation of the IL-4 receptor and association of PI 3-kinase to the IL-4 receptor in the mouse T-cell line HT2.[1219] Since the IL-4 receptor does not possess tyrosine kinase activity, IL-4-induced phosphorylation of tyrosine residues must depend on the action of tyrosine kinases which could include, at least in part, products of the Src family.

IL-4 may be involved in the regulation of gene expression. A gene induced by IL-4 in cytotoxic T lymphocytes codes for a lipase.[1220] The role of IL-4 in the regulation of proto-oncogene expression is little understood. No consistent effect of IL-4 on c-*myc* mRNA levels was detected in mouse B cells stimulated to proliferate by Fab'2 fragments or rabbit anti-mouse Ig antibodies.[1221] IL-4 inhibits the accumulation of c-*fos* and c-*jun* mRNA, as well as AP-1 protein levels, in LPS-stimulated human monocytes.[1222]

E. ROLE OF IL-4 IN NEOPLASTIC PROCESSES

IL-4 alone has a direct inhibitory effect on the growth of human melanoma and renal cell carcinoma cell lines.[1223] High-affinity IL-4 receptors are expressed by primary cultures of human renal carcinoma cells, and the growth of these cells is inhibited by IL-4 through downregulation of IL-4 receptor expression.[1224] Gastric carcinoma cell lines express IL-4 receptors and are even more sensitive to the growth-inhibitory effects of IL-4.[1225] The levels of responsiveness of tumor cells to IL-4 are related to the presence of IL-4 receptors on the cell surface, but the mechanism of IL-4-mediated inhibition of tumor cell growth is unknown. A wide range of human cancers express IL-4 receptors and it has been proposed that these tumors may be targeted with chimeric toxin composed of IL-4 and *Pseudomonas* exotoxin.[1226]

VII. INTERLEUKIN 5

A soluble factor of T-cell origin involved in the regulation of immunoglobulin synthesis is a glycoprotein termed BCGF-II, or IL-5.[1227,1228] While BSF-1/IL-4 acts in the initial stages leading to the functional activation of B cells, IL-5 is crucially required for the T-cell-dependent final maturation process of B cells and for the induction of Ig production.[1229-1234] IL-5 was previously referred to as T-cell replacing factor or killer-helper factor. This factor was shown to induce terminal differentiation of B cells, rather than to augment B cell proliferation. IL-5 does not affect resting B cells, but acts late in the G_1 phase of the cycle and induces Ig secretion in naturally occurring large B cells. Stimulation of B cells *in vitro* (CH12LX cell line) with recombinant IL-4 induces membrane Ig expression with only minimal secretion, whereas IL-5 induces IgA secretion without increasing the proportion of membrane IgA-bearing cells.[1159] IL-1 can synergize with IL-5 for primary antibody responses; whereas IL-1 acts in the early phases of B-cell activation, IL-5 acts primarily during the later phases of this activation.[68] Moreover, IL-1 may induce or increase the expression of IL-5 receptors on B cells. Thus, IL-1 or IL-4 and IL-5 may act in a stepwise fashion to stimulate B-cell differentiation. In addition, IL-5 is involved in the generation of cytotoxic T lymphocytes from thymocytes.[1235] Human IL-5 can stimulate a human NK cell line (YT cells), murine thymocytes, and some EBV-transformed B-cell lines, but not peripheral blood T cells.[1236]

IL-5 regulates the production of eosinophils in human bone marrow cultures and selectively stimulates cells of the eosinophil lineage.[1237] IL-5 is responsible for the production of eosinophils from bone marrow cells and for their survival and functional activation.[1238,1239] IL-3 and CSF-2 also stimulate the production of eosinophils, but IL-5 induces the greatest production of these cells in human bone marrow culture, probably through its action on a smaller population of committed precursors. Whereas CSF-2 acts on early stages of eosinophilopoiesis, IL-5 stimulates the growth and terminal differentiation of the eosinophilic cells.[1240] Increased production of IL-5, concomitantly with eosinophilia, is observed in patients with malignant diseases, helminth infections, and allergic diseases, as well as in patients with the idiopathic hypereosinophilic syndrome. Eosinophilia occurs in transgenic mice expressing an IL-5 gene.[1241] In addition to its potent action of eosinophils, IL-5 may be considered as a basophilopoietin, since it has important effects in basophil generation and function.[1242] Human eosinophils and basophils have been shown to share a common hematopoietic progenitor.

A. THE IL-5 GENE AND IL-5 STRUCTURE

The IL-5 gene is located on human chromosome region 5q31.[1243] The genes coding for IL-3, IL-4, CSF-1, CSF-2, the CSF-1 receptor, and the PDGF receptor are located on the same chromosome region, which is deleted in patients with the 5q-syndrome.[987] Human and murine cDNA clones coding for IL-5 have been isolated from concanavalin A-stimulated T cells and T-cell lines.[1142,1244,1245] The coding sequence for human IL-5 was synthesized chemically.[1246] Expression of human and murine cDNA clones in various eukaryotic systems results in the synthesis of mature, biologically active IL-5 proteins. The human IL-5 gene encodes a precursor polypeptide of 134 amino acids that contains an amino-terminal signal sequence. The mature IL-5 protein is glycosylated, and its biological activity depends on the formation of 40- to 50-kDa homodimers, linked together by disulfide bridges. Recombinant IL-5 is active on human B cells and is capable of inducing Ig synthesis in B lymphocytes stimulated by *Staphylococcus aureus* mitogen.

The gene encoding IL-5 maps to the same locus of that for IL-3 on mouse chromosome 11, at band B1, near its proximal interface with band A5.[975] A cDNA clone encoding mouse IL-5 was isolated from the 2.19 murine T-cell line.[1247] The putative IL-5 polypeptide encoded by this clone has a molecular weight of 12,300 Da and is 133 amino acids long. It is distantly related in its primary structure to IL-3, CSF-2, and IFN-γ. Recombinant murine IL-5 translated in *Xenopus laevis* oocytes is a dimeric protein of 45 to 50 kDa.[1248]

B. THE IL-5 RECEPTOR

IL-5 stimulates a pattern of functional responses similar to those of IL-3 and CSF-2. In normal human myeloid cells, cell-surface IL-5 receptors are expressed by eosinophils and basophils but not neutrophils or monocytes, and IL-3 and CSF-2 cross-compete with IL-5 for binding to the receptor.[1249,1250]

Murine IL-5-binding activity can be expressed on the surface of *Xenopus laevis* oocytes injected with mRNA derived from murine IL-5-dependent cells.[1251] IL-5-dependent early B-cell lines of murine origin express both high-affinity and low-affinity IL-5 binding sites.[1252,1253] The number of high-affinity IL-5 receptors is upregulated by LPS and downregulated by IL-5. The murine receptor precipitated by a rat monoclonal antibody is a glycoprotein of 60 kDa.[1254] Analysis of a cDNA indicates that the murine IL-5 receptor is a protein of 415 amino acid residues which includes a glycosylated extracellular domain, a single transmembrane domain, and a cytoplasmic tail of 54 amino acids.[1255] The murine IL-5 receptor shows homology in its extracellular domain with the receptors for several cytokines, growth hormone, and prolactin. In contrast to conserved features of the extracellular domain, the cytoplasmic domain of the IL-5 receptor is unique and exhibits no consensus sequences for protein kinases, either tyrosine-specific or nontyrosine-specific. COS7 cells transfected with the cDNA encoding the murine IL-5 receptor expressed a 60-kDa protein that bound IL-5 with a single class of affinity. However, binding and cross-linking studies suggest a two-chain model for the IL-5 receptor: an α chain represented by the 60-kDa component and corresponding to the low affinity IL-5 binding site, and a β chain of 130 kDa that associates with the α chain to form the high-affinity binding site.[1253]

Low-affinity IL-5 receptors present on the surface of human eosinophils are represented by a 60-kDa protein.[1256] The receptor is a member of the cytokine receptor superfamily and contains three fibronectin type III (FBN III) modules.[1257] The high-affinity IL-5 receptor is a dimer composed of a 60-kDa α chain, which is a soluble polypeptide with antagonistic properties, and a 130-kDa β chain which is identical to the β chain of the CSF-2 receptor.[1258] The finding that IL-5 and CSF-2 share a receptor subunit provides a molecular basis for the observation that these cytokines can partially interfere with each others binding and have overlapping biological activities on eosinophils. The gene encoding the IL-5 receptor α subunit has been mapped to human chromosome region 3p24-p26.[1259]

C. POSTRECEPTOR MECHANISMS OF ACTION OF IL-5

The postreceptor mechanisms of action of IL-5 are little known but may be associated with changes in phosphoinositide metabolism, resulting in the generation of inositol trisphosphate and intracellular redistribution of Ca^{2+}.[1260] However, the results obtained with a clone of the murine B-cell line BCL_1, in which IL-5 induces a process of differentiation, suggest that an increased mobilization of Ca^{2+} is probably not involved in the cellular response to IL-5.[1261] Phosphorylation of cellular proteins on serine and tyrosine residues is stimulated by IL-5. In the IL-5-dependent murine early B-lineage cell line T88-M, the proteins phosphorylated by the action of IL-5 are similar or identical, at least in part, to those whose phosphorylation is stimulated by IL-3, suggesting that these proteins may play an important role in signal transduction of both IL-5 and IL-3.[1262] The possible role of proto-oncogene products in the postreceptor mechanisms of IL-5 action is unknown. In the IL-5-dependent murine early B-cell line J6, IL-5 induces expression of c-*myb*, c-*fos,* and c-*fms* RNA.[1263] IL-5-induced differentiation of the murine chronic leukemia B-cell line BCL_1-B20 is associated with increased expression of the c-*myc* proto-oncogene.

VIII. INTERLEUKIN 6

Interleukin 6 (IL-6) is a cytokine with multiple biological activities which was first described as a product of stimulated fibroblasts. However, IL-6 production can be induced by a variety of agents in a wide diversity of cells. IL-6 plays a central role in host defense mechanisms and may function as a messenger among cells both inside and outside the immune system.[1264-1270] It contributes in important ways to the regulation of hematopoiesis, immune responses, and acute phase reactions. IL-6 plays an important role in the normal developmental process.[1271] It is also involved in malignancies such as plasma cell neoplasias.[1272]

IL-6 is identical with a murine and human protein with B-cell differentiation-inducing activity, termed B-cell-stimulating factor 2 (BSF-2), as well as with IFN-β_2.[1273,1274] Moreover, BSF-2/IL-6/IFN-β_2 is identical to a monocyte-derived growth factor, the hepatocyte-stimulating factor, which plays a central role in the development of the acute phase response to inflammation by the liver.[1275-1277] IL-6 is also identical to a growth factor referred to as B-cell hybridoma growth factor.[1278]

A. BIOLOGICAL EFFECTS OF IL-6

IL-6 has important effects on B and T lymphoid cells. It induces the final maturation of B cells into Ig-secreting lymphocytes. The activation of T lymphocytes by IL-6 is mediated by the production of IL-2.[1279] IL-6 functions as a signal for IL-2 production by mature T cells and is capable of stimulating the proliferation of mature thymic and peripheral murine cells in the presence of either PHA or anti-T-cell receptor antibodies.[1280-1282] IL-6 is present in concanavalin A-induced T-cell supernatants and is able to enhance the proliferative response of IL-4/PMA-stimulated thymocytes.[1283] In addition, IL-6 enhances the cytotoxic activity of human NK cells via IL-2.[1284] IL-6, either alone or in combination with IL-1, is not involved in the induction of CSF production by human marrow stromal cells or fibroblasts.[1285]

In cooperation with other HGFs, IL-6 may exert important effects in hematopoietic cells not pertaining to the lymphoid lineage, including megakaryocytic, myeloid, erythroid, and multipotential progenitor cells.[1286] IL-6, in concert with IL-3, CSF-2, and other HGFs, is involved in the control of megakaryocytopoiesis.[1287-1292] Both IL-6 and its receptor are expressed in human megakaryocytes, and IL-6-induced regulation of megakaryopoiesis may occur by an IL-6 autocrine loop.[1293] IL-6 is a potent stimulator of murine and primate megakaryopoiesis *in vivo*, and appears to act early in megakaryocyte differentiation.[1294,1295] However, the effects of IL-6 on megakaryopoiesis may be indirect.

IL-6 contributes to support the growth and differentiation of human and murine hematopoietic precursors.[1296,1297] The effects of IL-6 on hematopoietic stem cells have been verified *in vivo*. Continuous perfusion of IL-6 into mice results in a marked increase in the number of CFUs in the spleen, which represent pluripotent stem cells.[1298] Injection of IL-6 into rats causes biphasic neutrophilia, mild lymphopenia, and reticulocytosis, indicating that IL-6 can act as a stimulus for myelopoiesis and erythropoiesis.[1299] However, these results do not necessarily implicate a direct effect of IL-6 on hematopoietic stem cells. In general, IL-6 requires the presence of serum, or factors present in serum, for displaying *in vitro* its effects on hematopoietic progenitor cells. IL-3, which is a multi-CSF, acts synergistically with IL-6 in supporting the proliferation of murine multipotential progenitor cells in culture.[1300] In murine systems, IL-6 enhances the sensitivity of multipotential hematopoietic progenitors to IL-3.[1301] IL-6 would indirectly support the formation of several types of hematopoietic colonies, including those derived from early blast cells, and would directly support the proliferation of granulocyte/macrophage progenitors.[1302] IL-6 may enhance CSF-1-induced monocyte-macrophage colony formation in cultures of highly enriched progenitor cells from human bone marrow.[1303] Human CSF-2 at suboptimal doses interacts synergistically with IL-6 in supporting the proliferation of human myeloid hematopoietic progenitor cells.[1304] The granulocytic differentiation of these cells is directly induced by IL-6. In addition, IL-6 functions as an activator of polymorphonuclear neutrophils, enhancing the antibody-dependent cytotoxicity of these cells.[1305]

Cells not pertaining to the hematopoietic system may also be targets for IL-6 action, which indicates a role for IL-6 in the regulation of a wide diversity of biological phenomena. TNF-α-induced expression of class I HLA gene expression in human fibroblasts may be mediated by IL-6.[1306] IL-6 exerts important metabolic effects in the liver and is involved in the development of an acute phase response to noxious agents. It is a hepatocyte-stimulating factor and has endogenous pyrogen activity, and is necessary, in addition to IL-1, TNF-α, and glucocorticoids, for the development of an optimal hepatic acute phase response both *in vitro* and *in vivo*.[96,1307] IL-6 is a potent regulator of acute phase protein synthesis in adult human liver cells.[1308] In fact, IL-6 appears to be the major effector factor in the hepatic acute phase response.[1309] Whereas IL-1 and TNF-α induce only a partial and weak response to factors inducing the acute phase response, IL-6 is capable of inducing the same spectrum of acute phase proteins as that found in humans during inflammation.[1310] IL-6 is capable of stimulating hepatic lipogenesis, and the lipogenic effects of TNF-α are mediated by IL-6.[1311] Liver-specific genes regulated at the transcriptional level by IL-6 during the acute phase response include those coding for haptoglobin and complement factor B.[97] The 5'-flanking regions of these genes contain information for the IL-6-specific induction of the acute phase response. TGF-β and EGF modulate basal and IL-6-induced amino acid uptake and acute phase protein synthesis in rat hepatocytes.[1312]

IL-6 may have important effects on endocrine cells and may be involved in the complex interactions that occur between the neuroendocrine and immune system. IL-6, possibly induced by IL-1β in the pituitary gland, stimulates the release of gonadotropins and prolactin.[1313] In conscious rats, IL-6 stimulates the secretion of ACTH through the release of CRH by the hypothalamus.[1314] Sertoli cells in the testis produce and secrete IL-6, which may have a role in the paracrine regulation of spermatogenesis.[1315]

IL-6 can affect insulin secretion and glucose metabolism of rat pancreatic islets *in vitro*.[1316] Inhibition of insulin secretion from rat islets of Langerhans by IL-6 is an effect distinct from that of IL-1.[1317] Pancreatic β cells produce IL-6, and this production is stimulated by IFN-γ and TNF-α.[1318] In addition to a possible role in the physiologic regulation of β-cell function, IL-6 may be a co-stimulator for autoreactive B and T lymphocytes in type I, autoimmune diabetes mellitus.

Osteoclasts, the cells involved in bone resorption, develop from hematopoietic precursor cells of bone marrow under the control of growth factors present in the microenvironment. IL-6 may have an important function in osteoclastogenesis. Production of IL-6 by marrow stromal cells and osteoblastic cells, both of which influence osteoclastogenesis, can be inhibited by 17β-estradiol, and 17β-estradiol as well as a neutralizing antibody to IL-6 can suppress osteoclast development in cultures of mouse marrow cells. Estrogen loss (ovariectomy) in mice results in an increase in the number of CFU-GM, enhancement in osteoclast development in *ex vivo* cultures of bone marrow, and an increase in the number of osteoclasts in trabecular bone.[1319] These changes can be prevented by estradiol or an antibody to IL-6, suggesting that estrogen loss may result in IL-6-mediated stimulation of osteoclastogenesis. The osteopenia and osteoporosis observed in clinical conditions associated with estrogen deficiency, such as the menopause, may occur by a mechanism involving the action of IL-6 on bone cells.

IL-6 may function as a nerve cell differentiation factor. Transcripts of the IL-6 gene are expressed in glioblastoma and astrocytoma cell lines, and IL-6 is capable of inducing neuronal differentiation of the PC12 rat pheochromocytoma cell line.[1320] The IL-6-stimulated PC12 cells express the c-*fos* gene transiently and exhibit a morphological change to neurite-extending cells after several days. The number of voltage-dependent Na$^+$ channels is increased in IL-6-treated PC12 cells. These effects are similar to those produced by NGF, but IL-6 is not able to support long-term culture of neuronal cells.

B. IL-6 GENE AND THE STRUCTURE OF IL-6

The IL-6 gene is located on human chromosome 7.[1321] Full-length cDNAs corresponding to the human IL-6 gene have been produced and expressed in heterologous systems.[1322-1325] These cDNAs encode a 23.7-kDa polypeptide of 212 amino acid residues which is posttranslationally modified by glycosylation, sialylation, and phosphorylation.[1326] Human fibroblasts and monocytes stimulated with TNF-α, IL-1, bacterial LPS (endotoxin), or virus infection secrete IL-6 in the form of a glycoprotein constituted by a doublet of 25 kDa or a triplet of 30 kDa, which are phosphorylated on serine residues.[1327] Phosphorylation of IL-6 at Ser-54 is an early event in the secretory pathway in human fibroblasts.[1328] Differential phosphorylation of IL-6 may be a mechanism to modulate the functions of IL-6 in a tissue-specific manner.

Expression of the IL-6 gene promoter in HeLa cells is repressed by the wild-type, but not mutant, protein products of the tumor suppressor genes p53 and RB.[1329] Modulation of IL-6 gene expression by the p53 and RB proteins may have important implications for the regulation of cell growth and differentiation as well as for the origin and development of tumors.

The murine IL-6 gene is located on the proximal region of chromosome 5.[1330] A complete cDNA sequence for the murine IL-6 protein was isolated from a library prepared by using mRNA from a murine helper T-cell clone activated with a clonotypic antibody.[1331] The murine IL-6 cDNA predicts a mature polypeptide of 187 amino acids and a molecular weight of 21,710 Da. Studies with another murine IL-6 cDNA clone indicate that IL-6 exhibits significant homology to human IL-6 in its amino acid sequence, and that IL-6 expression is inducible in IL-1-treated bone marrow stromal cells as well as in activated helper T-cell and macrophage cell lines.[1332]

The structure and sequence of the rat IL-6 gene, as well as the amino acid sequence of rat IL-6, have been reported.[1333] A rat macrophage-derived cell line was used as a source of mRNA and as a tool for studies of the expression of the IL-6 gene. Murine and human cell lines can express and secrete functionally active recombinant rat IL-6. Two distinct IL-6 mRNA species derive from the single-copy rat IL-6 gene by alternative polyadenylation.

C. PRODUCTION OF IL-6

IL-6 is produced by lymphocytic cells as well as by cells of the mononuclear phagocyte lineage.[1334] IL-2 induces IL-6 production by human monocytes.[1335] Locally secreted IL-6 can stimulate Ig secretion by B cells invading sites of inflammation, and both IL-6 and TNF-α are synthesized and secreted by normal tonsillar B cells after stimulation with IL-2.[1336] IL-6 and TNF-α may be involved in autocrine/paracrine regulation of B-cell differentiation.

Production of IL-6 by human B cells is stimulated by IL-4.[1163] However, IL-4 downregulates IL-6 production by human peripheral blood mononuclear cells.[1164] Synthesis of IL-6 declines during the course of monocyte maturation into macrophages. Monocytes are the main source of circulating IL-6, whereas IL-6 present at various tissue sites may be provided by resident macrophages and/or fibroblasts. Freshly isolated, unstimulated human peripheral blood monocytes do not usually express IL-6 mRNA, but activation of monocytes by either adherence *in vitro* or the action some factors (CSF-1, CSF-2, IL-1α, and IFN-γ) induces high levels of IL-6 mRNA.[1337] Adherence *in vitro* mimics monocyte migration through the vascular endothelium into the site of infection, as it occurs during the initial stage of the inflammatory response.

Certain leukemic cell lines synthesize and secrete IL-6 when they are treated with differentiation inducers. IL-6 is not produced by unstimulated U-937 or HL-60 human leukemia cell lines, but IL-6 mRNA is rapidly detected after treatment of these cell lines with PMA.[1337] IL-6 is also produced by M1 mouse myeloid leukemia cells when they are induced to differentiate into macrophages by treatment with calcitriol or the differentiation-inducing factor, D-factor.[1338]

In addition to lymphocytes and monocytes, IL-6 is produced and secreted by a diversity of other cell types, including endothelial and fibroblastoid cells as well as trophoblasts.[1339] Proliferating or IL-1-activated human vascular smooth-muscle cells secrete copious IL-6.[1340] In contrast, no expression of IL-6 mRNA occurs in the regenerating liver of the rat.[1341]

A complex network of growth factor interactions is involved in the control of endogenous IL-6 production and secretion.[1342,1343] Factors involved in such interactions include TNF-α, PDGF, IL-1, IL-2, and IFN-β-1. Freshly explanted human endometrial stromal cells secrete biologically active IL-6 in response to IL-1α, IL-1β, TNF-α, and IFN-γ, and this secretion can be inhibited by estrogens at concentrations within the physiologic range.[1344] Expression of the IL-6 gene in freshly explanted human endothelial cells is rapidly enhanced by IL-1α and TNF-α as well as by LPS.[1345,1346] Recombinant IL-6 inhibits the incorporation of labeled thymidine by the human endothelial cells, suggesting that IL-6 is not only produced by these cells but may also affect their proliferation. Cytokine-induced regulation of IL-6 secretion is also observed *in vivo*. Administration of TNF-α or IL-2, but not IFN-α, to cancer patients rapidly induces the appearance of circulating, biologically active IL-6.[1347]

IL-1 stimulates the synthesis and secretion of IL-6 by human chondrocytes and stromal cells.[1348] TGF-β stimulates production of IL-6 by cultured normal human fibroblasts, and this effect is exerted at the level of increased IL-6 gene transcription.[1349] TGF-β also enhances IL-6 secretion by intestinal epithelial cells.[1350] Production of IL-6 by human fibroblasts and the MG-63 human osteosarcoma cell line is stimulated by small amounts of IL-1.[1278] IL-1 induces a rapid and sustained increase in IL-6 gene transcription in cultures of diploid human FS-4 fibroblasts.[1351] The effect of IL-1 on IL-6 gene expression requires new protein synthesis. TNF-α also stimulates in FS-4 cells the transcriptional expression of the IL-6 gene, but this effect is not influenced by cycloheximide. Both IL-1 and TNF-α stimulate IL-6 production by FS-4 cells, and this effect is partially mediated by activation of cAMP-dependent protein kinase.[329] Regulation of IL-6 gene expression by different agents may occur through mechanisms that may involve the activation of protein kinase C or the elevation of $[Ca^{2+}]_i$.[1352]

DNA sequences contained in the 5′-flanking side of the IL-6 gene may play an important role in the regulation of IL-6 gene expression in different types of cells. Studies with a plasmid vector carrying 5′-flanking sequences of the human IL-6 gene transfected into human HeLa cells indicate that activation of the IL-6 gene promoter by cytokines and growth factors (IL-1, TNF-α, and EGF), second-messenger agonists (diacylglycerol and calcium ionophore A23187), and viruses (pseudorabies and Sendai viruses) depends on a DNA sequence of 113 bp situated between nucleotides −225 and −113.[1353] In an independent study it was determined that the human IL-6 gene contains on its 5′-flanking side (positions −72 to −62) a sequence which shares 90% homology with an enhancer element of the gene encoding the Ig light-chain kappa. In human fibroblasts, TNF-α- and IL-1-stimulated synthesis of IL-6 is related to binding of a nuclear factor (NF-κB-like factor) to the specific kappa-B-like sequence contained in the IL-6 gene.[1354] This pathway for IL-6 induction is different, in part, from that of IL-6 induction by agents that increase cAMP levels and induce activation of protein kinase A, as demonstrated by the effects of forskolin.

The IL-6 gene promoter of human liver cells contains an IL-6 responsive element which is necessary and sufficient for the IL-6-dependent activation of transcription.[1355] The IL-6 effect does not require *de novo* protein synthesis and is mediated by a liver-specific nuclear protein (IL-6DBP) which binds to the

IL-6 promoter as well as to similar sequences present in the promoters of genes encoding hemopexin and other proteins activated in the acute phase response. The IL-6DBP DNA-binding activity is induced by IL-6 via a posttranslational mechanism.

D. THE IL-6 RECEPTOR

Cloning, characterization, and functional expression of the rat liver IL-6 receptor gene has been reported.[1356] The cell surface IL-6 receptor is a dimeric protein consisting of a ligand-binding α chain of 80 kDa (IL-6Rα) and a β-chain glycoprotein of 130 kDa (IL-6Rβ), which has an essential role in transmembrane signaling. The human gene for IL-6Rα is localized on chromosome band 1q21.[1357] The β chain associates with the ligand-binding chain only after binding of IL-6. The IL-6 receptor ligand-binding chains are similar in leukocytes and hepatocytes and the differences observed in the responses of different cells to IL-6 are related to cell-type-specific components of the IL-6 transduction machinery. Binding sites with high affinity for IL-6 detected in human lymphoblastoid cells are not competed for by other cytokines.[1358]

IL-6 receptor expression in different types of cells is subjected to complex regulatory mechanisms. Expression of the IL-6 receptor β chain in human epithelial cells is enhanced by IL-6, IL-1, and TNF-α.[1359] High-affinity IL-6 receptors are upregulated by glucocorticoids in human epithelial cells.[1360] LIF induces downregulation of IL-6 receptors in murine myelomonocytic leukemia cells.[1361]

E. POSTRECEPTOR MECHANISMS OF ACTION OF IL-6

The postreceptor transductional mechanisms of action of IL-6 remain poorly understood. Some of the effects of IL-6 on its target cells are exerted at the transcriptional level. IL-6 regulates metallothionein gene expression in the liver.[1362] The responses of cultured hepatocytes to IL-6 require the presence of glucocorticoid. The transcriptional effects of IL-6 may include proto-oncogenes. IL-6 modulates c-sis/PDGF-B gene expression in cultured human endothelial cells.[1363] It also stimulates DNA synthesis and proliferation of cultured vascular smooth muscle cells, and this effect is preceded by a rapid, dose-dependent induction of c-*myc* mRNA expression.[1364]

F. ROLE OF IL-6 IN NEOPLASIA

IL-6 is expressed by a diversity of tumors. Most types of human tumors stain positively for the presence of IL-6 protein, as shown in an immunohistochemical study on frozen samples of human tumors of epithelial and mesenchymal origin using a polyclonal antiserum raised against human IL-6.[1365] The tumor cells, and not just the supporting stromal tissues, expressed IL-6 immunoreactivity. Human normal and transformed bronchial epithelial cells express and release both biologically and immunologically intact IL-6 *in vitro*.[1366] Release of IL-6 is a general property of human glioblastomas.[1367] Prostatic carcinomas express IL-6 receptors and secrete IL-6, which raises the possibility that IL-6 is involved in the growth of these tumors through autocrine mechanisms.[1368] Serum levels of IL-6 correlate with tumor burden, clinical disease status, and survival in patients with epithelial ovarian cancer.[1369] Increased serum IL-6 levels have been detected in patients with myelodysplastic syndromes.[1370] Since IL-6 is a major mediator of the host response to injury, IL-6 could be implicated in some of the systemic manifestations of cancer, including fever, increased erythrocyte sedimentation rate, and alterations in plasma protein composition. In addition, IL-6 could mediate local effects of the tumor such as alterations in cellular proliferation, increased tumor cell motility, and decreased intercellular adhesions between the tumor cells. IL-6 may also alter the immunologic status of the host.

Kaposi sarcoma lesions, which are very frequent in AIDS patients, produce different types of cytokines and growth factors, including ECGF, IL-1β, and basic FGF. Cell lines derived from these lesions produce IL-6 and contain IL-6 receptors.[1371] IL-6 is required for optimal growth of Kaposi sarcoma cells, suggesting that it may act as an autocrine growth factor for Kaposi sarcoma.

The possible role of IL-6 in the origin and development of leukemias and lymphomas *in vivo* is unknown. IL-6 appears to have little or no effect, by itself, on the proliferation of blast precursors present in the peripheral blood of patients with AML.[1372] However, IL-6 synergizes with CSF-2 and IL-3 in the stimulation of AML blast colony formation. Serum IL-6 levels are elevated in some patients with lymphoma and may correlate with survival in advanced Hodgkin's disease.[1373]

Activation of the c-*myc* proto-oncogene by juxtaposition to an Ig locus and introduction of the v-*abl* oncogene acts synergistically in generating murine plasmacytoma. IL-6 may have a role in the development of murine plasmacytomas, and the v-Abl oncoprotein could act on plasmacytomagenesis by stimulating the endogenous production of IL-6. However, v-*abl* gene expression does not abolish IL-6 requirement by plasmacytoma cells.[1374]

IL-6 exerts antiproliferative and differentiation-inducing effects on several human and murine myeloid leukemic cells, including the U-937, THP-1, and M1 cell lines, which undergo differentiation into macrophage-like cells.[395,1375,1376] Treatment of these leukemic cells with both IL-6 and IL-1 may result in either an additive or a synergistic inhibition of growth. The human KU812 leukemic cell line is characterized by both a capacity for self-renewal and the ability to differentiate spontaneously along erythroid and basophilic cell lineages. IL-6 and its specific receptor are expressed in KU812 cells. Addition of antibody against IL-6 to these cells weakly inhibits their proliferation but strongly inhibits their differentiation, and this effect is reversed by the addition of human IL-6.[1377] In contrast, IL-1 and IL-6, whether alone or in combination, do not influence the growth and differentiation of HL-60 human promyelocytic leukemia cells. Human melanoma cells obtained from early-stage, metastatically incompetent primary lesions are sensitive to the growth-inhibitory effects of IL-6, but the cells obtained from the more advanced, metastatically competent lesions or from metastases are resistant or growth stimulated by IL-6.[1378] It may be concluded that the effects of IL-6 on the proliferation and differentiation of neoplastic cells are variable and depend on the specific type of cells and their state of genetic alteration.

IX. INTERLEUKIN 7

Interleukin 7 (IL-7) was initially called lymphopoietin 1 or pre-B-cell growth factor because of its growth-promoting activity for cells early in the B-lymphocyte lineage.[1379] The use of factor-dependent B-cell precursors obtained from long-term bone marrow cultures (Witte-Whitlock cultures) allowed the detection of the IL-7 factor active on precursor B cells.[1380] A clonal cell line (I×N/A6) secretes IL-7 in serum-free medium.

A. IL-7 GENE AND THE STRUCTURE OF IL-7

IL-7 is represented by a 25-kDa protein and is distinct from previously described HGFs. A cDNA encoding biologically active murine IL-7 was isolated from a bone marrow stroma cell cDNA library and expressed in COS-7 cells.[1381] The molecular cloning of human IL-7 and the activity of IL-7 on human and murine B-lineage cells was reported.[1382] The gene for IL-7 is located on the long arm of human chromosome 8, at region 8q12-q13.[1383]

B. BIOLOGICAL EFFECTS OF IL-7

IL-7 rapidly induces a proliferation of B-cell precursors (pre-B cells) in cells freshly isolated from mouse bone marrow, and this proliferative function is inhibited by TGF-β and IL-α.[1384,1385] In addition to its effects on cells from long-term marrow cultures, IL-7 stimulates cell growth in cultures of fresh bone marrow. A combination of IL-7 and SCGF co-stimulates proliferation of pre-B cells after they have differentiated by the action of molecules produced by stromal cells.[1386] IL-7 may be essential in the normal process of B-cell proliferation and differentiation in the marrow.

IL-7 displays effects on developing T lymphocytes and is also a potent stimulator of the growth of mature T cells, provided they are activated.[1387] Addition of IL-7 to cultures of purified T cells together with concanavalin A results in expression of IL-2 receptors and production of IL-2, with stimulation of T-cell proliferation. IL-7 may be involved in the generation of immunocompetent T cells in the thymus in concert with IL-2.[1388] Recent evidence suggests that, at least in some cases, IL-7 can directly stimulate T-cell proliferation independently of other cytokines.[1389-1391] However, IL-7-supported generation of cytotoxic T lymphocytes from thymocytes requires the presence of other interleukins, in particular IL-2 and IL-6.[1392] IL-7 is a potent initial stimulus for multiple cytokine production by human T lymphocytes. Highly purified T cells stimulated with IL-7, in the absence of co-mitogen, secrete IL-2, IL-4, IL-6, and IFN-γ upon restimulation with phorbol ester and ionomycin.[1393]

In addition to its effects on lymphocyte proliferation and differentiation, IL-7 may have important effects on cells of the monocytic lineage.[1394] Administration of human IL-7 to mice alters the frequency and number of myeloid progenitor cells in the bone marrow and spleen.[1395] IL-7 is a potent inducer of the secretion of IL-6, IL-1α, IL-1β, and TNF-α by human peripheral blood mononuclear cells. The full range of IL-7 target cells and biological activities remains to be established, but present evidence indicates that IL-7 is involved in both the regulation of immune processes and lymphopoiesis.[1379]

C. THE IL-7 RECEPTOR

IL-7 exerts its effects on its target cells through binding to specific surface receptors. The murine cell line IxN/2b, which depends on IL-7 for continued growth, has been used to define the functional and structural characteristics of the murine IL-7 receptor.[1396] The cells express about 2000 to 2500 IL-7 binding sites and the receptors are represented by a 75- to 79-kDa protein. Structural analysis and expression of cDNA clones encoding the human and murine IL-7 receptor has been reported.[1397,1398] The human and murine IL-7 receptor gene consists of 8 exons, spanning 23 and 19 kb, respectively, and its 5' region contains consensus binding sequences for several transcription factors as well as an IFN-regulatory element (IRE). The IL-7 receptor exhibits in its extracellular domain homology to several known cytokine receptors as well as to the receptors for growth hormone and prolactin. All these receptors are members of the hematopoietin receptor family. The IL-7 receptor forms noncovalently associated dimers in the plasma membrane. The IL-7 receptor is expressed on pre-B cells, but not on mature B-cell lines or primary mature B cells. It is also expressed on murine thymocytes, some T lineage cell lines, and bone marrow-derived macrophages. The gene for the IL-7 receptor is located on human chromosome region 5p13.[1399]

D. POSTRECEPTOR MECHANISMS OF IL-7 ACTION

The postreceptor mechanisms of IL-7 action are little known but may include alterations in phosphoinositide metabolism and protein phosphorylation. Binding of IL-7 to its receptor on the surface of human B-lymphocyte precursors results in stimulation of tyrosine phosphorylation, phosphoinositide turnover, and clonal cell proliferation, as well as selective differentiation to the CD4 lineage of human fetal thymocytes.[1400,1401] The IL-2 receptor mediates activation of PI 3-kinase in human B-cell precursors.[1402] The Fyn tyrosine kinase may have an important role in the mechanism of IL-7 action. In pre-B cells, the IL-7 receptor may function by recruiting the Fyn tyrosine kinase through a segment of its cytoplasmic tail, which may lead to activation of the PI 3-kinase.[1403] The possible role of proto-oncogene products in the cellular mechanisms of IL-2 action is not understood, but there is evidence that IL-7 induces c-*myc* and N-*myc* gene expression in normal B-lymphocyte precursors.[1404]

E. ROLE OF IL-7 IN NEOPLASIA

The possible role of IL-7 in neoplastic processes is unknown, but IL-7 could be involved, in concert with other cytokines and growth factors, in the reaction of the organism against various types of tumors. It can induce monocyte/macrophage tumoricidal activity against human melanoma cells. IL-7 enhances the proliferation and effector function of tumor-infiltrating lymphocytes from renal cell carcinoma.[1405]

IL-7 may be involved in the complex mechanisms associated with leukemogenesis and lymphomagenesis. The IL-7 gene is transcribed in leukemic cell subsets of individuals with CLL.[1406] IL-7 induces a growth response in malignant cells from B-cell precursor ALL and immature T-cell ALL.[1407] The ALL cells would contain both high- and low-affinity IL-7 receptors. Purified neoplastic cells of various differentiation stages express receptors for IL-7, and IL-7 can provide a strong stimulatory signal to these cells, including cells of the nonlymphoid lineage.[1408] The proliferation of malignant cells of ALL patients with the CD7$^+$, CD4$^-$, CD8$^-$ phenotype can be supported by exogenous IL-7.[1409] This phenotype corresponds to a syndrome of pluripotent lymphohematopoietic cells which are capable of multilineage differentiation *in vitro*.

Endogenous IL-7 expression may not be necessary for transformation of pre-B cells.[1410] The expression is not sufficient to explain the malignant phenotype of v-*abl*-oncogene-transformed cells. However, upregulation of IL-7 expression in transformed pre-B cells may be one of several synergistic events which can lead to malignant conversion. Expression of a retroviral vector carrying the IL-7 gene induced neoplastic transformation in an immortal IL-7-dependent pre-B cell line.[1411] The infected cells produced variable quantities of IL-7 and their proliferation was inhibited by a neutralizing antibody directed against IL-7, indicating that an autocrine mechanism was responsible for their transformation. In contrast to the parental cells, the infected cells were acutely tumorigenic in syngeneic hosts. However, an autocrine loop involving IL-7 does not exist in A-MuLV-transformed pre-B cells.

X. INTERLEUKIN 8

Interleukin 8 (IL-8) is a cytokine which was first isolated from LPS-stimulated human peripheral blood monocytes.[1412] It is a potent chemotactic agent for neutrophils and T cells and is a major mediator of inflammation.[1413,1414] IL-8 was previously designated monocyte-derived neutrophil chemotactic factor

(MDNCF), granulocyte chemotactic protein (GCP), or neutrophil-activating peptide-1 (NAP-1). A soluble leukocyte adhesion inhibitor (LAI), which acts on leukocytes to attenuate a hyperadhesive interaction, is identical to IL-8.[1415] The IL-8/LAI factor acts as a protective agent in neutrophil-mediated endothelial injury. A factor similar or identical to IL-8 is produced by human dermal fibroblasts stimulated by IL-1 or TNF-α.[85]

A. PRODUCTION AND BIOLOGICAL EFFECTS OF IL-8

The largest amounts of IL-8 are produced by monocytes, but other types of cells also produce IL-8. Expression of IL-8 mRNA occurs in human T cells stimulated with a combination of phorbol ester (PMA) and ionomycin, or PMA and PHA, and is specific to the CD4+ T-cell subset.[1416] However, the stimulated cells do not secrete IL-8, even in the presence of accessory monocytes. By contrast, human CD3– large granular lymphocytes can be induced to express IL-8 mRNA and secrete IL-8 protein upon specific stimulation with IL-2 and ligand for the NK-cell receptor for IgG-Fc, or upon nonspecific stimulation with PMA. Expression of the IL-8 gene in human synovial cells is stimulated by IL-1.[370]

Human peripheral blood neutrophils synthesize and secrete IL-8 in response to LPS, TNF-α, and IL-1β.[1417] IL-8 exerts potent chemotactic activity for neutrophils *in vitro* and provokes a rapid granulocytosis on i.v. injection into rabbits. On intradermal injection in rabbit skin, picomole amounts of human IL-8 were found to induce neutrophil accumulation that was fast in onset, short in duration, and associated with a parallel time course of plasma leakage and edema formation.[1418] Movement of neutrophils from the bloodstream to inflamed tissue depends on the activation of both the neutrophil and the endothelial cell. Production of a 77-amino acid variant of IL-8 by endothelial cells may be required for transendothelial neutrophil migration during acute inflammatory processes.[1419] Macrophage-derived IL-8 may act as a mediator of angiogenesis in wound repair as well as in disorders such as rheumatoid arthritis and tumorigenesis.[1420] IL-4 may inhibit IL-8 expression from stimulated human monocytes, but has no effect on IL-8 expression from nonimmune cells such as fibroblasts and endothelial cells.[1184,1185]

B. THE IL-8 GENE AND IL-8 STRUCTURE

IL-8 was originally purified from lymphocytes as a 72-amino acid peptide.[1421] The molecular cloning of a human gene encoding IL-8 was subsequently reported.[1422] IL-8 is a member of a superfamily of genes including melanoma growth stimulatory activity (MGSA), macrophage inflammatory protein 2, platelet factor 4 (PF-4), platelet basic protein and its cleavage products, connective tissue-activating peptide, and neutrophil-activating peptide 2. The genes encoding the members of this protein superfamily are closely linked on the long arm of chromosome 4.[1423]

C. THE IL-8 RECEPTOR

cDNA clones encoding the human and rabbit IL-8 receptor have been isolated.[1424-1427] The amino acid sequence shows that the IL-8 receptor is a member of the superfamily of receptors that couple to G proteins. More recently, analysis of cDNA clones has shown the existence of two distinct high-affinity IL-8 receptors, termed IL-8R-A or α (IL-8R type 1) and IL-8R-B or β (IL-8R type 2).[1428] These two receptors have 77% amino acid identity and are members of the G protein-coupled superfamily of receptors, which is characterized by the presence of seven transmembrane domains. The receptor affinities for the IL-8-related protein, melanocyte growth-stimulatory activity/Gro (MGSA) are different — whereas IL-8R-A binds MGSA with low affinity, IL-8R-B binds MGSA with high affinity. The genes encoding IL-8R-A and IL-8R-B have been mapped to human chromosome region 2q35.[1429,1430]

IL-8 regulates the expression of its own receptor.[1431] Ligand-associated IL-8 receptors are internalized but can be rapidly recycled to the neutrophil surface. The reappearance of IL-8 receptors on the cell surface may be essential for the neutrophil chemotactic response to IL-8.

D. POSTRECEPTOR MECHANISMS OF ACTION OF IL-8

Signal transduction of the activated IL-8 receptor are coupled to activation of G protein-associated pathways.[1432] IL-8 receptors appear to interact with pertussis toxin-sensitive heterotrimeric G proteins, which results in release of βγ subunits that activate phospholipase-$β_2$. The effects of IL-8 on the migration of human peripheral blood lymphocytes are associated with receptor-mediated increases in $[Ca^{2+}]_i$, G protein stimulation, and protein kinase C activation.[1433] Phosphoinositide metabolism has an important role in the postreceptor mechanism of IL-8 action. IL-8 stimulates phosphatidylinositol 4-phosphate kinase activity in human polymorphonuclear leukocytes.[1434]

E. ROLE OF IL-8 IN NEOPLASIA

Cellular inflammatory responses are frequently observed at the site of malignant tumors and may be associated with the action of specific cytokines and chemotactic factors. IL-8, a potent chemoattractant for T lymphocytes as well as for neutrophils and basophils, may be secreted by certain human tumors, including primary and metastatic brain tumors, and may be involved in leukocyte infiltration occurring in these tumors.[1435] IL-8 may have an important role in the development of cerebrospinal fluid pleocytosis in infectious diseases such as meningoencephalitis.

XI. INTERLEUKIN 9

Interleukin-9 (IL-9) is a lymphokine identified in the mouse as a factor, termed P40, which is capable of supporting the growth of certain T cell clones, but not of fresh T cells.[1436] IL-9 derived from T cells is a glycoprotein of 32 to 39 kDa. Analysis of cDNA clones encoding murine IL-9 showed that IL-9 is synthesized as a precursor of 144 amino acids including a signal peptide of 18 residues.[1437,1438] The cloning and expression of cDNAs coding for human IL-9 have been reported.[1439-1441] The human gene encoding IL-9 consists of 5 exons and 4 introns and is localized on human chromosome region 5q31-q35. Expression of IL-9 in human T cells depends on IL-2.[1442]

IL-9 may be involved in normal hematopoiesis. It has synergistic effects with CSF-2 and IL-3 for the maturation of hematopoietic progenitors and may act on both lymphoid and myeloid lineages.[1443] It can also support maturation of fetal and adult erythroid progenitors. IL-9 stimulates the colony growth of early erythroid progenitor cells (BFU-E) in the presence of erythropoietin and, in combination with CSF-2, has an additive effect on BFU-E growth.[1444] Mature blood cells may respond to IL-9. Saturable and specific IL-9 binding sites have been detected in a variety of murine blood cells including T cells, mast cells, and macrophages, but not in B cells or fibroblasts.[1445] Expression of IL-9 is a physiologic event during the antigenic stimulation of normal T cells.

Expression cloning and sequence of a cDNA encoding the human and murine IL-9 receptor predicts that it is a protein of 52 kDa containing a signal peptide and a transmembrane domain.[1446] The IL-9 receptor belongs to the superfamily of hematopoietic receptors and is expressed, as the other receptors of this family, in membrane-bound and soluble forms. The mechanism of IL-9 signal transduction is unknown.

IL-9 may have an important role in neoplastic processes. It is produced by some neoplastic hematopoietic cell lines and is present in conditioned medium from the human T-cell leukemia cell line C5MJ2, which can support growth of the human megakaryoblastic leukemia cell line MO7E. Expression of IL-9 receptors correlates with IL-9 responsiveness on a variety of T cell lines. IL-9 is expressed by primary and cultured Reed-Sternberg cells.[1447] It may act as an autocrine factor in Hodgkin's disease and large cell anaplastic lymphoma, but apparently not in B- and T-cell lymphomas.[1448] Transfection of a murine T helper cell clone with IL-9 DNA results in autonomous growth and tumorigenicity.[1449]

XII. INTERLEUKIN 10

The product of the long-term mouse T-cell clone $T_H 2$ is the cytokine synthesis inhibitory factor (CSIF).[1450,1451] This factor, now called interleukin 10 (IL-10), displays a wide diversity of biological effects.[1452-1454] A factor termed B-cell-derived T-cell growth factor (B-TCGF) is identical with IL-10.[1455]

Both B and T lymphocytes produce IL-10, and IL-10 functions as a cofactor for mature and immature T cells and plays a role in T-cell development in the thymus. IL-10 impairs the ability of macrophages to provide costimulatory signals for resting T cell proliferation, and this suppression is primarily mediated by inhibition of IL-2 production.[1456,1457] IL-10 inhibits the synthesis of cytokines such as IL-1, TNF-α, and IFN-γ by stimulated helper T cells.[1458] In turn, IFN-γ can inhibit the production of IL-10 by monocytes.[1459] In addition to its effects on T cells, IL-10 has a stimulatory effect on B lymphocytes. IL-10 is a potent growth and differentiation factor for activated human B lymphocytes, upregulates their class II MHC antigens, and enhances B-cell viability.[1460,1461] IL-10 alone is not able to support the growth of mast cell lines or mast cell progenitors, but IL-10 markedly enhances the growth of these cells when combined with IL-3 or IL-4.[1462] A combination of IL-3, IL-4, and IL-10 may be required for optimal mast cell growth. Epstein-Barr virus (EBV)-induced transformation stimulates human B cells to produce IL-10.[1463] Murine keratinocytes can also produce IL-10 mRNA and protein, and this production is stimulated by application of hapten to the skin.[1464] IL-10 protects mice from lethal endotoxemia.[1465]

IL-10 is an acid-labile protein of 35 to 40 kDa. Isolation and analysis of cDNA clones encoding mouse IL-10 predicts a protein of 18.7 kDa and 160 amino acids. IL-10 cDNA clones prepared from RNA of cultured OX8-OX22 rat thoracic duct cells have also been synthesized and characterized.[1466] The cellular actions of the IL-10 protein are mediated by its binding to a specific receptor located on the cell surface, but the cellular and molecular mechanisms of IL-10 action remain poorly characterized.

The possible role of IL-10 in human malignant diseases is unknown, but the IL-10 protein exhibits extensive homology with the product of an uncharacterized ORF (BCRFI or BCRF1) present in the EBV.[1467] BCRFI may represent the viral homolog of the cellular IL-10 gene. It is conceivable that EBV exploits the biological activity of a captured cytokine sequence to manipulate the immune response against the cells infected by the virus, therefore promoting its survival in the host. However, the BCRFI protein can enhance *in vitro* B-cell viability but does not upregulate class II MHC antigen.[1460] Human B-cell lines derived from patients with AIDS or Burkitt's lymphoma constitutively secrete large quantities of IL-10.[1468] Malignant cells from AIDS-associated lymphomas also produce IL-10 *in vivo*.[1469]

XIII. INTERLEUKIN 11

Interleukin 11 is a pleiotropic hematopoietin with stimulatory effects on hematopoietic progenitor cells.[1470,1471] IL-11 is a 199-amino acid polypeptide of 23 kDa, initially derived from the primate bone marrow cell line PU-34. It can support long-term hematopoiesis by human and nonhuman primate progenitor cells in culture.[1472] The cloning of a cDNA encoding IL-11 and its expression in COS cells showed that IL-11 is unrelated to other known cytokines. The cDNA sequence contains a single ORF encoding an IL-11 protein of 199 amino acids. The predicted amino acid sequence of the mature IL-11 protein does not contain cysteine residues and has a net positive charge, suggesting a protein with an unusually high isoelectric point. The genomic sequences of human IL-11 have been determined and the gene has been mapped to chromosome region 19q13.3-q13.4.[1473] The 5'-flanking region of the IL-11 gene contains sequences similar to those present in the 5'-regulatory regions of other cytokine genes.

IL-11 has varied biological activities. It can support the growth of plasmacytoma cells and stimulates T-cell-dependent development of B cells in cultures of spleen cells. IL-11 can promote accessory cell-dependent B-cell differentiation in humans.[1474] IL-4 interacts with IL-11 to stimulate the growth of multipotent hematopoietic progenitors.[1475] IL-11 can influence myelopoiesis in intact mice.[1476] It can also stimulate multiple phases of erythropoiesis *in vitro*,[1477] as well as IL-3-dependent development of megakaryocyte colonies in bone marrow cell clonal culture.[1478] IL-11 acts as an autocrine factor for human megakaryoblastic cell lines.[1479] It stimulates megakaryocytopoiesis and increases peripheral platelets in normal and splenectomized mice.[1480] Such diverse biological properties suggest that IL-11 may function as a regulator in both hematopoiesis and lymphopoiesis. In addition to its activities in the hematopoietic system, IL-11 may have other functions. IL-11 induces the secretion of acute phase proteins in the liver in a manner similar to that of IL-6.[1481] Molecular cloning of a cDNA encoding an adipogenesis inhibitory factor showed its identity with IL-11.[1482] It is thus clear that IL-11 has a wide range of physiological effects.

The cellular mechanism of IL-11 action is initiated by its interaction with a cell surface receptor protein of 151 kDa.[1471] This interaction results in a rapid activation of tyrosine kinase activity, although the IL-11 receptor does not possess this type of activity.[1483] Stimulation of 3T3-LI and C3H10T1/2 cells with IL-11 results in the appearance of tyrosine-phosphorylated proteins of 150, 97, 47, and 44 kDa. In H-35 cells, IL-11 induces the expression of tyrosine-phosphorylated proteins of 97 and 44 kDa. Expression of early response genes such as *jun*-B and *tis*-11 is activated by IL-11. The adipogenesis inhibitory activity of IL-11 on 3T3-L1 cells is associated with inhibition of lipoprotein lipase activity at a posttranscriptional level. In general, the biological effects of IL-11 and IL-6 on different types of cells are similar, which may be explained, at least in part, by the fact that both cytokines as well as LIF, oncostatin M, and the ciliary neurotrophic factor (CNTF) utilize the gp130 signal transducer protein in their cellular mechanism of action.

The possible role of IL-11 in neoplastic diseases is unknown. IL-11 alone has little effect on human leukemic cells isolated from patients with AML.[1484] However, in combination with other growth factors, including IL-3, CSF-2, and Steel factor, IL-11 frequently enhances the proliferation of leukemic cell populations.

XIV. INTERLEUKIN 12

Interleukin 12 (IL-12) is a cytokine capable of inducing the proliferation of PHA-activated T cells and synergizing with IL-2 in the induction of LAK cells.[1485-1487] IL-12, originally called NK cell stimulatory factor (NKSF) or cytotoxic lymphocyte maturation factor (CLMF), is a 75-kDa heterodimeric glycoprotein composed of two disulfide-bonded subunits of 40 and 35 kDa, respectively. cDNA clones coding for each IL-12 subunit have been isolated and characterized. IL-12 induces IFN-γ production by resting peripheral blood mononuclear cells and enhances NK activity. In the presence of cortisol, IL-12 synergizes with IL-2 to induce LAK cells. IL-12 acts as a growth factor for PHA-activated human lymphoblasts independently of IL-2 and IL-2 receptor. IL-12 and IL-4 have synergistic effects on NK cell proliferation.[1488]

IL-12 is a heterodimer composed of two unrelated disulfide-linked chains: a 35-kDa (p35) A (or α) chain and a 40-kDa (p40) B (or β) chain. The A chain of IL-12 is a member of the cytokine receptor family, most closely related to the IL-6 receptor, and forming a subgroup with this receptor and the G-CSF/CSF-3 receptor. The B chain of IL-12 is related to ligands of the cytokine receptor family. The gene for the A chain of IL-12 is located on human chromosome region 5q31-q33, whereas the gene for the B chain is located on human chromosome region 3p12-3q13.2.[1489]

The IL-12 receptor expressed by PHA-activated human lymphoid cells is represented by a single protein of 110 kDa.[1490] Activation of T cells or NK cells, but not B cells, results in upregulation of IL-12 receptor expression on the cell surface.[1491] Antibodies to the B subunit of IL-12 block IL-12 receptor binding and IL-12 biologic activity on activated human lymphoblasts.[1492] These results suggest that the B subunit has no direct contact points with the IL-12 receptor, or needs to assume a specific configuration with the A subunit to properly bind the receptor.

XV. INTERLEUKIN 13

Interleukin 13 (IL-13) is a human T-cell-derived cytokine involved in the regulation of human monocyte and B-cell function and in inflammatory and immune responses.[1493-1495] The human IL-13 gene is localized on chromosome region 5q23-q31, closely linked to the IL-4 gene. The cloning and expression of the human IL-13 gene predicts a nonglycosylated polypeptide of 134 amino acids and 12,397 Da. Expression of IL-13 cDNA in COS cells results in the synthesis of a secreted protein of 17 kDa which may represent a glycosylated form of IL-13. The IL-13 protein sequence shows limited homology with IL-4, but exhibits approximately 60% sequence identity with a protein, P600, expressed by the Th2 subset of mouse T helper lymphocytes. The Th2 lymphocyte subset also expresses IL-3, IL-4, CSF-2, and IL-10, whereas the Th1 lymphocyte subset expresses IL-2, IL-3, and IFN-γ.

Recombinant IL-13 inhibits LPS-induced inflammatory cytokine production by human peripheral blood monocytes. IL-13 synergizes with IL-2 in regulating IFN-γ synthesis in large granular lymphocytes. It is capable of increasing the proliferation of B lymphocytes and induces IL-4-independent IgG4 and IgE synthesis and CD23 expression by human B cells. The action of IL-13 may be associated with a generalized inhibition of inflammatory cytokine synthesis, including the synthesis of IL-1β, TNF-α, and IL-8. It may be concluded that IL-13 behaves as a pleiotropic, antiinflammatory cytokine that exhibits properties similar, but not identical, to those of IL-4 and IL-10. However, the cellular and molecular mechanisms of IL-13 action remain to be elucidated.

XVI. LEUKEMIA INHIBITORY FACTOR

A differentiation-inducing factor (DIF), the D-factor, which induces differentiation of mouse myeloid leukemia M1 cells into macrophages, was purified from serum-free conditioned medium of mouse L929 cells.[1495] The D-factor can inhibit pluripotential embryonic stem cell differentiation.[1496] It is identical to a factor purified from the conditioned medium of Krebs ascites tumor cells and called leukemia inhibitory factor (LIF). The LIF suppresses the clonogenicity and induces the differentiation of the M1 murine leukemia cell line.[1497] The M1 cells can also be induced to differentiation into macrophages by treatment with calcitriol, which results in the production of IL-6, although this production is not responsible for the D-factor- or calcitriol-induced M1 cell differentiation.[1498] The differentiation inducer DIF-A, purified from human monocytic leukemia THP-1 cells, is a human counterpart or the murine LIF/D-factor.[1499] A factor similar or identical to LIF is present in the serum of patients with CML.[1500] Analysis of a cDNA clone coding for LIF showed that it is identical with a myeloid factor termed human interleukin for DA cells (HILDA).[1501] LIF is also identical with the hepatocyte-stimulating factor III (HSF-III), which was purified from conditioned medium of COLO-16 human tumor cells.[1502] Furthermore, LIF is identical with a cholinergic neuronal differentiation factor (CNDF) secreted by cultured rat heart cells that can direct the choice of neurotransmitter phenotype.[1503] CNDF is a 45-kDa glycoprotein which acts on postmitotic sympathetic neurons to induce the expression of acetylcholine synthesis and cholinergic function, while suppressing catecholamine synthesis and noradrenergic function.

A. THE LIF GENE AND LIF STRUCTURE

The molecular cloning and heterologous expression of cDNAs encoding murine and human LIF has been reported.[1504-1506] The murine and human clones predict a sequence of 179 amino acid residues for the mature protein. The reported molecular weights of LIF range from 38 to 67 kDa, but this heterogeneity can be attributed to variable degrees of glycosylation of the polypeptide. The LIF gene is localized on human chromosome at region 22q12.q12.2, in close proximity to the gene of oncostatin M.[1507,1508]

B. CELLULAR MECHANISMS OF LIF ACTION

Little is known of the mechanisms of action of LIF, but LIF receptors have been detected in various types of cells at different stages of development, including hematopoietic cells as well as cells of bone, liver, and neural origin. The number of LIF receptors per cell is higher in adult hepatocytes than in bone marrow monocytes. A major binding protein for LIF contained in normal mouse serum is represented by a soluble form of the cellular LIF receptor.[1509]

C. BIOLOGICAL PROPERTIES OF LIF

LIF can be considered as a pleiotropic cytokine involved in the regulation of the proliferation, differentiation, and specific functions of a wide diversity of cell types.[1510,1511] Through the induction of cytokines, LIF can modulate inflammation, immune responses, and connective tissue metabolism, and can act as a pathogenetic mediator in different disease states.[1512]

LIF shows specific binding to macrophages, monocytes, and their precursors, suggesting that it may play a role in the generation and/or functional regulation of cells of the macrophage lineage. LIF plays an important role, along with IL-6 and CSF-3, in the regulation of hematopoietic stem cell growth and differentiation. It is necessary for the maintenance of hematopoietic stem cells and thymocyte stimulation.[1513] LIF is as effective as either IL-6 or CSF-3 in the enhancement of IL-3-dependent formation of colonies by very primitive blast hematopoietic cells.[1514] Normal human bone marrow stromal cells express LIF mRNA, and this expression is enhanced by IL-1α, IL-1β, TNF-α, and TGF-β, but not IFN-α.[1515] Constitutive expression of LIF mRNA in marrow stromal cells from some patients with CML is highly increased. LIF may participate, either alone or through interaction with other cytokines, in the bone marrow microenvironment-mediated influence of normal and neoplastic hematopoietic processes. Both LIF and IL-11 are capable of promoting the maturation of murine and human megakaryocytes *in vitro*.[1516] Injection of LIF into adult mice results in elevation in the numbers of megakaryocytes and platelets but has no effect on mature neutrophils, monocytes, or eosinophils.[1517]

LIF is a potent cachexia-inducing agent and may have marked effects on bone metabolism.[1518-1522] LIF is involved in the normal regulation of bone cell function and is able to stimulate bone resorption in a manner similar or identical to a factor called osteoclast-activating factor (OAF), and may play a role in regulating the function of osteoblasts. There is evidence that osteoblasts may be involved in osteoclastic bone resorption, and expression of LIF in osteoblasts may occur in response to local bone-resorbing agents such as IL-1α, IL-1β, and TNF-α. In the liver, LIF can induce a similar set of acute phase plasma proteins as IL-6, although IL-6 and LIF bind to distinct receptors. In the nervous system, LIF may be involved in the development of peripheral neurons from their precursors in the embryonic neural crest as well as in a diversity of nervous functions.

LIF has a role in the regulation of early developmental processes. It is expressed in mouse blastocyst prior to hematopoiesis and may be involved in the regulation of the growth and development of trophoblasts or embryonic stem cells.[1523] LIF is also synthesized in the extraembryonic part of the mouse embryo and acts on the embryonic tissues during mouse development.[1524] It is involved in intertissue relationships during early mouse embryogenesis. The study of LIF and other similar factors reinforces the concept that the distinction between growth-promoting, growth-inhibiting, and differentiation-inducing activities is largely determined by the target cell type and its stage of differentiation.

REFERENCES

1. **Grossman, Z.,** The stem cell concept revisited: self-renewal capacity is a dynamic property of hemopoietic cells, *Leukemia Res.,* 10, 937, 1986.
2. **Kasakura, S. and Lowenstein, L.,** A factor stimulating DNA synthesis derived from the medium of leukocyte cultures, *Nature,* 208, 794, 1965.

3. **Gordon, J. and Maclean, L.D.,** A lymphocyte-stimulating factor produced in vitro, *Nature,* 208, 795, 1965.
4. **Dinarello, C.A. and Mier, J.W.,** Interleukins, *Annu. Rev. Med.,* 37, 173, 1986.
5. **Strober, W. and James, S.P.,** The interleukins, *Pediatr. Res.,* 24, 549, 1988.
6. **Mizel, S.B.,** The interleukins, *FASEB J.,* 3, 2379, 1989.
7. **Arai, K., Lee, F., Miyajima, A., Miyatake, S., Arai, N., and Yokota, T.,** Cytokines: coordinators of immune and inflammatory responses, *Annu. Rev. Biochem.,* 59, 783, 1990.
8. **Kennedy, R.L. and Jones, T.H.,** Cytokines in endocrinology — their roles in health and disease, *J. Endocrinol.,* 129, 167, 1991.
9. **Aggarwal, B.B. and Pocsik, E.,** Cytokines: from clone to clinic, *Arch. Biochem. Biophys.,* 292, 335, 1992.
10. **Andus, T., Palitzsch, K.-D., Gross, V., and Schölmerich, J.,** Metabolische und endokrine Funktionen der Zytokine, *Dtsch. Med. Wochesnschr.,* 118, 306, 1993.
11. **Mitchell, M.D., Trautman, M.S., and Dudley, D.J.,** Cytokine networking in the placenta, *Placenta,* 14, 249, 1993.
12. **Paul, W.E.,** Lymphokine nomenclature, *Immunol. Today,* 9, 366, 1988.
13. **Larsson, E.L., Iscove, N.N., and Coutinho, A.,** Two distinct factors are required for induction of T-cell growth, *Nature,* 283, 664, 1980.
14. **Smith, K.A., Lachman, L.B., Oppenheim, J.J., and Favata, M.F.,** The functional relationship of the interleukins, *J. Exp. Med.,* 151, 1551, 1980.
15. **Maizel, A.L. and Mehta, S.R.,** Effect of interleukin 1 on human thymocytes and purified human T cells, *J. Exp. Med.,* 153, 470, 1980.
16. **Houssiau, F.A., Coulie, P.G., and Van Snick, J.,** Distinct roles of IL-1 and IL-6 in human T cell activation, *J. Immunol.,* 143, 2520, 1989.
17. **Cardell, S. and Sander, B.,** Interleukin-2, interleukin-4 and interleukin-5 are sequentially produced in mitogen-stimulated murine spleen cell cultures, *Eur. J. Immunol.,* 20, 389, 1990.
18. **Suda, T., Murray, R., Guidos, C., and Zlotnik, A.,** Growth-promoting activity of IL-1α, IL-6, and tumor necrosis factor-α in combination with IL-2, IL-4, or IL-7 on murine thymocytes. Differential effects on CD4/CD8 subsets and on CD3$^+$/CD3$^-$ double-negative thymocytes, *J. Immunol.,* 144, 3039, 1990.
19. **Tabibzadeh, S.,** Human endometrium: an active site of cytokine production and action, *Endocrine Rev.,* 12, 272, 1991.
20. **Arzt, E., Buric, R., Stelzer, G., Stalla, J., Sauer, J., Renner, U., and Stalla, G.K.,** Interleukin involvement in anterior pituitary cell growth regulation: effects of IL-2 and IL-6, *Endocrinology,* 132, 459, 1993.
21. **Sabharwal, P., Glaser, R., Lafuse, W., Varma, S., Liu, Q., Arkins, S., Rooijman, R., Kutz, L., Kelley, K.W., and Malarkey, W.B.,** Prolactin synthesized and secreted by human peripheral blood mononuclear cells: an autocrine growth factor for lymphoproliferation, *Proc. Natl. Acad. Sci. U.S.A.,* 89, 7713, 1992.
22. **O'Neal, K.D., Montgomery, D.W., Truong, T.M., and Yu-Lee, L.,** Prolactin gene expression in human thymocytes, Mol. Cell. Endocrinol., 87, R19, 1992.
23. **Cosman, D.,** The hematopoietin receptor superfamily, *Cytokine,* 5, 95, 1993.
24. **Miyajima, A.,** Molecular structure of the IL-3, GM-CSF and IL-5 receptors, *Int. J. Cell Cloning,* 10, 126, 1992.
25. **Guy, G.R., Bee, N.S., and Peng, C.S.,** Lymphokine signal transduction, *Cell. Signal.,* 2, 415, 1990.
26. **Chiba, T., Nagata, Y., Machide, M., Kishi, A., Amanuma, H., Sugiyama, M., and Todokoro, K.,** Tyrosine kinase activation through the extracellular domains of cytokine receptors, *Nature,* 362, 646, 1993.
27. **Lange, W., Brugger, W., Rosenthal, F.M., Kanz, L., and Lindemann, A.,** The role of cytokines in oncology, *Int. J. Cell Cloning,* 9, 252, 1991.
28. **Männel, D.N. and Jänicke, R.,** Induction of monokine production by tumor cells, *Lymphokine Res.,* 8, 257, 1989.
29. **Black, R.J. and Friedman, R.M.,** Cytokines and oncogene activity, *Cancer Surv.,* 8, 725, 1989.
30. **Hock, H., Dorsch, M., Kunzendorf, U., Qin, Z., Diamantstein, T., and Blankenstein, T.,** Mechanisms of rejection induced by tumor cell-targeted gene transfer of interleukin 2, interleukin 4, interleukin 7, tumor necrosis factor, or interferon γ, *Proc. Natl. Acad. Sci. U.S.A.,* 90, 2774, 1993.

31. **Hock, H., Dorsch, M., Kunzendorf, U., Überla, K., Qin, Z., Diamantstein, T., and Blankenstein, T.,** Vaccinations with tumor cells genetically engineered to produce different cytokines: effectivity not superior to a classical adjuvant, *Cancer Res.,* 53, 714, 1993.
32. **Dinarello, C.A. and Savage, N.,** Interleukin-1 and its receptor, *Crit. Rev. Immunol.,* 9, 1, 1989.
33. **Fuhlbrigge, R.C., Hogquist, K.A., Unanue, E.R., and Chaplin, D.D.,** Molecular biology and genetics of interleukin-1, *Yearb. Immunol.,* 5, 21, 1989.
34. **Fibbe, W.E., Schaafsma, M.R., Falkenburg, J.H.F., and Willemze, R.,** The biological activities of interleukin-1, *Blut,* 59, 147, 1989.
35. **Flad, H.-D., Kirchner, H., and Resch, K.,** Interleukin 1 and related cytokines, *Lymphokine Res.,* 8, 227, 1989.
36. **Bagby, G.C., Jr.,** Interleukin-1 and hematopoiesis, *Blood Rev.,* 3, 152, 1989.
37. **Krakauer, T.,** Biochemical characterization of interleukin 1 from a human monocytic cell line, *J. Leukocyte Biol.,* 37, 511, 1985.
38. **Doyle, M.V., Brindley, L., Kawasaki, E., and Larrick, J.,** High level human interleukin 1 production by a hepatoma cell line, *Biochem. Biophys. Res. Commun.,* 130, 768, 1985.
39. **March, C.J., Mosley, B., Larsen, A., Cerretti, D.P., Braedt, G., Price, V., Gillis, S., Henney, C.S., Kronheim, S.R., Grabstein, K., Conlon, P.J., Hopp, T.P., and Cosman, D.,** Cloning, sequence and expression of two distinct human interleukin-1 complementary DNAs, *Nature,* 315, 641, 1985.
40. **Kurt-Jones, E.A., Beller, D.I., Mizel, S., and Unanue, E.R.,** Identification of a cell surface associated interleukin 1, *Proc. Natl. Acad. Sci. U.S.A.,* 82, 1204, 1985.
41. **Kurt-Jones, E.A., Fiers, W., and Pober, J.S.,** Membrane interleukin 1 induction on human endothelial cells and dermal fibroblasts, *J. Immunol.,* 139, 2317, 1987.
42. **Fryling, C., Dombalagian, M., Burgess, W., Hollander, N., Schereiber, A.B., and Haimovich, J.,** Purification and characterization of tumor inhibitory factor-2: its identity to interleukin 1, *Cancer Res.,* 49, 3333, 1989.
43. **Dinarello, C.A.,** Interleukin-1 and the pathogenesis of the acute-phase response, *N. Engl. J. Med.,* 311, 1413, 1984.
44. **Maury, C.P.J.,** Interleukin 1 and the pathogenesis of inflammatory diseases, *Acta Med. Scand.,* 220, 291, 1986.
45. **Fey, G.H. and Fuller, G.M.,** Regulation of acute phase gene expression by inflammatory mediators, *Mol. Biol. Med.,* 4, 323, 1987.
46. **Murphy, P.A., Simon, P.L., and Willoughby, W.F.,** Endogenous pyrogens made by the rabbit peritoneal exudate cells are identical with lymphocyte activating factor made by rabbit alveolar macrophages, *J. Immunol.,* 124, 2498, 1980.
47. **Le, J. and Vilcek, J.,** Tumor necrosis factor and interleukin 1: cytokines with multiple overlapping biological activities, *Lab. Invest.,* 56, 234, 1987.
48. **Dinarello, C.A.,** The biology of interleukin 1 and comparison to tumor necrosis factor, *Immunol. Lett.,* 16, 227, 1987.
49. **Dinarello, C.A.,** Interleukins, tumor necrosis factors (cachetin), and interferons as endogenous pyrogens and mediators of fever, *Lymphokines,* 14, 1 1987.
50. **Okusawa, S., Gelfand, J.A., Ikejima, T., Connolly, R.J., and Dinarello, C.A.,** Interleukin 1 induces shock-like state in rabbits. Synergism with tumor necrosis factor and the effect of cyclooxygenase inhibition, *J. Clin. Invest.,* 81, 1162, 1988.
51. **Bot, F.J., Schipper, P., Broeders, L., Delwel, R., Kaushansky, K., and Löwenberg, B.,** Interleukin-1α also induces granulocyte-macrophage colony-stimulating factor in immature normal bone marrow cells, *Blood,* 76, 307, 1990.
52. **Fibbe, W.E., van Damme, J., Billiau, A., Goselink, H.M., Voogt, P.J., van Eeden, G., Ralph, P., Altrock, B.W., and Falkenburg, J.H.,** Interleukin 1 induces human marrow stromal cells in long-term culture to produce granulocyte colony-stimulating factor and macrophage colony-stimulating factor, *Blood,* 71, 430, 1988.
53. **Kauma, S.W.,** Interleukin-1β stimulates colony-stimulating factor 1 production in human term placenta, *J. Clin. Endocrinol. Metab.,* 76, 701, 1993.
54. **Yang, Y.-C., Tsai, S., Wong, G.G., and Clark, S.C.,** Interleukin-1 regulation of hematopoietic growth factor production by human stromal fibroblasts, *J. Cell. Physiol.,* 134, 292, 1988.
55. **Neta, R., Sztein, M.B., Oppenheim, J.J., Gillis, S., and Douches, S.D.,** The in vivo effects of interleukin 1. I. Bone marrow cells are induced to cycle after administration of interleukin 1, *J. Immunol.,* 139, 1861, 1987.

56. Zucali, B.R., Broxmeyer, H.E., Dinarello, C.A., Gross, M.A., and Weiner, R.S., Regulation of early human hematopoietic (BFU-E and CFU-GEMM) progenitor cells in vitro by interleukin 1-induced fibroblast-conditioned medium, *Blood,* 69, 33, 1987.
57. Larsson, E.L., Iscove, N.N., and Coutinho, A., Two distinct factors are required for induction of T-cell growth, *Nature,* 283, 664, 1980.
58. Pike, B.L. and Nossal, G.J.V., Interleukin 1 can act as a B-cell growth and differentiation factor, *Proc. Natl. Acad. Sci. U.S.A.,* 82, 8153, 1985.
59. Chiplunkar, S., Langhorne, J., and Kauffman, S.H.E., Stimulation of B cell growth and differentiation by murine recombinant interleukin 1, *J. Immunol.,* 137, 3753, 1986.
60. Zucali, J.R., Elfenbein, G.J., Barth, K.C., and Dinarello, C.A., Effects of human interleukin 1 and human tumor necrosis factor on human T lymphocyte colony formation, *J. Clin. Invest.,* 80, 772, 1987.
61. McMannis, J.D. and Plate, J.M.D., Xenogeneic antiserum to soluble products from activated lymphoid cells inhibits interleukin 1-mediated functions in the helper pathway of cytolytic-effector-cell differentiation, *Proc. Natl. Acad. Sci. U.S.A.,* 82, 1513, 1985.
62. Koide, S.I., Inaba, K., and Steinman, R.M., Interleukin 1 enhances T-dependent immune responses by amplifying the function of dendritic cells, *J. Exp. Med.,* 165, 515, 1987.
63. Houssiau, F.A., Coulie, P.G., and Van Snick, J., Distinct roles of IL-1 and IL-6 in human T cell activation, *J. Immunol.,* 143, 2520, 1989.
64. Novak, T.J., Chen, D., and Rothenberg, E.V., Interleukin-1 synergy with phosphoinositide pathway agonists for induction of interleukin-2 gene expression: molecular basis of costimulation, *Mol. Cell. Biol.,* 10, 6325, 1990.
65. Lowenthal, J.W., Cerottini, J.-C., and MacDonald, H.R., Interleukin 1-dependent induction of both interleukin 2 secretion and interleukin 2 receptor expression by thymoma cells, *J. Immunol.,* 137, 1226, 1986.
66. Lacey, D.L., Chappel, J.C., and Teitelbaum, S.L., Interleukin 1 stimulates proliferation of a nontransformed T lymphocyte line in the absence of a co-mitogen, *J. Immunol.,* 139, 2649, 1987.
67. Swendeman, S. and Thorley-Lawson, D.A., The activation antigen BLAST-2, when shed, is an autocrine BCGF for normal and transformed B cells, *EMBO J.,* 6, 1637, 1987.
68. Koyama, N., Harada, N., Takahashi, T., Mita, S., Okamura, H., Tominaga, A., and Takatsu, K., Role of recombinant interleukin-1 compared to recombinant T-cell replacing factor/interleukin-5 in B-cell differentiation, *Immunology,* 63, 277, 1988.
69. Fotedar, R. and Diener, E., The role of recombinant IL-2 and IL-1 in murine B cell differentiation, *Lymphokine Res.,* 7, 393, 1988.
70. Peschel, C., Green, I., Ohara, J., and Paul, W.E., Role of B cell stimulatory factor 1/interleukin 4 in clonal proliferation of B cells, *J. Immunol.,* 139, 3338, 1987.
71. Freedman, A.S., Freeman, G., Whitman, J., Segil, J., Daley, J., and Nadler, L.M., Pre-exposure of human B cells to recombinant IL-1 enhances subsequent proliferation, *J. Immunol.,* 141, 3398, 1988.
72. Bagby, G.C., Jr., Dinarello, C.A., Wallace, P., Wagner, C., Hefeneider, S., and McCall, E., Interleukin 1 stimulates granulocyte macrophage colony-stimulating activity release by vascular endothelial cells, *J. Clin. Invest.,* 78, 1316, 1986.
73. Gallicchio, V.S., Watts, T.D., and DellaPuca, R., Synergistic action of recombinant-derived murine interleukin-1 on the augmentation of colony-stimulating activity on murine granulocyte-macrophage hematopoietic stem cells in vitro, *Exp. Cell Biol.,* 55, 83, 1987.
74. Schaafsma, M.R., Falkenburg, J.H.F., Duinkerken, N., Van Damme, J., Altrock, B.W., Willemze, R., and Fibbe, W.E., Interleukin-1 synergizes with granulocyte-macrophage colony-stimulating factor on granulocytic colony formation by intermediate production of granulocyte colony-stimulating factor, *Blood,* 74, 2398, 1989.
75. Van Damme, J., Opdenakker, G., de Ley, M., Heremans, H., and Billiau, A., Pyrogeneic and haematological effects of the interferon-inducing 22K factor (interleukin 1β) from human leukocytes, *Clin. Exp. Immunol.,* 66, 303, 1986.
76. Smith, R.J., Speziale, S.C., and Bowman, B.J., Properties of interleukin-1 as a complete secretagogue for human neutrophils, *Biochem. Biophys. Res. Commun.,* 130, 1233, 1985.
77. Parker, K.P., Benjamin, W.R., Kaffka, K.L., and Kilian, P.L., Presence of IL-1 receptors on human and murine neutrophils. Relevance to IL-1-mediated effects in inflammation, *J. Immunol.,* 142, 537, 1989.

78. **Moser, R., Schleiffenbaum, B., Groscurth, P., and Fehr, J.,** Interleukin 1 and tumor necrosis factor stimulate human vascular endothelial cells to promote transendothelial neutrophil passage, *J. Clin. Invest.,* 83, 444, 1989.
79. **Schooley, J.C., Kullgren, B., and Allison, A.C.,** Inhibition by interleukin-1 of the action of erythropoietin on erythroid precursors and its possible role in the pathogenesis of hypoplastic anaemias, *Br. J. Haematol.,* 67, 11, 1987.
80. **Hoang, T., Haman, A., Goncalves, O., Letendre, F., Mathieu, M., Wong, G.G., and Clark, S.C.,** Interleukin 1 enhances growth factor-dependent proliferation of the clonogenic cells in acute myeloblastic leukemia and of normal human primitive hematopoietic precursors, *J. Exp. Med.,* 168, 463, 1988.
81. **Lotem, J. and Sachs, L.,** Indirect induction of differentiation of normal and leukemic myeloid cells by recombinant interleukin 1, *Leukemia Res.,* 13, 13, 1989.
82. **Johnson, C.S., Keckler, D.J., Topper, M.I., Braunschweiger, P.G., and Furmanski, P.,** In vivo hematopoietic effects of recombinant interleukin-1α in mice: stimulation of granulocytic, monocytic, megakaryocytic, and early erythroid progenitors, suppression of late-stage erythropoiesis, and reversal of erythroid suppression with erythropoietin, *Blood,* 73, 678, 1989.
83. **Onozaki, K., Matsushima, K., Kleinerman, E.S., Saito, T., and Oppenheim, J.J.,** Role of interleukin 1 in promoting human monocyte-mediated tumor cytotoxicity, *J. Immunol.,* 135, 314, 1985.
84. **Lovett, D., Kozan, B., Hadam, M., Resch, K., and Gemsa, D.,** Macrophage cytotoxicity: interleukin 1 is a mediator of tumor cytostasis, *J. Immunol.,* 136, 340, 1986.
85. **Larsen, C.G., Zachariae, C.O.C., Oppenheim, J.J., and Matsushima, K.,** Production of monocyte chemotactic and activating factor (MCAF) by human fibroblasts in response to interleukin 1 or tumor necrosis factor, *Biochem. Biophys. Res. Commun.,* 160, 1403, 1989.
86. **Ramadori, G., Sipe, J.D., Dinarello, C.A., Mizel, S.B., and Colten, H.R.,** Pretranslational modulation of acute phase hepatic protein synthesis by murine recombinant interleukin 1 (IL-1) and purified human IL-1, *J. Exp. Med.,* 162, 930, 1985.
87. **Gauldie, J., Sauder, D.N., McAdam, K.P.W.J., and Dinarello, C.A.,** Purified interleukin-1 (IL-1) from human monocytes stimulates acute-phase protein synthesis by rodent hepatocytes *in vitro, Immunology,* 60, 203, 1987.
88. **Hill, M.R., Stith, R.D., and McCallum, R.E.,** Interleukin 1: a regulatory role in glucocorticoid-regulated hepatic metabolism, *J. Immunol.,* 137, 858, 1986.
89. **Sipe, J.D., Vogel, S.N., Douches, S., and Neta, R.,** Tumor necrosis factor/cachectin is a less potent inducer of serum amyloid A synthesis than interleukin 1, *Lymphokine Res.,* 6, 93, 1987.
90. **Mortensen, R.F., Shapiro, J., Lin, B.-F., Douches, S., and Neta, R.,** Interaction of recombinant IL-1 and recombinant tumor necrosis factor in the induction of mouse acute phase proteins, *J. Immunol.,* 140, 2260, 1988.
91. **Perlmutter, D.H., Goldberger, G., Dinarello, C.A., Mizel, S.B., and Colten, H.R.,** Regulation of class III major histocompatibility complex gene products by interleukin-1, *Science,* 232, 850, 1986.
92. **Darlington, G.J., Wilson, D.R., and Lachman, L.B.,** Monocyte-conditioned medium, interleukin-1, and tumor necrosis factor stimulate the acute phase response in human hepatoma cells in vitro, *J. Cell Biol.,* 103, 787, 1986.
93. **Bauer, J., Weber, W., Tran-Thi, T.-A., Northoff, G.-H., Decker, K., Gerok, W., and Heinrich, P.C.,** Murine interleukin 1 stimulates α_2-macroglobulin synthesis in rat hepatocyte primary cultures, *FEBS Lett.,* 190, 271, 1985.
94. **Roh, M.S., Moldawer, L.L., Ekman, L.G., Dinarello, C.A., Bistrian, B.R., Jeevanandam, M., and Brennan, M.F.,** Stimulatory effect of interleukin-1 upon hepatic metabolism, *Metabolism,* 35, 419, 1986.
95. **Warren, R.S., Donner, D.B., Starnes, H.F., Jr., and Brennan, M.F.,** Modulation of endogenous hormone action by recombinant human necrosis factor, *Proc. Natl. Acad. Sci. U.S.A.,* 84, 8619, 1987.
96. **Baumann, H., Richards, C., and Gauldie, J.,** Interaction among hepatocyte-stimulating factors, interleukin 1, and glucocorticoids for regulation of acute phase plasma proteins in human hepatoma (HepG2) cells, *J. Immunol.,* 139, 4122, 1987.
97. **Morrone, G., Ciliberto, G., Oliviero, S., Arcone, R., Dente, L., Content, J., and Cortese, R.,** Recombinant interleukin 6 regulates the transcriptional activation of a set of human acute phase genes, *J. Biol. Chem.,* 263, 12554, 1988.
98. **Nakamura, T., Arakaki, R., and Ichihara, A.,** Interleukin-1β is a potent growth inhibitor of adult rat hepatocytes in primary culture, *Exp. Cell Res.,* 179, 488, 1988.

99. **Woloski, B.M.R.N.J. and Fuller, G.M.,** Identification and partial characterization of hepatocyte-stimulating factor from leukemia cell lines: comparison with interleukin 1, *Proc. Natl. Acad. Sci. U.S.A.,* 82, 1443, 1985.
100. **Northoff, H., Andus, T., Tran-Thi, T.-A., Bauer, J., Decker, K., Kubanek, B., and Heinrich, P.C.,** The inflammation mediators interleukin 1 and hepatocyte-stimulating factor are differentially regulated by human monocytes, *Eur. J. Immunol.,* 17, 707, 1987.
101. **Okumura, T., Uehara, A., Okamura, K., Takasugi, Y., and Namiki, M.,** Inhibition of gastric pepsin secretion by peripherally or centrally injected interleukin-1 in rats, *Biochem. Biophys. Res. Commun.,* 167, 956, 1990.
102. **Dewhirst, F.E., Stashenko, P., Mole, J.E., and Tsuramachi, T.,** Purification and partial sequence of human osteoclast-acting factor: identity with interleukin-1β, *J. Immunol.,* 135, 2262, 1985.
103. **Sabatini, M., Boyce, B., Aufdemorte, T., Bonewald, L., and Mundy, G.R.,** Infusions of recombinant human interleukins 1α and 1β cause hypercalcemia in normal mice, *Proc. Natl. Acad. Sci. U.S.A.,* 85, 5235, 1988.
104. **Wano, Y., Hattori, T., Matsuoka, M., Takatsuki, K., Chua, A.O., Gubler, U., and Greene, W.C.,** Interleukin 1 gene expression in adult T cell leukemia, *J. Clin. Invest.,* 80, 911, 1987.
105. **Sato, K., Fujii, Y., Ono, M., Nomura, H., and Shizume, K.,** Production of interleukin 1α-like factor and colony-stimulating factor by a squamous cell carcinoma of the thyroid (T3M-5) derived from a patient with hypercalcemia and leukocytes, *Cancer Res.,* 47, 6474, 1987.
106. **Stashenko, P., Dewhirst, F.E., Peros, W.J., Kent, R.L., and Ago, J.M.,** Synergistic interactions between interleukin 1, tumor necrosis factor, and lymphotoxin in bone marrow resorption, *J. Immunol.,* 138, 1464, 1987.
107. **Lorenzo, J.A., Sousa, S.L., and Centrella, M.,** Interleukin-1 in combination with transforming growth factor-α produces enhanced bone resorption in vitro, *Endocrinology,* 123, 2194, 1988.
108. **Thomson, B.M., Saklatvala, J., and Chambers, T.J.,** Osteoblasts mediate interleukin 1 stimulation of bone resorption by rat osteoclasts, *J. Exp. Med.,* 164, 104, 1986.
109. **Hanazawa, S., Ohmori, Y., Amano, S., Miyoshi, T., Kumegawa, M., and Kitano, S.,** Spontaneous production of interleukin-1-like cytokine from a mouse osteoblastic cell line (MC3T3-E1), *Biochem. Biophys. Res. Commun.,* 131, 774, 1985.
110. **Canalis, E.,** Interleukin-1 has independent effects on deoxyribonucleic acid and collagen synthesis in cultures of rat calvariae, *Endocrinology,* 118, 74, 1986.
111. **Sato, K., Fujii, Y., Kasono, K., Saji, M., Tsushima, T., and Shizume, K.,** Stimulation of prostaglandin E_2 and bone resorption by recombinant human interleukin 1α in fetal mouse bones, *Biochem. Biophys. Res. Commun.,* 138, 618, 1986.
112. **Dedhar, S.,** Regulation of expression of the cell adhesion receptors, integrins, by recombinant human interleukin-1β in human osteosarcoma cells: inhibition of cell proliferation and stimulation of alkaline phosphatase activity, *J. Cell. Physiol.,* 138, 291, 1989.
113. **Heino, J. and Heinonen, T.,** Interleukin-1β prevents the stimulatory effect of transforming growth factor-β on collagen gene expression in human skin fibroblasts, *Biochem. J.,* 271, 827, 1990.
114. **Goto, M., Sasano, M., Yamanaka, H., Miyasaka, N., Kamatani, N., Inoue, K., Nishioka, K., and Miyamoto, T.,** Spontaneous production of an interleukin 1-like factor by cloned rheumatoid synovial cells in long-term culture, *J. Clin. Invest.,* 80, 786, 1987.
115. **Pujol, J.-P. and Loyau, G.,** Interleukin-1 and osteoarthritis, *Life Sci.,* 41, 1187, 1987.
116. **Bocquet, J., Daireaux, M., Langris, M., Jouis, V., Pujol, J.-P., Beliard, R., and Loyau, G.,** Effect of a interleukin-1 factor (mononuclear cell factor) on proteoglycan synthesis in cultured human articular chondrocytes, *Biochem. Biophys. Res. Commun.,* 134, 539, 1986.
117. **Bender, S., Haubeck, H.D., Vandeleur, E., Dufhues, G., Schiel, X., Lauwerijns, J., Greiling, H., and Heinrich, P.C.,** Interleukin-1β induces synthesis and secretion of interleukin-6 in human chondrocytes, *FEBS Lett.,* 263, 321, 1990.
118. **Lacey, D.L., Grosso, L.E., Moser, S.A., Erdmann, J., Tan, H.L., Pacifici, R., and Villareal, D.T.,** IL-1-induced osteoblast IL-6 production is mediated by the type-1 receptor and is increased by 1,25-dihydroxyvitamin D_3, *J. Clin. Invest.,* 91, 1731, 1993.
119. **Sato, K., Fujii, Y., Asano, S., Ohtsuki, T., Kawakami, M., Kasono, K., Tsuchima, T., and Shizume, K.,** Recombinant human interleukin 1 α and β stimulate mouse osteoblast-like cells (MC3T3-E1) to produce macrophage-colony stimulating activity and prostaglandin E_2, *Biochem. Biophys. Res. Commun.,* 141, 285, 1986.

120. **Sato, K., Kasono, K., Fujii, Y., Kawakami, M., Tsuhima, T., and Shizume, K.,** Tumor necrosis factor type α (cachectin) stimulates mouse osteoblast-like cells (MC3T3-E1) to produce macrophage-colony stimulating activity and prostaglandin E_2, *Biochem. Biophys. Res. Commun.,* 145, 323, 1987.
121. **Kähäri, V.-M., Heino, J., and Vuorio, E.,** Interleukin-1 increases collagen production and mRNA levels in cultured skin fibroblasts, *Biochim. Biophys. Acta,* 929, 142, 1987.
122. **Austgulen, R., Hammerstrom, J., and Nissen-Meyer, J.,** In vitro cultured human monocytes release fibroblast proliferation factor(s) different from interleukin 1, *J. Leukocyte Biol.,* 42, 1, 1987.
123. **Singh, J.P., Adams, L.D., and Bonin, P.D.,** Mode of fibroblast growth enhancement by human interleukin-1, *J. Cell Biol.,* 106, 813, 1988.
124. **Raines, E.W., Dower, S.K., and Ross, R.,** Interleukin-1 mitogenic activity for fibroblasts and smooth muscle cells is due to PDGF-AA, *Science,* 243, 393, 1989.
125. **Lee, M., Segal, G.M., and Bagby, G.C.,** Interleukin-1 induces human bone marrow-derived fibroblasts to produce multilineage hematopoietic growth factors, *Exp. Hematol.,* 15, 983, 1987.
126. **Zucali, J.R., Dinarello, C.A., Oblon, D.J., Gross, M.A., Anderson, L., and Weiner, R.S.,** Interleukin-1 stimulates fibroblasts to produce granulocyte macrophage colony-stimulating activity and prostaglandin-E_2, *J. Clin. Invest.,* 77, 1857, 1986.
127. **Van Damme, J., De Ley, M., Opdenakker, G., Billiau, A., De Somer, P., and Van Beeumen, J.,** Homogeneous interferon-inducing 22K factor is related to endogenous pyrogen and interleukin-1, *Nature,* 314, 266, 1985.
128. **Montesano, R., Orci, L., and Vassalli, P.,** Human endothelial cell cultures: phenotypic modulation by leukocyte interleukins, *J. Cell. Physiol.,* 122, 424, 1985.
129. **Norioka, K., Hara, M., Kitani, A., Hirose, T., Hirose, W., Hiragai, M., Suzuki, K., Kawakami, M., Tabata, H., Kawagoe, M., and Nakamura, H.,** Inhibitory effect of human recombinant interleukin-1 α and β on growth of human vascular endothelial cells, *Biochim. Biophys. Res. Commun.,* 145, 969, 1987.
130. **Seelentag, W.K., Mermod, J.-J., Montesano, R., and Vassalli, P.,** Additive effects of interleukin 1 and tumour necrosis factor-α on the accumulation of the three granulocyte and macrophage colony-stimulating factor mRNAs in human endothelial cells, *EMBO J.,* 6, 2261, 1987.
131. **Fibbe, W.E., Daha, M.R., Hiemstra, P.S., Duinkerken, N., Lurvink, E., Ralph, P., Altrock, B.W., Kaushansky, K., Willemze, R., and Falkenburg, J.H.F.,** Interleukin 1 and poly(rI)poly(rC) induce production of granulocyte CSF, macrophage CSF, and granulocyte-macrophage CSF by human endothelial cells, *Exp. Hematol.,* 17, 229, 1989.
132. **Gay, C.G. and Winkles, J.A.,** Interleukin-1 regulates heparin-binding growth factor-2 gene expression in vascular smooth muscle cells, *Proc. Natl. Acad. Sci. U.S.A.,* 88, 296, 1991.
133. **Hauser, C., Saurat, J.-H., Schmitt, A., Jaunin, F., and Dayer, J.-M.,** Interleukin 1 as present in normal human epidermis, *J. Immunol.,* 136, 3317. 1986.
134. **Hauser, C., Dayer, J.-M., Jaunin, F., de Rochemonteix, B., and Saurat, J.-H.,** Intracellular epidermal interleukin 1-like factors in the human epidermoid carcinoma cell line A431, *Cell. Immunol.,* 100, 89, 1986.
135. **Ristow, H.-J.,** A major factor contributing to epidermal proliferation in inflammatory skin diseases appears to be interleukin 1 or a related protein, *Proc. Natl. Acad. Sci. U.S.A.,* 84, 1940, 1987.
136. **Besedovsky, H., del Rey, A., Sorkin, E., and Dinarello, C.A.,** Immunoregulatory feedback between interleukin-1 and glucocorticoid hormones, *Science,* 233, 652, 1986.
137. **Uehara, A., Gottschalk, P.E., Dahl, R.R., and Arimura, A.,** Interleukin-1 stimulates ACTH release by an indirect action which requires endogenous corticotropin releasing factor, *Endocrinology,* 121, 1580, 1987.
138. **Watanabe, T., Morimoto, A., Sakata, Y., and Murakami, N.,** ACTH response induced by interleukin-1 is mediated by CRF secretion by hypothalamic PGE, *Experientia,* 46, 481, 1990.
139. **Suda, T., Tozawa, F., Ushiyama, T., Sumitomo, T., Yamada, M., and Demura, H.,** Interleukin-1 stimulates corticotropin-releasing factor gene expression in rat hypothalamus, *Endocrinology,* 126, 1223, 1990.
140. **Brown, S.L., Smith, L.R., and Blalock, J.E.,** Interleukin 1 and interleukin 2 enhance proopiomelanocortin gene expression in pituitary cells, *J. Immunol.,* 139, 3181, 1987.
141. **Fagarasan, M.O., Axelrod, J., and Catt, K.J.,** Interleukin-1 potentiates agonist-induced secretion of β-endorphin in anterior pituitary cells, *Biochem. Biophys. Res. Commun.,* 173, 988, 1990.
142. **Bernton, E.W., Beach, J.E., Holaday, J.W., Smallridge, R.C., and Fein, H.G.,** Release of multiple hormones by a direct action of interleukin-1 on pituitary cells, *Science,* 238, 519, 1987.

143. Beach, J.E., Smallridge, R.C., Kinzer, C.A., Bernton, E.W., Holaday, J.W., and Fein, H.G., Rapid release of multiple hormones from rat pituitaries perifused with recombinant interleukin-1, *Life Sci.,* 44, 1, 1989.
144. Gwosdow, A.R., Spencer, J.A., O'Connell, N.A., and Abou-Samra, A.B., Interleukin-1 activates protein kinase A and stimulates adrenocorticotropic hormone release from AtT-20 cells, *Endocrinology,* 132, 710, 1993.
145. Steele, G.L., Currie, W.D., Leung, E.H., Yuen, B.H., and Leung, P.C.K., Rapid stimulation of human chorionic gonadotropin secretion by interleukin-1β from perifused first trimester trophoblast, *J. Clin. Endocrinol. Metab.,* 75, 783, 1992.
146. Mine, M., Tramontano, D., Chin, W.W., and Ingbar, S.H., Interleukin-1 stimulates thyroid cell growth and increases the concentration of the c-myc proto-oncogene mRNA in thyroid follicular cells in culture, *Endocrinology,* 120, 1212, 1987.
147. Kawabe, Y., Eguchi, K., Shimomura, C., Mine, M., Otsubo, T., Ueki, Y., Tezuka, H., Nakao, H., Kawakami, A., Migita, K., Yamashita, S., Matsunaga, M., Ishikawa, N., Ito, K., and Nagataki, S., Interleukin-1 production and action in thyroid tissue, *J. Clin. Endocrinol. Metab.,* 68, 1174, 1989.
148. Bendtzen, K., Mandrup-Poulsen, T., Nerup, J., Nielsen, J.H., Dinarello, C.A., and Svenson, M., Cytotoxicity of human interleukin-1 for pancreatic islets of Langerhans, *Science,* 232, 1545, 1986.
149. Zawalich, W.S. and Diaz, V.A., Interleukin 1 inhibits insulin secretion from isolated perifused rat islets, *Diabetes,* 35, 1119, 1986.
150. Comens, P.G., Wolf, B.A., Unanue, E.R., Lacy, P.E., and McDaniel, M.L., Interleukin 1 is potent modulator of insulin secretion from isolated rt islets of Langerhans, *Diabetes,* 36, 963, 1987.
151. McDaniel, M.L., Hughes, J.H., Wolf, B.A., Easom, R.A., and Turk, J.W., Descriptive and mechanistic considerations of interleukin 1 and insulin secretion, *Diabetes,* 37, 1311, 1988.
152. Hammonds, P., Beggs, M., Beresford, G., Espinal, J., Clarke, J., and Mertz, R.J., Insulin-secreting β-cells possess specific receptors for interleukin-1β, *FEBS Lett.,* 261, 97, 1990.
153. Zawalich, W.S. and Zawalich, K.C., Interleukin 1 is a potent stimulator of islet insulin secretion and phosphoinositide hydrolysis, *Am. J. Physiol.,* 256, E19, 1989.
154. Zawalich, W.S., Zawalich, K.C., and Rasmussen, H., Interleukin-1α exerts glucose-dependent stimulatory and inhibitory effects on islet cell phosphoinositide hydrolysis and insulin secretion, *Endocrinology,* 124, 2350, 1989.
155. Welsh, N., Nilsson, T., Hallberg, A., Arkhammar, P., Berggren, P.-O., and Sandler, S., Human interleukin 1β stimulates islet insulin release by a mechanism not dependent on changes in phospholipase C and protein kinase C activities or Ca^{2+} handling, *Acta Endocrinol.,* 121, 698, 1989.
156. Sandler, S., Andersson, A., and Hellerström, C., Inhibitory effects of interleukin 1 on insulin secretion, insulin biosynthesis, and oxidative metabolism of isolated rat pancreatic islets, *Endocrinology,* 121, 1424, 1987.
157. Rabinovitch, A., Pukel, C., and Baquerizo, H., Interleukin-1 inhibits glucose-modulated insulin and glucagon secretion in rat islet monolayer cultures, *Endocrinology,* 122, 2393, 1988.
158. Khan, S.A., Khan, S.J., and Dorrington, J.H., Interleukin-1 stimulates deoxyribonucleic acid synthesis in immature rat Leydig cells *in vitro, Endocrinology,* 131, 1853, 1992.
159. Calkins, J.H., Sigel, M.M., Nankin, H.R., and Lin, T., Interleukin-1 inhibits Leydig cell steroidogenesis in primary culture, *Endocrinology,* 123, 1605, 1988.
160. Calkins, J.H., Guo, H., Sigel, M.M., and Lin, T., Tumor necrosis factor-α enhances inhibitory effects of interleukin-1 on Leydig cell steroidogenesis, *Biochem. Biophys. Res. Commun.,* 166, 1313, 1990.
161. Lin, T., Wang, D., Napgal, M.L., Chang, W., and Calkins, J.H., Down-regulation of Leydig cell insulin-like growth factor-I gene expression by interleukin-1, *Endocrinology,* 130, 1217, 1992.
162. Gottschall, P.E., Uehara, A., Hoffmann, S.T., and Arimura, A., Interleukin-1 inhibits follicle stimulating hormone-induced differentiation in rat granulosa cells in vitro, *Biochem. Biophys. Res. Commun.,* 149, 502, 1987.
163. Fukuoka, M., Yasuda, K., Taii, S., Takakura, K., and Mori, T., Interleukin-1 stimulates growth and inhibits progesterone secretion in cultures of porcine granulosa cells, *Endocrinology,* 124, 884, 1989.
164. Gottschall, P.E., Katsuura, G., and Arimura, A., Interleukin-β 1 is more potent than interleukin-1α in suppressing follicle-stimulating hormone-induced differentiation of ovarian granulosa cells, *Biochem. Biophys. Res. Commun.,* 163, 764, 1989.

165. Kalra, P.S., Sahu, A., and Kalra, S.P., Interleukin-1 inhibits the ovarian steroid-induced luteinizing hormone surge and release of hypothalamic luteinizing hormone-releasing hormone in rats, *Endocrinology,* 126, 2145, 1990.
166. Giulian, D., Baker, T.J., Shih, L.-C.N., and Lachman, L.B., Interleukin 1 on the central nervous system is produced by ameboid microglia, *J. Exp. Med.,* 164, 594, 1986.
167. Breder, C.D., Dinarello, C.A., and Saper, C.B., Interleukin-1 immunoreactive innervation of the human hypothalamus, *Science,* 240, 321, 1988.
168. Lindholm, D., Heumann, R., Hengerer, B., and Thoenen, H., Interleukin 1 increases stability and transcription of mRNA encoding nerve growth factor in cultured rat fibroblasts, *J. Biol. Chem.,* 263, 16348, 1988.
169. Lindholm, D., Heumann, R., Meyer, M., and Thoenen, H., Interleukin-1 regulates synthesis of nerve growth factor in nonneuronal cells of rat sciatic nerve, *Nature,* 330, 658, 1987.
170. Lomedico, P.T., Gubler, U., Hellmann, C.P., Dukovich, M., Giri, J.G., Pan, Y.-C.E., Collier, K., Semionov, R., Chua, A.O., and Mizel, S.B., Cloning and expression of murine interleukin-1 cDNA in *Escherichia coli, Nature,* 312, 458, 1984.
171. Auron, P.E., Webb, A.C., Rosenwasser, L.J., Mucci, S.F., Rich, A., Wolff, S.M., and Dinarello, C.A., Nucleotide sequence of human monocyte interleukin 1 precursor cDNA, *Proc. Natl. Acad. Sci. U.S.A.,* 81, 7907, 1984.
172. Huang, J.J., Newton, R.C., Rutledge, S.J., Horuk, R., Matthew, J.B., Covington, M., and Lin, Y., Characterization of murine IL-1β: isolation, expression, and purification, *J. Immunol.,* 140, 3838, 1988.
173. Nishida, T., Nishino, N., Takano, M., Sekiguchi, Y., Kawai, K., Mizuno, K., Nakai, S., Masui, Y., and Hirai, Y., Molecular cloning and expression of rat interleukin-1α cDNA, *J. Biochem.,* 105, 351, 1989.
174. Cameron, P., Limjuco, G., Rodkey, J., Bennett, C., and Schmidt, J.A., Amino acid sequence analysis of human interleukin 1 (IL-1): evidence for biochemically distinct forms of IL-1, *J. Exp. Med.,* 162, 790, 1985.
175. Cameron, P.M., Limjuco, G.A., Chin, J., Silberstein, L., and Schmidt, J.A., Purification to homogeneity and amino acid sequence analysis of two anionic species of human interleukin 1, *J. Exp. Med.,* 164, 237, 1986.
176. Hopp, T.P., Dower, S.K., and March, C.J., The molecular forms of interleukin-1, *Immunol. Res.,* 5, 271, 1986.
177. Webb, A.C., Collins, K.L., Auron, P.E., Eddy, R.L., Nakai, H., Byers, M.G., Haley, L.L., Henry, W.M., and Shows, T.B., Interleukin-1 gene (IL1) assigned to long arm of human chromosome 2, *Lymphokine Res.,* 5, 77, 1986.
178. Mochizuki, D.Y., Eisenman, J.R., Conlon, P.J., Larsen, A.D., and Tushinski, R.J., Interleukin 1 regulates hematopoietic activity, a role previously ascribed to hemopoietin 1, *Proc. Natl. Acad. Sci. U.S.A.,* 84, 5267, 1987.
179. Bird, T.A. and Saklatvala, J., Identification of a common class of high affinity receptors for both types of porcine interleukin-1 on connective tissue cells, *Nature,* 324, 263, 1986.
180. Gray, P.W., Glaister, D., Chen, E., Goeddel, D.V., and Pennica, D., Two interleukin 1 genes in the mouse: cloning and expression of the cDNA for murine interleukin 1β, *J. Immunol.,* 137, 3644, 1986.
181. Lafage, M., Maroc, N., Dubreuil, D., Malefijt, R.D., Pébusque, M.J., Carcassonne, Y., and Mannoni, P., The human interleukin-1α gene is located on the long arm of chromosome 2 at band q13, *Blood,* 73, 104, 1989.
182. Furutani, Y., Notake, M., Fukui, T., Ohue, M., Nomura, H., Yamada, M., and Nakamura, S., Complete nucleotide sequence of the gene for human interleukin 1α, *Nucleic Acids Res.,* 14, 3167, 1986.
183. Clark, B.D., Collins, K.L., Gandy, M.S., Webb, A.C., and Auron, P.E., Genomic sequence for human prointerleukin 1β: possible evolution from a reverse transcribed prointerleukin 1α gene, *Nucleic Acids Res.,* 14, 7897, 1986.
184. Wingfield, P., Payton, M., Tavernier, J., Barnes, M., Shaw, A., Rose, K., Simona, M.G., Demczuk, S., Williamson, K., and Dayer, J.-M., Purification and characterization of human interleukin-1β expressed in recombinant *Escherichia coli, Eur. J. Biochem.,* 160, 491, 1986.
185. Bensi, G., Raugei, G., Palla, E., Carinci, V., Buonamasa, D.T., and Melli, M., Human interleukin-1β gene, *Gene,* 52, 95, 1987.

186. **Kikumoto, Y., Hong, Y.-M., Nishida, T., Nakai, S., Masui, Y., and Hirai, Y.,** Purification and characterization of recombinant human interleukin-1β produced in *Escherichia coli*, *Biochem. Biophys. Res. Commun.*, 147, 315, 1987.
187. **Rosenwasser, L.J., Webb, A.C., Clark, B.D., Irie, S., Chang, L., Dinarello, C.A., Gehrke, L., Wolff, S.M., Rich, A., and Auron, P.E.,** Expression of biologically active human interleukin 1 subpeptides by transfected simian COS cells, *Proc. Natl. Acad. Sci. U.S.A.*, 83, 5243, 1986.
188. **Cerretti, D.P., Kozlowky, C.J., Mosley, B., Nelson, N., Van Ness, K., Greenstreet, T.A., March, C.J., Kronheim, S.R., Druck, T., Cannizzaro, L.A., Huebner, K., and Black, R.A.,** Molecular cloning of the interleukin-1β converting enzyme, *Science*, 256, 97, 1992.
189. **Jobling, S.A., Auron, P.E., Gurka, G., Webb, A.C., McDonald, B., Rosenwasser, L.J., and Gehrke, L.,** Biological activity and receptor binding of human prointerleukin-1β and subpeptides, *J. Biol. Chem.*, 263, 16372, 1988.
190. **Hazuda, D., Webb, R.L., Simon, P., and Young, P.,** Purification and characterization of human recombinant precursor interleukin 1β, *J. Biol. Chem.*, 264, 1689, 1989.
191. **Meyers, C.A., Johanson, K.O., Miles, L.M., McDevitt, P.J., Simon, P.L., Webb, R.L., Chen, M.-J., Holskin, B.P., Lillquist, J.S., and Young, P.R.,** Purification and characterization of human recombinant interleukin-1β, *J. Biol. Chem.*, 262, 11176, 1987.
192. **Tocci, M.J., Hutchinson, N.I., Cameron, P.M., Kirk, K.E., Norman, D.J., Chin, J., Rupp, E.A., Limjuco, G.A., Bonilla-Agudo, V.M., and Schmidt, J.A.,** Expression in *Escherichia coli* of fully active recombinant human IL 1β: comparison with native human IL 1β, *J. Immunol.*, 138, 1109, 1987.
193. **Palaszynski, E.W.,** Synthetic C-terminal peptide of IL-1 functions as a binding domain as well as an antagonist for the IL-1 receptor, *Biochem. Biophys. Res. Commun.*, 147, 204, 1987.
194. **DeChiara, T.M., Young, D., Semionow, R., Stern, A.S., Batula-Bernardo, C., Fiedler-Nagy, C., Kaffka, K.L., Kilian, P.L., Yamazaki, S., Mizel, S.B., and Lomedico, P.T.,** Structure-function analysis of murine interleukin 1: biologically active polypeptides are at least 127 amino acids long and are derived from the carboxyl terminus of a 270-amino acid precursor, *Proc. Natl. Acad. Sci. U.S.A.*, 83, 8303, 1986.
195. **Silver, A.R.J., Masson, W.K., George, A.M., Adam, J., and Cox, R.,** The IL-1α gene and IL-1β gene are closely linked (less than 70-kb) on mouse chromosome 2, *Somat. Cell Mol. Genet.*, 16, 549, 1990.
196. **Telford, J.L., Macchia, G., Massone, A., Carinci, V., Palla, E., and Melli, M.,** The murine interleukin 1β gene: structure and evolution, *Nucleic Acids Res.*, 14, 9955, 1986.
197. **MacDonald, H.R., Wingfield, P., Schmeissner, U., Shaw, A., Clore, G.M., and Gronenborn, A.M.,** Point mutations of human interleukin-1 with decreased receptor binding affinity, *FEBS Lett.*, 209, 295, 1986.
198. **Mosley, B., Dower, S.K., Gillis, S., and Cosman, D.,** Determination of the minimum polypeptide lengths of the functionally active sites of human interleukins 1α and 1β, *Proc. Natl. Acad. Sci. U.S.A.*, 84, 4572, 1987.
199. **Gehrke, L., Jobling, S.A., Paik, L.S.K., McDonald, B., Rosenwasser, L.J., and Auron, P.E.,** A point mutation uncouples human interleukin-1β biological activity and receptor binding, *J. Biol. Chem.*, 265, 5922, 1990.
200. **Baldari, C.T. and Telford, J.L.,** The intracellular precursor of IL-1β is associated with microtubules in activated U937 cells, *J. Immunol.*, 142, 785, 1989.
201. **Mosley, B., Urdal, D.L., Prickett, K.S., Larsen, A., Cosman, D., Conlon, P.J., Gillis, S., and Dower, S.K.,** The interleukin-1 receptor binds the human interleukin-1α precursor but not the interleukin-1β precursor, *J. Biol. Chem.*, 262, 2941, 1987.
202. **Conlon, P.J., Grabstein, K.H., Alpert, A., Prickett, K.S., Hopp, T.P., and Gillis, S.,** Localization of human mononuclear cell interleukin 1, *J. Immunol.*, 139, 98, 1987.
203. **Beuscher, H.U., Günther, C., and Röllinghoff, M.,** IL-1β is secreted by activated murine macrophages as biologically inactive precursor, *J. Immunol.*, 144, 2179, 1990.
204. **Kobayashi, Y., Appella, E., Yamada, M., Copeland, T.D., Oppenheim, J.J., and Matsushima, K.,** Phosphorylation of intracellular precursors of human IL-1, *J. Immunol.*, 140, 2279, 1988.
205. **Gallagher, G., Christie, J.F., and Stimson, W.H.,** Interleukin-1α, but not interleukin-1β, can induce S-phase entry in human B-CLL B-cells, *IRCS Med. Sci. Biochem.*, 14, 770, 1986.
206. **Garcia-Welsh, A., Schneiderman, J.S., and Baly, D.L.,** Interleukin-1 stimulates glucose transport in rat adipose cells. Evidence for receptor discrimination between IL-1β and IL-1α, *FEBS Lett.*, 269, 421, 1990.

207. **Uehara, A., Gottschalk, P.E., Dahl, R.R., and Arimura, A.,** Stimulation of ACTH release by human interleukin-1β, but not interleukin-1α, in conscious, freely-moving rats, *Biochem. Biophys. Res. Commun.*, 146, 1286, 1987.
208. **Lachman, L.B., Dinarello, C.A., Llansa, N.D., and Fidler, I.J.,** Natural and recombinant human interleukin 1β is cytotoxic for human melanoma cells, *J. Immunol.*, 136, 3098, 1986.
209. **Huang, J.J., Newton, R.C., Horuk, R., Matthew, J.B., Covington, M., Pezzella, K., and Lin, Y.,** Muteins of human interleukin-1 that show enhanced bioactivities, *FEBS Lett.*, 223, 294, 1987.
210. **Köck, A., Danner, M., Stadler, B.M., and Luger, T.A.,** Characterization of a monoclonal antibody directed against the biologically active site of human interleukin 1, *J. Exp. Med.*, 163, 463, 1986.
211. **Valentine, M., Lotz, M., Dinarello, C.A., Carson, D.A., and Vaughan, J.H.,** Lymphoblastoid B cell lines produce an interleukin-1-like activity that can be serologically distinct from macrophage interleukin-1, *Lymphokine Res.*, 5, 173, 1986.
212. **Kimball, E.S., Pickeral, S.F., Oppenheim, J.J., and Rossio, J.L.,** Interleukin 1 activity in normal human urine, *J. Immunol.*, 133, 256, 1984.
213. **Koide, S. and Steinman, R.M.,** Induction of murine interleukin 1: stimuli and responsive primary cells, *Proc. Natl. Acad. Sci. U.S.A.*, 84, 3802, 1987.
214. **Arend, W.P., Gordon, D.F., Wood, W.M., Janson, R.W., Joslin, F.G., and Jameel, S.,** IL-1β production in cultured human monocytes is regulated at multiple levels, *J. Immunol.*, 143, 118, 1989.
215. **Sandborg, C.I., Berman, M.A., Imfeld, K.L., Zaldivar, F., Jr., Masada, M.P., and Kenney, J.S.,** Modulation of IL-1α, IL-1β, and 25 K non-IL-1 activity released by human mononuclear cells, *J. Leukocyte Biol.*, 46, 117, 1989.
216. **Tartakovsky, B., Finnegan, A., Muegge, K., Brody, D.T., Kovacs, E.J., Smith, M.R., Berzofsky, J.A., Young, H.A., and Durum, S.K.,** IL-1 is an autocrine growth factor for T cell clones, *J. Immunol.*, 141, 3863, 1988.
217. **Bertoglio, J.H.,** B-cell-derived human interleukin 1, *Crit. Rev. Immunol.*, 8, 299, 1988.
218. **Gerard, N., Syed, V., Bardin, W., Genetet, N., and Jegou, B.,** Sertoli cells are the site of interleukin-1α synthesis in rat testis, *Mol. Cell. Endocrinol.*, 82, R13, 1991.
219. **Takcs, L., Kovacs, E.J., Smith, M.R., Young, H.A., and Durum, S.K.,** Detection of IL-1α and IL-1β gene expression by in situ hybridization. Tissue localization of IL-1 mRNA in the normal C57BL/6 mouse, *J. Immunol.*, 141, 3081, 1988.
220. **Tamatani, T., Tsunoda, H., Iwasaki, H., Kaneko, M., Hashimoto, T., and Onozaki, K.,** Existence of both IL-1 α and β in normal human amniotic fluid: unique high molecular weight form of IL-1β, *Immunology*, 65, 337, 1988.
221. **Ollivierre, F., Gubler, U., Towle, C.A., Laurencin, C., and Treadwell, B.V.,** Expression of IL-1 genes in human and bovine chondrocytes: a mechanism for autocrine control of cartilage matrix degradation, *Biochem. Biophys. Res. Commun.*, 141, 904, 1986.
222. **Kupper, T.S., Ballard, D.W., Chua, A.O., McGuire, J.S., Flood, P.M., Horowitz, M.C., Langdon, R., Lightfoot, L., and Gubler, U.,** Human keratinocytes contain mRNA indistinguishable from monocyte interleukin 1 α and β mRNA, *J. Exp. Med.*, 164, 2095, 1986.
223. **Ansel, J.C., Luger, T.A., Lowry, D., Perry, P., Roop, D.R., and Mountz, J.D.,** The expression and modulation of IL-1α in murine keratinocytes, *J. Immunol.*, 140, 2274, 1988.
224. **Rath, N.C., Oronsky, A.L., and Kerwar, S.S.,** Synthesis of interleukin-1-like activity by normal rat chondrocytes in culture, *Clin. Immunol. Immunopathol.*, 47, 39, 1988.
225. **Bingel, M., Lonnemann, G., Koch, K.M., Dinarello, C.A., and Shaldon, S.,** Enhancement of in-vitro human interleukin-1 production by sodium acetate, *Lancet*, 1, 14, 1987.
226. **Nishida, T., Takano, M., Kawakami, T., Nishino, N., Nakai, S., and Hirai, Y.,** The transcription of the interleukin 1β gene is induced with PMA and inhibited with dexamethasone in U937 cells, *Biochem. Biophys. Res. Commun.*, 156, 269, 1988.
227. **Griffin, J.D., Rambaldi, A., Vellenga, E., Young, D.C., Ostapovicz, D., and Cannistra, S.A.,** Secretion of interleukin-1 by acute myeloblastic leukemia cells in vitro induces endothelial cells to secrete colony stimulating factors, *Blood*, 70, 1218, 1987.
228. **Bagby, G.C., Jr., Dinarello, C.A., Neerhout, R.C., Ridgway, D., and McCall, E.,** Interleukin 1-dependent paracrine granulopoiesis in chronic granulocytic leukemia of the juvenile type, *J. Clin. Invest.*, 82, 1430, 1988.

229. **Ree, H.J., Crowley, J.P., and Dinarello, C.A.**, Anti-interleukin-1 reactive cells in Hodgkin's disease, *Cancer,* 59, 1717, 1987.
230. **Hsu, S.-M. and Zhao, X.**, Expression of interleukin-1 in Reed-Sternberg cells and neoplastic cells from the histiocytic malignancies, *Am. J. Pathol.,* 125, 221, 1986.
231. **Spear, G.T., Paulnock, D.M., Helgeson, D.O., and Borden, E.C.**, Requirement of differentiative signals of both interferon-γ and 1,25-dihydroxyvitamin D_3 for induction and secretion of interleukin-1 by HL-60 cells, *Cancer Res.,* 48, 1740, 1988.
232. **Nishida, T., Nishino, N., Takano, M., Kawai, K., Bando, K., Masui, Y., Nakai, S., and Hirai, Y.**, cDNA cloning of IL-1α and IL-1β from mRNA of U937 cell line, *Biochem. Biophys. Res. Commun.,* 143, 345, 1987.
233. **Knudsen, P.J., Dinarello, C.A., and Strom, T.B.**, Purification and characterization of a unique human interleukin 1 from the tumor cell line U937, *J. Immunol.,* 136, 3311, 1986.
234. **Lee, S.W., Tsou, A.-P., Chan, H., Thomas, J., Petrie, K., Eugui, E.M., and Allison, A.C.**, Glucocorticoids selectively inhibit the transcription of the interleukin 1β gene and decrease the stability of interleukin 1β mRNA, *Proc. Natl. Acad. Sci. U.S.A.,* 85, 1204, 1988.
235. **Noma, T., Nakamura, T., Maeda, M., Masafumi, O., Taniguchi, Y., Tagaya, Y., Yaoita, Y., Yodoi, J., and Honjo, T.**, Interleukin 1α mRNA in virus-transformed T and B cells, *Biochem. Biophys. Res. Commun.,* 139, 353, 1986.
236. **Wakasugi, H., Rimsky, L., Mahe, Y., Kamel, A.M., Fradelizi, D., Tursz, T., and Bertoglio, J.**, Epstein-Barr virus-containing B-cell line produces an interleukin 1 that it uses as a growth factor, *Proc. Natl. Acad. Sci. U.S.A.,* 84, 804, 1987.
237. **Busson, P., Braham, K., Ganem, G., Thomas, F., Grausz, D., Lipinski, M., Wakasugi, H., and Tursz, T.**, Epstein-Barr virus-containing epithelial cells from nasopharyngeal carcinoma produce interleukin 1α, *Proc. Natl. Acad. Sci. U.S.A.,* 84, 6262, 1987.
238. **Köck, A., Schwarz, T., Urbanski, A., Peng, Z., Vetterlein, M., Micksche, M., Ansel, J.C., Kung, H.F., and Luger, T.A.**, Expression and release of interleukin-1 by different human melanoma cell lines, *J. Natl. Cancer Inst.,* 81, 36, 1989.
239. **Bennicelli, J.L., Elias, J., Kern, J., and Guerry, D., IV,** Production of interleukin 1 activity by cultured human melanoma cells, *Cancer Res.,* 49, 930, 1989.
240. **Warner, S.J.C., Auger, K.R., and Libby, P.**, Interleukin 1 induces interleukin 1. II. Recombinant human interleukin 1 induces interleukin 1 production by adult human vascular endothelial cells, *J. Immunol.,* 139, 1911, 1987.
241. **Lord, P.C.W., Wilmoth, L.M.G., Mizel, S.B., and McCall, C.E.**, Expression of interleukin-1 α and β genes by human blood polymorphonuclear leukocytes, *J. Clin. Invest.,* 87, 1312, 1991.
242. **Wang, D.L., Nagpal, M.L., Calkins, J.H., Chang, W.W., Sigel, M.M., and Tu, L.**, Interleukin-1β induces interleukin-1α messenger ribonucleic acid expression in primary cultures of Leydig cells, *Endocrinology,* 129, 2862, 1991.
243. **Mauviel, A., Temine, N., Charron, D., Loyau, G., and Pujol, J.-P.**, Interleukin-1 α and β induce interleukin-1β gene expression in human dermal fibroblasts, *Biochem. Biophys. Res. Commun.,* 156, 1209, 1988.
244. **Demczuk, S., Baumberger, C., Mach, B., and Dayer, J.-M.**, Expression of human IL-1 α and β messenger RNAs and IL 1 activity in human peripheral blood mononuclear cells, *J. Mol. Cell. Immunol.,* 3, 255, 1987.
245. **Numerof, R.P., Aronson, F.R., and Mier, J.W.**, IL-2 stimulates the production of IL-1α and IL-1β by human peripheral blood mononuclear cells, *J. Immunol.,* 141, 4250, 1988.
246. **Kovacs, E.J., Brock, B., Varesio, L., and Young, H.A.**, IL-2 induction of IL-1β mRNA expression in monocytes. Regulation by agents that block second messenger pathways, *J. Immunol.,* 143, 3532, 1989.
247. **Palkama, T., Matikainen, S., and Hurme, M.**, Tyrosine kinase activity is involved in the protein kinase C-induced expression of interleukin 1β gene in monocytic cells, *FEBS Lett.,* 319, 100, 1993.
248. **Donnelly, R.P., Fenton, M.J., Kaufman, J.D., and Gerrard, T.L.**, IL-1 expression in human monocytes is transcriptionally and posttranscriptionally regulated by IL-4, *J. Immunol.,* 146, 3431, 1991.
249. **Weaver, C.T. and Unanue, E.R.**, T cell induction of membrane IL 1 on macrophages, *J. Immunol.,* 137, 3868, 1986.

250. **Merluzzi, V.J., Faanes, R.B., Czajkowski, M., Last-Barney, K., Harrison, P.C., Kahn, J., and Rothlein, R.,** Membrane-associated interleukin 1 activity on human U937 tumor cells: stimulation of PGE_2 production by human chondrosarcoma cells, *J. Immunol.,* 139, 166, 1987.
251. **Kovacs, E.J., Oppenheim, J.J., Carter, D.B., and Young, H.A.,** Enhanced interleukin-1 production by human monocyte cell lines following treatment with 5-azacytidine, *J. Leukocyte Biol.,* 41, 40, 1987.
252. **Libby, P., Ordovas, J.M., Auger, K.R., Robbins, A.H., Birinyi, L.K., and Dinarello, C.A.,** Endotoxin and tumor necrosis factor induce interleukin-1 gene expression in adult human vascular endothelial cells, *Am. J. Pathol.,* 124, 179, 1986.
253. **Libby, P., Ordovas, J.M., Birinyi, L.K., Auger, K.R., and Dinarello, C.A.,** Inducible interleukin-1 gene expression in human vascular smooth muscle cells, *J. Clin. Invest.,* 78, 1432, 1986.
254. **Hiro, D., Ito, A., Matsuta, K., and Mori, Y.,** Hyaluronic acid is an endogenous inducer of interleukin-1 production by human monocytes and rabbit macrophages, *Biochem. Biophys. Res. Commun.,* 140, 715, 1986.
255. **Phadke, K.,** Fibroblast growth factor enhances the interleukin-1-mediated chondrocytic protease release, *Biochem. Biophys. Res. Commun.,* 142, 448, 1987.
256. **Gupta, S., Vayuvegula, B., Ruhling, M., and Thornton, M.,** Interleukin 1 and interleukin 12 production in the acquired immune deficiency syndrome (AIDS) and AIDS-related complex, *J. Clin. Lab. Immunol.,* 22, 113, 1987.
257. **Singer, I.I., Scott, S., Hall, G.L., Limjuco, G., Chin, J., and Schmidt, J.A.,** Interleukin 1β is localized in the cytoplasmic ground substance but is largely absent from the Golgi apparatus and plasma membranes of stimulated human monocytes, *J. Exp. Med.,* 167, 389, 1988.
258. **Brandwein, S.R.,** Regulation of interleukin 1 production by mouse peritoneal macrophages: effects of arachidonic acid metabolites, cyclic nucleotides, and interferons, *J. Biol. Chem.,* 261, 8624, 1986.
259. **Collart, M.A., Belin, D., Vassalli, J.-D., de Kossodo, S., and Vasalli, P.,** γ Interferon enhances macrophage transcription of the tumor necrosis factor/cachectin, interleukin 1, and urokinase genes, which are controlled by short-lived repressors, *J. Exp. Med.,* 164, 2113, 1986.
260. **Newton, R.C.,** Lack of a central role for calcium in the induction and release of human interleukin-1, *Biochem. Biophys. Res. Commun.,* 147, 1027, 1987.
261. **Gerrard, T.L., Siegel, J.P., Dyer, D.R., and Zoon, K.C.,** Differential effects of interferon-α and interferon-γ on interleukin secretion by monocytes, *J. Immunol.,* 138, 2535, 1987.
262. **Le, J., Weinstein, D., Gubler, U., and Vilcek, J.,** Induction of membrane-associated interleukin 1 by tumor necrosis factor in human fibroblasts, *J. Immunol.,* 138, 2137, 1987.
263. **Hoffman, M.K.,** The effects of tumor necrosis factor on the production of interleukin-1 by macrophages, *Lymphokine Res.,* 5, 255, 1986.
264. **Bachwich, P.R., Chensue, S.W., Larrick, J.W., and Kunkel, S.L.,** Tumor necrosis factor stimulates interleukin-1 and prostaglandin E_2 production in resting macrophages, *Biochem. Biophys. Res. Commun.,* 136, 94, 1986.
265. **Knudsen, P.J., Dinarello, C.A., and Strom, T.B.,** Prostaglandins posttranscriptionally inhibit monocyte expression of interleukin 1 activity by increasing intracellular cyclic adenosine monophosphate, *J. Immunol.,* 137, 3189, 1986.
266. **Katakami, Y., Nakao, Y., Matsui, T., Koizumi, T., Kaibuchi, K., Takai, Y., and Fujita, T.,** Possible involvement of protein kinase C in interleukin-1 production by mouse peritoneal macrophages, *Biochem. Biophys. Res. Commun.,* 135, 355, 1986.
267. **Strulovici, b., Daniel-Issakani, S., Oto, E., Nestor, J., Jr., Chan, H., and Tsou, A.-P.,** Activation of distinct protein kinase C isozymes by phorbol esters: correlation with induction of interleukin 1β expression, *Biochemistry,* 28, 3569, 1989.
268. **Herman, J. and Rabson, A.R.,** Tumor cells stimulate interleukin 1 (IL-1) production from enriched large granular lymphocytes, *Clin. Immunol. Immunopathol.,* 38, 282, 1986.
269. **Evans, R. and Duffy, T.M.,** Activation of the IL-1 pathway during amplification of immune responses in tumor-bearing mice, *Cell. Immunol.,* 105, 86, 1987.
270. **Larrick, J.W.,** Native interleukin 1 inhibitors, *Immunol. Today,* 10, 61, 1989.
271. **Tiku, K., Tiku, M.L., Liu, S., and Skosey, J.L.,** Normal human neutrophils are a source of a specific interleukin 1 inhibitor, *J. Immunol.,* 136, 3686, 1986.

272. **Schwarz, T., Urbanska, A., Gschnait, F., and Luger, T.A.,** UV-irradiated epidermal cells produce a specific inhibitor of interleukin 1 activity, *J. Immunol.,* 138, 1457, 1987.
273. **Liao, Z., Grimshaw, R.S., and Rosenstreich, D.L.,** Identification of a specific interleukin-1 inhibitor in the urine of febrile patients, *J. Exp. Med.,* 159, 126, 1984.
274. **Liao, Z., Haimovitz, Y., Chen, Y., Chan, J., and Rosenstreich, D.L.,** Characterization of a human interleukin 1 inhibitor, *J. Immunol.,* 134, 3882, 1985.
275. **Seckinger, P., Williamson, K., Balavoine, J.-F., Mach, B., Mazzei, G., Shaw, A., and Dayer, J.-M.,** A urine inhibitor of interleukin 1 activity affects both interleukin 1α and 1β but not tumor necrosis factor α, *J. Immunol.,* 139, 1541, 1987.
276. **Muchmore, A.V. and Decker, J.M.,** Uromodulin. An immunosuppressive 85-kilodalton glycoprotein isolated from human pregnancy urine is a high affinity ligand for recombinant interleukin 1α, *J. Biol. Chem.,* 261, 13404, 1986.
277. **Brown, K.M., Muchmore, A.V., and Rosenstreich, D.L.,** Uromodulin, an immunosuppressive protein derived from pregnancy urine, is an inhibitor of interleukin 1, *Proc. Natl. Acad. Sci. U.S.A.,* 83, 9119, 1986.
278. **Muchmore, A.V. and Decker, J.M.,** Evidence that recombinant IL-1α exhibits lectin-like specificity and binds to homogeneous uromodulin via N-linked oligosaccharides, *J. Immunol.,* 138, 2541, 1987.
279. **Muchmore, A.V., Shifrin, S., and Decker, J.M.,** In vitro evidence that carbohydrate moieties derived from uromodulin, an 85,000 dalton immunosuppressive glycoprotein isolated from human pregnancy urine, are immunosuppressive in the absence of intact protein, *J. Immunol.,* 138, 2547, 1987.
280. **Cannon, J.G., Tatro, J.B., Reichlin, S., and Dinarello, C.A.,** α Melanocyte stimulating hormone inhibits immunostimulatory and inflammatory actions of interleukin 1, *J. Immunol.,* 137, 2232, 1986.
281. **Daynes, R.A., Robertson, B.A., Cho, B.-H., Burnham, D.K., and Newton, R.,** α-Melanocyte stimulating hormone exhibits target cell selectivity in its capacity to affect interleukin 1-inducible responses in vivo and in vitro, *J. Immunol.,* 139, 103, 1987.
282. **Cianciolo, G.J., Copeland, T.D., Oroszlan, S., and Snyderman, R.,** Inhibition of lymphocyte proliferation by a synthetic peptide homologous to retroviral envelope proteins, *Science,* 230, 453, 1985.
283. **Gottlieb, R.A., Lennarz, W.J., Knowles, R.D., Cianciolo, G.J., Dinarello, C.A., Lachman, L.B., and Kleinerman, E.S.,** Synthetic peptide corresponding to a conserved domain of the retroviral protein p15E blocks IL-1-mediated signal transduction, *J. Immunol.,* 142, 4321, 1989.
284. **Kleinerman, E.S., Lachman, L.B., Knowles, R.D., Snyderman, R., and Cianciolo, G.J.,** A synthetic peptide homologous to the envelope proteins of retroviruses inhibits monocyte-mediated killing by inactivating interleukin 1, *J. Immunol.,* 139, 2329, 1987.
285. **Arend, W.P., Joslin, F.G., Thompson, R.C., and Hannum, C.H.,** An IL-1 inhibitor from human monocytes. Production and characterization of biologic properties, *J. Immunol.,* 143, 1851, 1989.
286. **Hannum, C.H., Wilcox, C.J., Arend, W.P., Joslin, F.G., Dripps, D.J., Heimdal, P.L., Armes, L.G., Sommer, A., Eisenberg, S.P., and Thompson, R.C.,** Interleukin-1 receptor antagonist activity of a human interleukin-1 inhibitor, *Nature,* 343, 336, 1990.
287. **Bienkowski, M.J., Eessalu, T.E., Berger, A.E., Truesdell, S.E., Shelly, J.A., Laborde, A.L., Zurcher-Neely, H.A., Reardon, I.M., Heinrikson, R.L., Chosay, J.G., and Tracey, D.E.,** Purification and characterization of interleukin 1 receptor level antagonist proteins from THP-1 cells, *J. Biol. Chem.,* 265, 14505, 1990.
288. **Arend, W.P.,** Interleukin 1 receptor antagonist. A new member of the interleukin 1 family, *J. Clin. Invest.,* 88, 1445, 1991.
289. **Eisenberg, S.P., Evans, R.J., Arend, W.P., Verderber, E., Brewer, M.T., Hannum, C.H., and Thompson, R.C.,** Primary structure and functional expression from complementary DNA of a human interleukin-1 receptor antagonist, *Nature,* 343, 341, 1990.
290. **Carter, D.B., Delbel, M.R., Jr., Dunn, C.J., Tomich, C.-S.C., Laborde, A.L., Slightom, J.L., Berger, A.E., Bienkowski, M.J., Sun, F.F., McEwan, R.N., Harris, P.K.W., Yem, A.W., Waszak, G.A., Chosay, J.G., Sieu, L.C., Hardee, M.M., Zurcher-Neely, H.A., Reardon, I.M., Heinrikson, R.L., Truesdell, S.E., Shelly, J.A., Eessalu, T.E., Taylor, B.M., and Tracey, D.E.,** Purification, cloning, expression and biological characterization of an interleukin-1 receptor antagonist protein, *Nature,* 344, 633, 1990.
291. **Eisenberg, S.P., Brewer, M.T., Verderber, E., Heimdal, P., Brandhuber, B.J., and Thompson, R.C.,** Interleukin 1 receptor antagonist is a member of the interleukin 1 gene family: evolution of a cytokine control mechanism, *Proc. Natl. Acad. Sci. U.S.A.,* 88, 5232, 1991.

292. **Steinkasserer, A., Spurr, N.K., Cox, S., Jeggo, P., and Sim, R.B.,** The human IL-1 receptor antagonist gene *(IL1RN)* maps to chromosome 2q14-q21, in the region of the IL-1α and IL-1β loci, *Genomics,* 13, 654, 1992.
293. **Patterson, D., Jones, C., Hart, I., Bleskan, J., Berger, R., Geyer, D., Eisenberg, S.P., Smith, M.F., and Arend, W.P.,** The human interleukin-1 receptor antagonist *(IL1RN)* gene is located in the chromosome 2q14 region, *Genomics,* 15, 173, 1993.
294. **Martel-Pelletier, J., McCollum, R., and Pelletier, J.P.,** The synthesis of IL-1 receptor antagonist (IL-1RA) by synovial fibroblasts is markedly increased by the cytokines TNF-α and IL-1, *Biochim. Biophys. Acta,* 1175, 302, 1993.
295. **Dower, S.K., Kronheim, S.R., March, C.J., Conlon, P.J., Hopp, T.P., Gillis, S., and Urdal, D.L.,** Detection and characterization of high affinity plasma membrane receptors for human interleukin 1, *J. Exp. Med.,* 162, 501, 1985.
296. **Sims, J.E., Acres, R.B., Grubin, C.E., McMahan, C.J., Wignall, J.M., March, C.J., and Dower, S.K.,** Cloning the interleukin 1 receptor from human T cells, *Proc. Natl. Acad. Sci. U.S.A.,* 86, 8946, 1989.
297. **Lowenthal, J.W. and MacDonald, H.R.,** Expression of interleukin 1 receptors is restricted to the L3T4+ subset of mature T lymphocytes, *J. Immunol.,* 138, 1, 1987.
298. **Sujita, K., Okuno, F., Tanaka, Y., Hirano, Y., Inamoto, Y., Eto, S., and Arai, M.,** Effect of interleukin-1 (IL-1) on the levels of cytochrome P-450 involving IL-1 receptor on the isolated hepatocytes of rat, *Biochem. Biophys. Res. Commun.,* 168, 1217, 1990.
299. **Hamby, B.A., Huggins, E.M., Jr., Lachman, L.B., Dinarello, C.A., and Sigel, M.M.,** Fish lymphocytes respond to human IL-1, *Lymphokine Res.,* 5, 157, 1986.
300. **Lowenthal, J.W. and MacDonald, H.R.,** Binding and internalization of interleukin 1 by T cells. Direct evidence for high- and low-affinity classes of interleukin 1 receptor, *J. Exp. Med.,* 164, 1060, 1986.
301. **Chin, J., Cameron, P.M., Rupp, E., and Schmidt, J.A.,** Identification of a high-affinity receptor for native human interleukin 1β and interleukin 1α on normal human lung fibroblasts, *J. Exp. Med.,* 165, 70, 1987.
302. **Qwarnstrom, E.E., Page, R.C., Gillis, S., and Dower, S.K.,** Binding, internalization, and intracellular localization of interleukin-1β in human diploid fibroblasts, *J. Biol. Chem.,* 263, 8261, 1988.
303. **Dower, S.K., Call, S.M., Gillis, S., and Urdal, D.L.,** Similarity between the interleukin 1 receptors on a murine T-lymphoma cell line and on a murine fibroblast cell line, *Proc. Natl. Acad. Sci. U.S.A.,* 83, 1060, 1986.
304. **Bomsztyk, K., Sims, J.E., Stanto, T.H., Slack, J., McMahan, C.J., Valentine, M.A., and Dower, S.K.,** Evidence for different interleukin 1 receptors in murine B- and T-cell lines, *Proc. Natl. Acad. Sci. U.S.A.,* 86, 8034, 1989.
305. **Horuk, R., Huang, J.J., Covington, M., and Newton, R.C.,** A biochemical and kinetic analysis of the interleukin-1 receptor, *J. Biol. Chem.,* 262, 16275, 1987.
306. **Bron, C. and MacDonald, H.R.,** Identification of the plasma membrane receptor for interleukin-1 on mouse thymoma cells, *FEBS Lett.,* 219, 365, 1987.
307. **Urdal, D.L., Call, S.M., Jackson, J.L., and Dower, S.K.,** Affinity purification and chemical analysis of the interleukin-1 receptor, *J. Biol. Chem.,* 263, 2870, 1988.
308. **Matsushima, K., Akahoshi, T., Yamada, M., Furutani, Y., and Oppenheim, J.J.,** Properties of a specific interleukin 1 (IL 1) receptor on human Epstein Barr virus-transformed B lymphocytes: identity of the receptor for IL 1-α and IL 1-β, *J. Immunol.,* 136, 4496, 1986.
309. **Benjamin, D., Wormsley, S., and Dower, S.K.,** Heterogeneity in interleukin (IL)-1 receptors expression on human B cell lines. Differences in the molecular properties of IL-1α and IL-1β binding sites, *J. Biol. Chem.,* 265, 1990.
310. **McMahan, C.J., Slack, J.L., Mosley, B., Cosman, D., Lupton, S.D., Brunton, L.L., Grubin, C.E., Wignall, J.M., Jenkins, N.A., Brannan, C.I., Copeland, N.G., Huebner, K., Croce, C.M., Cannizzaro, L.A., Benjamin, D., Dower, S.K., Spriggs, M.K., and Sims, J.E.,** A novel IL-1 receptor, cloned from B cells by mammalian expression, is expressed in many cell types, *EMBO J.,* 10, 2821, 1991.
311. **Chizzonite, R., Truitt, T., Kilian, P.L., Stern, A.S., Nunes, P., Parker, K.P., Kaffka, K.L., Chua, A.O., Lugg, D.K., and Gubler, U.,** Two high-affinity interleukin 1 receptors represent separate gene products, *Proc. Natl. Acad. Sci. U.S.A.,* 86, 8029, 1989.

312. **Slack, J., McMahan, C.J., Waugh, S., Schooley, K., Spriggs, M.K., Sims, J.E., and Dower, S.K.,** Independent binding of interleukin-1α and interleukin-1β to type-I and type-II interleukin-1 receptors, *J. Biol. Chem.*, 268, 2513, 1993.
313. **Stylianou, E., O'Neill, L.A.J., Rawlison, L., Edbrooke, M.R., Woo, P., and Saklatvala, J.,** Interleukin-1 induces NF-kB through its type-I but not its type-II receptor in lymphocytes, *J. Biol. Chem.*, 267, 15836, 1992.
314. **Akahoshi, T., Oppenheim, J.J., and Matsushima, K.,** Interleukin 1 stimulates its own receptor expression on human fibroblasts through the endogenous production of prostaglandin(s), *J. Clin. Invest.*, 82, 1219, 1988.
315. **Matsushima, K., Yodoi, J., Tagaya, Y., and Oppenheim, J.J.,** Down-regulation of interleukin 1 (IL 1) receptor expression by IL 1 and fate of internalized ^{125}I-labeled IL 1β in a human large granular lymphocyte cell line, *J. Immunol.*, 137, 3183, 1986.
316. **Giri, J.G., Newton, R.C., and Horak, R.,** Identification of soluble interleukin-1 protein in cell-free supernatants. Evidence for soluble interleukin-1 receptor, *J. Biol. Chem.*, 265, 17416, 1990.
317. **Matsushima, K., Kobayashi, Y., Copeland, T.D., Akahoshi, T., and Oppenheim, J.J.,** Phosphorylation of a cytosolic 65-kDa protein induced by interleukin 1 in glucocorticoid pretreated normal human peripheral blood mononuclear leukocytes, *J. Immunol.*, 139, 3367, 1987.
318. **Shieh, J.-H., Peterson, R.H.F., and Moore, M.A.S.,** Granulocyte colony-stimulating factor modulation of cytokine receptors on murine bone marrow cells. In vivo and in vitro studies, *J. Immunol.*, 147, 2984, 1991.
319. **Harvey, A.K., Hrubey, P.S., and Chandrasekhar, S.,** Transforming growth factor-β inhibition of interleukin-1 activity involves down-regulation of interleukin-1 receptor on chondrocytes, *Exp. Cell Res.*, 195, 376, 1991.
320. **Chandrasekhar, S. and Harvey, A.K.,** Induction of interleukin-1 receptors on chondrocytes by fibroblast growth factor: a possible mechanism for modulation of interleukin-1 activity, *J. Cell. Physiol.*, 138, 236, 1989.
321. **Bonin, P.D. and Singh, J.P.,** Modulation of interleukin-1 receptor expression and interleukin-1 response in fibroblasts by platelet-derived growth factor, *J. Biol. Chem.*, 263, 11052, 1988.
322. **Chiou, W.J., Bonin, P.D., Harris, P.K.W., Carter, D.B., and Singh, J.P.,** Platelet-derived growth factor induces interleukin-1 receptor gene expression in Balb/c 3T3 fibroblasts, *J. Biol. Chem.*, 264, 21442, 1989.
323. **Bonin, P.D., Chiou, W.J., McGee, J.E., and Singh, J.P.,** Two signal transduction pathways mediate interleukin-1 receptor expression in Balb/c3T3 fibroblasts, *J. Biol. Chem.*, 265, 18643, 1990.
324. **Curtis, B.M., Widmer, M.B., DeRoos, P., and Quarnstrom, E.E.,** IL-1 and its receptor are translocated to the nucleus, *J. Immunol.*, 144, 1295, 1990.
325. **Grenfell, S., Smithers, N., Miller, K., and Solari, R.,** Receptor-mediated endocytosis and nuclear transport of human interleukin 1α, *Biochem. J.*, 264, 813, 1989.
326. **Heguy, A., Baldari, C., Bush, K., Nagele, R., Newton, R.C., Robb, R.J., Horuk, R., Telford, J.L., and Melli, M.,** Internalization and nuclear localization of interleukin 1 are not sufficient for function, *Cell Growth Differ.*, 2, 311, 1991.
327. **Porat, R., Clark, B.D., Wolff, S.M., and Dinarello, C.A.,** Enhancement of growth of virulent strains of *Escherichia coli* by interleukin-1, *Science*, 254, 430, 1991.
328. **Bird, T.A., Davies, A., Baldwin, S.A., and Saklatvala, J.,** Interleukin 1 stimulates hexose transport in fibroblasts by increasing the expression of glucose transporters, *J. Biol. Chem.*, 265, 13578, 1990.
329. **Turunen, J.P., Mattila, P., and Kenkonen, R.,** cAMP mediates IL-1-induced lymphocyte penetration through endothelial monolayers, *J. Immunol.*, 145, 4192, 1990.
330. **Weitzmann, M.N. and Savage, N.,** Cyclic 3′,5′-monophosphate, a second messenger in interleukin-1 mediated K562 cytostasis, *Biochem. Biophys. Res. Commun.*, 190, 564, 1993.
331. **Zhang, Y., Lin, J.-X., and Vilcek, J.,** Enhancement of cAMP levels and protein kinase activity by tumor necrosis factor and interleukin 1 in human fibroblasts: role in the induction of interleukin 6, *Proc. Natl. Acad. Sci. U.S.A.*, 85, 6802, 1988.
332. **Burch, R.M., White, M.F., and Connor, J.R.,** Interleukin 1 stimulates prostaglandin synthesis and cyclic AMP accumulation in Swiss 3T3 fibroblasts: interactions between two second messenger systems, *J. Cell. Physiol.*, 139, 29, 1989.

333. **Kasahara, T., Yagisawa, H., Yamashita, K., Yamaguchi, Y., and Akiyama, Y.,** IL-1 induces proliferation and IL6 mRNA expression in a human astrocytoma cell line: positive and negative modulation by cholera toxin and cAMP, *Biochem. Biophys. Res. Commun.*, 167, 1242, 1990.
334. **Pfeilschifter, J. and Schwarzenbach, H.,** Interleukin-1 and tumor necrosis factor stimulate cGMP formation in rat renal mesangial cells, *FEBS Lett.*, 273, 185, 1990.
335. **O'Neill, L.A.J., Bird, T.A., Gearing, A.J.H., and Saklatvala, J.,** Interleukin-1 signal transduction. Increased GTP binding and hydrolysis in membranes of a murine thymoma cell line (EL4), *J. Biol. Chem.*, 265, 3146, 1990.
336. **Stanton, T.H., Maynard, M., and Bomsztyk, K.,** Effect of interleukin-1 on intracellular concentration of sodium, calcium, and potassium in 70Z/3 cells, *J. Biol. Chem.*, 261, 5699, 1986.
337. **Ostrowski, J., Meier, K.E., Stanton, T.H., Smith, L.L., and Bomsztyk, K.,** Interferon-γ and interleukin-1α induce transient translocation of protein kinase C activity to membranes in a B lymphoid cell line. Evidence for a protein kinase C-independent pathway in lymphokine-induced cytoplasmic alkalinization, *J. Biol. Chem.*, 263, 13786, 1988.
338. **Civitelli, R., Teitelbaum, S.L., Hruska, K.A., and Lacey, D.L.,** IL-1 activates the Na^+/H^+ antiport in a murine T cell, *J. Immunol.*, 143, 4000, 1989.
339. **Calalb, M.B., Stanton, T.H., Smith, L., Cragoe, E.J., Jr., and Bomsztyk, K.,** Recombinant human interleukin 1-stimulated Na^+/H^+ exchange is not required for differentiation in pre-B lymphocytic cell line, 70Z/3, *J. Biol. Chem.*, 262, 3680, 1987.
340. **Georgilis, K., Schaefer, C., Dinarello, C.A., and Klempner, M.S.,** Human recombinant interleukin 1β has no effect on intracellular calcium or on functional responses of human neutrophils, *J. Immunol.*, 138, 3403, 1987.
341. **Kester, M., Simonson, M.S., Mené, P., and Sedor, J.R.,** Interleukin-1 generates transmembrane signals from phospholipids through novel pathways in cultured rat mesangial cells, *J. Clin. Invest.*, 83, 718, 1989.
342. **Yu, H.S. and Ferrier, J.,** Interleukin-1α induces a sustained increase in cytosolic free calcium in cultured rabbit osteoclasts, *Biochem. Biophys. Res. Commun.*, 191, 343, 1993.
343. **Endo, Y., Matsushima, K., Onozaki, K., and Oppenheim, J.J.,** Role of ornithine decarboxylase in the regulation of cell growth by IL-1 and tumor necrosis factor, *J. Immunol.*, 141, 2342, 1989.
344. **Bristol, L.A., Smith, M.R., Bhat, N.K., and Durum, S.K.,** IL-1 induces ornithine decarboxylase in normal lymphocytes-T, *J. Immunol.*, 146, 1509, 1991.
345. **Pfeilschifter, J., Pignat, W., Vosbeck, K., and Märki, F.,** Interleukin 1 and tumor necrosis factor synergistically stimulate prostaglandin synthesis and phospholipase A2 release from rat mesangial cells, *Biochem. Biophys. Res. Commun.*, 159, 385, 1989.
346. **Kerr, J.S., Stevens, T.M., Davis, G.L., McLaughlin, J.A., and Harris, R.R.,** Effects of recombinant interleukin-1β on phospholipase A_2 activity, phospholipase A_2 mRNA levels, and eicosanoid formation in rabbit chondrocytes, *Biochem. Biophys. Res. Commun.*, 165, 1079, 1989.
347. **Maier, J.A.M., Hia, T., and Maciag, T.,** Cyclooxygenase is an immediate-early gene induced by interleukin-1 in human endothelial cells, *J. Biol. Chem.*, 265, 10805, 1990.
348. **Postlethwaite, A.E., Raghow, R., Stricklin, G.P., Poppleton, H., Seyer, J.M., and Kang, A.H.,** Modulation of fibroblast functions by interleukin 1: increased steady-state accumulation of type I procollagen messenger RNAs and stimulation of other functions but not chemotaxis by human recombinant interleukin 1α and β, *J. Cell Biol.*, 106, 311, 1988.
349. **Chiou, W.J., Bonin, P.D., and Singh, J.P.,** Obligatory action of polypeptide growth factors for the IL-1-mediated prostaglandin E_2 production in fibroblasts. Potential role of growth factors in modulation of tissue response to IL-1, *J. Immunol.*, 145, 2155, 1990.
350. **Hoffmann, O., Klaushofer, K., Gleispach, H., Leis, H.J., Luger, T., Koller, K., and Peterlik, M.,** Gamma interferon inhibits basal and interleukin 1-induced prostaglandin production and bone marrow resorption in neonatal mouse calvaria, *Biochem. Biophys. Res. Commun.*, 143, 38, 1987.
351. **Newton, R.C. and Covington, M.,** The activation of human fibroblast prostaglandin E production by interleukin 1, *Cell. Immunol.*, 110, 338, 1987.
352. **Kawakami, M., Ishibashi, S., Ogawa, H., Murase, T., Takaku, F., and Shibata, S.,** Cachectin/TNF as well as interleukin-1 induces prostacyclin synthesis in cultured vascular endothelial cells, *Biochem. Biophys. Res. Commun.*, 141, 482, 1986.

353. **Raz A., Wyche, A., Siegel, N., and Needleman, P.,** Regulation of fibroblast cyclooxygenase synthesis by interleukin-1, *J. Biol. Chem.*, 263, 3022, 1988.
354. **Martin, M., Lovett, D., and Resch, K.,** Interleukin 1 induces specific phosphorylation of a 41 kDa plasma membrane protein from the human tumor cell line K 562, *Immunobiology*, 171, 165, 1986.
355. **Resch, K., Martin, M., Lovett, D.H., Kyas, U., and Gemsa, D.,** The receptor for interleukin 1 in plasma membranes of the human leukemia cell K 562: biological and biochemical characterization, *Immunobiology*, 172, 336, 1986.
356. **Gallis, B., Prickett, K.S., Jackson, J., Slack, J., Schooley, K., Sims, J.E., and Dower, S.K.,** IL-1 induces rapid phosphorylation of the IL-1 receptor, *J. Immunol.*, 143, 3235, 1989.
357. **Williams, J.M., Dinarello, C.A., Rosenwasser, L.J., Kelley, V., Reddish, M., and Strom, T.B.,** Phorbol myristate acetate-protein complex mimics bioactivity of human IL-1, *Lymphokine Res.*, 4, 275, 1985.
358. **Bird, T.A., Woodward, A., Jackson, J.L., Dower, S.K., and Sims, J.E.,** Phorbol ester induces phosphorylation of the 80 kilodalton murine interleukin 1 receptor at a single threonine residue, *Biochem. Biophys. Res. Commun.*, 177, 61, 1991.
359. **Fagarasan, M.O., Bishop, J.F., Rinaudo, M.S., and Axelrod, J.,** Interleukin 1 induces early protein phosphorylation and requires only a short exposure for late induced secretion of β-endorphin in a mouse pituitary cell line, *Proc. Natl. Acad. Sci. U.S.A.*, 87, 2555, 1990.
360. **Qwarnström, E.E., MacFarlane, S.A., Page, R.C., and Dower, S.K.,** Interleukin 1β induces rapid phosphorylation and redistribution of talin: a possible mechanism for modulation of fibroblast focal adhesion, *Proc. Natl. Acad. Sci. U.S.A.*, 88, 1232, 1991.
361. **Mukaida, N., Kasahara, T., Yagisawa, H., Shiori-Nakano, K., and Kawai, T.,** Signal requirement for interleukin 1-dependent interleukin 2 production by a human leukemia-derived HSB.2 subclone, *J. Immunol.*, 139, 3321, 1987.
362. **Macchia, G., Baldari, C.T., Massone, A., and Telford, J.L.,** A role for protein kinase C activity in interleukin-1 (IL-1) induction of IL-2 gene expression but not in IL-1 signal transduction, *Mol. Cell. Biol.*, 10, 2731, 1990.
363. **Hulkower, K.I., Georgescu, H.I., and Evans, C.H.,** Evidence that responses of articular chondrocytes to interleukin-1 and basic fibroblast growth factor are not mediated by protein kinase C, *Biochem. J.*, 276, 157, 1991.
364. **Godfrey, R.W., Johnson, W.J., and Hoffstein, S.T.,** Recombinant tumor necrosis factor and interleukin-1 both stimulate human synovial cell arachidonic acid release and phospholipid metabolism, *Biochem. Biophys. Res. Commun.*, 142, 235, 1987.
365. **Suffys, P., Van Roy, F., and Fiers, W.,** Tumor necrosis factor and interleukin 1 activate phospholipase in rat chondrocytes, *FEBS Lett.*, 232, 24, 1988.
366. **Ballou, L.R., Barker, S.C., Postlethwaite, A.E., and Kang, A.H.,** Interleukin-1 stimulates phosphatidylinositol kinase activity in human fibroblasts, *J. Clin. Invest.*, 87, 299, 1991.
367. **Rosoff, P.M., Savage, N., and Dinarello, C.A.,** Interleukin-1 stimulates diacylglycerol production in T lymphocytes by a novel mechanism, *Cell*, 54, 73, 1988.
368. **Didier, M., Aussel, C., Pelassy, C., and Fehlmann, M.,** IL-1 signaling for IL-2 production in T cells involves a rise in phosphatidylserine synthesis, *J. Immunol.*, 141, 3078, 1988.
369. **Beresini, M.H., Lempert, M.J., and Epstein, L.B.,** Overlapping polypeptide induction in human fibroblasts in response to treatment with interferon-α, interferon-β, interleukin 1α, interleukin 1β, and tumor necrosis factor, *J. Immunol.*, 140, 485, 1988.
370. **Hagiwara, H., Huang, H.-J.S., Arai, N., Herzenberg, L.A., Arai, K.-I., and Zlotnik, A.,** Interleukin 1 modulates messenger RNA levels of lymphokines and of other molecules associated with T cell activation in the T cell lymphoma LBRM33-1A5, *J. Immunol.*, 138, 2514, 1987.
371. **DeMarco, D., Kunkel, S.L., Strieter, R.M., Basha, M., and Zurier, R.B.,** Interleukin-1 induced gene expression of neutrophil activating protein (interleukin-8) and monocyte chemotactic peptide in human synovial cells, *Biochem. Biophys. Res. Commun.*, 174, 411, 1991.
372. **Bomsztyk, K., Rooney, J.W., Iwasaki, T., Rachie, N.A., Dower, S.K., and Sibley, C.J.,** Evidence that interleukin-1 and phorbol esters activate NF-kappa B by different pathways; role of protein kinase C, *Cell Regul.*, 2, 329, 1991.
373. **Bethea, J.R., Gillespie, G.Y., and Benveniste, E.N.,** Interleukin-1β induction of TNF-α gene expression — involvement of protein kinase C, *J. Cell. Physiol.*, 152, 264, 1992.

374. Weitzmann, M.N. and Savage, N., Nuclear internalisation and DNA binding activities of interleukin-1, interleukin-1 receptor and interleukin-1/receptor complexes, *Biochem. Biophys. Res. Commun.,* 187, 1166, 1992.
375. Kovacs, E.J., Oppenheim, J.J., and Young, H.A., Induction of c-fos and c-myc expression in T lymphocytes after treatment with recombinant interleukin 1α, *J. Immunol.,* 137, 3649, 1986.
376. Fagarasan, M.O., Aiello, F., Muegge, K., Durum, S., and Axelrod, J., Interleukin 1 induces β-endorphin secretion via *Fos* and *Jun* in AtT-20 pituitary cells, *Proc. Natl. Acad. Sci. U.S.A.,* 87, 7871, 1990.
377. Lin, J.-X. and Vilcek, J., Tumor necrosis factor and interleukin-1 cause a rapid and transient stimulation of c-*fos* and c-*myc* mRNA levels in human fibroblasts, *J. Biol. Chem.,* 262, 11908, 1987.
378. Kessler, D.J., Duyao, M.P., Spicer, D.B., and Sonenshein, G.E., NF-kappa B-like factors mediate interleukin-1 induction of c-*myc* gene transcription in fibroblasts, *J. Exp. Med.,* 176, 787, 1992.
379. Libby, P., Warner, S.J.C., and Friedman, G.B., Interleukin-1: a mitogen for human vascular smooth muscle cells that induces the release of growth-inhibitory prostanoids, *J. Clin. Invest.,* 81, 487, 1988.
380. Hughes, J.H., Watson, M.A., Easom, R.A., Turk, J., and McDaniel, M.L., Interleukin-1 induces rapid and transient expression of the c-fos proto-oncogene in isolated pancreatic islets and in purified β cells, *FEBS Lett.,* 266, 33, 1990.
381. Eizirik, D.L., Björklund, A., and Welsh, N., Interleukin-1-induced expression of nitric oxide synthase in insulin-producing cells is preceded by c-*fos* induction and depends on gene transcription and protein synthesis, *FEBS Lett.,* 317, 62, 1993.
382. Tsai, S.-C. and Gaffney, E.V., Inhibition of cell proliferation by interleukin-1 derived from monocytic leukemic cells, *Cancer Res.,* 46, 1471, 1986.
383. Vanle, L., Oh, S.T., Anners, J.A., Rinehart, C.A., and Halme, J., Interleukin-1 inhibits growth of normal human endometrial stromal cells, *Obstet. Gynecol.,* 80, 405, 1992.
384. Morinaga, Y., Hayashi, H., Takeuchi, A., and Onozaki, K., Antiproliferative effect of interleukin 1 (IL-1) on tumor cells: $G_0 + G_1$ arrest of a human melanoma cell line by IL-1, *Biochem. Biophys. Res. Commun.,* 173, 186, 1990.
385. Li, B.Y., Mohanraj, D., Olson, M.C., Moradi, M., Twiggs, L., Carson, L.F., and Ramakrishnan, S., Human ovarian epithelial cancer cells cultured in vitro express both interleukin 1α and 1β genes, *Cancer Res.,* 52, 2248, 1992.
386. Gaffney, E.V. and Tsai, S.-C., Lymphocyte-activating and growth-inhibitory activities for several sources of native and recombinant interleukin 1, *Cancer Res.,* 46, 3834, 1986.
387. Gaffney, E.V., Koch, G., Tsai, S.-C., Louks, T., and Lingenfelter, S.E., Correlation between human cell growth response to interleukin 1 and receptor binding, *Cancer Res.,* 48, 5455, 1988.
388. Paciotti, G.F. and Tamarkin, L., Interleukin-1 directly regulates hormone-dependent human breast cancer cell proliferation *in vitro, Mol. Endocrinol.,* 2, 459, 1988.
389. Cozzolino, F., Rubartelli, A., Aldinucci, D., Sitia, R., Torcia, M., Shaw, A., and Di Guglielmo, R., Interleukin 1 as an autocrine growth factor for acute myeloid leukemia cells, *Proc. Natl. Acad. Sci. U.S.A.,* 86, 2369, 1989.
390. Murohashi, I., Tohda, S., Suzuki, T., Nagata, K., Yamashita, Y., and Nara, N., Mechanism of action of interleukin 1 on the progenitors of blast cells in acute myeloblastic leukemia, *Exp. Hematol.,* 18, 133, 1990.
391. Delwel, R., van Buitenen, C., Salem, M., Bot, F., Gillis, S., Kaushansky, K., Altrock, B., and Löwenberg, B., Interleukin-1 stimulates proliferation of acute myeloblastic leukemia cells by induction of granulocyte-macrophage colony-stimulating factor release, *Blood,* 74, 586, 1989.
392. Bradbury, D., Bowen, G., Kozlowski, R., Reilly, I., and Russell, N., Endogenous interleukin-1 regulates the autonomous growth of the blast cells of acute myeloblastic leukemia by inducing autocrine secretion of GM-CSF, *Leukemia,* 4, 44, 1990.
393. Lovett, D., Kozan, B., Hadam, M., Resch, K., and Gemsa, D., Macrophage cytotoxicity: interleukin 1 is a mediator of tumor cytostasis, *J. Immunol.,* 136, 340, 1986.
394. Onozaki, K., Tamatani, T., Hashimoto, T., and Matsushima, K., Growth inhibition and augmentation of mouse myeloid leukemic cell line differentiation by interleukin 1, *Cancer Res.,* 47, 2397, 1987.
395. Onozaki, K., Akiyama, Y., Okano, A., Hirano, T., Kishimoto, T., Hashimoto, T., Yoshizawa, K., and Taniyama, T., Synergistic regulatory effects of interleukin 6 and interleukin 1 on the growth and differentiation of human and mouse myeloid leukemic cell lines, *Cancer Res.,* 49, 3602, 1989.

396. **Tamatani, T., Urawa, H., Hashimoto, T., and Onozaki, K.,** Tumor necrosis factor as an interleukin 1-dependent differentiation inducing factor (D-factor) for mouse myeloid leukemic cells, *Biochem. Biophys. Res. Commun.,* 143, 390, 1987.
397. **Endo, Y., Matsushima, K., and Oppenheim, J.J.,** Mechanism of *in vitro* antitumor effects of interleukin 1 (IL 1), *Immunobiology,* 172, 316, 1986.
398. **Ruggiero, V. and Baglioni, C.,** Synergistic anti-proliferative activity of interleukin 1 and tumor necrosis factor, *J. Immunol.,* 138, 661, 1987.
399. **Morinaga, Y., Suzuki, H., Takatsuki, F., Akiyama, Y., Taniyama, T., Matsushima, K., and Onozaki, K.,** Contribution of IL-6 to the antiproliferative effect of IL-1 and tumor necrosis factor on tumor cell lines, *J. Immunol.,* 143, 3538, 1989.
400. **Tsai, S.-C.J. and Gaffney, E.V.,** Modulation of cell proliferation by human recombinant interleukin-1 and immune interferon, *J. Natl. Cancer Inst.,* 79, 77, 1987.
401. **Sakai, K., Hattori, T., Matsuoka, M., Asou, N., Yamamoto, S., Sagawa, K., and Takatsuki, K.,** Autocrine stimulation of interleukin 1β in acute myelogenous leukemia cells, *J. Exp. Med.,* 166, 1597, 1987.
402. **Hamburger, A.W., Lurie, K.A., and Condon, M.E.,** Stimulation of anchorage-independent growth of human tumor cells by interleukin 1, *Cancer Res.,* 47, 5612, 1987.
403. **Gong, J.-H., Renz, H., Nain, M., and Gemsa, D.,** Interleukin 1 as a tumor cytostatic mediator released from tumor ascites-treated macrophages, *Immunobiology,* 177, 339, 1988.
404. **Orr, F.W., Buchanan, M.R., Tron, V.A., Guy, D., Lauri, D., and Sauder, D.N.,** Chemotactic activity of endothelial cell-derived interleukin 1 for human tumor cells, *Cancer Res.,* 48, 6758, 1988.
405. **Evans, R., Duffy, T.M., Blake, S.S., and Lin, H.-S.,** Regulation of systemic macrophage *IL-1* gene transcription: the involvement of tumor-derived macrophage growth factor, CSF-1, *J. Leukocyte Biol.,* 46, 428, 1989.
406. **Morgan, D.A., Ruscetti, F.W., and Gallo, R.C.,** Selective in vitro growth of T lymphocytes from normal human bone marrows, *Science,* 193, 107, 1976.
407. **Ruscetti, F.W. and Gallo, R.C.,** Human T-lymphocyte growth factor: regulation of growth and function of T lymphocytes, *Blood,* 57, 379, 1981.
408. **Sarin, P.S. and Gallo, R.C.,** Human T-cell growth factor (TCGF), *Crit. Rev. Immunol.,* 4, 279, 1984.
409. **Smith, K.A.,** Interleukin 2, *Annu. Rev. Immunol.,* 2, 319, 1984.
410. **Robb, R.J.,** Human interleukin 2, *Methods Enzymol.,* 116, 493, 1985.
411. **Fletcher, M. and Goldstein, A.L.,** Recent advances in the understanding of the biochemistry and clinical pharmacology of interleukin 2, *Lymphokine Res.,* 6, 45, 1987.
412. **Smith, K.A.,** Interleukin 2: inception, impact, and implications, *Science,* 240, 1169, 1988.
413. **Semenzato, G., Pizzolo, G., and Zambello, R.,** The interleukin-2/interleukin-2 receptor system. Structural, immunological, and clinical features, *Int. J. Clin. Lab. Res.,* 22, 133, 1992.
414. **Lattime, E.C., Bykowsky, M.J., and Stutman, O.,** Natural cytotoxic (NC) activity: a multi-lineage system regulated by IL-2, *Immunol. Res.,* 5, 5, 1986.
415. **Owen-Schaub, L.B., Crump, W.L., III, Morin, G.I., and Grimm, E.A.,** Regulation of lymphocyte tumor necrosis factor receptors by IL-2, *J. Immunol.,* 143, 2236, 1989.
416. **Malkovsky, M., Loveland, B., North, M., Asherson, G.L., Gao, L., Ward, P., and Fiers, W.,** Recombinant interleukin-2 directly augments the cytotoxicity of human monocytes, *Nature,* 325, 262, 1987.
417. **Kupper, T.S., Coleman, D.L., McGuire, J., Goldsmitz, D., and Horowitz, M.C.,** Keratinocyte-derived T-cell growth factor: a T-cell growth factor functionally distinct from interleukin 2, *Proc. Natl. Acad. Sci. U.S.A.,* 83, 4451, 1986.
418. **Coleman, D.L., Kupper, T.S., Flood, P.M., Fultz, C.C., and Horowitz, M.C.,** Characterization of a keratinocyte-derived T cell growth factor distinct from interleukin 2 and B cell stimulatory factor 1, *J. Immunol.,* 138, 3314, 1987.
419. **Mosmann, T., Cherwinski, H., Bond, M.W., Geidlen, M., and Coffman, R.L.,** Two types of murine T helper cell. I. Definition according to profile of lymphokine activities and secreted proteins, *J. Immunol.,* 136, 2348, 1986.
420. **Zlotnik, A., Ransom, J., Frank, G., Fischer, M., and Howard, M.,** Interleukin 4 is a growth factor for activated thymocytes: possible role in T-cell ontogeny, *Proc. Natl. Acad. Sci. U.S.A.,* 84, 3856, 1987.
421. **Kupper, T., Flood, P., Coleman, D., and Horowitz, M.,** Growth of an interleukin 2/interleukin 4-dependent T cell line induced by granulocyte-macrophage colony-stimulating factor (GM-CSF), *J. Immunol.,* 138, 4288, 1987.

422. **Laing, T.J. and Weiss, A.,** Evidence for IL-2 independent proliferation in human T cells, *J. Immunol.,* 140, 1056, 1988.
423. **Ogata, M., Sato, S., Sano, H., Hamaoka, T., Doi, H., Nakanishi, K., Asano, Y., Itoh, T., and Fujiwara, H.,** Thymic stroma-derived T cell growth factor (TSTGF). I. Functional distinction of TSTGF from interleukins 2 and 4 and its preferential growth-promoting effect on helper T cell clones, *J. Immunol.,* 139, 1987.
424. **Lakhanpal, S., Gonchoroff, N.J., and Handwerger, B.S.,** Interleukin 2 induces proliferation of normal "resting" human T cells in the absence of other known external stimulation, *Cell. Immunol.,* 106, 62, 1987.
425. **Cantrell, D.A. and Smith, K.A.,** The interleukin-2 T-cell system: a new cell growth model, *Science,* 224, 1312, 1984.
426. **London, L., Perussia, B., and Trinchieri, G.,** Induction of proliferation in vitro of resting human natural killer cells: IL 2 induces into cell cycle most peripheral blood NK cells, but only a minor subset of low density T cells, *J. Immunol.,* 137, 3845, 1986.
427. **Ben Aribia, M.-H., Leroy, E., Lantz, O., Métivier, D., Autran, B., Charpentier, B., Hercend, T., and Senik, A.,** rIL 2-induced proliferation of human circulating NK cells and T lymphocytes: synergistic effects of IL 1 and IL 2, *J. Immunol.,* 139, 443, 1987.
428. **Gullberg, M. and Smith, K.A.,** Regulation of T cell autocrine growth. T4+ cells become refractory to interleukin 2, *J. Exp. Med.,* 163, 270, 1986.
429. **Kurasuyama, H., Tohyama, N., and Tada, T.,** Autocrine growth and tumorigenicity of interleukin 2-dependent helper T cells transfected with IL-2 gene, *J. Exp. Med.,* 169, 13, 1989.
430. **Tsuchida, T. and Sakane, T.,** Intracellular activation signal requirements for the induction of IL-2 responsiveness in resting T cell subsets in humans, *J. Immunol.,* 140, 3446, 1988.
431. **Stern, J.B. and Smith, K.A.,** Interleukin-2 induction of T-cell G_1 progression and c-*myb* expression, *Science,* 233, 203, 1986.
432. **Kupper, T., Horowitz, M., Lee, F., Robb, R., and Flood, P.M.,** Autocrine growth of T cells independent of interleukin 1: identification of interleukin 4 ((L 4, BSF-1) as an autocrine growth factor for a cloned antigen-specific helper T cell, *J. Immunol.,* 138, 4280, 1987.
433. **Gallagher, G., Wilcox, F., and Al-Azzawi, F.,** Interleukin-3 and interleukin-4 each strongly inhibit the induction and function of human LAK cells, *Clin. Exp. Immunol.,* 74, 166, 1988.
434. **Gray, J.D. and Horwitz, D.A.,** Lymphocytes expressing type 3 complement receptors proliferate in response to interleukin 2 and are the precursors of lymphokine-activated killer cells, *J. Clin. Invest.,* 81, 1247, 1988.
435. **Sayers, T.J., Mason, A.T., and Ortaldo, J.R.,** Regulation of human natural killer cell activity by interferon-γ: lack of a role in interleukin 2-mediated augmentation, *J. Immunol.,* 136, 2176, 1986.
436. **Hoyer, M., Meineke, T., Lewis, W., Zwilling, B., and Rinehart, J.,** Characterization and modulation of human lymphokine (interleukin 2) activated killer cell induction, *Cancer Res.,* 46, 2843, 1986.
437. **Talmadge, J.E., Wiltrout, R.H., Counts, D.F., Herberman, R.B., McDonald, T., and Ortaldo, J.R.,** Proliferation of human peripheral blood lymphocytes induced by recombinant human interleukin 2: contribution of large granular lymphocytes and T lymphocytes, *Cell. Immunol.,* 102, 261, 1986.
438. **Yamada, S., Ruscetti, F.W., Overton, W.R., Herberman, R.B., Birchenall-Sparks, M.C., and Ortaldo, J.R.,** Regulation of human large granular lymphocyte and T cell growth and function by recombinant interleukin 2: induction of interleukin 2 receptor and promotion of growth of cells with enhanced cytotoxicity, *J. Leukocyte Biol.,* 41, 505, 1987.
439. **Hattori, M., Sudo, T., Iizuka, M., Kobayashi, S., Nishio, S., Kano, S., and Minato, N.,** Generation of continuous large granular lymphocyte lines by interleukin 2 from the spleen cells of mice infected with Moloney leukemia virus, *J. Exp. Med.,* 166, 833, 1987.
440. **Itoh, K., Tilden, A.B., and Balch, C.M.,** Interleukin 2 activation of cytotoxic T-lymphocytes infiltrating into human metastatic melanomas, *Cancer Res.,* 46, 3011, 1986.
441. **Espevik, T., Figari, I.S., Ranges, G.E., and Palladino, M.A., Jr.,** Transforming growth factor-β_1 (TGF-β_1) and recombinant human tumor necrosis factor-α reciprocally regulate the generation of lymphokine-activated killer cell activity. Comparison between natural porcine platelet-derived TGF-β_1 and TGF-β_2, and recombinant human TGF-β_1, *J. Immunol.,* 140, 2312, 1988.
442. **Moldwin, R.L., Lancki, D.W., Herold, K.C., and Fitch, F.W.,** An antigen receptor-driven interleukin 2-independent pathway for proliferation of murine cytolytic T lymphocyte clones, *J. Exp. Med.,* 163, 1566, 1986.

443. **Milanese, C., Siciliano, R.F., Schmidt, R.E., Ritz, J., Richardson, N.E., and Reinherz, E.L.,** A lymphokine that activates the cytolytic program of both cytotoxic T lymphocyte and natural killer cell clones, *J. Exp. Med.,* 163, 1583, 1986.
444. **Miglioratti, G., Cannarile, L., Herberman, R.B., Bartocci, A., Stanley, E.R., and Riccardi, C.,** Role of interleukin 2 (IL 2) and hemopoietin-1 (H-1) in the generation of mouse natural killer (NK) cells from primitive bone marrow precursors, *J. Immunol.,* 138, 3618, 1987.
445. **Ostensen, M.E., Thiele, D.L., and Lipsky, P.E.,** Tumor necrosis factor-α enhances cytolytic activity of human natural killer cells, *J. Immunol.,* 138, 4185, 1987.
446. **Santoli, D., Clark, S.C., Kreider, B.L., Maslin, P.A., and Rovera, G.,** Amplification of IL-2-driven T cell proliferation by recombinant human IL-3 and granulocyte-macrophage colony-stimulating factor, *J. Immunol.,* 141, 519, 1988.
447. **Farrar, W.L., Birchenall-Sparks, M.C., and Young, H.B.,** Interleukin 2 induction of interferon-γ mRNA synthesis, *J. Immunol.,* 137, 3836, 1986.
448. **Russell, J.K., Torres, B.A., and Johnson, H.M.,** Phospholipase A_2 treatment of lymphocytes provides helper signal for interferon-γ induction. Evidence for second messenger role of endogenous arachidonic acid, *J. Immunol.,* 139, 3442, 1987.
449. **Brunda, M.J., Tarnowski, D., and Davatelis, V.,** Interaction of recombinant interferons with recombinant interleukin-2: differential effects on natural killer cell activity and interleukin-2-activated killer cells, *Int. J. Cancer,* 37, 787, 1986.
450. **Ythier, A.A., Abbud-Filho, M., Williams, J.M., Lertscher, R., Schuster, M.W., Nowill, A., Hansen, J.A., Maltezos, D., and Strom, T.B.,** Interleukin 2-dependent release of interleukin 3 activity by T4+ human T-cell clones, *Proc. Natl. Acad. Sci. U.S.A.,* 82, 7020, 1985.
451. **Cook, W.D., Fazekas de St. Groth, B., Miller, J.F.A.P., MacDonald, H.R., and Gabathuler, R.,** Abelson virus transformation of an interleukin 2-dependent antigen-specific T-cell line, *Mol. Cell. Biol.,* 7, 2631, 1987.
452. **Bichthuy, L.T. and Fauci, A.S.,** Recombinant interleukin-2 and γ-interferon act synergistically on distinct steps of in vitro terminal human B-cell maturation, *J. Clin. Invest.,* 77, 1173, 1986.
453. **Mond, J.J., Thompson, C., Finkelman, F.D., Farrar, J., Schaefer, M., and Robb, R.J.,** Affinity-purified interleukin 2 induces proliferation of large but not small B cells, *Proc. Natl. Acad. Sci. U.S.A.,* 82, 1518, 1985.
454. **Romagnani, S., Delprete, G., Giudizi, M.G., Biagiotti, R., Almerigogna, F., Tiri, A., Alessi, A., Mazzetti, M., and Ricci, M.,** Direct induction of human B-cell differentiation by recombinant interleukin-2, *Immunology,* 58, 31, 1986.
455. **Weyand, C.M., Goronzy, J., Dallman, M.J., and Fathman, C.G.,** Administration of recombinant interleukin 2 in vivo induces a polyclonal IgM response, *J. Exp. Med.,* 163, 1607, 1986.
456. **Weyand, C., Goronzy, J., Fathman, C.G., and O'Hanyley, P.,** Administration in vivo of recombinant interleukin 2 protects mice against septic death, *J. Clin. Invest.,* 79, 1756, 1987.
457. **Emilie, D., Karray, S., Crevon, M.-C., Vazquez, A., and Galanaud, P.,** B cell differentiation and interleukin 2 (IL2): corticosteroid interact with monocytes to enhance the effect of IL2, *Eur. J. Immunol.,* 17, 791, 1987.
458. **Torigoe, T., Saragovi, H.U., and Reed, J.C.,** Interleukin-2 regulates the activity of the *lyn* protein-tyrosine kinbase in a B-cell line, *Proc. Natl. Acad. Sci. U.S.A.,* 89, 2674, 1992.
459. **Finkelman, F.D., Malek, T.R., Shevach, E.M., and Mond, J.J.,** In vivo and in vitro expression of an interleukin 2 receptor by murine B and T lymphocytes, *J. Immunol.,* 137, 2252, 1986.
460. **Julius, M.H., Paige, C.J., Leanderson, T., and Cambier, J.C.,** Neither interleukin 2 nor γ interferon directly promote growth and differentiation of mouse B cells, *Scand. J. Immunol.,* 25, 195, 1987.
461. **Punnonen, J. and Eskola, J.,** Recombinant interleukin 2 induces proliferation and differentiation of human B lymphocytes, *Acta Pathol. Microbiol. Scand.,* C95, 167, 1987.
462. **Herrmann, F., Cannistra, S.A., Lindemann, A., Blohm, D., Rambaldi, A., Mertelsmann, R.H., and Griffin, J.D.,** Functional consequences of monocyte IL-2 receptor expression. Induction of IL-1β secretion by IFN γ and IL-2, *J. Immunol.,* 142, 139, 1989.
463. **Talmadge, J.E., Schneider, M., Keller, J., Ruscetti, F., Longo, D., Pennington, R., Bowersox, O., and Tribble, H.,** Myelostimulatory activity of recombinant human interleukin-2 in mice, *Blood,* 73, 1458, 1989.
464. **Burdach, S., Shatsky, M., Wagenhorst, B., and Levitt, L.,** Receptor-specific modulation of myelopoiesis by recombinant DNA-derived interleukin 2, *J. Immunol.,* 139, 452, 1987.

465. **Guo, H., Calkins, H., Sigel, M.M., and Lin, T.,** Interleukin-2 is a potent inhibitor of Leydig cell steroidogenesis, *Endocrinology,* 127, 1234, 1990.
466. **Fowlkes, B.J. and Pardoll, D.M.,** Molecular and cellular events of T cell development, *Adv. Immunol.,* 44, 207, 1989.
467. **Teh, H.S., Kisielow, P., Scott, B., Kishi, H., Uematsu, Y., Blüthmann, H., and von Boehmer, H.,** Thymic major histocompatibility complex antigens and the αβ T-cell receptor determine the CD4/CD8 phenotype of T cells, *Nature,* 335, 229, 1988.
468. **Weiss, A., Imboden, J., Hardy, K., Manger, B., Terhorst, C., and Stobo, J.,** The role of the T3/antigen receptor in T-cell activation, *Annu. Rev. Immunol.,* 4, 593, 1986.
469. **Gallatin, M., John, T.P.S., Siegelman, M., Reichert, R., Butcher, E.C., and Weissman, I.L.,** Lymphocyte homing receptors, *Cell,* 44, 673, 1986.
470. **Reinherz, E.L., Kung, P.C., Goldstein, G., Levy, R.H., and Schlossman, S.F.,** Discrete stages of human intrathymic differentiation: analysis of normal thymocytes and leukemic lymphoblasts on T-cell lineage, *Proc. Natl. Acad. Sci. U.S.A.,* 77, 1588, 1980.
471. **Smith, L.,** CD4$^+$ murine T cells develop from CD8$^+$ precursors in vivo, *Nature,* 326, 798, 1987.
472. **Hood, L., Kronenberg, M., and Hunkapiller, T.,** T cell antigen receptors and the immunoglobulin supergene family, *Cell,* 40, 225, 1985.
473. **June, C.H., Fletcher, M.C., Ledbetter, J.A., Schieven, G.L., Siegel, J.N., Phillips, A.F., and Samelson, L.E.,** Inhibition of tyrosine phosphorylation prevents T-cell receptor-mediated signal transduction, *Proc. Natl. Acad. Sci. U.S.A.,* 87, 7722, 1990.
474. **Rudd, C.E., Trevillyan, J.M., Dasgupta, J.D., Wong, L.L., and Schlossman, S.F.,** The CD4 receptor is complexed in detergent lysates to a protein-tyrosine kinase (pp58) from human T lymphocytes, *Proc. Natl. Acad. Sci. U.S.A.,* 85, 5190, 1988.
475. **Straus, D.B. and Weiss, A.,** Genetic evidence for the involvement of the lck tyrosine kinase in signal transduction through the T-cell antigen receptor, *Cell,* 70, 585, 1992.
476. **Shaw, A.S., Amrein, K.E., Hammond, C., Stern, C.F., Sefton, B.M., and Rose, J.K.,** The *lck* tyrosine protein kinase interacts with the cytoplasmic tail of the CD4 glycoprotein through its unique amino-terminal domain, *Cell,* 59, 627, 1989.
477. **Turner, J.M., Brodsky, M.H., Irving, B.A., Levin, S.D., Perlmutter, R.M., and Littman, D.R.,** Interaction of the unique N-terminal region of tyrosine kinase p56^{lck} with cytoplasmic domains of CD4 and CD8 is mediated by cysteine motifs, *Cell,* 60, 755, 1990.
478. **Glaichenhaus, N., Shastri, N., Littman, D.R., and Turner, J.M.,** Requirement for association of p56^{lck} with CD4 in antigen-specific signal transduction in T cells, *Cell,* 64, 511, 1991.
479. **Telfer, J.C. and Rudd, C.E.,** A 32-kD GTP-binding protein associated with the CD4-p56^{lck} and CD8-p56^{lck} T cell receptor complexes, *Science,* 254, 439, 1991.
480. **Luo, K.X. and Sefton, B.M.,** Activated *lck* tyrosine protein kinase stimulates antigen-independent interleukin-2 production in T cells, *Mol. Cell. Biol.,* 12, 4724, 1992.
481. **Cooke, M.P., Abraham, K.M., Forbush, K.A., and Perlmutter, R.M.,** Regulation of T cell receptor signaling by a *src* family protein-tyrosine kinase (p59^{fyn}), *Cell,* 65, 281, 1991.
482. **Shiroo, M., Goff, L., Biffen, M., Shivnan, E., and Alexander, D.,** CD45 tyrosine phosphatase-activated p59^{fyn} couples the T cell antigen receptor to pathways of diacylglycerol production, protein kinase C activation and calcium influx, *EMBO J.,* 11, 4887, 1992.
483. **Furue, M., Katz, S.I., Kawakami, Y., and Kawakami, T.,** Coordinate expression of src family protooncogenes in T cell activation and its modulation by cyclosporine, *J. Immunol.,* 144, 736, 1990.
484. **Baldari, C.T., Heguy, A., and Telford, J.L.,** Ras protein activity is essential for T-cell antigen receptor signal transduction, *J. Biol. Chem.,* 268, 2693, 1993.
485. **Rayter, S.I., Woodrow, M., Lucas, S.C., Cantrell, D.A., and Downward, J.,** p21^{ras} mediates control of *IL-2* gene promoter function in T cell activation, *EMBO J.,* 11, 4549, 1992.
486. **Klatzmann, D., Champagne, E., Chamaret, S., Gruest, J., Guétard, D., Hercend, T., Gluckman, J.C., and Montagnier, L.,** T-lymphocyte T4 molecule behaves as the receptor for human retrovirus LAV, *Nature,* 312, 767, 1984.
487. **Isobe, M., Huebner, K., Maddon, P.J., Littman, D.R., Axel, R., and Croce, C.M.,** The gene encoding the T-cell surface protein T4 is located on human chromosome 12, *Proc. Natl. Acad. Sci. U.S.A.,* 83, 4399, 1986.
488. **Minden, M.D. and Mak, T.W.,** The structure of the T-cell antigen receptor genes in normal and malignant T cells, *Blood,* 68, 327, 1986.

489. **Allison, J.P. and Lanier, L.L.,** Structure, function, and serology of the T-cell antigen receptor complex, *Annu. Rev. Immunol.,* 5, 503, 1987.
490. **Ashwell, J.D. and Klausner, R.D.,** Genetic and mutational analysis of the T-cell antigen receptor, *Annu. Rev. Immunol.,* 8, 139, 1990.
491. **Klausner, R.D., Lippincott-Schwartz, J., and Bonifacio, J.S.,** The T-cell antigen receptor. Insights into organelle biology, *Annu. Rev. Cell Biol.,* 6, 403, 1990.
492. **Croce, C.M., Isobe, M., Palumbo, A., Puck, J., Ming, J., Tweardy, D., Erikson, J., Davis, M., and Rovera, G.,** Gene for α-chain of human T-cell receptor: location on chromosome 14 region involved in T-cell neoplasms, *Science,* 227, 1044, 1985.
493. **Murre, C., Waldmann, R.A., Morton, C.C., Bongiovanni, K.F., Waldmann, T.A., Shows, T.B., and Seidman, J.G.,** Human γ-chain genes are rearranged in leukaemic T cells and map to the short arm of chromosome 7, *Nature,* 316, 549, 1985.
494. **Ho, I.-C., Bhat, N.K., Gottschalk, L.R., Lindsten, T., Thompson, C.B., Papas, T.S., and Leiden, J.M.,** Sequence-specific binding of human Ets-1 to the T cell receptor α gene enhancer, *Science,* 250, 814, 1990.
495. **Alt, F.W., Blackwell, T.K., DePinho, R.A., Reth, M.G., and Yancopoulos, G.D.,** Regulation of genome rearrangement events during lymphocyte differentiation, *Immunol. Rev.,* 89, 5, 1986.
496. **Korsmeyer, S.J.,** Antigen receptor genes as molecular markers of lymphoid neoplasms, *J. Clin. Invest.,* 79, 1291, 1987.
497. **Toyonaga, B. and Mak, T.W.,** Genes of the T-cell antigen receptor in normal and malignant T cells, *Annu. Rev. Immunol.,* 5, 585, 1987.
498. **Cossman, J., Uppenkamp, M., Sundeen, J., Coupland, R., and Raffeld, M.,** Molecular genetics and the diagnosis of lymphoma, *Arch. Pathol. Lab. Med.,* 112, 117, 1988.
499. **Chien, Y., Iwashima, M., Kaplan, K.B., Elliott, J.F., and Davis, M.M.,** A new T-cell receptor gene located within the α locus and expressed early in T-cell differentiation, *Nature,* 327, 677, 1987.
500. **Epplen, J.T., Bartels, F., Becker, A., Nerz, G., Prester, M., Rinaldy, A., and Simon, M.M.,** Change in antigen specificity of cytotoxic T lymphocytes is associated with the rearrangement and expression of a T-cell receptor β-chain gene, *Proc. Natl. Acad. Sci. U.S.A.,* 83, 4441, 1986.
501. **Ikuta, K., Hattori, M., Wake, K., Kano, S., Honjo, T., Yodoi, J., and Minato, N.,** Expression and rearrangement of the, α, β, and γ chain genes of the T cell receptor in cloned murine large granular lymphocyte lines, *J. Exp. Med.,* 164, 428, 1986.
502. **Calman, A.F. and Peterlin, B.M.,** Expression of T cell receptor genes in human B cells, *J. Exp. Med.,* 164, 1940, 1986.
503. **Morinaga, T., Fotedar, A., Singh, B., Wegmann, T.G., and Tamaoki, T.,** Isolation of cDNA clones encoding a T-cell receptor β-chain from a beef insulin-specific hybridoma, *Proc. Natl. Acad. Sci. U.S.A.,* 82, 8163, 1985.
504. **Tillinghast, J.P., Behlke, M.A., and Loh, D.Y.,** Structure and diversity of the human T-cell receptor β-chain variable region genes, *Science,* 233, 879, 1986.
505. **Waldmann, T.A., Longo, D.L., Leonard, W.J., Depper, J.M., Thompson, C.B., Krönke, M., Goldman, C.K., Sharrow, S., Bongiovanni, K., and Greene, W.C.,** Interleukin 2 receptor (Tac antigen) expression in HTLV-I-associated adult T-cell leukemia, *Cancer Res.,* 45, 4559s, 1985.
506. **Gold, D.P., Puck, J.M., Pettey, C.L., Cho, M., Coligan, J., Woody, J.N., and Terhorst, C.,** Isolation of cDNA clones encoding the 20K non-glycosylated polypeptide chain of the human T-cell receptor complex, *Nature,* 321, 431, 1986.
507. **Brenner, M.B., Trowbridge, I.S., and Strominger, J.L.,** Cross-linking of human T cell receptor proteins: association between the T cell idiotype β subunit and the T3 glycoprotein heavy subunit, *Cell,* 40, 183, 1985.
508. **van den Elsen, P., Shepley, B.-A., Borst, J., Coligan, J.E., Markham, A.F., Orkin, S., and Terhorst, C.,** Isolation of cDNA clones encoding the 20K T3 glycoprotein of human T-cell receptor complex, *Nature,* 312, 413, 1984.
509. **Reiser, H., Coligan, J., Benacerraf, B., and Rock, K.L.,** Biosynthesis, glycosylation, and partial N-terminal amino acid sequence of the T-cell activating protein TAP, *Proc. Natl. Acad. Sci. U.S.A.,* 84, 3370, 1987.
510. **Weiss, A., Kortzky, G., Schatzman, R.C., and Kadlecek, T.,** Functional activation of the T-cell antigen receptor induces tyrosine phosphorylation of phospholipase C-γ1, *Proc. Natl. Acad. Sci. U.S.A.,* 88, 5484, 1991.

511. Secrist, J.P., Karnitz, L., and Abraham, R.T., T-cell antigen receptor ligation induces tyrosine phosphorylation of phospholipase C-γ1, *J. Biol. Chem.,* 266, 12135, 1991.
512. Cantrell, D.A., Davies, A.A., and Crumpton, M.J., Activation of protein kinase C down-regulate and phosphorylate the T3/T-cell antigen receptor complex of human T lymphocytes, *Proc. Natl. Acad. Sci. U.S.A.,* 82, 8158, 1985.
513. Davies, A.A., Cantrell, D.A., Hexham, J.M., Parker, P.J., Rothbard, J., and Crumpton, M.J., The human T3 γ chain is phosphorylated at serine 126 in response to T lymphocyte activation, *J. Biol. Chem.,* 262, 10918, 1987.
514. Samelson, L.E., Patel, M.D., Weissman, A.M., Harford, J.B., and Klausner, R.D., Antigen activation of murine T cells induces tyrosine phosphorylation of a polypeptide associated with the T-cell antigen receptor, *Cell,* 46, 1083, 1986.
515. Samelson, L.E., Davidson, W.F., Morse, H.C., III, and Klausner, R.D., Abnormal tyrosine phosphorylation on T-cell receptor in lymphoproliferative disorders, *Nature,* 324, 674, 1986.
516. Ledbetter, J.A., Gentry, L.E., June, C.H., Rabinovitch, P.S., and Purchio, A.F., Stimulation of T cells through the CD3/T-cell receptor complex: role of cytoplasmic calcium, protein kinase C translocation, and phosphorylation of pp60^{c-src} in the activation pathway, *Mol. Cell. Biol.,* 7, 650, 1987.
517. O'Rourke, A.M. and Mescher, M.F., T cell receptor-mediated signalling occurs in the absence of inositol phosphate production, *J. Biol. Chem.,* 263, 18594, 1988.
518. Boehm, T. and Rabbitts, T.H., The human T cell receptor genes are targets for chromosomal abnormalities, *FASEB J.,* 3, 2344, 1989.
519. Reis, M.D., Grieser, H., and Mak, T.W., Antigen receptor genes in hemopoietic malignancies, *Biochim. Biophys. Acta,* 1072, 177, 1991.
520. Pittaluga, S., Uppenkamp, M., and Cossman, J., Development of T3/T cell receptor gene expression in human pre-T neoplasms, *Blood,* 69, 1062, 1987.
521. **Van Dongen, J.J.M., Quertermous, T., Bartram, C.R., Gold, D.P., Wolvers-Tettero, I.L.M., Comans-Bitter, W.M., Hooijkaas, H., Adriaansen, H.J., de Klein, A., Raghavachar, A., Ganser, A., Duby, A.D., Seidman, J.G., Van den Elsen, P., and Terhorst, C.,** T-cell receptor-CD3 complex during early T-cell differentiation. Analysis of immature T-cell acute lymphoblastic leukemias (T-ALL) at DNA, RNA, and cell membrane level, *J. Immunol.,* 138, 1260, 1987.
522. Waldmann, T.A., Davis, M.M., Bongiovanni, K.F., and Korsmeyer, S.J., Rearrangements of genes for the antigen receptor on T cells as markers of lineage and clonality in human lymphoid neoplasms, *N. Engl. J. Med.,* 313, 776, 1985.
523. **Williams, M.E., Innes, D.J., Jr., Borowitz, M.J., Lovell, M.A., Swerdlow, S.H., Hurtubise, P.E., Byrnes, R.K., Chan, W.C., Byrne, G.E., Jr., Whitcomb, C.C., and Thomas, C.Y., IV,** Immunoglobulin and T cell receptor gene rearrangements in human lymphoma and leukemia, *Blood,* 69, 79, 1987.
524. **Foroni, L., Foldi, J., Matutes, E., Catovsky, D., O'Connor, N.J., Baer, R., Forster, A., Rabbitts, T.H., and Luzzatto, L.,** α, β, and γ T-cell receptor genes: rearrangements correlate with haematological phenotype in T cell leukemias, *Br. J. Haematol.,* 67, 307, 1987.
525. Le Paslier, D., Chen, Z., Loiseau, P., Cohen, D., and Sigaux, F., T cell rearranging gene γ: diversity and mRNA expression in fresh cells from T cell acute lymphoblastic leukemia, *Blood,* 70, 637, 1987.
526. **Furley, A.J., Mizutani, S., Weilbaecher, K., Dhaliwal, H.S., Ford, A.M., Chan, L.C., Molgaard, H.V., Toyonaga, B., Mak, T., van den Elsen, P., Gold, D., Terhorst, C., and Greaves, M.F.,** Developmentally regulated rearrangement and expression of genes encoding the T-cell receptor-T3 complex, *Cell,* 46, 75, 1986.
527. Pelicci, P.-G., Knowles, D.M., II, and Dalla Favera, R., Lymphoid tumors displaying rearrangements of both immunoglobulin and T cell receptor genes, *J. Exp. Med.,* 162, 1015, 1985.
528. **Davey, M.P., Bongiovanni, K.F., Kaulfersch, W., Quertermous, T., Seidman, J.G., Hershfeld, M.S., Kurtzberg, J., Haynes, B.F., Davis, M.M., and Waldmann, T.A.,** Immunoglobulin and T-cell receptor gene rearrangement and expression in human lymphoid leukemia cells at different stages of maturation, *Proc. Natl. Acad. Sci. U.S.A.,* 83, 8759, 1986.
529. Baer, R., Chen, K.-C., Smith, S.D., and Rabbitts, T.H., Fusion of an immunoglobulin variable gene and a T-cell receptor constant gene in the chromosome 14 inversion associated with T cell tumors, *Cell,* 43, 705, 1985.
530. **Malissen, M., McCoy, C., Blanc, D., Trucy, J., Devaux, C., Schmitt-Verhulst, A.-M., Fitch, F., Hood, L., and Malissen, B.,** Direct evidence for chromosomal inversion during T-cell receptor β-gene rearrangements, *Nature,* 319, 28, 1986.

531. Shima, E.A., Le Beau, M.M., McKeithan, T.W., Minowada, J., Showe, L.C., Mak, T.W., Minden, M.D., Rowley, J.D., and Diaz, M.O., Gene encoding the α chain of the T-cell receptor is moved immediately downstream of c-*myc* in a chromosomal 8:14 translocation in a cell line from a human T-cell leukemia, *Proc. Natl. Acad. Sci. U.S.A.*, 83, 3439, 1986.
532. Erikson, J., Finger, L., Sun, L., ar-Rushdi, A., Nishikura, K., Minowada, J., Finan, J., Emanuel, B.S., Nowell, P.C., and Croce, C.M., Deregulation of c-*myc* by translocation of the α-locus of the T-cell receptor in T-cell leukemias, *Science*, 232, 884, 1986.
533. Cheng, G.Y., Minden, M.D., Toyonaga, B., Mak, T.W., and McCulloch, E.A., T-cell receptor and immunoglobulin gene rearrangements in acute myeloblastic leukemia, *J. Exp. Med.*, 163, 414, 1986.
534. Boehm, T.L.J., Werle, A., and Drahovsky, D., Immunoglobulin heavy chain and T-cell receptor γ and β chain gene rearrangements in acute myeloid leukemias, *Mol. Biol. Med.*, 4, 51, 1987.
535. Bellgrau, D. and Talmadge, D.W., T cells can be cytotoxic without making interleukin 2: a model of separate pathways of induction, *Proc. Natl. Acad. Sci. U.S.A.*, 83, 3412, 1986.
536. Chen, L,-K., Mathieu-Mahul, D., Bach, F.H., Dausset, J., Bensussan, A., and Sasportes, M., Recombinant interferon α can induce rearrangement of T-cell antigen receptor α-chain genes and maturation to cytotoxicity in T-lymphocyte clones *in vitro, Proc. Natl. Acad. Sci. U.S.A.*, 83, 4887, 1986.
537. Lichtman, A.H., Kurt-Jones, E.A., and Abbas, A.K., B-cell stimulatory factor 1 and not interleukin 2 is the autocrine growth factor for some helper T lymphocytes, *Proc. Natl. Acad. Sci. U.S.A.*, 84, 824, 1987.
538. Mier, J.W. and Gallo, R.C., Purification and characteristics of human T-cell growth factor, *Proc. Natl. Acad. Sci. U.S.A.*, 77, 6134, 1980.
539. Robb, R.J., Kutny, R.M., Panico, M., Morris, H.R., and Chowdhry, V., Amino acid sequence and post-translational modification of human interleukin 2, *Proc. Natl. Acad. Sci. U.S.A.*, 81, 6486, 1984.
540. Liang, S.-M., Thatcher, D.R., Liang, C.-M., and Allet, B., Studies of structure-activity relationships of human interleukin-2, *J. Biol. Chem.*, 261, 334, 1986.
541. Wang, A., Lu, S.-D., and Mark, D.F., Site-specific mutagenesis of the human interleukin-2 gene: structure-function analysis of the cysteine residues, *Science*, 224, 1431, 1984.
542. Kuo, L.-M. and Robb, R.J., Structure-function relationships for the IL 2-receptor system. I. Localization of a receptor binding site on IL 2, *J. Immunol.*, 137, 1538, 1986.
543. Cohen, F.E., Kosen, P.A., Kuntz, I.D., Epstein, L.B., Ciardelli, T.L., and Smith, K.A., Structure-activity studies of interleukin-2, *Science*, 234, 349, 1986.
544. Ju, G., Collins, L., Kaffka, K.L., Tsien, W.-H., Chizzonite, R., Crowl, R., Bhatt, R., and Kilian, P.L., Structure-function analysis of human interleukin-2: identification of amino acid residues required for biological activity, *J. Biol. Chem.*, 262, 5723, 1987.
545. Conradt, H.S., Hauser, H., Lorenz, C., Mohr, H., and Plessing, A., Posttranslational modification of interleukin-2 is a late event during activation of human T lymphocytes by ionophore A23187 and phorbol ester, *Biochem. Biophys. Res. Commun.*, 150, 97, 1988.
546. Shows, T., Eddy, R., Haley, L., Byers, M., Henry, M., Fujita, T., Matsui, H., and Tanaguchi, T., Interleukin 2 *(IL2)* is assigned to human chromosome 4, *Somat. Cell Mol. Genet.*, 10, 315, 1984.
547. Seigel, L.J., Harper, M.E., Wong-Staal, F., Gallo, R.C., Nash, W.G., and O'Brien, S.J., Gene for T-cell growth factor: location on human chromosome 4q and feline chromosome B1, *Science*, 223, 175, 1984.
548. Holbrook, N.J., Smith, K.A., Fornace, A.J., Jr., Comeau, C.M., Wiskocil, R.L., and Crabtree, G.R., T-cell growth factor: complete nucleotide sequence and organization of the gene in normal and malignant cells, *Proc. Natl. Acad. Sci. U.S.A.*, 81, 1634, 1984.
549. Clark, S.C., Arya, S.K., Wong-Staal, F., Matsumoto-Kobayashi, M., Kay, R.M., Kaufman, R.J., Brown, E.L., Shoemaker, C., Copeland, T., Oroszlan, S., Smith, K., Sarngadharan, M.G., Lindner, S.G., and Gallo, R.C., Human T-cell growth factor: partial amino acid sequence, cDNA cloning, and organization and expression in normal and leukemic cells, *Proc. Natl. Acad. Sci. U.S.A.*, 81, 2543, 1984.
550. Fuse, A., Fujita, T., Yasumitsu, H., Kashima, N., Hasegawa, K., and Taniguchi, T., Organization and structure of the mouse interleukin-2 gene, *Nucleic Acids Res.*, 12, 9323, 1984.
551. Kato, K., Yamada, T., Kawahara, K., Onda, H., Asano, T., Sugino, H., and Kakinuma, A., Purification and characterization of recombinant human interleukin-2 produced in *Escherichia coli*, *Biochem. Biophys. Res. Commun.*, 130, 692, 1985.

552. **Ishida, N., Kanomori, H., Noma, T., Nikaido, T., Sabe, H., Suzuki, N., Shimizu, A., and Honjo, T.,** Molecular cloning and structure of the human interleukin 2 gene, *Nucleic Acids Res.,* 13, 7579, 1985.
553. **Lindenmaier, W., Dittmar, K.E.J., Hauser, H., Necker, A., and Sebald, W.,** Isolation of a functional human interleukin 2 gene from a cosmid library by recombination in vivo, *Gene,* 39, 33, 1985.
554. **Mita, S., Maeda, S., and Shimada, K.,** Characterization of human genomic DNA sequences homologous to the interleukin-2 cDNA, *Biochem. Biophys. Res. Commun.,* 138, 966, 1986.
555. **Weir, M.P. and Sparks, J.,** Purification and renaturation of recombinant human interleukin-2, *Biochem. J.,* 245, 85, 1987.
556. **Sano, C., Ishikawa, K., Nagashima, N., Tsuji, T., Kawakita, T., Fukuhara, K., Mitsui, Y., and Iitaka, Y.,** Crystallization and preliminary X-ray studies of human recombinant interleukin-2, *J. Biol. Chem.,* 262, 4766, 1987.
557. **Muñoz, A., Perez-Aranda, A., and Barbero, J.L.,** Cloning and expression of human interleukin 2 in *Streptomyces lividans* using the *Escherichia coli* consensus promoter, *Biochem. Biophys. Res. Commun.,* 133, 511, 1985.
558. **Kashima, N., Nishi-Takaoka, C., Fujita, T., Taki, S., Yamada, G., Hamuro, J., and Taniguchi, T.,** Unique structure of murine interleukin-2 as deduced from cloned cDNAs, *Nature,* 313, 402, 1985.
559. **Cerretti, D.P., McKereghan, K., Larsen, A., Cantrell, M.A., Anderson, D., Gillis, S., Cosman, D., and Baker, P.E.,** Cloning, sequence, and expression of bovine interleukin 2, *Proc. Natl. Acad. Sci. U.S.A.,* 83, 3223, 1986.
560. **Serfling, E., Barthelmäs, R., Pfeuffer, I., Schenck, B., Zarius, S., Swoboda, R., Mercurio, F., and Karin, M.,** Ubiquitous and lymphocyte-specific factors are involved in the induction of the mouse interleukin 2 gene in T lymphocytes, *EMBO J.,* 8, 465, 1989.
561. **Chen, D. and Rothenberg, E.V.,** Molecular basis for developmental changes in interleukin-2 gene inducibility, *Mol. Cell. Biol.,* 13, 228, 1993.
562. **Ullman, K.S., Flanagan, W.M., Edwards, C.A., and Crabtree, G.R.,** Activation of early gene expression in T lymphocytes by Oct-1 and an inducible protein, OAP[40], *Science,* 254, 558, 1991.
563. **Baldari, C.T., Macchia, G., and Telford, J.L.,** Interleukin-2 promoter activation in T-cells expressing activated Ha-ras, *J. Biol. Chem.,* 267, 4289, 1992.
564. **Shaw, J., Meerovitch, K., Bleackley, R.C., and Paetkau, V.,** Mechanisms regulating the level of IL-2 mRNA in T lymphocytes, *J. Immunol.,* 140, 2243, 1988.
565. **Fujita, T., Shibuya, H., Ohashi, T., Yamanishi, K., and Taniguchi, T.,** Regulation of human interleukin-2 gene: functional DNA sequences in the 5′ flanking region for the gene expression in activated T lymphocytes, *Cell,* 46, 401, 1986.
566. **Hardy, K.J., Peterlin, B.M., Atchison, R.E., and Stobo, J.D.,** Regulation of expression of the human interferon γ gene, *Proc. Natl. Acad. Sci. U.S.A.,* 82, 8173, 1985.
567. **Holbrook, N.J., Lieber, M., and Crabtree, G.R.,** DNA sequence of the 5′ flanking region of the human interleukin 2 gene: homologies with adult T-cell leukemia virus, *Nucleic Acids Res.,* 12, 5005, 1984.
568. **Wong-Staal, F. and Gallo, R.C.,** Human T-lymphotropic retroviruses, *Nature,* 317, 395, 1985.
569. **Hunsmann, G. and Hinuma, Y.,** Human adult T-cell leukemia virus and its association with disease, *Adv. Viral Oncol.,* 5, 147, 1985.
570. **Yoshida, M.,** Expression of the HTLV-1 genome and its association with a unique T-cell malignancy, *Biochim. Biophys. Acta,* 907, 145, 1987.
571. **Hjelle, B.,** Human T-cell leukemia/lymphoma viruses, *Arch. Pathol. Lab. Med.,* 115, 440, 1991.
572. **Essex, M.,** Immunopathogenesis of HTLV, *AIDS Res. Hum. Retrovirus,* 8, 719, 1992.
573. **Palker, T.J.,** Human T-cell lymphotropic viruses: review and prospects for antiviral therapy, *Antiviral Chem. Chemother.,* 3, 127, 1992.
574. **Chen, S.J., Holbrook, N.J., Mitchell, K.F., Vallone, C.A., Greengard, J.S., Crabtree, G.R., and Lin, Y.,** A viral long terminal repeat in the interleukin 2 gene of a cell line that constitutively produces interleukin 2, *Proc. Natl. Acad. Sci. U.S.A.,* 82, 7284, 1985.
575. **Renan, M.J.,** Sequence homologies in the control regions of c-*myc,* c-*fos,* HTLV and the interleukin 2 receptor, *Cancer Lett.,* 28, 69, 1985.
576. **McGuire, K.L. and Rothenberg, E.V.,** Inducibility of interleukin-2 RNA expression in individual mature and immature T lymphocytes, *EMBO J.,* 6, 939, 1987.

577. **Stanley, J.B., Gorczynski, R., Huang, C.-K., Love, J., and Mills, G.B.,** Tyrosine phosphorylation is an obligatory event in IL-2 secretion, *J. Immunol.,* 145, 2189, 1990.
578. **Cardenas, J.M., Marshall, P., Henderson, B., and Altman, A.,** Human interleukin 2. Quantitation by a sensitive radioimmunoassay, *J. Immunol. Methods,* 89, 181, 1986.
579. **Weiss, A., Shields, R., Newton, M., Manger, B., and Imboden, J.,** Ligand-receptor interactions required for commitment to the activation of the interleukin 2 gene, *J. Immunol.,* 138, 2169, 1987.
580. **Croll, A.D., Siggins, K.W., Morris, A.G., and Pither, J.M.,** The induction of IFN-γ production and m-RNAs of interleukin 2 and IFN-γ by phorbol esters and a calcium ionophore, *Biochem. Biophys. Res. Commun.,* 146, 927, 1987.
581. **Grabstein, K., Dower, S., Gillis, S., Urdal, D., and Larsen, A.,** Expression of interleukin 2, interferon-γ, and the IL 2 receptor by human peripheral blood lymphocytes, *J. Immunol.,* 136, 4503, 1986.
582. **Efrat, S. and Kaempfer, R.,** Control of biologically active interleukin 2 messenger RNA formation in induced human lymphocytes, *Proc. Natl. Acad. Sci. U.S.A.,* 81, 2601, 1984.
583. **Taira, S., Matsui, M., Hayakawa, K., Yokoyama, T., and Nariuchi, H.,** Interleukin secretion by B cell lines and splenic B cells stimulated with calcium ionophore and phorbol ester, *J. Immunol.,* 139, 2957, 1987.
584. **Boehm, K.D., Kelley, M.F., and Ilan, J.,** The interleukin 2 gene is expressed in the syncytiotrophoblast of human placenta, *Proc. Natl. Acad. Sci. U.S.A.,* 86, 656, 1989.
585. **Modiano, J.F., Kolp, R., Lamb, R.J., and Nowell, P.C.,** Protein kinase C regulates both production and secretion of interleukin-2, *J. Biol. Chem.,* 266, 10552, 1991.
586. **Lugo, J.P., Krishnan, S.N., Sailor, R.D., and Rothenberg, E.V.,** Early precursor thymocytes can produce interleukin 2 upon stimulation with calcium ionophore and phorbol ester, *Proc. Natl. Acad. Sci. U.S.A.,* 83, 1862, 1986.
587. **Mohr, H., Monner, D., and Plessing, A.,** Calcium ionophore A23187 in the presence of phorbol ester PMA: a potent inducer of interleukin 2 and interferon-γ synthesis by human blood cells, *Immunobiology,* 171, 195, 1986.
588. **Arya, S.K. and Gallo, R.C.,** Transcriptional modulation of human T-cell growth factor gene by phorbol ester and interleukin 1, *Biochemistry,* 23, 6685, 1984.
589. **Truneh, A., Simon, P., and Schmitt-Verhulst, A.-M.,** Interleukin 1 and protein kinase C activator are dissimilar in their effects on the IL-2 receptor expression and IL-2 secretion by T lymphocytes, *Cell. Immunol.,* 103, 365, 1986.
590. **Kelleher, D., Pandol, S.J., and Kagnoff, M.F.,** Phorbol myristate acetate induces IL-2 secretion by HUT 78 cells by a mechanism independent of protein kinase C translocation, *Immunology,* 63, 351, 1988.
591. **Harrison, J.R., Lynch, K.R., and Sando, J.J.,** Phorbol esters induce interleukin 2 mRNA in sensitive but not in resistant EL4 cells, *J. Biol. Chem.,* 262, 234, 1987.
592. **Goodwin, J.S., Atluru, D., Sierakowski, S., and Llanos, E.A.,** Mechanism of action of glucocorticoids. Inhibition of T-cell proliferation and interleukin 2 production by hydrocortisone is reversed by leukotriene B_4, *J. Clin. Invest.,* 77, 1244, 1986.
593. **Matsui, T., Takanashi, R., Nakao, Y., Koizumi, T., Katakami, Y., Mihara, K., Sugiyama, T., and Fujita, T.,** 1,25-dihydroxyvitamin D_3-regulated expression of genes involved in human T-lymphocyte proliferation and differentiation, *Cancer Res.,* 46, 5827, 1986.
594. **Ye, R.D., Prossnitz, E.R., Zou, A.H., and Cochrane, C.G.,** Characterization of a human cDNA that encodes a functional receptor for platelet activating factor, *Biochem. Biophys. Res. Commun.,* 180, 105, 1991.
595. **Sugimoto, T., Tsuchimochi, H., McGregor, C.G.A., Mutoh, H., Shimizu, T., and Kurachi, Y.,** Molecular cloning and characterization of the platelet-activating factor receptor gene expressed in the human heart, *Biochem. Biophys. Res. Commun.,* 189, 617, 1992.
596. **Schulam, P.G., Kuruvilla, A., Putcha, G., Mangus, L., Franklin-Johnson, J., and Shearer, W.T.,** Platelet-activating factor induces phospholipid turnover, calcium influx, arachidonic acid liberation, eicosanoid generation, and oncogene expression in a human B cell line, *J. Immunol.,* 146, 1642, 1991.
597. **Gomez-Cambronero, J., Wang, E., Johnson, G., Huang, C.-K., and Sha'afi, R.I.,** Platelet-activating factor induces tyrosine phosphorylation in human neutrophils, *J. Biol. Chem.,* 268, 6240, 1991.
598. **Dhar, A. and Shukla, S.D.,** Involvement of $pp60^{c-src}$ in platelet-activating factor-stimulated platelets. Evidence for translocation from cytosol to membrane, *J. Biol. Chem.,* 266, 18797, 1991.

599. **Tripathi, Y.B., Lim, R., Fernandez-Gallardo, S., Kandala, J.C., Guntaka, R.V., and Shukla, S.D.,** Involvement of tyrosine kinase and protein kinase C in platelet-activating factor-induced c-*fos* gene expression in A-431 cells, *Biochem. J.,* 286, 527, 1992.
600. **Rola-Pleszczynski, M., Pignol, B., Pouliot, C., and Braquet, P.,** Inhibition of human lymphocyte proliferation and interleukin 2 production by platelet activating factor (PAF-acether); reversal by a specific antagonist, BN 5201, *Biochem. Biophys. Res. Commun.,* 142, 754, 1987.
601. **Negoro, S., Hara, H., Miyata, S., Saiki, O., Tanaka, T., Yoshizaki, K., Igarashi, T., and Kishimoto, S.,** Mechanisms of age-related decline in antigen-specific T-cell proliferative response: IL-2 receptor expression and recombinant IL-2 induced proliferative response of purified Tac-positive T cells, *Mech. Ageing Dev.,* 36, 223, 1986.
602. **Nagel, J.E., Chopra, R.K., Chrest, F.J., McCoy, M.T., Schneider, E.L., Holbrook, N.J., and Adler, W.H.,** Decreased proliferation, interleukin 2 synthesis, and interleukin 2 receptor expression are accompanied by decreased mRNA expression in phytohemagglutinin-stimulated cells from elderly donors, *J. Clin Invest.,* 81, 1096, 1988.
603. **Bruley-Rosset, M. and Payelle, B.,** Deficient tumor-specific immunity in old mice: *in vivo* mediation by suppressor cells, and correction of the defect by interleukin 2 supplementation *in vitro* but not *in vivo, Eur. J. Immunol.,* 17, 307, 1987.
604. **Proust, J.J., Kittur, D.S., Buchholz, M.A., and Nordin, A.A.,** Restricted expression of mitogen-induced high affinity IL-2 receptors in aging mice, *J. Immunol.,* 141, 4209, 1988.
605. **Wu, W., Pahlavani, M., Cheung, H.T., and Richardson, A.,** The effect of aging on the expression of interleukin 2 messenger ribonucleic acid, *Cell. Immunol.,* 100, 224, 1986.
606. **Holbrook, N.J., Chopra, R.K., McCoy, M.T., Nagel, J.E., Powers, D.C., Adler, W.H., and Schneider, E.L.,** Expression of interleukin and interleukin 2 receptor in aging rats, *Cell. Immunol.,* 120, 1, 1989.
607. **Holbrook, N.J., Gulino, A., Durand, D., Lin, Y., and Crabtree, G.R.,** Transcriptional activity of the gibbon ape leukemia virus in the interleukin 2 gene of MLA 144 cells, *Virology,* 159, 178, 1987.
608. **O'Shea, J.J., Ashwell, J.D., Bailey, T.L., Cross, S.L., Samelson, L.E., and Klausner, R.D.,** Expression of v-*src* in a murine T-cell hybridoma results in constitutive T-cell receptor phosphorylation and interleukin 2 production, *Proc. Natl. Acad. Sci. U.S.A.,* 88, 1741, 1991.
609. **Kucharz, E.J. and Goodwin, J.S.,** Serum inhibitors of interleukin-2, *Life Sci.,* 42, 1485, 1988.
610. **Kucharz, E.J., Sierakowski, S., and Goodwin, J.S.,** Decreased activity of interleukin-2 inhibitor in plasma of patients with systemic lupus erythematosus, *Clin. Rheumatol.,* 6, 87, 1987.
611. **Greene, W.C. and Leonard, W.J.,** The human interleukin-2 receptor, *Annu. Rev. Immunol.,* 4, 69, 1986.
612. **Waldmann, T.A.,** The structure, function, and expression of interleukin-2 receptors on normal and malignant lymphocytes, *Science,* 232, 727, 1986.
613. **Smith, K.A.,** The interleukin 2 receptor, *Annu. Rev. Cell Biol.,* 5, 397, 1989.
614. **Kuziel, W.A. and Greene, W.C.,** Interleukin-2 and the IL-2 receptor: new insights into structure and function, *J. Invest. Dermatol.,* 84, 27S, 1990.
615. **Waldmann, T.A.,** The interleukin-2 receptor, *J. Biol. Chem.,* 266, 2681, 1991.
616. **Minami, Y., Kono, T., Yamada, K., and Taniguchi, T.,** The interleukin-2 receptors. Insights into a complex signalling mechanism, *Biochim. Biophys. Acta,* 1114, 163, 1992.
617. **Minami, Y., Kono, T., Miyazaki, T., and Taniguchi, T.,** The IL-2 receptor complex. Its structure, function, and target tissues, *Annu. Rev. Immunol.,* 11, 245, 1993.
618. **Urdal, D.L., March, C.J., Gillis, S., Larsen, A., and Dower, S.K.,** Purification and chemical characterization of the receptor for interleukin 2 from activated human T lymphocytes and from a human T-cell lymphoma cell line, *Proc. Natl. Acad. Sci. U.S.A.,* 81, 6481, 1984.
619. **Rand, T.H., Silberstein, D.S., Kornfeld, H., and Weller, P.F.,** Human eosinophils express functional interleukin-2 receptors, *J. Clin. Invest.,* 88, 825, 1991.
620. **Saito, Y., Tada, H., Sabe, H., and Honjo, T.,** Biochemical evidence for a third chain of the interleukin-2 receptor, *J. Biol. Chem.,* 266, 22186, 1991.
621. **Noguchi, M., Adelstein, S., Caoi, X.Q., and Leonard, W.J.,** Characterization of the human interleukin-2 receptor γ-chain gene, *J. Biol. Chem.,* 268, 13601, 1993.
622. **Leonard, W.J., Donlon, T.A., Lebo, R.V., and Greene, W.C.,** Localization of the gene encoding the human interleukin-2 receptor on chromosome 10, *Science,* 228, 1547, 1985.

623. Leonard, W.J., Depper, J.M., Kanehisa, M., Krönke, M., Peffer, N.J., Svetlik, P.B., Sullivan, M., and Greene, W.C., Structure of the human interleukin-2 receptor gene, *Science*, 230, 633, 1985.
624. Ferrari, S., Cannizzaro, L.A., Battini, R., Huebner, K., and Baserga, R., The gene encoding human vimentin is located on the short arm of chromosome 10, *Am. J. Hum. Genet.*, 41, 616, 1987.
625. Kaczmarek, L., Calabretta, B., and Baserga, R., Effect of interleukin-2 on the expression of cell cycle genes in human T lymphocytes, *Biochem. Biophys. Res. Commun.*, 133, 410, 1985.
626. Suzuki, N., Matsunami, N., Kanamori, H., Ishida, N., Shimizu, A., Yaoita, Y., Nikaido, T., and Honjo, T., The human IL-2 receptor gene contains a positive regulatory element that functions in cultured cells and cell-free extracts, *J. Biol. Chem.*, 262, 5079, 1987.
627. Nikaido, T., Shimizu, A., Ishida, N., Sabe, H., Teshigawara, K., Maeda, M., Uchiyama, T., Yodoi, J., and Honjo, T., Molecular cloning of cDNA encoding human interleukin-2 receptor, *Nature*, 311, 631, 1984.
628. Leonard, W.J., Depper, J.M., Crabtree, G.R., Rudikoff, S., Pumphrey, J., Robb, R.J., Krönke, M., Svetlik, P.B., Peffer, N.J., Waldmann, T.A., and Greene, W.C., Molecular cloning and expression of cDNAs for the human interleukin-2 receptor, *Nature*, 311, 626, 1984.
629. Cosman, D., Cerretti, D.P., Larsen, A., Park, L., March, C., Dower, S., Gillis, S., and Urdal, D., Cloning, sequence and expression of human interleukin-2 receptor, *Nature*, 312, 768, 1984.
630. Greene, W.C., Robb, R.J., Svetlik, P.B., Rusk, C.M., Depper, J.M., and Leonard, W.J., Stable expression of cDNA encoding the human interleukin 2 receptor in eukaryotic cells, *J. Exp. Med.*, 162, 363, 1985.
631. Kondo, S., Shimizu, A., Maeda, M., Tagaya, Y., Yodoi, J., and Honjo, T., Expression of functional human interleukin-2 receptor in mouse T cells by cDNA transfection, *Nature*, 320, 75, 1986.
632. Chanda, P.K., Chen, G.-F.T., Baine, Y., Leonard, W.J., Greene, W.C., Chang, T.W., and Chang, N.T., Expression of human interleukin-2 receptor cDNA in E. coli, *Biochem. Biophys. Res. Commun.*, 141, 804, 1986.
633. Hakimi, J., Seals, C., Anderson, L.E., Podlaski, F.J., Lin, P., Danho, W., Jenson, J.C., Perkins, A., Donadio, P.E., Familletti, P.C., Pan, Y.-C.E., Tsien, W.-H., Chizzonite, R.A., Casabo, L., Nelson, D.L., and Cullen, B.R., Biochemical and functional analysis of soluble human interleukin-2 receptor produced in rodent cells. Solid-phase reconstitution of a receptor-ligand binding reaction, *J. Biol. Chem.*, 262, 17336, 1987.
634. Kuo, L.-M., Rusk, C.M., and Robb, R.J., Structure-function relationships for the IL 2-receptor system. II. Localization of an IL 2 binding site on high and low affinity receptors, *J. Biol. Chem.*, 137, 1544, 1986.
635. Shackelford, D.A. and Trowbridge, I.S., Evidence for two extracellular domains in the human interleukin-2 receptor: localization of IL-2 binding, *EMBO J.*, 5, 3275, 1986.
636. Miedel, M.C., Hulmes, J.D., and Pan, Y.-C.E., Limited proteolysis of recombinant human soluble interleukin-2 receptor. Identification of an interleukin-2 binding core, *J. Biol. Chem.*, 264, 21097, 1989.
637. Cullen, B.R., Podlaski, F.J., Peffer, N.J., Hosking, J.B., and Greene, W.C., Sequence requirements for ligand binding and cell surface expression of the Tac antigen, a human interleukin-2 receptor, *J. Biol. Chem.*, 263, 4900, 1988.
638. Miedel, M.C., Hulmes, J.D., Weber, D.V., Bailon, P., and Pan, Y.-C.E., Structural analysis of recombinant soluble human interleukin-2 receptor, *Biochem. Biophys. Res. Commun.*, 154, 372, 1988.
639. Gallis, B., Lewis, A., Wignall, J., Alpert, A., Mochizuki, D.Y., Cosman, D., Hopp, T., and Urdal, D., Phosphorylation of the human interleukin-2 receptor and a synthetic peptide identical to its C-terminal, cytoplasmic domain, *J. Biol. Chem.*, 261, 5075, 1986.
640. Hatakeyama, M., Doi, T., Kono, T., Maruyama, M., Minamoto, S., Mori, H., Kobayashi, M., Uchiyama, T., and Taniguchi, T., Transmembrane signaling of interleukin 2 receptor. Conformation and function of human interleukin 2 receptor (p55)/insulin receptor chimeric molecules, *J. Exp. Med.*, 166, 362, 1987.
641. Sharon, M., Klausner, R.D., Cullen, B.R., Chizzonite, R., and Leonard, W.J., Novel interleukin-2 receptor subunit detected by cross-linking under high-affinity conditions, *Science*, 234, 859, 1986.
642. Tsudo, M., Kozak, R.W., Goldman, C.K., and Waldmann, T.A., Demonstration of a non-Tac peptide that binds interleukin 2: a potential participant in a multichain interleukin 2 receptor complex, *Proc. Natl. Acad. Sci. U.S.A.*, 83, 9694, 1986.

643. **Teshigawara, K., Wang, H.-M., Kato, K., and Smith, K.A.,** Interleukin 2 high-affinity receptor expression requires two distinct binding proteins, *J. Exp. Med.,* 165, 223, 1987.
644. **Robb, R.J., Rusk, C.M., Yodoi, J., and Greene, W.C.,** Interleukin 2 binding molecule distinct from the Tac protein: analysis of its role in formation of high-affinity receptors, *Proc. Natl. Acad. Sci. U.S.A.,* 84, 2002, 1987.
645. **Robb, R.J. and Greene, W.C.,** Internalization of interleukin 2 is mediated by the β chain of the high-affinity of the high-affinity interleukin 2 receptor, *J. Exp. Med.,* 165, 1201, 1987.
646. **Dukovich, M., Wano, Y., Thuy, L.B., Katz, P., Cullen, B.R., Kehrl, J.H., and Greene, W.C.,** A second human interleukin-2 binding protein that may be a component of high-affinity interleukin-2 receptors, *Nature,* 327, 518, 1987.
647. **Lowenthal, J.W. and Greene, W.C.,** Contrasting interleukin 2 binding properties of the α (p55) and β (p70) protein subunits of the human high-affinity interleukin 2 receptor, *J. Exp. Med.,* 166, 1156, 1987.
648. **Tsudo, M., Kozak, R.W., Goldman, C.K., and Waldmann, T.A.,** Contribution of a p75 interleukin 2 binding peptide to a high-affinity interleukin 2 receptor complex, *Proc. Natl. Acad. Sci. U.S.A.,* 84, 4215, 1987.
649. **Hatakeyama, M., Tsudo, M., Minamoto, S., Kono, T., Doi, T., Miyata, T., Miyasaka, M., and Taniguchi, T.,** Interleukin-2 receptor β chain gene: generation of three receptor forms by cloned human α and β chain cDNAs, *Science,* 244, 551, 1989.
650. **Shibuya, H., Yoneyama, M., Nakamura, Y., Harada, H., Hatakeyama, M., Minamoto, S., Kono, T., Doi, T., White, R., and Taniguchi, T.,** The human interleukin-2 receptor β-chain gene: genomic organization, promoter analysis and chromosomal assignment, *Nucleic Acids Res.,* 18, 3697, 1990.
651. **Tsudo, M., Goldman, C.K., Bongiovanni, K.F., Chan, W.C., Winton, E.F., Yagita, M., Grimm, E.A., and Waldmann, T.A.,** The p75 peptide is the receptor for interleukin 2 expressed on large granular lymphocytes and is responsible for the interleukin 2 activation of these cells, *Proc. Natl. Acad. Sci. U.S.A.,* 84, 5394, 1987.
652. **Siegel, J.P., Sharon, M., Smith, P.L., and Leonard, W.J.,** The IL-2 receptor β chain (p70): role in mediating signals for LAK, NK, and proliferative activities, *Science,* 238, 75, 1987.
653. **Tanaka, T., Saiki, O., Doi, S., Negoro, S., and Kishimoto, S.,** Interleukin 2 functions through novel interleukin 2 binding molecules in T cells, *J. Immunol.,* 140, 470, 1988.
654. **Saiki, O., Tanaka, T., Doi, S., and Kishimoto, S.,** Expression and the functional role of a p70/75 interleukin 2-binding molecule in human B cell, *J. Immunol.,* 140, 853, 1988.
655. **Tanaka, T., Saiki, O., Doi, S., Fuji, M., Sugamura, K., Hara, H., Negoro, S., and Kishimoto, S.,** Novel receptor-mediated internalization 2 in B cells, *J. Immunol.,* 140, 866, 1988.
656. **Saltzman, E.M., Luhowskyj, S.M., and Casnellie, J.E.,** The 75,000-dalton interleukin-2 receptor transmits a signal for the activation of a tyrosine protein kinase, *J. Biol. Chem.,* 264, 19979, 1989.
657. **Hatakeyama, M., Mori, H., Doi, T., and Taniguchi, T.,** A restricted cytoplasmic region of IL-2 receptor β chain is essential for growth signal transduction but not for ligand binding and internalization, *Cell,* 59, 837, 1989.
658. **Liang, S.-M., Lee, N., Zoon, K.C., Manischewitz, J.F., Chollet, A., Liang, C.-M., and Quinnan, G.V.,** Biological characterization of human interleukin-2 mutant proteins: structure-activity relationship studies, *J. Biol. Chem.,* 263, 4768, 1988.
659. **Wang, H.-M. and Smith, K.A.,** The interleukin 2 receptor: functional consequences of its biomolecular structure, *J. Exp. Med.,* 166, 1055, 1987.
660. **Mills, G.B., Cragoe, E.J., Jr., Gelfand, E.W., and Grinstein, S.,** Interleukin 2 induces a rapid increase in intracellular pH through activation of a Na^+/H^+ antiport. Cytoplasmic alkalinization is not required for lymphocyte proliferation, *J. Biol. Chem.,* 260, 12500, 1985.
661. **Espinoza-Delgado, I., Ortaldo, J.R., Winkler-Pickett, R., Sugamura, K., Varesio, L., and Longo, D.L.,** Expression and role of p75 interleukin 2 receptor on human monocytes, *J. Exp. Med.,* 171, 1821, 1990.
662. **Jankovic, D.L., Rebollo, A., Kumar, A., Gilbert, M., and Theze, J.,** IL-2-dependent proliferation of murine T cells requires expression of both the p55 and p70 subunits of the IL-2 receptor, *J. Immunol.,* 145, 4136, 1990.
663. **Benedict, S.H., Mills, G.B., and Gelfand, E.W.,** Interleukin 2 activates a receptor-associated protein kinase, *J. Immunol.,* 139, 1694, 1987.

664. **Farrar, W.L. and Ferris, D.K.,** Two-dimensional analysis of interleukin 2-regulated tyrosine kinase activation mediated by the p70-75 β subunit of the interleukin 2 receptor, *J. Biol. Chem.,* 264, 12562, 1989.
665. **Mills, G.B., May, C., McGill, M., Fung, M., Baker, M., Sutherland, R., and Greene, W.C.,** Interleukin 2-induced tyrosine phosphorylation. Interleukin 2 receptor β is tyrosine phosphorylated, *J. Biol. Chem.,* 265, 3561, 1990.
666. **Hatakeyama, M., Kono, T., Kobayashi, N., Kawahara, A., Levin, S.D., Perlmutter, R.M., and Taniguchi, T.,** Interaction of the IL-2 receptor with the *src*-family kinase p56[lck]: identification of novel intermolecular association, *Science,* 252, 1523, 1991.
667. **Minami, Y., Kono, T., Yamada, K., Kobayashi, N., Kawahara, A., Perlmutter, R.M., and Taniguchi, T.,** Association of p56[lck] with IL-2 receptor is critical for the IL-2-induced activation of p56[lck], *EMBO J.,* 12, 759, 1993.
668. **Maslinski, W., Remillard, B., Tsudo, M., and Strom, T.B.,** Interleukin-2 (IL-2) induces tyrosine kinase-dependent translocation of active Raf-1 from the IL-2 receptor into the cytosol, *J. Biol. Chem.,* 267, 15281, 1992.
669. **Kawamura, H., Sharrow, S.O., Alling, D.W., Stephany, D., York-Jolley, J., and Berzofsky, J.A.,** Interleukin 2 receptor expression in unstimulated murine splenic T cells: localization to L3T4[+] cells and regulation by non-H-2-linked genes, *J. Exp. Med.,* 86, 1376, 1986.
670. **Smith, K.A. and Cantrell, D.A.,** Interleukin 2 regulates its own receptors, *Proc. Natl. Acad. Sci. U.S.A.,* 82, 864, 1985.
671. **Ceredig, R., Lowenthal, J.W., Nabholz, M., and MacDonald, H.R.,** Expression of interleukin-2 receptors as a differentiation marker on intrathymic stem cells, *Nature,* 314, 98, 1985.
672. **Raulet, D.H.,** Expression and function of interleukin-2 receptors on immature thymocytes, *Nature,* 314, 101, 1985.
673. **Sztein, M.B., Serrate, S.A., and Goldstein, A.L.,** Modulation of interleukin 2 receptor expression on normal human lymphocytes by thymic hormones, *Proc. Natl. Acad. Sci. U.S.A.,* 83, 6107, 1986.
674. **Gauchat, J.-F., Khandjian, E.W., and Weil, R.,** Cyclosporin A prevents induction of the interleukin 2 receptor gene in cultured murine thymocytes, *Proc. Natl. Acad. Sci. U.S.A.,* 83, 6430, 1986.
675. **Duprez, V., Cornet, V., and Dautry-Varsat, A.,** Down-regulation of high affinity IL-2 receptors in a human tumor T-cell line. Interleukin 2 increases the rate of surface receptor decay, *J. Biol. Chem.,* 263, 12860, 1988.
676. **Narumiya, S., Hirata, M., Nanba, T., Nikaido, T., Taniguchi, Y., Tagaya, Y., Okada, M., Mitsuya, H., and Yodoi, J.,** Activation of interleukin-2 receptor gene by forskolin and cyclic AMP analogs, *Biochem. Biophys. Res. Commun.,* 143, 753, 1987.
677. **Patarca, R., Schwartz, J., Singh, R.P., Kong, Q.-T., Murthy, E., Anderson, Y., Sheng, F.-Y.W., Singh, P., Johnson, K.A., Guarnagia, S.M., Durfee, T., Blattner, F., and Cantor, H.,** Protein rpt-1, an intracellular protein from helper/inducer T cells that regulates gene expression of interleukin 2 receptor and human immunodeficiency virus type 1, *Proc. Natl. Acad. Sci. U.S.A.,* 85, 2733, 1988.
678. **Hardt, C., Sato, N., and Wagner, H.,** Functional and biochemical characteristics of a murine interleukin 2 receptor-inducing factor, *Eur. J. Immunol.,* 17, 209, 1987.
679. **Hardt, C.,** Activation of murine Cd8[+] lymphocytes: two distinct signals regulate c-*myc* and interleukin 2 receptor RNA expression, *Eur. J. Immunol.,* 17, 1711, 1987.
680. **Ashwell, J.D., Robb, R.J., and Malek, T.R.,** Proliferation of T lymphocytes in response to interleukin 2 varies with their state of activation, *J. Immunol.,* 137, 2572, 1986.
681. **Palacios, R. and von Boehmer, H.,** Requirements for growth of immature thymocytes from fetal and adult mice *in vitro, Eur. J. Immunol.,* 16, 12, 1986.
682. **Gullberg, M.,** Structural analysis of high- vs. low-affinity interleukin-2 receptors by means of selective expression of distinct receptor classes, *EMBO J.,* 5, 2171, 1986.
683. **Weissman, A.M., Harford, J.B., Svetlik, P.B., Leonard, W.L., Depper, J.M., Waldmann, T.A., Greene, W.C., and Klausner, R.D.,** Only high-affinity receptors for interleukin 2 mediate internalization of the ligand, *Proc. Natl. Acad. Sci. U.S.A.,* 83, 1463, 1986.
684. **Robb, R.J. and Rusk, C.M.,** High and low affinity receptors for interleukin 2: implications of pronase, phorbol ester, and cell membrane studies upon the basis for differential ligand affinities, *J. Immunol.,* 137, 142, 1986.

685. **Kondo, S., Shimizu, A., Saito, Y., Kinoshita, M., and Honjo, T.,** Molecular basis for two different affinity states of the interleukin 2 receptor: affinity conversion model, *Proc. Natl. Acad. Sci. U.S.A.,* 83, 9026, 1986.
686. **Feldman, R.D., Hunninghake, G.W., and McArdle, W.L.,** β-Adrenergic receptor-mediated suppression of interleukin 2 receptors in human lymphocytes, *J. Immunol.,* 139, 3355, 1987.
687. **Mingari, M.C., Gerosa, F., Carra, G., Accolla, R.S., Moretta, A., Zubler, R.H., Waldmann, T.A., and Moretta, L.,** Human interleukin-2 promotes proliferation of activated B cells via surface receptors similar to those of activated T cells, *Nature,* 312, 641, 1984.
688. **Sauerwein, R.W., Van der Meer, W.G.J., Dräger, A., and Aarden, L.A.,** Interleukin 2 induces T cell dependent IgM production in human B cells, *Eur. J. Immunol.,* 15, 611, 1985.
689. **Rambaldi, A., Young, D.C., Herrmann, F., Cannistra, S.A., and Griffin, J.D.,** Interferon-γ induces expression of the interleukin 2 receptor gene in human monocytes, *Eur. J. Immunol.,* 17, 153, 1987.
690. **Fujii, M., Sugamura, K., Sano, K., Nakai, M., Sugita, K., and Hinuma, Y.,** High-affinity receptor-mediated internalization and degradation of interleukin 2 in human T cells, *J. Exp. Med.,* 163, 550, 1986.
691. **Lowenthal, J.W., MacDonald, H.R., and Iacopetta, B.J.,** Intracellular pathway of interleukin 2 following receptor-mediated endocytosis, *Eur. J. Immunol.,* 16, 1461, 1986.
692. **Duprez, V. and Dautry-Varsat, A.,** Receptor-mediated endocytosis of interleukin 2 in a human tumor T-cell line. Degradation of interleukin 2 and evidence for the absence of recycling of interleukin receptors, *J. Biol. Chem.,* 261, 15450, 1986.
693. **Duprez, V., Ferrer, M., and Dautry-Varsat, A.,** High-affinity interleukin-2 receptor α and β chains are internalized and remain associated inside the cells after interleukin-2 endocytosis, *J. Biol. Chem.,* 267, 18639, 1992.
694. **Pui, C.-H.,** Serum interleukin-2 receptor: clinical and biological implications, *Leukemia,* 3, 323, 1989.
695. **Rubin, L.A.,** The soluble interleukin-2 receptor: biology, function, and clinical application, *Ann. Intern. Med.,* 113, 619, 1990.
696. **Zerler, B.,** The soluble interleukin-2 receptor as a marker for human neoplasia and immune status, *Cancer Cells,* 3, 471, 1991.
697. **Schirrmacher, V., Josimovic-Alasevic, O., Osawa, H., and Diamantstein, T.,** Determination of cell-free interleukin 2 receptor level in the serum of normal animals and of animals bearing IL-2 receptor positive tumours with high or low metastatic capacity, *Br. J. Cancer,* 55, 583, 1987.
698. **Rubin, L.A., Kurman, C.C., Fritz, M.E., Biddison, W.E., Boutin, B., Yarchoan, R., and Nelson, D.L.,** Soluble interleukin 2 receptors are released from activated human lymphoid cells in vitro, *J. Immunol.,* 135, 3172, 1985.
699. **Nelson, D.L., Kurman, C.C., Fritz, M.E., Boutin, B., and Rubin, L.A.,** The production of soluble and cellular interleukin-2 receptors by cord blood mononuclear cells following in vitro activation, *Pediatr. Res.,* 20, 136, 1986.
700. **Pui, C.-H., Ip, S.H., Iflah, S., Behm, F.G., Grose, B.H., Dodge, R.K., Crist, W.M., Furman, W.L., Murphy, S.B., and Rivera, G.K.,** Serum interleukin 2 receptor levels in childhood acute lymphoblastic leukemia, *Blood,* 71, 1135, 1988.
701. **Steiss, R.G., Marcon, L., Clark, J., Urba, W., Longo, D.L., Nelson, D.L., and Maluish, A.E.,** Serum soluble IL-2 receptor as a tumor marker in patients with hairy cell leukemia, *Blood,* 71, 1304, 1988.
702. **Kloster, B.E., John, P.A., Miller, L.E., Rubin, L.A., Nelson, D.L., Blair, D.C., and Tomar, R.H.,** Soluble interleukin 2 receptors are elevated in patients with AIDS or at risk of developing AIDS, *Clin. Immunol. Immunopathol.,* 45, 440, 1987.
703. **Prince, H.E., Kleinman, S., and Williams, A.E.,** Soluble IL-2 receptor levels in serum from blood donors seropositive for HIV, *J. Immunol.,* 140, 1139, 1988.
704. **Reddy, M.M. and Grieco, M.H.,** Elevated soluble interleukin-2 receptor levels in serum of human immunodeficiency virus infected populations, *AIDS Res. Hum. Retrovirus,* 4, 115, 1988.
705. **Reem, G.H. and Yeh, N.-H.,** Interleukin 2 regulates expression of its receptor and synthesis of γ interferon by human lymphocytes, *Science,* 225, 429, 1984.
706. **Reem, G.H., Yeh, N.-H., Urdal, D.L., Kilian, P.L., and Farrar, J.J.,** Induction and upregulation by interleukin 2 of high-affinity interleukin 2 receptors on thymocytes and T cells, *Proc. Natl. Acad. Sci. U.S.A.,* 82, 8663, 1985.

707. **Reske-Kunz, A.B., von Steldern, D., Rüde, E., and Diamantstein, T.,** Regulation of interleukin 2 receptor expression by interleukin 2, *Scand. J. Immunol.,* 23, 693, 1986.
708. **Depper, J.M., Leonard, W.J., Drogula, C., Krönke, M., Waldmann, T.A., and Greene, W.C.,** Interleukin 2 (IL-2) augments transcription of the IL-2 receptor gene, *Proc. Natl. Acad. Sci. U.S.A.,* 82, 4230, 1985.
709. **Leonard, W.J., Krönke, M., Peffer, N.J., Depper, J.M., and Greene, W.C.,** Interleukin 2 receptor expression in normal human T lymphocytes, *Proc. Natl. Acad. Sci. U.S.A.,* 82, 6281, 1985.
710. **Katzen, D., Chu, E., Terhost, C., Leung, D.Y., Gesner, M., Miller, R.A., and Geha, R.S.,** Mechanisms of human T cell response to mitogens: IL 2 receptor expression and proliferation but not IL 2 synthesis in PHA-stimulated T cells, *J. Immunol.,* 135, 1840, 1985.
711. **Swift, A.M., Davidson, S.O., and Berger, A.E.,** Phosphorylation of a M_r 70,000 protein is associated with interleukin 2 receptor expression, *J. Biol. Chem.,* 263, 2389, 1988.
712. **Lee, J.C., Truneh, A., Smith, M.F., Jr., and Tsang, K.Y.,** Induction of interleukin 2 receptor (Tac) by tumor necrosis factor in YT cells, *J. Immunol.,* 139, 1935, 1987.
713. **Birchnall-Sparks, M.C., Farrar, W.L., Rennick, D., Kilian, P.L., and Ruscetti, F.W.,** Regulation of the interleukin-2 receptor on hemopoietic cells by interleukin 3, *Science,* 233, 455, 1986.
714. **Shackelford, D.A., Smith, A.V., and Trowbridge, I.S.,** Changes in gene expression induced by a phorbol diester: expression of IL 2 receptor, T3, and T cell antigen receptor, *J. Immunol.,* 138, 613, 1987.
715. **Reed, J.C., Abidi, A.H., Alpers, J.D., Hoover, R.G., Robb, R.J., and Nowell, P.C.,** Effect of cyclosporin A and dexamethasone on interleukin 2 receptor gene expression, *J. Immunol.,* 137, 150, 1986.
716. **Northrop, J.P., Crabtree, G.R., and Mattila, P.S.,** Negative regulation of interleukin-2 transcription by the glucocorticoid receptor, *J. Exp. Med.,* 175, 1235, 1992.
717. **Honda, M., Chan, C., and Shevach, E.M.,** Characterization and partial purification of a specific interleukin-2 inhibitor, *J. Immunol.,* 135, 1834, 1985.
718. **Maki, T., Satomi, S., Gotoh, M., and Monaco, A.P.,** Contra-IL 2; a suppressor lymphokine that inhibits IL 2 activity, *J. Immunol.,* 136, 3298, 1986.
719. **Pruett, S.B. and Lackey, A.,** Apparent interleukin 2 (IL-2) inhibitory activity of human serum is due to rapid killing of IL-2-dependent mouse cells, *Clin. Exp. Immunol.,* 69, 624, 1987.
720. **Imboden, J.B., Weiss, A., and Stobo, J.D.,** Transmembrane signalling by the T-cell antigen receptor complex generates inositol phosphates and releases calcium ions from intracellular sites, *Immunol. Today,* 6, 328, 1985.
721. **Cantrell, D.A., Collins, M.K.L., and Crumpton, M.J.,** Autocrine regulation of T-lymphocyte proliferation: differential induction of IL-2 and IL-2 receptor, *Immunology,* 65, 343, 1988.
722. **Tan, T.-H., Huang, G.P., Sica, A., Ghosh, P., Young, H.A., Longo, D.L., and Rice, N.R.,** kB site-dependent activation of the interleukin-2 receptor α-chain gene promoter by human c-Rel, *Mol. Cell. Biol.,* 12, 4067, 1992.
723. **Rosolen, A., Nakanishi, M., Poplack, D.G., Cole, D., Quinones, R., Reaman, G., Trepel, J.B., Cotelingam, J.D., Sausville, E.A., Marti, G.E., Jaffe, E.S., Neckers, L.M., and Colamonici, O.R.,** Expression of interleukin-2 receptor β subunit in hematopoietic malignancies, *Blood,* 73, 1968, 1989.
724. **Kono, T., Doi, T., Yamada, G., Hatakeyama, M., Minamoto, S., Tsudo, M., Miyasawa, M., Miyata, T., and Taniguchi, T.,** Murine interleukin 2 receptor β chain: dysregulated gene expression in lymphoma cell line EL-4 caused by a promoter insertion, *Proc. Natl. Acad. Sci. U.S.A.,* 87, 1806, 1990.
725. **Giglia, J.S., Ovak, G.M., Yoshida, M.A., Twist, C.J., Jeffery, A.R., and Pauly, J.L.,** Isolation of mouse T-cell lymphoma lines from different long-term interleukin 2-dependent cultures, *Cancer Res.,* 45, 5027, 1985.
726. **Sodroski, J.,** The human T-cell leukemia virus (HTLV) transactivator (Tax) protein, *Biochim. Biophys. Acta,* 1114, 19, 1992.
727. **Uchiyama, T., Hori, T., Tsudo, M., Wano, Y., Umadome, H., Tamori, S., Yodoi, J., Maeda, M., Sawami, H., and Uchino, H.,** Interleukin-2 receptor (Tac antigen) expressed on adult T-cell leukemia cells, *J. Clin. Invest.,* 76, 446, 1985.
728. **Shirakawa, F., Yamashita, U., Oda, S., Chiba, S., Eto, S., and Suzuki, H.,** Calcium dependency in the growth of adult T-cell leukemia cells *in vitro, Cancer Res.,* 46, 658, 1986.

729. **Waldmann, T.,** The interleukin-2 receptor on malignant cells: a target for diagnosis and therapy, *Cell. Immunol.,* 99, 53, 1986.
730. **Reinherz, E.L., Kung, P.C., Goldstein, G., Levy, R.H., and Schlossman, S.F.,** Discrete stages of human intrathymic differentiation: analysis of normal thymocytes and leukemic lymphoblasts on T-cell lineage, *Proc. Natl. Acad. Sci. U.S.A.,* 77, 1588, 1980.
731. **Tsudo, M., Uchiyama, T., Umadone, H., Wano, Y., Hori, T., Tamori, S., Uchino, H., Kita, K., Chiba, S., Mitsutani, S., and Nesumi, N.,** Expression of interleukin-2 receptor on T cell chronic lymphocytic leukemia cells and their response to interleukin-2, *Blood,* 67, 316, 1986.
732. **Rossi, J.-F., Klein, B., Commes, T., and Jourdan, M.,** Interleukin 2 production in B cell chronic lymphocytic leukemia, *Blood,* 66, 840, 1985.
733. **Foa, R., Giovarelli, M., Jemma, C., Fierro, M.T., Lusso, P., Ferrando, M.L., Lauria, F., and Forni, G.,** Interleukin 2 (IL 2) and interferon-γ production by T lymphocytes from patients with B-chronic lymphocytic leukemia: evidence that normally released IL 2 is absorbed by the neoplastic B cell population, *Blood,* 66, 614, 1985.
734. **Touw, I. and Löwenberg, B.,** Interleukin 2 stimulates chronic lymphocytic leukemia colony formation in vitro, *Blood,* 66, 237, 1985.
735. **de Paoli, P. and Santini, G.F.,** Well-differentiated B cell lymphomas/leukemias express IL-2 receptors identified by immunofluorescence and flow cytometry, *Clin. Exp. Immunol.,* 68, 223, 1987.
736. **Korsmeyer, S.J., Greene, W.C., Cossman, J., Hsu, S.M., Jensen, J.P., Neckers, L.M., Marshall, S.L., Bakhshi, A., Depper, J.M., Leonard, W.J., Jaffe, E.S., and Waldmann, T.A.,** Rearrangement and expression of immunoglobulin genes and expression of Tac antigen in hairy cell leukemia, *Proc. Natl. Acad. Sci. U.S.A.,* 80, 4522, 1983.
737. **Touw, I., Delwel, R., Bolhuis, R., van Zanen, G., and Löwenberg, B.,** Common and pre-B acute lymphoblastic leukemia cells express interleukin 2 receptors, and interleukin 2 stimulates in vitro colony formation, *Blood,* 66, 556, 1985.
738. **Pui, C.-H., Ip, S.H., Kung, P., Dodge, R.K., Berard, C.W., Crist, W.M., and Murphy, S.B.,** High serum interleukin-2 receptor levels are related to advanced disease and a poor outcome in childhood non-Hodgkin's lymphoma, *Blood,* 70, 624, 1987.
739. **Harrington, D.S., Patil, K., Lai, P.K., Yasuda, N.N., Armitage, J.O., Ip, S.H., Weisenburger, D.P., Linder, J., and Purtilo, D.T.,** Soluble interleukin 2 receptors in patients with malignant lymphoma, *Arch. Pathol. Lab. Med.,* 112, 597, 1988.
740. **Pizzolo, G., Chilosi, M., Vinante, F., Dazzi, F., Lestani, M., Perona, G., Benedetti, F., Godeschini, G., Vincenzi, C., Trentin, L., and Semenzato, G.,** Soluble interleukin-2 receptors in the serum of patients with Hodgkin's disease, *Br. J. Cancer,* 55, 427, 1987.
741. **Visani, G., Delwel, R., Touw, I., Bot, F., and Löwenberg, B.,** Membrane receptors for interleukin 2 on hematopoietic precursors in chronic myeloid leukemia, *Blood,* 69, 1182, 1987.
742. **Löwenberg, B. and Touw, I.P.,** Interleukin 2: its role in the proliferation of neoplastic T and B cells, *J. Pathol.,* 149, 15, 1986.
743. **Georgoulias, V., Triebel, F., Kosmatopoulos, C., Allouche, M., Gluckman, J.C., Mathe, G., and Jasmin, C.,** T-cell colony formation in patients with T-cell malignancies: growth factor requirements for *in-vitro* proliferation of peripheral blood T-cell colony-forming cells, *Leukemia Res.,* 10, 419, 1986.
744. **Haas, M., Altman, A., Rothenberg, E., Bogart, M.H., and Jones, O.W.,** Mechanism of T-cell lymphomagenesis: transformation of growth-factor-dependent T-lymphoblastoma cells to growth-factor-independent T-lymphoma cells, *Proc. Natl. Acad. Sci. U.S.A.,* 81, 1742, 1984.
745. **Duprez, V., Lenoir, G., and Dautry-Varsat, A.,** Autocrine growth stimulation of a human T-cell lymphoma line by interleukin 2, *Proc. Natl. Acad. Sci. U.S.A.,* 82, 6932, 1985.
746. **Sugamura, K., Fujii, M., Kobayashi, N., Sakitani, M., Hatanaka, M., and Hinuma, Y.,** Retrovirus-induced expression of interleukin 2 receptors on cells of human B-cell lineage, *Proc. Natl. Acad. Sci. U.S.A.,* 81, 7441, 1984.
747. **Broder, S., Bunn, P.A., Jr., Jaffe, E.S., Blattner, W., Gallo, R.C., Wong-Staal, F., Waldmann, T.A., and DeVita, V.T.,** T-cell lymphoproliferative syndrome associated with human T-cell leukemia/lymphoma virus, *Ann. Intern. Med.,* 100, 543, 1984.
748. **Touw, I., Delwel, R., van Zanen, G., and Löwenberg, B.,** Acute lymphoblastic leukemia and non-Hodgkin's lymphoma of T lineage: colony-forming cells retain growth factor (interleukin 2) dependence, *Blood,* 68, 1088, 1986.

749. **Shackelford, D.A. and Trowbridge, I.S.,** Induction of expression and phosphorylation of the human interleukin 2 receptor by a phorbol diester, *J. Biol. Chem.,* 259, 11706, 1984.
750. **Kosmatopoulos, C., Allouche, M., Triebel, F., Zanti, M., Clemenceau, C., Gluckman, J.-C., Jasmin, C., and Georgoulias, V.,** Media conditioned by human leukemic T-cells induce expression of IL2 receptors and proliferation of normal T lymphocytes, *Int. J. Cancer,* 37, 247, 1986.
751. **Farrar, W.L., Cleveland, J.L., Beckner, S.K., Bonvini, E., and Evans, S.W.,** Biochemical and molecular events associated with interleukin 2 regulation of lymphocyte proliferation, *Immunol. Rev.,* 92, 49, 1986.
752. **LeGrue, S.J.,** Does interleukin 2 stimulus-response coupling result in generation of intracellular second messengers?, *Lymphokine Res.,* 7, 187, 1988.
753. **Morla, A.O., Schereurs, J., Miyajima, A., and Wang, J.Y.J.,** Hematopoietic growth factors activate the tyrosine phosphorylation of distinct sets of proteins in interleukin-3-dependent murine cell lines, *Mol. Cell. Biol.,* 8, 2214, 1988.
754. **Saltzman, E.M., Thom, R.R., and Casnellie, J.E.,** Activation of a tyrosine protein kinase as an early event in the stimulation of T lymphocytes by interleukin-2, *J. Biol. Chem.,* 263, 6956, 1988.
755. **Beckner, S.K. and Farrar, W.L.,** Inhibition of adenylate cyclase by IL 2 in human T lymphocytes is mediated by protein kinase C, *Biochem. Biophys. Res. Commun.,* 145, 176, 1987.
756. **Johnson, K.W., Davis, B.H., and Smith, K.A.,** cAMP antagonizes interleukin 2-promoted T-cell cycle progression at a discrete point in early G_1, *Proc. Natl. Acad. Sci. U.S.A.,* 85, 6072, 1988.
757. **Beckner, S.K. and Farrar, W.L.,** Potentiation of lymphokine-activated killer cell differentiation and lymphocyte proliferation by stimulation of protein kinase C or inhibition of adenylate cyclase, *J. Immunol.,* 140, 208, 1988.
758. **Evans, S.W., Beckner, S.K., and Farrar, W.L.,** Stimulation of specific GTP binding and hydrolysis activities in lymphocyte membrane by interleukin-2, *Nature,* 325, 166, 1987.
759. **Farrar, W.L. and Anderson, W.B.,** Interleukin-2 stimulates association of protein kinase C with plasma membrane, *Nature,* 315, 233, 1985.
760. **Mire, A.R., Wickremasinghe, R.G., Michalevicz, R., and Hoffbrand, A.V.,** Interleukin-2 induces rapid phosphorylation of an 85 kilodalton protein in permeabilized lymphocytes, *Biochim. Biophys. Acta,* 847, 159, 1985.
761. **Kohno, M., Kuwata, S., Namba, Y., and Hanaoka, M.,** Interleukin 2 induces rapid phosphorylation of cellular proteins in murine T lymphocytes, *FEBS Lett.,* 198, 33, 1986.
762. **Ishii, T., Sugamura, K., Nakamura, M., and Hinuma, Y.,** Interleukin 2 (IL-2) rapidly induces phosphorylation of a cellular protein, pp67, in an IL-2 dependent murine cell line, *Biochem. Biophys. Res. Commun.,* 135, 487, 1986.
763. **Farrar, W.L. and Taguchi, M.,** Interleukin 2 stimulation of protein kinase C membrane association: evidence for IL-2 receptor phosphorylation, *Lymphokine Res.,* 4, 87, 1985.
764. **Polke, C.R., Lowenthal, J.W., Roth, S.A., Rohwer, P., MacDonald, H.R., and Kalden, J.R.,** Phorbol ester enhances both interleukin 2 receptor expression and immunoglobulin secretion in human Epstein-Barr virus-immortalized B cells, *Eur. J. Immunol.,* 16, 146, 1986.
765. **Clark, R.B., Love, J.T., Jr., Sgroi, D., Lingenheld, E.G., and Sha'afi, R.I.,** The protein kinase C inhibitor, H-7, inhibits antigen and IL-2-induced proliferation of murine T-cell lines, *Biochem. Biophys. Res. Commun.,* 145, 666, 1987.
766. **Mills, G.B., Girard, P., Grinstein, S., and Gelfand, E.W.,** Interleukin-2 induces proliferation of T-lymphocyte mutants lacking protein kinase C, *Cell,* 55, 91, 1988.
767. **Isakov, N. and Altman, A.,** Human T lymphocyte activation by tumor promoters: role of protein kinase C, *J. Immunol.,* 138, 3100, 1987.
768. **Taguchi, M., Thomas, T.P., Andersen, W.B., and Farrar, W.L.,** Direct phosphorylation of the IL-2 receptor Tac antigen epitope by protein kinase C, *Biochem. Biophys. Res. Commun.,* 135, 239, 1986.
769. **Berridge, M.J.,** Inositol trisphosphate and diacylglycerol as second messengers, *Biochem. J.,* 220, 345, 1984.
770. **Donnelly, T.E., Jr., Sittler, R., and Scholar, E.M.,** Relationship between membrane-bound protein kinase C activity and calcium-dependent proliferation of BALB/c 3T3 cells, *Biochem. Biophys. Res. Commun.,* 126, 741, 1985.
771. **Remillard, B., Petrillo, R., Maslinkski, W., Tsudo, M., Strom, T.B., Cantley, L., and Varticovski, L.,** Interleukin-2 receptor regulates activation of phosphatidylinositol 3-kinase, *J. Biol. Chem.,* 266, 14167, 1991.
772. **Merida, I., Diez, E., and Gaulton, G.N.,** IL-2 binding activates a tyrosine-phosphorylated phosphatidylinositol-3-kinase, *J. Immunol.,* 147, 2202, 1991.

773. **Larsen, C.S., Knudsen, T.E., and Johnsen, H.E.,** The role of calcium in stimulation of activated T lymphocytes with interleukin 2, *Scand. J. Immunol.,* 24, 689, 1986.
774. **Cassatella, M.A., Anegón, I., Cuturi, M.C., Griskey, P., Trinchieri, G., and Perusia, B.,** FcγR (CD16) interaction with ligand induces Ca^{2+} mobilization and phosphoinositide turnover in human natural killer cells, *J. Exp. Med.,* 169, 549, 1989.
775. **Rossio, J.L., Ruscetti, F.W., and Farrar, W.L.,** Ligand-specific calcium mobilization in IL 2 and IL 3 dependent cell lines, *Lymphokine Res.,* 5, 163, 1986.
776. **LeGrue, S.J.,** Interleukin-2 stimulus-response coupling is calcium independent, *Lymphokine Res.,* 6, 1, 1987.
777. **Trunch, A., Albert, F., Golstein, P., and Schmitt-Verhulst, A.-M.,** Early steps of lymphocyte activation bypassed by synergy between calcium ionophores and phorbol ester, *Nature,* 313, 318, 1985.
778. **Koyasu, S., Suzuki, G., Asano, Y., Osawa, H., Diamantstein, T., and Yahar, I.,** Signals for activation and proliferation of murine T lymphocyte clones, *J. Biol. Chem.,* 262, 4689, 1987.
779. **Harris, D.T., Kozumbo, W.J., Cerutti, P., and Cerottini, J.-C.,** Molecular mechanisms involved in T-cell activation. I. Evidence for independent signal-transducing pathways in lymphokine production vs. proliferation in cloned cytotoxic T lymphocytes, *J. Immunol.,* 138, 600, 1987.
780. **Kozumbo, W.J., Harris, D.T., Gromkowski, S., Cerottini, J.-C., and Cerutti, P.A.,** Molecular mechanisms involved in T-cell activation. II. The phosphatidylinositol signal-transducing mechanism mediates antigen-induced lymphokine production but not interleukin 2-induced proliferation in cloned cytotoxic T lymphocytes, *J. Immunol.,* 138, 606, 1987.
781. **Mueller, D.L., Jenkins, M.K., Chiodetti, L., and Schwartz, R.H.,** An intracellular calcium increase and protein kinase C activation fail to initiate T-cell proliferation in the absence of a costimulatory signal, *J. Immunol.,* 144, 3701, 1990.
782. **Ebeling, J.G., Vandenbark, G.R., Kuhn, L.J., Ganong, B.R., Bell, R.M., and Niedel, J.E.,** Diacylglycerols mimic phorbol diester induction of leukemic cell differentiation, *Proc. Natl. Acad. Sci. U.S.A.,* 82, 815, 1985.
783. **Finke, J.H., Yen-Lieberman, B., Scott, J.W., Proffitt, M.R., and Orosz, C.G.,** Phorbol ester-inactivation of cloned cytotoxic T lymphocytes: restoration of lytic activity by interleukin 2 and induction of interferon production are separable events, *Lymphokine Res.,* 4, 299, 1985.
784. **Mills, G.B., Cragoe, E.J., Jr., Gelfand, E.W., and Grinstein, S.,** Interleukin 2 induces a rapid increase in intracellular pH through activation of a Na^+/H^+ antiport. Cytoplasmic alkalinization is not required for lymphocyte proliferation, *Proc. Natl. Acad. Sci. U.S.A.,* 260, 12500, 1985.
785. **Redondo, J.M., López Rivas, A., and Fresno, M.,** Activation of the Na^+/K^+-ATPase by interleukin-2, *FEBS Lett.,* 206, 199, 1986.
786. **Mills, G.B. and May, C.,** Binding of interleukin 2 to its 75-kDa intermediate affinity receptor is sufficient to activate Na^+/H^+ exchange, *J. Immunol.,* 139, 4083, 1987.
787. **Bowlin, T.L., McKown, B.J., Babcock, G.F., and Sunkara, P.S.,** Intracellular polyamine biosynthesis is required for interleukin 2 responsiveness during lymphocyte mitogenesis, *Cell. Immunol.,* 106, 420, 1987.
788. **Ziegler, I., Schwulera, U., and Ellwart, J.,** Pteridines are produced during interleukin-2-induced proliferation and modulate transmission of this signal, *Exp. Cell Res.,* 167, 531, 1986.
789. **Horak, I.D., Gress, R.E., Lucas, P.J., Horak, E.M., Waldmann, T.A., and Bolen, J.B.,** T-lymphocyte interleukin 2-dependent tyrosine protein kinase signal transduction involves the activation of p56^{lck}, *Proc. Natl. Acad. Sci. U.S.A.,* 88, 1996, 1991.
790. **Kim, Y.H., Buchholz, M.J., and Nordin, A.A.,** Murine T-lymphocyte proliferation induced by interleukin-2 correlates with a transient increase in p56^{lck} kinase activity and the tyrosine phosphorylation of a 97-kDa protein, *Proc. Natl. Acad. Sci. U.S.A.,* 90, 3187, 1993.
791. **Shackelford, D.A. and Trowbridge, I.S.,** Ligand-stimulated tyrosine phosphorylation of the IL-2 receptor β chain and receptor-associated proteins, *Cell Regul.,* 2, 73, 1991.
792. **Siliciano, J.D., Morrow, T.A., and Desideris, S.V.,** *itk,* A T-cell-specific tyrosine kinase gene inducible by interleukin-2, *Proc. Natl. Acad. Sci. U.S.A.,* 89, 11194, 1992.
793. **Fung, M.R., Scearce, R.M., Hoffman, J.A., Peffer, N.J., Hammes, S.R., Hosking, J.B., Schmandt, R., Kuziel, W.A., Haynes, B.F., Mills, G.B., and Greene, W.C.,** A tyrosine kinase physically associates with the β-subunit of the human IL-2 receptor, *J. Immunol.,* 147, 1253, 1991.
794. **Garcia, G.G., Evans, G.A., Michiel, D.F., and Farrar, W.L.,** Characterization of a tyrosine kinase activity associated with the high-affinity interleukin 2 receptor complex, *Biochem. J.,* 285, 851, 1992.

795. **Ferris, D.K., Willette-Brown, J., Ortaldo, J.R., and Farrar, W.L.,** IL-2 regulation of tyrosine kinase activity is mediated through the p70-75 β-subunit of the IL-2 receptor, *J. Immunol.,* 143, 870, 1989.
796. **Saltzman, E.M., White, K., and Casnellie, J.E.,** Stimulation of the antigen and interleukin-2 receptors on T lymphocytes activates distinct tyrosine protein kinases, *J. Biol. Chem.,* 265, 10138, 1990.
797. **Evans, S.W. and Farrar, W.L.,** Identity of common phosphoprotein substrates stimulated by interleukin 2 and diacylglycerol suggests a role of protein kinase C for signal transduction, *J. Cell. Biochem.,* 34, 47, 1987.
798. **Zu, Y., Kohno, M., Kubota, I., Nishida, E., Hanaoka, M., and Namba, Y.,** Characterization of interleukin 2 stimulated 65-kilodalton phosphoprotein in human T cells, *Biochemistry,* 29, 1055, 1990.
799. **Zu, Y., Shigesada, K., Nishida, E., Kubota, I., Kohno, M., Hanaoka, M., and Namba, Y.,** 65-Kilodalton protein phosphorylated by interleukin 2 stimulation bears two putative actin-binding sites and two calcium-binding sites, *Biochemistry,* 29, 8319, 1990.
800. **Turner, B., Rapp, U., App, H., Greene, M., Dobashi, K., and Reed, J.,** Interleukin 2 induces tyrosine phosphorylation and activation of p72-74 Raf-1 kinase in a T-cell line, *Proc. Natl. Acad. Sci. U.S.A.,* 88, 1227, 1991.
801. **Rayhel, E.J., Fields, T.J., Albright, J.W., Diamantstein, T., and Hughes, J.P.,** Interleukin 2 and a lactogen regulate proliferation and protein phosphorylation in Nb2 cells, *Biochem. J.,* 249, 333, 1988.
802. **Sabath, D.E., Podolin, P.L., Comber, P.G., and Prystowsky, M.B.,** cDNA cloning and characterization of interleukin 2-induced genes in a cloned T-helper lymphocyte, *J. Biol. Chem.,* 265, 12671, 1990.
803. **Kaczmarek, L., Calabretta, B., and Baserga, R.,** Effect of interleukin-2 on the expression of cell cycle genes in human T lymphocytes, *Biochem. Biophys. Res. Commun.,* 133, 410, 1985.
804. **Blackman, M.A., Tigges, M.A., Minie, M.E., and Koshland, M.E.,** A model system for peptide hormone action in differentiation: interleukin 2 induces a B lymphoma to transcribe the J chain gene, *Cell,* 47, 609, 1986.
805. **Arima, N., Kuziel, W.A., Grdina, T.A., and Greene, W.C.,** IL-2-induced signal transduction involves the activation of nuclear NF-kB expression, *J. Immunol.,* 149, 83, 1992.
806. **Ghosh, P., Tan, T.-H., Rice, N.R., Sica, A., and Young, H.A.,** The interleukin 2 CD28-responsive complex contains at least three members of the NF kB family: c-Rel, p50, and p65, *Proc. Natl. Acad. Sci. U.S.A.,* 90, 1696, 1993.
807. **Beadling, C., Johnson, K.W., and Smith, K.A.,** Isolation of interleukin-2-induced immediate-early genes, *Proc. Natl. Acad. Sci. U.S.A.,* 90, 2719, 1993.
808. **Cleveland, J.L., Rapp, U.R., and Farrar, W.L.,** Role of c-*myc* and other genes in interleukin 2 regulated CT6 lymphocytes and their malignant variants, *J. Immunol.,* 138, 3495, 1987.
809. **Kelly, K., Cochran, B.H., Stiles, C.D., and Leder, P.,** Cell-specific regulation of the c-*myc* gene by lymphocyte mitogens and platelet-derived growth factor, *Cell,* 35, 603, 1983.
810. **Schneider-Schaulies, J., Hünig, T., Schimpl, A., and Wecker, E.,** Kinetics of cellular oncogene expression in mouse lymphocytes. I. Expression of c-myc and c-ras[Ha] in T lymphocytes induced by various mitogens, *Eur. J. Immunol.,* 16, 312, 1986.
811. **Persson, H., Hennighausen, L., Taub, R., DeGrado, W., and Leder, P.,** Antibodies to human c-*myc* oncogene product: evidence of an evolutionary conserved protein induced during cell proliferation, *Science,* 225, 687, 1984.
812. **Reed, J.C., Sabath, D.E., Hoover, R.G., and Prystowsky, M.B.,** Recombinant interleukin 2 regulates levels of c-*myc* mRNA in a cloned murine T lymphocyte, *Mol. Cell. Biol.,* 5, 3361, 1985.
813. **Reed, J.C., Nowell, P.C., and Hoover, R.G.,** Regulation of c-*myc* mRNA levels in normal human lymphocytes by modulators of cell proliferation, *Proc. Natl. Acad. Sci. U.S.A.,* 82, 4221, 1985.
814. **Gravekamp, C., van den Bulck, L.P., Vijg, J., van de Griend, R.J., and Bolhuis, R.L.H.,** c-myc Gene expression and interleukin-2 receptor levels in cloned human CD2+,CD3+ and CD2+, CD3- lymphocytes, *Nat. Immunol. Cell Growth Regul.,* 6, 28, 1987.
815. **Reed, J.C., Alpers, J.D., Scherle, P.A., Hoover, R.G., Nowell, P.C., and Prystowsky, M.B.,** Protooncogene expression in cloned T lymphocytes: mitogens and growth factors induce different patterns of expression, *Oncogene,* 1, 223, 1987.
816. **Carding, S. and Reem, G.H.,** C-MYC gene expression and activation of human thymocytes, *Thymus,* 10, 219, 1987.

817. **Churilla, A.M., Braciale, T.J., and Braciale, V.L.,** Regulation of T lymphocyte proliferation. Interleukin 2-mediated induction of c-*myb* gene expression is dependent on T-lymphocyte activation state, *J. Exp. Med.,* 170, 105, 1989.
818. **Reed, J.C., Alpers, J.D., Nowell, P.C., and Hoover, R.G.,** Sequential expression of proto-oncogenes during lectin-stimulate mitogenesis of normal human lymphocytes, *Proc. Natl. Acad. Sci. U.S.A.,* 83, 3982, 1986.
819. **Pauza, C.D.,** Regulation of human T-lymphocyte gene expression by interleukin 2: immediate-response genes include the proto-oncogene c-*myb, Mol. Cell. Biol.,* 7, 342, 1987.
820. **Espinoza-Delgado, I., Longo, D.L., Gusella, G.L., and Varesio, L.,** IL-2 enhances c-fms expression in human monocytes, *J. Immunol.,* 145, 1137, 1990.
821. **Zmuidzinas, A., Mamon, H.J., Roberts, T.M., and Smith, K.A.,** Interleukin-2-triggered Raf-1 expression, phosphorylation, and associated kinase activity increase through G_1 and S in CD3-stimulated primary human T cells, *Mol. Cell. Biol.,* 11, 2794, 1991.
822. **Turner, B.C., Tonks, N.K., Rapp, U.R., and Reed, J.C.,** Interleukin-2 regulates Raf-1 kinase activity through a tyrosine phosphorylation-dependent mechanism in a T-cell line, *Proc. Natl. Acad. Sci. U.S.A.,* 90, 5544, 1993.
823. **Satoh, T., Minami, Y., Kono, T., Yamada, K., Kawahara, A., Taniguchi, T., and Kaziro, Y.,** Interleukin 2-induced activation of Ras requires two domains of interleukin 2 receptor β subunit, the essential region for growth stimulation and Lck binding domain, *J. Biol. Chem.,* 267, 25423, 1992.
824. **Reed, J.C., Tsujimoto, Y., Alpers, J.D., Croce, C.M., and Nowell, P.C.,** Regulation of *bcl*-2 proto-oncogene expression during normal human lymphocyte proliferation, *Science,* 236, 1295, 1987.
825. **Mercer, W.E. and Baserga, R.,** Expression of the p53 protein during the cell cycle of human peripheral blood lymphocytes, *Exp. Cell Res.,* 160, 31, 1985.
826. **Fresa, K., Hameed, M., and Cohen, S.,** Intracellular mechanisms of lymphoid cell activation, *Clin. Immunol. Immunopathol.,* 50, 8, 1989.
827. **Elliott, L., Brooks, W., and Roszman, T.,** Role of interleukin-2 (IL-2) and IL-2 receptor expression in the proliferative defect observed in mitogen-stimulated lymphocytes from patients with gliomas, *J. Natl. Cancer Inst.,* 78, 919, 1987.
828. **Yodoi, J. and Uchiyama, T.,** IL-2 receptor dysfunction and adult T-cell leukemia, *Immunol. Rev.,* 92, 135, 1986.
829. **Shimoyama, M., Kagami, Y., Shimotohno, K., Miwa, M., Minato, K., Tobinai, K., Suemasu, K., and Sugimura, T.,** Adult T-cell leukemia/lymphoma not associated with human T-cell leukemia virus type I, *Proc. Natl. Acad. Sci. U.S.A.,* 83, 4524, 1986.
830. **Feuer, G. and Chen, I.S.Y.,** Mechanisms of human T-cell leukemia virus-induced leukemogenesis, *Biochim. Biophys. Acta,* 1114, 223, 1992.
831. **Su, I.-J. and Kadin, M.E.,** Expression of growth factor/receptor genes in post-thymic T-cell malignancies, *Am. J. Pathol.,* 135, 439, 1989.
832. **Froehlich, C.J. and Guiffaut, S.,** Lysis of human T-cell leukemia virus infected T and B lymphoid cells by interleukin 2-activated killer cells, *J. Immunol.,* 139, 3637, 1987.
833. **Popovic, M., Lange-Wantzin, G., Sarin, P.S., Mann, D., and Gallo, R.C.,** Transformation of human umbilical cord blood T cells by human T-cell leukemia/lymphoma virus, *Proc. Natl. Acad. Sci. U.S.A.,* 80, 5402, 1983.
834. **Maeda, M., Shimizu, A., Ikuta, K., Okamoto, H., Kashihara, M., Uchiyama, T., Honjo, T., and Yodoi, J.,** Origin of human T-lymphotrophic virus I-positive T-cell lines in adult T-cell leukemia: analysis of T-cell receptor gene rearrangement, *J. Exp. Med.,* 162, 2169, 1985.
835. **Maeda, M., Arima, N., Daitoku, Y., Kashihara, M., Okamoto, H., Uchiyama, T., Shirono, K., Matsuoka, M., Takatsuki, K., Ikuta, K., Shimizu, A., Honjo, T., and Yodoi, J.,** Evidence for the interleukin-2 dependent expansion of leukemic cells in adult T-cell leukemia, *Blood,* 70, 1407, 1987.
836. **Kohtz, D.S., Altman, A., Kohtz, J.D., and Puszkin, S.,** Immunological and structural homology between human T-cell leukemia virus type I envelope glycoprotein and a region of human interleukin-2 implicated in binding the β receptor, *J. Virol.,* 62, 659, 1988.
837. **Arya, S.K., Wong-Staal, F., and Gallo, R.C.,** T-cell growth factor gene: lack of expression in human T-cell leukemia-lymphoma virus-infected cells, *Science,* 223, 1086, 1984.
838. **Dodon, M.D. and Gazzolo, L.,** Loss of interleukin-2 requirement for the generation of T colonies defines an early event of human T-lymphotropic virus type I infection, *Blood,* 69, 12, 1987.

839. **Arima, N., Daitoku, Y., Yamamoto, Y., Fujimoto, K., Ohgaki, S., Kojima, K., Fukumori, J., Matsushita, K., Tanaka, H., and Onoue, K.,** Heterogeneity in response to interleukin 2 and interleukin 2-producing ability of adult T-cell leukemic cells, *J. Immunol.,* 138, 3069, 1987.
840. **Poiesz, B.J., Ruscetti, F.W., Mier, J.W., Woods, A.M., and Gallo, R.C.,** T-cell lines from human T-lymphocytic neoplasias by direct response to T-cell growth factor, *Proc. Natl. Acad. Sci. U.S.A.,* 77, 6815, 1980.
841. **Hori, T., Uchiyama, T., Umadome, H., Tamori, S., Tsudo, M., Araki, K., and Uchino, H.,** Dissociation of interleukin-2-mediated cell proliferation and interleukin-2 receptor upregulation in adult T-cell leukemia cells, *Leukemia Res.,* 10, 1447, 1986.
842. **Georgoulias, V., Allouche, M., Salvatore, A., Clemenceau, C., and Jasmin, C.,** Interleukin 2 responsiveness of immature T-cell colony-forming cells (T-CFC) from patients with acute T-cell lymphoblastic leukemias, *Cell. Immunol.,* 105, 317, 1987.
843. **Yodoi, J., Okada, M., Tagawa, Y., Teshigawara, K., Fukui, K., Ishida, N., Ikuta, K.-I., Maeda, M., Honjo, T., Osawa, H., Diamantstein, T., Tateno, M., and Yoshiki, T.,** Rat lymphoid cell lines producing human T-cell leukemia virus. II. Constitutive expression of rat interleukin 2 receptor, *J. Exp. Med.,* 161, 924, 1985.
844. **Krönke, M., Leonard, W.J., Depper, J.M., and Greene, W.C.,** Deregulation of interleukin-2 receptor gene expression in HTLV-I-induced adult T-cell leukemia, *Science,* 228, 1275, 1985.
845. **Inoue, J., Seiki, M., Taniguchi, T., Tsuru, S., and Yoshida, M.,** Induction of interleukin 2 receptor gene expression by p40^x encoded by human T-cell leukemia virus type I, *EMBO J.,* 5, 2883, 1986.
846. **Siekevitz, M., Feinberg, M.B., Holbrook, N., Wong-Staal, F., and Greene, W.C.,** Activation of interleukin 2 and interleukin 2 receptor (Tac) promoter expression by the trans-activator *(tat)* gene product of human T-cell leukemia virus, type I, *Proc. Natl. Acad. Sci. U.S.A.,* 84, 5389, 1987.
847. **Marriott, S.J., Trinh, D., and Brady, J.N.,** Activation of interleukin-2 receptor-α expression by extracellular HTLV-I tax1 protein. A potential role in HTLV-I pathogenesis, *Oncogene,* 7, 1749, 1992.
848. **Arima, N., Daitoku, Y., Ohgaki, J., Tanaka, H., Yamamoto, Y., Fujimoto, K., and Onoue, K.,** Autocrine growth or interleukin 2-producing leukemic cells in a patient with adult T-cell leukemia, *Blood,* 68, 779, 1986.
849. **Katoh, T., Harada, T., Morikawa, S., and Wakutani, T.,** IL-2- and IL-2-R-independent proliferation of T-cell lines from adult T-cell leukemia/lymphoma patients, *Int. J. Cancer,* 38, 265, 1986.
850. **Greene, W.C., Leonard, W.J., Wano, Y., Svetlik, P.B., Peffer, N.J., Sodroski, J.G., Rosen, C.A., Goh, W.C., and Haseltine, W.A.,** *Trans*-activator gene of HTLV-II induces IL-2 receptor and IL-2 cellular gene expression, *Science,* 232, 877, 1986.
851. **Tomita, S., Ambrus, J.L., Jr., Volkman, D.J., Longo, D.L., Mitsuya, H., Reitz, M.S., Jr., and Fauci, A.S.,** Human T-cell leukemia/lymphoma virus I infection and subsequent cloning of normal human B cells: direct responsiveness of cloned cells to recombinant interleukin 2 by differentiation in the absence of enhanced proliferation, *J. Exp. Med.,* 162, 393, 1985.
852. **Barnett, D., Wilson, G.A., Lawrence, A.C.K., and Buckley, G.A.,** The interleukin-2 receptor and its expression in the acute leukaemias and lymphoproliferative disorders, *Dis. Markers,* 6, 133, 1988.
853. **Bentaboulet, M., Allouche, M., Tsapis, A., Jasmin, C., and Georgoulias, V.,** Characterization of interleukin-2 receptors expressed on acute leukemic B cells, *Blood,* 70, 954, 1987.
854. **Malkovska, V., Murphy, J., Hudson, L., and Bevan, D.,** Direct effect of interleukin 2 on chronic lymphocytic leukemia B-cell functions and morphology, *Clin. Exp. Immunol.,* 68, 677, 1987.
855. **Morishima, Y., Morishita, Y., Adachi, K., Tanimoto, M., Ohno, R., and Saito, H.,** Phorbol ester induces interleukin-2 receptor on the cell surface of precursor thymocyte leukemia with no rearrangement of T-cell receptor β and γ genes, *Blood,* 70, 1291, 1987.
856. **Strauchen, J.A. and Breakstone, B.A.,** IL-2 receptor expression in human lymphoid lesions: immunohistochemical study of 166 cases, *Am. J. Pathol.,* 126, 506, 1987.
857. **Hargett, S., Wanebo, H.J., Pace, R., Katz, D., Sando, J., and Cantrell, R.,** Interleukin-2 production in head and neck cancer patients, *Am. J. Surg.,* 150, 456, 1985.
858. **Rimoldi, D., Salvi, L.S., Hartamann, F., Schreyer, M., Blum, S., Zografos, L., Plaisance, S., Azzarone, B., and Carrei, S.,** Expression of IL-2 receptors in human melanoma cells, *Anticancer Res.,* 13, 555, 1993.
859. **Fauci, A.S., Masur, H., Gelmann, E.P., Markham, P.D., Hahn, B.H., and Lane, H.C.,** The acquired immunodeficiency syndrome: an update, *Ann. Intern. Med.,* 102, 800, 1985.
860. **Curran, J.W., Morgan, W.M., Hardy, A.M., Jaffe, H.W., Darrow, W.W., and Dowdle, W.R.,** The epidemiology of AIDS: current status and future prospects, *Science,* 229, 1352, 1985.

861. **Gallo, R.C. and Wong-Staal, F.,** A human T-lymphotropic retrovirus (HTLV-III) as the cause of the acquired immunodeficiency syndrome, *Ann. Intern. Med.,* 103, 679, 1985.
862. **Montagnier, L.,** Lymphadenopathy associated virus: its role in the pathogenesis of AIDS and related diseases, *Prog. Allergy,* 37, 46, 1986.
863. **Ho, D.D., Pomerantz, R.J., and Kaplan, J.C.,** Pathogenesis of infection with human immunodeficiency virus, *N. Engl. J. Med.,* 317, 278, 1987.
864. **Friedland, G.H. and Klein, R.S.,** Transmission of the human immunodeficiency virus, *N. Engl. J. Med.,* 317, 1125, 1987.
865. **Novick, B.E. and Rubinstein, A.,** AIDS — the pediatric perspective, *AIDS,* 1, 3, 1987.
866. **Piot, P., Kreiss, J.K., Ndinya-Achola, J.O., Ngugi, E.N., Simonsen, J.N., Cameron, D.W., Taelman, H., and Plummer, F.A.,** Heterosexual transmission of HIV, *AIDS,* 1, 199, 1987.
867. **Piot, P., Plummer, F.A., Mhalu, F.S., Lamboray, J.-L., Chin, J., and Mann, J.M.,** AIDS: an international perspective, *Science,* 239, 573, 1988.
868. **Novello, A.C.,** The HIV/AIDS epidemic — a current picture, *AIDS Res. Hum. Retrovirus,* 8, 695, 1992.
869. **Waisman, J., Rotterdam, H., Niedt, G.N., Lewin, K., and Racz, P.,** AIDS: an overview of the pathology, *Pathol. Res. Pract.,* 182, 729, 1987.
870. **Geleziunas, R., Schipper, H.M., and Wainberg, M.A.,** Pathogenesis and therapy of HIV-1 infection of the central nervous system, *AIDS,* 6, 1411, 1992.
871. **Dorfman, R.F.,** Kaposi's sarcoma revisited, *Hum. Pathol.,* 15, 1013, 1984.
872. **Biggar, R.J., Horm, J., Goedert, J.J., and Melbye, M.,** Cancer in a group at risk of acquired immunodeficiency syndrome (AIDS) through 1984, *Am. J. Epidemiol.,* 126, 578, 1987.
873. **Alizon, M. and Montagnier, L.,** Lymphadenopathy/AIDS virus: genetic organization and relationship to animal lentiviruses, *Anticancer Res.,* 6, 403, 1986.
874. **Fauci, A.S.,** The human immunodeficiency virus: infectivity and mechanisms of pathogenesis, *Science,* 239, 617, 1988.
875. **Levy, J.A.,** Human immunodeficiency viruses and the pathogenesis of AIDS, *J. Am. Med. Assoc.,* 261, 2997, 1989.
876. **Hammarskjöld, M.-L. and Kerosh, D.,** The molecular biology of the human immunodeficiency virus, *Biochim. Biophys. Acta,* 989, 269, 1989.
877. **Greene, W.C.,** The molecular biology of human immunodeficiency virus type-1 infection, *N. Engl. J. Med.,* 324, 308, 1991.
878. **Clavel, F.,** HIV-2, the West African AIDS virus, *AIDS,* 1, 135, 1987.
879. **Greene, W.C.,** The molecular biology of human immunodeficiency virus type 1 infection, *N. Engl. J. Med.,* 324, 308, 1991.
880. **Haseltine, W.A.,** Molecular biology of the human immunodeficiency virus type 1, *FASEB J.,* 5, 2349, 1991.
881. **Cullen, B.R.,** Regulation of HIV-1 gene expression, *FASEB J.,* 5, 2361, 1991.
882. **Gallo, R.C.,** Mechanism of disease induction by HIV, *J. Acquired Immune Deficiency Syndr.,* 3, 380, 1990.
883. **Rosenberg, Z.F. and Fauci, A.S.,** Immunopathogenesis of HIV infection, *FASEB J.,* 5, 2382, 1991.
884. **Pantaleo, G., Graziosi, C., and Fauci, A.S.,** The immunopathogenesis of human immunodeficiency virus infection, *N. Engl. J. Med.,* 341, 327, 1993.
885. **Weiss, R.A.,** How does HIV cause AIDS?, *Science,* 260, 1273, 1993.
886. **Bukrinsky, M.I., Stanwick, T.L., Dempsey, M.P., and Stevenson, M.,** Quiescent T lymphocytes as an inducible virus reservoir in HIV-1 infection, *Science,* 254, 423, 1991.
887. **Arya, S.K. and Gallo, R.C.,** Human T-cell growth factor (interleukin 2) and γ-interferon genes: expression in human T-lymphotropic virus type III- and type I-infected cells, *Proc. Natl. Acad. Sci. U.S.A.,* 82, 8691, 1985.
888. **Antonen, J. and Krohn, K.,** Interleukin 2 production in HTLV-III/LAV infection: evidence of defective antigen-induced, but normal mitogen-induced IL-2 production, *Clin. Exp. Immunol.,* 65, 489, 1986.
889. **Reuben, J.M., Hersh, E.M., Murray, J.L., Munn, C.G., Mehta, S.R., and Mansell, P.W.A.,** IL-2 production and response in vitro by the leukocytes of patients with acquired immune deficiency syndrome, *Lymphokine Res.,* 4, 103, 1985.
890. **Shapiro, I.M., Meier, C., Vlach, V., McDonald, T.L., Wigzell, H., and Stevenson, M.,** Autonomous growth of lymphoid cells following IL-2 expression from retrovirus vectors containing HIV-1 *trans*-acting elements, *Somat. Cell Mol. Genet.,* 16, 1, 1990.

891. **Prince, H.E. and John, J.K.**, Abnormalities of interleukin 2 receptor expression associated with decreased antigen-induced lymphocyte proliferation in patients with AIDS and related disorders, *Clin. Exp. Immunol.*, 67, 59, 1987.
892. **Donnelly, R.P., La Via, M.F., and Tsang, K.Y.**, Humoral-mediated suppression of interleukin 2-dependent target cell proliferation in acquired immune deficiency syndrome (AIDS): interference with normal IL-2 receptor expression, *Clin. Exp. Immunol.*, 68, 488, 1987.
893. **Weigent, D.A., Hoeprich, P.D., Bost, K.L., Brunck, T.K., Reiher, W.E., III, and Blalock, J.E.**, The HTLV-III envelope protein contains a hexapeptide homologous to a region of interleukin-2 that binds to the interleukin-2 receptor, *Biochem. Biophys. Res. Commun.*, 139, 367, 1986.
894. **Reiher, W.E., III, Blalock, J.E., and Brunck, T.K.**, Sequence homology between acquired immunodeficiency syndrome virus envelope protein and interleukin 2, *Proc. Natl. Acad. Sci. U.S.A.*, 83, 9188, 1986.
895. **Böhnlein, E., Lowenthal, J.W., Siekiewitz, M., Ballard, D.W., Franza, B.R., and Greene, W.C.**, The same inducible nuclear proteins regulates mitogen activation of both the interleukin-2 receptor α gene and type 1 HIV, *Cell*, 53, 827, 1988.
896. **Samuel, K.P., Seth, A., Konopka, A., Lautenberger, J.A., and Papas, T.S.**, The 3′-orf protein of human immunodeficiency virus shows structural homology with the phosphorylation domain of human interleukin-2 receptor and the ATP-binding site of the protein kinase family, *FEBS Lett.*, 218, 81, 1987.
897. **Molina, J.-M., Scadden, D.T., Byrn, R., Dinarello, C.A., and Groopman, J.E.**, Production of tumor necrosis factor α and interleukin 1β by monocytic cells infected with human immunodeficiency virus, *J. Clin. Invest.*, 84, 733, 1989.
898. **Osborn, L., Kunkel, S., and Nabel, G.J.**, Tumor necrosis factor α and interleukin 1 stimulate the human immunodeficiency virus enhancer by activation of the nuclear factor kB, *Proc. Natl. Acad. Sci. U.S.A.*, 86, 2336, 1989.
899. **Rook, A.H., Hooks, J.J., Quinnan, G.U., Lane, H.C., Manischewitz, J.F., Macher, A.M., Masur, H., Fauci, A.S., and Djeu, J.Y.**, Interleukin-2 enhances the natural killer cell activity of acquired immunodeficiency syndrome patients through an interferon-independent mechanism, *J. Immunol.*, 134, 1503, 1985.
900. **Rinaldo, C., Piazza, P., Wang, Y., Armstrong, J., Gupta, P., Ho, M., Petteway, S., Reed, D., Lyter, D., and Kingsley, L.**, HIV-1-specific production of IFN-γ and modulation by recombinant IL-2 during early HIV-1 infection, *J. Immunol.*, 140, 3389, 1988.
901. **Volberding, P., Moody, D.J., Beardslee, D., Bradley, E.C., and Wofsy, C.B.**, Therapy of acquired immune deficiency syndrome with recombinant interleukin 2, *AIDS Res. Hum. Retrovirus*, 3, 115, 1987.
902. **Nakamura, S., Salahuddin, S.Z., Biberfeld, P., Ensoli, B., Markham, P.D., Wong-Staal, F., and Gallo, R.C.**, Kaposi's sarcoma cells: long-term culture with growth factor from retrovirus-infected CD4+ T cells, *Science*, 242, 426, 1988.
903. **Ensoli, B., Nakamura, S., Salahuddin, S.Z., Biberfeld, P., Larsson, L., Beaver, B., Wong-Staal, F., and Gallo, R.C.**, AIDS-Kaposi's sarcoma-derived cells express cytokines with autocrine and paracrine growth effects, *Science*, 243, 223, 1989.
904. **Lopez-Cepero, M., Specter, S., Matteucci, D., Friedman, H., and Bendinelli, M.**, Altered interleukin production during Friend leukemia virus infection, *Proc. Soc. Exp. Biol. Med.*, 188, 353, 1988.
905. **Rosenberg, S.A. and Lotze, M.T.**, Cancer immunotherapy using interleukin-2 and interleukin-2-activated lymphocytes, *Annu. Rev. Immunol.*, 4, 681, 1986.
906. **Cheever, M.A., Thompson, J.A., Peace, D.J., and Greenberg, P.D.**, Potential uses of interleukin 2 in cancer therapy, *Immunobiology*, 172, 193, 1986.
907. **Grimm, E.A.**, Human lymphokine-activated killer cells (LAK cells) as a potential immunotherapeutic modality, *Biochem. Biophys. Acta*, 865, 267, 1986.
908. **Kradin, R., Yamin, R., and Kurnick, J.**, Immunological effects of adoptive immunotherapy with IL-2: an overview, *Pathol. Immunopathol. Res.*, 7, 434, 1988.
909. **Parkinson, D.R.**, Interleukin-2 in cancer therapy, *Semin. Oncol.*, 15, 10, 1988.
910. **Kohler, P.C. and Sondel, P.M.**, The role of interleukin-2 in cancer therapy, *Cancer Surv.*, 8, 861, 1989.
911. **Foa, R., Guarini, A., and Gansbacher, B.**, IL2 treatment for cancer: from biology to gene therapy, *Br. J. Cancer*, 66, 992, 1992.

912. **Maas, R.A., Dullens, H.F.J., and Denotter, W.,** Interleukin-2 in cancer treatment: disappointing or (still) promising? A review, *Cancer Immunol. Immunother.,* 36, 141, 1993.
913. **Bubeník, J.,** Local immunotherapy of cancer with interleukin 2, *Immunol. Lett.,* 21, 267, 1989.
914. **Kaye, W.A., Adri, M.N.S., Soeldner, J.S., Rabinowe, S.L., Kaldany, A., Kahn, C.R., Bistrian, B., Srikanta, S., Ganda, O.P., and Eisenbarth, G.S.,** Acquired defect in interleukin-2 production in patients with type I diabetes mellitus, *N. Engl. J. Med.,* 315, 920, 1986.
915. **Feutren, G., Papoz, L., Assan, R., Vialettes, B., Pehuet, M., Vexiau, P., Durostu, H., Rodier, M., Sirmai, J., Lallemand, A., and Bach, J.-F.,** Induction de rémissions du diabète insulino-dépendant par la cyclosporine, *C. R. Acad. Sci. Paris,* 303, 295, 1986.
916. **Hamburger, J.,** Le diabète insulino-dépendant, maladie autoimmune, *C. R. Acad. Sci. Paris,* 303, 299, 1986.
917. **Saneto, R.P., Altman, A., Knobler, R.L., Johnson, H.M., and de Vellis, J.,** Interleukin 2 mediates the inhibition of oligodendrocyte progenitor cell proliferation *in vitro, Proc. Natl. Acad. Sci. U.S.A.,* 83, 9221, 1986.
918. **DeFreitas, E.C., Sandberg-Wollheim, M., Schonely, K., Boufal, M., and Koprowski, H.,** Regulation of interleukin 2 receptors on T cells from multiple sclerosis patients, *Proc. Natl. Acad. Sci. U.S.A.,* 83, 2637, 1986.
919. **Theofilopoulos, A.N. and Dixon, F.J.,** Etiopathogenesis of murine SLE, *Immunol. Rev.,* 55, 179, 1981.
920. **Rosenberg, Y.J., Malek, T.R., Schaeffer, D.E., Santoro, T.J., Mark, G.E., Steinberg, A.D., and Mountz, J.D.,** Unusual expression of IL 2 receptors and both the c-*myb* and c-*raf* oncogenes in T-cell lines and clones derived from autoimmune MRL-*lpr/lpr* mice, *J. Immunol.,* 134, 3120, 1985.
921. **Katagiri, K., Katagiri, T., Yokota, S., Eisenberg, R.A., Cohen, P.L., and Ting, J.P.-Y.,** Two different molecular pathways account for low Il-2 receptor and c-*myc* mRNA expression by *lpr* Lyt-2⁻ and L3T4-2⁻ T cells, *J. Immunol.,* 141, 2145, 1988.
922. **Umland, S.P., Smith, S.R., and Strausser, H.R.,** Production of and responsiveness to interleukin 2 in autoimmune BXSB mice, *Cell. Immunol.,* 107, 158, 1987.
923. **Tsokos, G.C., Smith, P.L., Christian, C.B., Lipnick, R.N., Balow, J.E., and Djeu, J.Y.,** Interleukin-2 restores the depressed allogeneic cell mediated lympholysis and natural killer cell activity in patients with systemic lupus erythematosus, *Clin. Immunol. Immunopathol.,* 34, 379, 1985.
924. **Kobayashi, K., Kasama, T., Fukushima, T., Kashara, K., Tabata, M., Sekine, F., Negishi, M., Ide, H., and Takahashi, T.,** Deficiency of interleukin 2 inhibitor activity in serum from autoimmune-prone mice, *Immunol. Invest.,* 16, 45, 1987.
925. **Diamantstein, T. and Osawa, H.,** The interleukin-2 receptor, its physiology and a new approach to a selective immunosuppressive therapy by anti-interleukin-2 receptor monoclonal antibodies, *Immunol. Rev.,* 92, 5, 1986.
926. **Waldmann, T.A.,** Multichain interleukin-2 receptor: a target for immunotherapy in lymphoma, *J. Natl. Cancer Inst.,* 81, 914, 1989.
927. **Ihle, J.N. and Askew, D.,** Origins and properties of hematopoietic growth factor-dependent cell lines, *Int. J. Cell Cloning,* 7, 68, 1989.
928. **Ihle, J.N.,** The molecular and cellular biology of interleukin-3, *Yearb. Immunol.,* 5, 59, 1989.
929. **Yang, Y.-C. and Clark, S.C.,** Human interleukin 3: analysis of the gene and its role in the regulation of hematopoiesis, *Int. J. Cell Cloning,* 8 (Suppl. 1), 121, 1990.
930. **Oster, W. and Schulz, G.,** Interleukin 3: biological and clinical effects, *Int. J. Cell Cloning,* 9, 5, 1991.
931. **Metcalf, D.,** Multi-CSF-dependent colony formation by cells of a murine hemopoietic cell line: specificity and action of multi-CSF, *Blood,* 65, 357, 1985.
932. **Iscove, N.N., Roitsch, C.A., Williams, N., and Guilbert, L.J.,** Molecules stimulating early red cell, granulocyte, macrophage, and megakaryocyte precursor in culture: similarity in size, hydrophobicity, and charge, *J. Cell. Physiol.,* Suppl. 1, 65, 1982.
933. **Miyatake, S., Yokota, T., Lee, F., and Arai, K.,** Structure of the chromosomal gene for murine interleukin 3, *Proc. Natl. Acad. Sci. U.S.A.,* 82, 316, 1985.
934. **Merchav, S., Nagler, A., Sahar, E., and Tatarsky, I.,** Production of human pluripotent progenitor cell colony stimulating activity (CFU-GEMM$_{CSA}$) in patients with myelodysplastic syndromes, *Leukemia Res.,* 11, 273, 1987.
935. **Guba, S.C., Stella, G., Turka, L.A., June, C.H., Thompson, C.B., and Emerson, S.G.,** Regulation of interleukin 3 gene induction in normal human T cells, *J. Clin. Invest.,* 84, 1701, 1989.

936. **Chang, M.-P., Utsuyama, M., Hirokawa, K., and Makinodan, T.,** Decline of the production of interleukin-3 with age in mice, *Cell. Immunol.,* 115, 1, 1988.
937. **Kimoto, M., Kindler, V., Higachi, M., Ody, C., Izui, S., and Vassalli, P.,** Recombinant murine IL-3 fails to stimulate T or B lymphopoiesis in vivo, but enhances immune responses to T-cell-dependent antigens, *J. Immunol.,* 140, 1889, 1988.
938. **Zupo, S., Perussia, B., Baldi, L., Corcione, A., Dono, M., Ferrarini, M., and Pistoia, V.,** Production of granulocyte-macrophage colony-stimulating factor but not IL-3 by normal and neoplastic human lymphocytes B, *J. Immunol.,* 148, 1423, 1992.
939. **Segal, G.M., McCall, E., Steve, T., and Bagby, G.C., Jr.,** Interleukin 1 stimulates endothelial cells to release multilineage human colony-stimulating activity, *J. Immunol.,* 138, 1772, 1987.
940. **Tanno, Y., Stadler, B., and Denburg, J.A.,** Human interleukin-3-like activity, basophil and eosinophil growth promoting activities and colony stimulating factor derived from several cell lines, *Int. Arch. Allergy Immunol.,* 83, 1, 1987.
941. **Lee, J.C., Hapel, A.J., and Ihle, J.N.,** Constitutive production of a unique lymphokine (IL-3) by the WEHI-3 cell line, *J. Immunol.,* 128, 2393, 1982.
942. **Ymer, S., Tucker, W.Q.J., Sanderson, C.J., Hapel, A.J., Campbell, H.D., and Young, I.G.,** Constitutive synthesis of interleukin-3 by leukaemia cell line WEHI-3B is due to retroviral insertion near the gene, *Nature,* 317, 255, 1985.
943. **Abe, J. Moriya, Y., Saito, M., Sugawara, Y., Suda, T., and Nishii, Y.,** Modulation of cell growth, differentiation, and production of interleukin-3 by $1\alpha,25$-dihydroxyvitamin D_3 in the murine myelomonocytic leukemia cell line WEHI-3, *Cancer Res.,* 46, 6316, 1986.
944. **Metcalf, D. and Nicola, N.A.,** Tissue localization and fate in mice of injected multipotential colony-stimulating factor, *Proc. Natl. Acad. Sci. U.S.A.,* 85, 3160, 1988.
945. **Leary, A.G., Yang, Y.-C., Clark, S.C., Gasson, J.C., Golde, D.W., and Ogawa, M.,** Recombinant gibbon interleukin 3 supports formation of human multilineage colonies and blast cell colonies in culture: comparison with recombinant human granulocyte-macrophage colony-stimulating factor, *Blood,* 70, 1343, 1987.
946. **London, L. and McKearn, J.P.,** Activation and growth of colony-stimulating factor-dependent cell lines is cell cycle stage dependent, *J. Exp. Med.,* 166, 1419, 1987.
947. **Keller, J.R. and Ihle, J.N.,** Unique pathway of IL-3-driven hemopoietic differentiation, *J. Immunol.,* 143, 4025, 1989.
948. **Lopez, A.F., Dyson, P.G., To, L.B., Elliott, M.J., Milton, S.E., Russell, J.A., Juttner, C.A., Yang, Y.-C., Clark, S.C., and Vadas, M.A.,** Recombinant human interleukin-3 stimulation of hematopoiesis in humans: loss of responsiveness with differentiation in the neutrophilic myeloid series, *Blood,* 72, 1797, 1988.
949. **Valent, P., Schmidt, G., Besemer, J., Mayer, P., Zenke, G., Liehl, E., Hinterberger, W., Lechner, K., Maurer, D., and Bettelheim, P.,** Interleukin-3 is a differentiation factor for human basophils, *Blood,* 73, 1763, 1989.
950. **Barton, B.E. and Mayer, R.,** IL-3 induces differentiation of bone marrow precursor cells to osteoclast-like cells, *J. Immunol.,* 143, 3211, 1989.
951. **Lord, B.I., Molineux, G., Testa, N.G., Kelly, M., Spooncer, E., and Dexter, T.M.,** The kinetic response of haemopoietic precursor cells, *in vivo,* to highly purified recombinant interleukin-3, *Lymphokine Res.,* 5, 97, 1986.
952. **Ulich, T.R., del Castillo, J., McNiece, I.K., Yin, S., Irwin, B., Busser, K., and Guo, K.,** Acute and subacute hematologic effects of multi-colony stimulating factor in combination with granulocyte colony-stimulating factor in vivo, *Blood,* 75, 48, 1990.
953. **Suda, T., Suda, J., Ogawa, M., and Ihle, J.N.,** Permissive role of interleukin 3 (IL-3) in proliferation and differentiation of multipotential hemopoietic progenitors in culture, *J. Cell. Physiol.,* 124, 182, 1985.
954. **Kelvin, D.J., Chance, S., Shreeve, M., Axelrad, A.A., Connolly, J.A., and McLeod, D.,** Interleukin 3 and cell cycle progression, *J. Cell. Physiol.,* 127, 403, 1986.
955. **Koike, K., Stanley, E.R., Ihle, J.N., and Ogawa, M.,** Macrophage colony formation supported by purified CSF-1 and/or interleukin 3 in serum-free culture: evidence for hierarchical difference in macrophage colony-forming cells, *Blood,* 67, 859, 1986.
956. **Jadus, M.R., Schmunk, G., Djeu, J.Y., and Parkman, R.,** Morphology and lytic mechanisms of interleukin 3-dependent natural cytotoxic cells: tumor necrosis factor as a possible mediator, *J. Immunol.,* 137, 2774, 1986.

957. **Cannistra, S.A., Vellenga, E., Groshek, P., Rambaldi, A., and Griffin, J.D.,** Human granulocyte-monocyte colony-stimulating factor and interleukin 3 stimulate monocyte cytotoxicity through a tumor necrosis factor-dependent mechanism, *Blood,* 71, 672, 1988.
958. **Kalland, T.,** Interleukin 3 is a major negative regulator of the generation of natural killer cells from bone marrow precursors, *J. Immunol.,* 137, 2268, 1986.
959. **Xia, X.L., and Choi, Y.S.,** Human recombinant IL-3 is a growth factor for normal B-cells, *J. Immunol.,* 148, 491, 1992.
960. **Palacios, R., Henson, G., Steinmetz, M., and McKearn, J.P.,** Interleukin-3 supports growth of mouse pre-B-cell clones *in vitro, Nature,* 309, 126, 1984.
961. **Palacios, R. and Steinmetz, M.,** IL3-dependent mouse clones that express B-220 surface antigen, contain Ig genes in germ-line configuration, and generate B lymphocytes in vivo, *Cell,* 41, 727, 1985.
962. **Burstein, S.A.,** Interleukin 3 promotes maturation of murine megakaryocytes in vitro, *Blood Cells,* 11, 469, 1986.
963. **Kavnoudias, H., Jackson, H., Ettlinger, K., Bertoncello, I., McNiece, I., and Williams, N.,** Interleukin-3 directly stimulates both megakaryocyte progenitor cells and immature megakaryocytes, *Exp. Hematol.,* 20, 43, 1992.
964. **Chen, B.D.-M. and Clark, C.R.,** Interleukin 3 (IL 3) regulates the in vitro proliferation of both blood monocytes and peritoneal exudate macrophages: synergism between a macrophage lineage-specific colony-stimulating factor (CSF-1) and IL 3, *J. Immunol.,* 137, 563, 1986.
965. **Miyauchi, J., Kelleher, C.A., Yang, Y.-C., Wong, G.G., Clark, S.C., Minden, M.D., Minkin, S., and McCulloch, E.A.,** The effects of three recombinant growth factors, IL-3, GM-CSF, and G-CSF, on the blast cells of acute myeloblastic leukemia maintained in short-term suspension culture, *Blood,* 70, 657, 1987.
966. **Bot, F.J., Dorssers, L., Wagemaker, G., and Löwenberg, B.,** Stimulating spectrum of human recombinant multi-CSF (IL-3) on human marrow precursors: importance of accessory cells, *Blood,* 71, 1609, 1988.
967. **Sonoda, Y., Yang, Y.-C., Wong, G.G., Clark, S.C., and Ogawa, M.,** Analysis in serum-free culture of the targets of recombinant human hemopoietic growth factors: interleukin 3 and granulocyte/macrophage-colony-stimulating factor are specific for early developmental stages, *Proc. Natl. Acad. Sci. U.S.A.,* 85, 4360, 1988.
968. **Goodman, J.W., Hall, E.A., Miller, K.L., and Shinpock, S.G.,** Interleukin 3 promotes erythroid burst formation in "serum-free" cultures without detectable erythropoietin, *Proc. Natl. Acad. Sci. U.S.A.,* 82, 3291, 1985.
969. **Suda, J., Suda, T., Kubota, K., Ihle, J.N., Saito, M., and Miura, Y.,** Purified interleukin-3 and erythropoietin support the terminal differentiation of hemopoietic progenitors in serum-free culture, *Blood,* 67, 1002, 1986.
970. **Lopez, A.F., To, L.B., Yang, Y.-C., Ganble, J.R., Shannon, M.F., Burns, G.F., Dyson, P.G., Juttner, C.A., Clark, S., and Vadas, M.A.,** Stimulation of proliferation, differentiation, and function of human cells by primate interleukin 3, *Proc. Natl. Acad. Sci. U.S.A.,* 84, 2761, 1987.
971. **Lopez, A.F., Eglinton, J.M., Gillis, D., Park, L.S., Clark, S., and Vadas, M.A.,** Reciprocal inhibition of binding between interleukin 3 and granulocyte-macrophage colony-stimulating factor to human eosinophils, *Proc. Natl. Acad. Sci. U.S.A.,* 86, 7022, 1989.
972. **Mazur, E.M., Cohen, J.L., Bogart, L., Mufson, R.A., Gesner, T.G., Yang, Y.-C., and Clark, S.C.,** Recombinant gibbon interleukin-3 stimulates megakaryocyte colony growth in vitro from human peripheral blood progenitor cells, *J. Cell. Physiol.,* 136, 439, 1988.
973. **Misago, M., Chiba, S., Kikuchi, M., Tsukada, J., Sato, T., Oda, S., and Eto, S.,** Effect of recombinant human interleukin 3, granulocyte-macrophage colony-stimulating factor and granulocyte colony-stimulating factor on human BFU-e in serum-free cultures, *Int. J. Cell Cloning,* 7, 37, 1989.
974. **Barlow, D.P., Bucan, M., Lehrach, H., Hogan, B.L.M., and Gough, N.M.,** Close genetic and physical linkage between the murine haemopoietic growth factor genes GM-CSF and multi-CSF (IL3), *EMBO J.,* 6, 617, 1987.
975. **Webb, G.C., Lee, J.S., Campbell, H.D., and Young, I.G.,** The genes for interleukins 3 and 5 map to the same locus on mouse chromosome 11, *Cytogenet. Cell Genet.,* 50, 107, 1989.
976. **Ihle, J.W., Keller, J., Henderson, L., Klein, F., and Palazinski, E.,** Procedure for the purification of interleukin-3 to homogeneity, *J. Immunol.,* 129, 2431, 1982.
977. **Clark-Lewis, I., Kent, S.B.H., and Schrader, J.W.,** Purification to apparent homogeneity of a factor stimulating the growth of multiple lineages of hemopoietic cells, *J. Biol. Chem.,* 259, 7488, 1984.

978. **Fung, M.C., Hapel, A.J., Ymer, S., Cohen, D.R., Johnson, R.M., Campbell, H.D., and Young I.G.,** Molecular cloning of cDNA for murine interleukin-3, *Nature,* 307, 233, 1984.
979. **Greenberger, J.S., Humphries, R.K., Messner, H., Reid, D.M., and Sakakeeny, M.A.,** Molecularly cloned and expressed murine T-cell gene product is similar to interleukin-3, *Exp. Hematol.,* 13, 249, 1985.
980. **Tsuchiya, T., Tojo, A., and Shibuya, M.,** Multi-copy introduction and high-level expression of interleukin-3 genes by retroviral vector superinfection, *Biochem. Biophys. Res. Commun.,* 158, 576, 1989.
981. **Cohen, D.R., Hapel, A.J., and Young, I.G.,** Cloning and expression of the rat interleukin-3 gene, *Nucleic Acids Res.,* 14, 3641, 1986.
982. **Yang, Y.-C., Ciarletta, A.B., Temple, P.A., Chung, M.P., Kovacic, S., Witek-Giannotti, J.S., Leary, A.C., Kriz, R., Donahue, R.E., Wong, G.G., and Clark, S.C.,** Human IL-3 (multi-CSF): identification by expression cloning of a novel hematopoietic growth factor related to murine IL-3, *Cell,* 47, 3, 1986.
983. **Otsuka, T., Miyajima, A., Brown, N., Otsu, K., Abrams, J., Saeland, S., Caux, C., de Waal Malefijt, R., de Vries, J., Meyerson, P., Yokota, K., Gemmel, L., Rennick, D., Lee, F., Arai, N., Arai, K.-I., and Yokota, T.,** Isolation and characterization of an expressible cDNA encoding human IL-3. Induction of IL-3 mRNA in human T-cell clones, *J. Immunol.,* 140, 2288, 1988.
984. **Le Beau, M.M., Epstein, N.D., O'Brien, S.J., Nienhuis, A.W., Yang, Y.-C., Clark, S.C., and Rowley, J.D.,** The interleukin 3 gene is located on human chromosome 5 and is deleted in myeloid leukemias with a deletion of 5q, *Proc. Natl. Acad. Sci. U.S.A.,* 84, 5913, 1987.
985. **Yang, Y.-C., Kovacic, S., Kriz, R., Wolf, S., Clark, S.C., Wellems, T.E., Nienhuis, A., and Epstein, N.,** The human genes for GM-CSF and IL 3 are closely linked in tandem on chromosome 5, *Blood,* 71, 958, 1988.
986. **Huebner, K., Nagarajan, L., Besa, E., Angert, E., Lange, B.J., Cannizzaro, L.A., van den Berghe, H., Santoli, D., Finan, J., Croce, C.M., and Nowell, P.C.,** Order of genes on human chromosome 5q with respect to 5q interstitial deletions, *Am. J. Hum. Genet.,* 46, 26, 1990.
987. **van den Berghe, H., Vermaelen, K., Mecucci, C., Barbieri, D., and Tricot, G.,** The 5q- anomaly, *Cancer Genet. Cytogenet.,* 17, 189, 1985.
988. **Kindler, V., Thorens, B., de Kossodo, S., Allet, B., Eliason, J.F., Thatcher, D., Farber, N., and Vassalli, P.,** Stimulation of hematopoiesis *in vivo* by recombinant bacterial murine interleukin 3, *Proc. Natl. Acad. Sci. U.S.A.,* 83, 1001, 1986.
989. **Clark-Lewis, I., Aebersold, R., Ziltener, H., Schrader, J.W., Hood, L.E., and Kent, S.B.H.,** Automated chemical synthesis of a protein factor for hemopoietic cells, interleukin 3, *Science,* 231, 134, 1986.
990. **Ziltener, H.J., Clark-Lewis, I., Hood, L.E., Kent, S.B.H., and Schrader, J.W.,** Antipeptide antibodies of predetermined specificity recognize and neutralize the bioactivity of the pan-specific hemopoietin interleukin 3, *J. Immunol.,* 138, 1099, 1987.
991. **Wodnar-Filipowitz, A. and Moroni, C.,** Regulation of interleukin 3 mRNA expression in mast cells occurs at the posttranscriptional level and is mediated by calcium ions, *Proc. Natl. Acad. Sci. U.S.A.,* 87, 777, 1990.
992. **Welte, K., Platzer, E., Lu, L., Gabrilove, J.L., Levi, E., Mertelsmann, R., and Moore, M.A.S.,** Purification and biochemical characterization of human pluripotent hematopoietic colony-stimulating factor, *Proc. Natl. Acad. Sci. U.S.A.,* 82, 1526, 1985.
993. **Frei, K., Bodmer, S., Schwerdel, C., and Fontana, A.,** Astrocytes of the brain synthesize interleukin 3-like factors, *J. Immunol.,* 135, 4044, 1985.
994. **Frei, K., Bodmer, S., Schwerdel, C., and Fontana, A.,** Astrocyte-derived interleukin 3 as a growth factor for microglia cells and peritoneal macrophages, *J. Immunol.,* 137, 3521, 1986.
995. **Li, C.L. and Johnson, G.R.,** Stimulation of multipotential, erythroid and other murine hematopoietic progenitor cells by adherent cell lines in the absence of detectable multi-CSF (IL-3), *Nature,* 316, 633, 1985.
996. **Gojobori, T., Aota, S., Inoue, T., and Shimotono, K.,** A sequence homology between the pX genes of HTLV-I/II and the murine IL-3 gene, *FEBS Lett.,* 208, 231, 1986.
997. **Palaszynski, E. and Ihle, J.N.,** Evidence for specific receptors for interleukin 3 on lymphokine-dependent cell lines established from long-term bone marrow cultures, *J. Immunol.,* 132, 1872, 1984.

998. **Palacios, R., Neri, T., and Brockhaus, M.,** Monoclonal antibodies specific for interleukin 3-sensitive murine cells, *J. Exp. Med.,* 163, 369, 1986.
999. **Nicola, N.A. and Metcalf, D.,** Binding of iodinated multipotential colony-stimulating factor (interleukin-3) to murine bone marrow cells, *J. Cell. Physiol.,* 128, 180, 1986.
1000. **Nicola, N.A. and Peterson, L.,** Identification of distinct receptors for two hemopoietic growth factors (granulocyte colony-stimulating factor and multipotential colony-stimulating factor) by chemical cross-linking, *J. Biol. Chem.,* 261, 12384, 1986.
1001. **Isfort, R.J., Stevens, D., May, W.S., and Ihle, J.N.,** Interleukin 3 binds to a 140-kDa phosphotyrosine-containing cell surface protein, *Proc. Natl. Acad. Sci. U.S.A.,* 85, 7982, 1988.
1002. **Budel, L.M., Elbaz, O., Hoogerbrugge, H., Delwel, R., Mahmoud, L.A., Löwenberg, B., and Touw, I.P.,** Common binding structure for granulocyte macrophage colony-stimulating factor and interleukin-3 on human acute myeloid leukemia cells and monocytes, *Blood,* 75, 1439, 1990.
1003. **Kitamura, T., Sato, N., Arai, K., and Miyajima, A.,** Expression cloning of the human IL-2 receptor cDNA reveals a shared β subunit for the human IL-3 and GM-CSF receptors, *Cell,* 66, 1165, 1991.
1004. **Lopez, A.F., Eglinton, J.M., Lyons, B., Tapley, P.M., To, L.B., Park, L.S., Clark, S.C., and Vadas, M.A.,** Human interleukin-3 inhibits the binding of granulocyte-macrophage colony-stimulating factor and interleukin-5 to basophils and strongly enhances their functional activity, *J. Cell. Physiol.,* 145, 69, 1990.
1005. **Mui, A.L.F., Kay, R.J., Humphries, R.K., and Krystal, G.,** Purification of the murine interleukin-3 receptor, *J. Biol. Chem.,* 267, 16523, 1992.
1006. **Hara, T. and Miyajima, A.,** Two distinct functional high affinity receptors for mouse interleukin-3 (IL-3), *EMBO J.,* 11, 1875, 1992.
1007. **Koyasu, S., Tojo, A., Miyajima, A., Akiyama, T., Kasuga, M., Urabe, A., Schreurs, J., Arai, K., Takaku, F., and Yahara, I.,** Interleukin 3-specific tyrosine phosphorylation of a membrane glycoprotein of M_r 150,000 in multi-factor-dependent myeloid cell lines, *EMBO J.,* 6, 3979, 1987.
1008. **Isfort, R., Huhn, R.D., Frackelton, A.R., Jr., and Ihle, J.N.,** Stimulation of factor-dependent myeloid cell lines with interleukin 3 induces tyrosine phosphorylation of several cellular substrates, *J. Biol. Chem.,* 263, 19203, 1988.
1009. **Wang, H.-M., Collins, M., Arai, K., and Miyajima, A.,** EGF induces differentiation of an IL-3-dependent cell line expressing the EGF receptor, *EMBO J.,* 8, 3677, 1989.
1010. **Schreurs, J., Sugawara, M., Arai, K.-I., Ohta, Y., and Miyajima, A.,** A monoclonal antibody with IL-3-like activity blocks IL-3 binding and stimulates tyrosine phosphorylation, *J. Immunol.,* 142, 819, 1989.
1011. **Sorensen, P., Mui, A.L.-F., and Krystal, G.,** Interleukin-3 stimulates the tyrosine phosphorylation of the 140-kilodalton interleukin-3 receptor, *J. Biol. Chem.,* 264, 19253, 1989.
1012. **Itoh, N., Yonehara, S., Schreurs, J., Gorman, D.M., Maruyama, K., Ishii, A., Yahara, I., Arai, K., and Miyajima, A.,** Cloning of an interleukin-3 receptor gene: a member of a distinct receptor gene family, *Science,* 247, 324, 1990.
1013. **Sakamaki, K., Miyajima, I., Kitamura, T., and Miyajima, A.,** Critical cytoplasmic domains of the common β subunit of the human GM-CSF, IL-3 and IL-5 receptors for growth signal transduction and tyrosine phosphorylation, *EMBO J.,* 11, 3541, 1992.
1014. **Duronio, V., Clark-Lewis, I., Federsppiel, B., Wieler, J.S., and Schrader, J.W.,** Tyrosine phosphorylation of receptor β subunits and common substrates in response to interleukin-3 and granulocyte-macrophage colony-stimulating factor, *J. Biol. Chem.,* 267, 21856, 1992.
1015. **Murthy, S.C., Sorensen, P.H.B., Mui, A.L.-F., and Krystal, G.,** Interleukin-3 down-regulates its own receptor, *Blood,* 73, 1180, 1989.
1016. **Akinsanya, A.A. and Whetton, A.D.,** Il-3 stimulated haemopoietic stem cell proliferation. Evidence for G-protein independent mitogenic signaling events, *J. Cell. Physiol.,* 152, 245, 1992.
1017. **Bradford, P.G., Jin, Y.Y., Hui, P., and Wang, X.H.,** IL-3 and GM-CSF induce the expression of the inositol trisphosphate receptor in K562 myeloblast cells, *Biochem. Biophys. Res. Commun.,* 187, 438, 1992.
1018. **Farrar, W.L., Thomas, T.P., and Anderson, W.B.,** Altered cytosol/membrane enzyme redistribution on interleukin-3 activation of protein kinase C, *Nature,* 315, 235, 1985.
1019. **Cook, P.P., Chen, J.M., and Ways, D.K.,** Interleukin-3 induces translocation and down-regulation of protein kinase C in human platelets, *Biochem. Biophys. Res. Commun.,* 185, 670, 1992.

1020. **Whetton, A.D., Heyworth, C.M., and Dexter, T.M.,** Phorbol esters activate protein kinase C and glucose transport and can replace the requirement for growth factor in interleukin-3-dependent multipotential stem cells, *J. Cell Sci.,* 84, 93, 1986.
1021. **Kraft, A.S., Wagner, F., and Housey, G.M.,** Overexpression of protein kinase C β1 is not sufficient to induce factor independence in the interleukin-3-dependent myeloid cell line FDC-P1, *Oncogene,* 5, 1243, 1990.
1022. **Klemm, D.J. and Elias, L.,** Purification and assay of a phosphatidylglycerol-stimulated protein kinase from murine leukemic cells and its perturbation in response to IL-3 and PMA treatment, *Exp. Hematol.,* 16, 855, 1988.
1023. **Whetton, A.D., Monk, P.N., Consalvey, S.D., and Downes, C.P.,** The haemopoietic growth factors interleukin 3 and colony-stimulating factor-1 stimulate proliferation but do not induce inositol lipid breakdown in murine bone-marrow-derived macrophages, *EMBO J.,* 5, 3281, 1986.
1024. **Barton, B.E., WoldeMussie, E., and Wheeler, L.,** The role of arachidonic acid metabolism in IL-3-induced proliferation, *Immunopharmacol. Immunotoxicol.,* 10, 35, 1988.
1025. **Duronio, V., Nip, L., and Pelech, S.L.,** Interleukin 3 stimulates phosphatidylcholine turnover in a mast/megakaryocyte cell line, *Biochem. Biophys. Res. Commun.,* 164, 804, 1989.
1026. **Garland, J.M., Ferris, D.K., and Farrar, W.L.,** Novel characteristics of a 33-kDa protein (pp33) rapidly phosphorylated in IL3 dependent cells by stimulation with IL3, *Biochem. Biophys. Res. Commun.,* 164, 520, 1989.
1027. **Ferris, D.K., Willet-Brown, J., Martensen, T., and Farrar, W.L.,** Interleukin 3 stimulation of tyrosine kinase activity in FDC-P1 cells, *Biochem. Biophys. Res. Commun.,* 154, 991, 1988.
1028. **Ferris, D.K., Willette-Brown, J., Martensen, T., and Farrar, W.L.,** Interleukin 3 and phorbol ester stimulate tyrosine phosphorylation of overlapping substrate proteins, *FEBS Lett.,* 246, 153, 1989.
1029. **Sorensen, P.H.B., Mui, A.L.-F., Murthy, S.C., and Krystal, G.,** Interleukin-3, GM-CSF, and TPA induce distinct phosphorylation events in an interleukin 3-dependent multipotential cell line, *Blood,* 73, 406, 1989.
1030. **Kanakura, Y., Druker, B., Wood, K.W., Mamon, H.J., Okuda, K., Roberts, T.M., and Griffin, J.D.,** Granulocyte-macrophage colony-stimulating factor and interleukin-3 induce rapid phosphorylation and activation of the proto-oncogene Raf-1 in a human factor-dependent myeloid cell line, *Blood,* 77, 243, 1991.
1031. **Tojo, A., Kasuga, M., Urabe, A., and Takaku, F.,** Vanadate can replace interleukin 3 for transient growth of factor-dependent cells, *Exp. Cell Res.,* 171, 16, 1987.
1032. **Kanakura, Y., Druker, B., Cannistra, S.A., Furukawa, Y., Torimoto, Y., and Griffin, J.D.,** Signal transduction of the human granulocyte-macrophage colony-stimulating factor and interleukin-3 receptors involves tyrosine phosphorylation of a common set of cytoplasmic proteins, *Blood,* 76, 706, 1990.
1033. **Torigoe, T., O'Connor, R., Santoli, D., and Reed, J.C.,** Interleukin-3 regulates the activity of the Lyn protein-tyrosine kinase in myeloid-committed leukemic cell lines, *Blood,* 80, 617, 1992.
1034. **Isfort, R.J.,** Frequency and mechanisms of factor independence in IL-3-dependent cell lines, *Somat. Cell Mol. Genet.,* 16, 109, 1990.
1035. **Serunian, L.A. and Rosenberg, N.,** Abelson virus potentiates long-term growth of mature B lymphocytes, *Mol. Cell. Biol.,* 6, 183, 1986.
1036. **Oliff, A., Agranovsky, O., McKinney, M.D., Murty, V.V.V.S., and Bauchwitz, R.,** Friend murine leukemia virus-immortalized myeloid cells are converted into tumorigenic cell lines by Abelson leukemia virus, *Proc. Natl. Acad. Sci. U.S.A.,* 82, 3306, 1985.
1037. **Cook, W.D., Metcalf, D., Nicola, N.A., Burgess, A.W., and Walker, F.,** Malignant transformation of a growth factor-dependent myeloid cell line by Abelson virus without evidence of an autocrine mechanism, *Cell,* 41, 677, 1985.
1038. **Pierce, J.H., Di Fiore, P.P., Aaronson, S.A., Potter, M., Pumphrey, J., Scott, A., and Ihle, J.N.,** Neoplastic transformation of mast cells by Abelson-Mu-LV: abrogation of IL-3 dependence by a nonautocrine mechanism, *Cell,* 41, 685, 1985.
1039. **Mathey-Prevot, B., Nabel, G., Palacios, R., and Baltimore, D.,** Abelson murine leukemia virus abrogation of interleukin 3 dependence in a lymphoid cell line, *Mol. Cell. Biol.,* 6, 4133, 1986.

1040. **Chung, S.W., Wong, P.M.C., Shen-Ong, G., Ruscetti, S., Ishizaka, T., and Eaves, C.J.,** Production of granulocyte-macrophage colony-stimulating factor by Abelson virus-induced tumorigenic mast cell lines, *Blood,* 68, 1074, 1986.

1041. **Rovera, G., Valtieri, M., Mavilio, F., and Reddy, E.P.,** Effect of Abelson murine leukemia virus on granulocytic differentiation and interleukin-3 dependence of a murine progenitor cell line, *Oncogene,* 1, 29, 1987.

1042. **Vogt, M., Lesley, J., Bogenberger, J.M., Haggblom, C., Swift, S., and Haas, M.,** The induction of growth factor-independence in murine myelocytes by oncogenes results in monoclonal cell lines and is correlated with cell crisis and karyotypic instability, *Oncogene Res.,* 2, 49, 1987.

1043. **Katzav, S., Martin-Zanca, D., Barbacid, M., Hedge, A.-M., Isfort, R., and Ihle, J.N.,** The *trk* oncogene abrogates growth factor requirements and transforms hematopoietic cells, *Oncogene,* 4, 1129, 1989.

1044. **Anderson, S.M., Carroll, P.M., and Lee, F.D.,** Abrogation of IL-3 dependent growth requires a functional v-*src* gene product: evidence for an autocrine growth cycle, *Oncogene,* 5, 317, 1990.

1045. **Rein, A., Keller, J., Schultz, A.M., Holmes, K.L., Medicus, R., and Ihle, J.N.,** Infection of immune mast cells by Harvey sarcoma virus: immortalization without loss of requirement for interleukin-3, *Mol. Cell. Biol.,* 5, 2257, 1985.

1046. **Andrejauskas, E. and Moroni, C.,** Reversible abrogation of IL-3 dependence by an inducible H-*ras* oncogene, *EMBO J.,* 8, 2575, 1989.

1047. **Uemura, N., Ozawa, K., Tojo, A., Takahashi, K., Okano, A., Karasuyama, H., Tani, K., and Asano, S.,** Acquisition of interleukin-3 independence in FDC-P2 cells after transfection with the activated c-H-*ras* gene using a bovine papillomavirus-based plasmid vector, *Blood,* 80, 3198, 1992.

1048. **Boswell, H.S., Harrington, M.A., Burgess, G.S., Nahreini, T.L., Derigs, H.G., Hodges, T.D., English, D., Crean, C.D., and Gabig, T.G.,** A mutant RAS gene acts through protein kinase C to augment interleukin-3 dependent proliferation in a fastidious immortal myeloid cell line, *Leukemia,* 3, 662, 1989.

1049. **Rapp, U.R., Cleveland, J.L., Brightman, K., Scott, A., and Ihle, J.N.,** Abrogation of IL-3 and IL-2 dependence by recombinant murine retroviruses expressing v-*myc* oncogenes, *Nature,* 317, 434, 1985.

1050. **Cleveland, J.L., Jansen, H.W., Bister, K., Fredrickson, T.N., Morse, H.C., III, Ihle, J.N., and Rapp, U.R.,** Interaction between *raf* and *myc* oncogenes in transformation in vivo and in vitro, *J. Cell. Biochem.,* 30, 195, 1986.

1051. **Hume, C.R., Nocka, K.H., Sorrentino, V., Lee, J.S., and Fleissner, E.,** Constitutive c-*myc* expression enhances the response of murine mast cells to IL-3, but does not eliminate their requirement for growth factors, *Oncogene,* 2, 223, 1988.

1052. **Dean, M., Cleveland, J.L., Rapp, U.R., and Ihle, J.N.,** Role of *myc* in the abrogation of IL3 dependence of myeloid FDC-P1 cells, *Oncogene Res.,* 1, 279, 1987.

1053. **Conscience, J.-F., Verrier, B., and Martin, G.,** Interleukin-3-dependent expression of the c-*myc* and c-*fos* proto-oncogenes in hemopoietic cell lines, *EMBO J.,* 5, 317, 1986.

1054. **Minks, M., Divinci, A., Bruno, S., Geido, E., Avignolo, C., and Giaretti, W.,** Interleukin 3 dependent c-*myc* protein expression during the cell cycle of murine mast cells, *Cancer Lett.,* 62, 243, 1992.

1055. **Mufson, R.A., Szabo, J., and Eckert, D.,** Human IL-3 induction of c-*jun* in normal monocytes is independent of tyrosine kinase and involves protein kinase C, *J. Immunol.,* 148, 1129, 1992.

1056. **Nahreini, T.S., Litz-Jacson, S., Burgess, G.S., Helvering, L.M., Manolagas, S.C., and Boswell, H.S.,** Interleukin-3 dependent mitogenesis in murine cells involves a predominant non-protein kinase C (pKC) dependent pathway for c-myc transcription. Role of a myc expression vector in rescuing pKC dependent mitogenesis, *Leukemia,* 5, 1099, 1991.

1057. **Gesner, T.G., Mufson, R.A., Nortonk C.R., Turner, K.J., Yang, Y.-C., and Clark, S.C.,** Specific binding, internalization, and degradation of human recombinant interleukin-3 by cells of the acute myelogenous leukemia line, KG-1, *J. Cell. Physiol.,* 136, 493, 1988.

1058. **Park, L.S., Waldron, P.E., Friend, D., Sassenfeld, H.M., Price, V., Anderson, D., Cosman, D., Andrews, R.G., Bernstein, I.D., and Urdal, D.L.,** Interleukin-3, GM-CSF, and G-CSF receptor expression on cell lines and primary leukemia cells: receptor heterogeneity and relationship to growth factor responsiveness, *Blood,* 74, 56, 1989.

1059. **Uckun, F.M., Gesner, T.G., Song, C.W., Myers, D.E., and Mufson, A.,** Leukemic B-cell precursors express functional receptors for human interleukin-3, *Blood,* 73, 533, 1989.

1060. **Clayberger, C., Luna-Fineman, S., Lee, J.E., Pillai, A., Campbell, M., Levy, R., and Krensky, A.M.,** Interleukin 3 is a growth factor for human follicular B-cell lymphomas, *J. Exp. Med.,* 175, 371, 1992.

1061. **Vellenga, E., Biesma, B., Meyer, C., Wagteveld, L., Esselink, M., and de Vries, E.G.E.,** The effects of five hematopoietic growth factors on human small cell lung carcinoma cell lines: interleukin 3 enhances the proliferation in one of the eleven cell lines, *Cancer Res.,* 51, 73, 1991.

1062. **Diamantis, I.D., Nair, A.P.K., Hirsch, H.H., and Moroni, C.,** Tumor suppression involves down-regulation of interleukin-3 expression in hybrids between autocrine mastocytoma and interleukin 3-dependent parental mast cells, *Proc. Natl. Acad. Sci. U.S.A.,* 86, 9299, 1989.

1063. **de Vries, E.G.E., van Gameren, M.M., and Willemse, P.H.B.,** Recombinant human interleukin 3 in clinical oncology, *Stem Cells,* 11, 72, 1993.

1064. **Keller, J.R., Ruscetti, S.K., and Ruscetti, F.W.,** Introduction of v-*abl* oncogene induces monocytic differentiation of an IL-3-dependent myeloid progenitor cell line, *Oncogene,* 5, 549, 1990.

1065. **Vaux, D.L., Cory, S., and Adams, J.M.,** Bcl-2 gene promotes haemopoietic cell survival and cooperates with c-*myc* to immortalize pre-B cells, *Nature,* 335, 440, 1988.

1066. **Nuñez, G., London, L., Hockenbery, D., Alexander, M., McKearn, J.P., and Korsmeyer, S.J.,** Deregulated Bcl-2 gene expression selectively prolongs survival of growth factor-deprived hemopoietic cell lines, *J. Immunol.,* 144, 3602, 1990.

1067. **Hapel, A.J., Vande Woude, G., Campbell, H.D., Young, I.G., and Robins, T.,** Generation of an autocrine leukemia using a retroviral expression vector carrying the interleukin-3 gene, *Lymphokine Res.,* 5, 249, 1986.

1068. **Jirik, F.R., Burstein, S.A., Treger, L., and Sorge, J.A.,** Transfection of a factor-dependent cell line with the murine interleukin-3 (IL-3) cDNA results in autonomous growth and tumorigenesis, *Leukemia Res.,* 11, 1127, 1987.

1069. **Chang, J.M., Metcalf, D., Lang, R.A., Gonda, T.J., and Johnson, G.R.,** Nonneoplastic hematopoietic myeloproliferative syndrome induced by dysregulated multi-CSF (IL-3) expression, *Blood,* 73, 1487, 1989.

1070. **Rolink, A. and Melchers, F.,** Molecular and cellular origins of B lymphocyte diversity, *Cell,* 66, 1081, 1991.

1071. **Korsmeyer, S.J. and Waldmann, T.A.,** Immunoglobulin genes: rearrangement and translocation in human lymphoid malignancy, *J. Clin. Immunol.,* 4, 1, 1984.

1072. **Waldmann, T.A., Korsmeyer, S.J., Bakhshi, A., Arnold, A., and Kirsch, I.R.,** Molecular genetic analysis of human lymphoid neoplasms: immunoglobulin genes and the c-*myc* oncogene, *Ann. Intern. Med.,* 102, 497, 1985.

1073. **Corcoran, L.M., Karvelas, M., Nossal, G.J.V., Ye, Z.-S., Jacks, T., and Baltimore, D.,** Oct-2 although not required for early B-cell development, is critical for later B-cell maturation and for postnatal survival, *Genes Develop.,* 7, 570, 1993.

1074. **Owens, T. and Zeine, R.,** The cell biology of T-dependent B cell activation, *Biochem. Cell Biol.,* 67, 481, 1989.

1075. **Rajasekar, R., Andersson, J., and Leanderson, T.,** Regulation of growth and differentiation of pre-activated B lymphocytes, *Scand. J. Immunol.,* 28, 509, 1988.

1076. **Muraguchi, A., Kehrl, J.H., Butler, J.L., and Fauci, A.S.,** Regulation of human B-cell activation, proliferation, and differentiation by soluble factors, *J. Clin. Immunol.,* 4, 337, 1984.

1077. **Grabstein, K., Mochizuki, D., Kronheim, S., Price, V., Cosman, D., Urdal, D., Gillis, S., and Conlon, P.,** Regulation of antibody production *in vitro* by granulocyte-macrophage colony stimulating factor, *J. Mol. Cell. Immunol.,* 2, 199, 1986.

1078. **del Guercio, P. and Katz, D.H.,** B cell-derived lymphokines: regulatory effects on the immune system, *Crit. Rev. Immunol.,* 6, 185, 1986.

1079. **Cambier, J.C., Justement, L.B., Newell, M.K., Chen, Z.Z., Harris, L.K., Sandoval, V.M., Klemsz, M.J., and Ransom, J.T.,** Transmembrane signals and intracellular "second messengers" in the regulation of quiescent B-lymphocyte activation, *Immunol. Rev.,* 95, 38, 1987.

1080. **Gold, M.R., Law, D.A., and DeFranco, A.L.,** Stimulation of protein tyrosine phosphorylation by the B-lymphocyte antigen receptor, *Nature,* 345, 810, 1990.

1081. **Defranco, A.L.,** Tyrosine phosphorylation and the mechanism of signal transduction by the B-lymphocyte antigen receptor, *Eur. J. Biochem.,* 210, 381, 1992.

1082. **Goodman, M.G., Speizer, L., Bakoch, G., Kanter, J., and Brunton, L.L.,** Activity of an intracellular lymphocyte stimulator is independent of G-protein interactions, $[Ca^{2+}]_i$ elevation, phosphoinositide hydrolysis, and protein kinase C translocation, *J. Biol. Chem.*, 265, 12248, 1990.
1083. **Hutchcroft, J.E., Harrison, M.L., and Geahlen, R.L.,** Lymphocyte-B activation is accompanied by phosphorylation of a 72-kDa protein-tyrosine kinase, *J. Biol. Chem.*, 266, 14846, 1991.
1084. **Butler, J.L., Falkoff, R.J.M., and Fauci, A.S.,** Development of a human T-cell hybridoma secreting separate B-cell growth and differentiation factors, *Proc. Natl. Acad. Sci. U.S.A.*, 81, 2475, 1984.
1085. **Takatsu, K.,** B-cell growth and differentiation factors, *Proc. Soc. Exp. Biol. Med.*, 188, 243, 1988.
1086. **Rennick, D., Hudak, S., Yang, G., and Jackson, J.,** Regulation of hemopoietic cell development by interleukins 4, 5 and 6, *Immunol. Res.*, 8, 215, 1989.
1087. **Bohjanen, P.R., Okajima, M., and Hodes, R.J.,** Differential regulation of interleukin 4 and interleukin 5 gene expression: a comparison of T-cell gene induction by anti-CD3 antibody or by exogenous lymphokines, *Proc. Natl. Acad. Sci. U.S.A.*, 87, 5283, 1990.
1088. **Ruuth, E., Praz, F., and Lundgren, E.,** Biochemical characterization of B cell stimulatory factors for lipopolysaccharide-preactivated B cell blasts: distinction from other known lymphokines, *Lymphokine Res.*, 7, 359, 1988.
1089. **Sharma, S., Mehta, S., Morgan, J., and Maizel, A.,** Molecular cloning and expression of a human B-cell growth factor gene in *Escherichia coli, Science,* 235, 1489, 1987.
1090. **Ennist, D.L., Greenblatt, D., Coffman, R., Sharma, S., Maizel, A., and Howard, M.,** Activity of a partially purified human BCGF on murine assays for B-cell stimulatory factors, *Cell. Immunol.*, 110, 77, 1987.
1091. **Ennist, D.L., Elkins, K.L., Cheng, S.C., and Howard, M.,** Activity of a partially purified human BCGF on murine assays for B cell stimulatory factors, *J. Immunol.*, 139, 1525, 1987.
1092. **Ambrus, J.L., Jr., Chesky, L., Chused, T., Young, K.R., Jr., McFarland, P., August, A., and Brown, E.J.,** Intracellular signaling events associated with the induction of proliferation of normal human B lymphocytes by two different antigenically related human B-cell growth factors (high molecular weight growth factor (HMW-BCGF) and the complement factor Bb), *J. Biol. Chem.*, 266, 3702, 1991.
1093. **Jelinek, D.F. and Lipsky, P.E.,** Comparative activation requirements of human peripheral blood, spleen, and lymph node B cells, *J. Immunol.*, 139, 1005, 1987.
1094. **Tseng, C.-T.K., Springgate, C.F., Piela, T.H., and Choi, Y.S.,** Development and characterization of a human B-cell line that responds to B cell growth factor but not interleukin 2, *J. Immunol.*, 138, 2554, 1987.
1095. **Jurgensen, C.H., Ambrus, J.L., Jr., and Fauci, A.S.,** Production of B-cell growth factor by normal B cells, *J. Immunol.*, 136, 4542, 1986.
1096. **Sahasrabuddhe, C.G., Martin, B., and Maizel, A.L.,** Purification and partial characterization of human intracellular B-cell growth factor, *Lymphokine Res.*, 5, 127, 1986.
1097. **Muraguchi, A., Nishimoto, H., Kawamura, N., Hori, A., and Kishimoto, T.,** B cell-derived BCGF functions as autocrine growth factor(s) in normal and transformed B lymphocytes, *J. Immunol.*, 137, 179, 1986.
1098. **Hutt-Fletcher, L.M.,** Synergistic activation of cells by Epstein-Barr virus and B-cell growth factor, *J. Virol.*, 61, 774, 1987.
1099. **Vazquez, A., Auffredou, M.-T., Gerard, J.-P., Delfraissy, J.-F., and Galanaud, P.,** Sequential effect of a high molecular weight B-cell growth factor and of interleukin 2 on activated human B cells, *J. Immunol.*, 139, 2344, 1987.
1100. **Muraguchi, A., Kehrl, J.H., Longo, D.L., Volkman, J., Smith, K.A., and Fauci, A.S.,** Interleukin 2 receptors on human B cells: implications for the role of interleukin 2 in human B cell function, *J. Exp. Med.*, 161, 181, 1985.
1101. **Kehrl, J.H., Grove, J.H., Goldsmith, P.K., and Fauci, A.S.,** B-cell growth factor and differentiation factors interact with receptors distinct from the interleukin 2 receptor, *Eur. J. Immunol.*, 16, 761, 1986.
1102. **Defrance, T., Aubry, J.-P., Vanbervliet, B., and Banchereau, J.,** Human interferon-γ acts as a B-cell growth factor in the anti-IgM antibody co-stimulatory assay but has no direct B-cell differentiation activity, *J. Immunol.*, 137, 3681, 1986.
1103. **Sidman, C.L., Marshall, J.D., Shultz, L.D., Gray, P.W., and Johnson, H.M.,** Gamma-interferon is one of several direct B-cell-maturing lymphokines, *Nature,* 309, 801, 1984.
1104. **Lee, G., Ellingsworth, L.R., Gillis, S., Wall, R., and Kincade, P.W.,** β Transforming growth factors are potential regulators of B lymphocytes, *J. Exp. Med.*, 166, 1290, 1987.

1105. Hirano, T., Taga, T., Nakano, N., Yasukawa, K., Kashiwamura, S., Shimizu, K., Nakajima, K., Pyun, K.H., and Kishimoto, T., Purification to homogeneity and characterization of human differentiation factor (BCDF or BSFp-2), *Proc. Natl. Acad. Sci. U.S.A.*, 82, 5490, 1985.

1106. Benjamin, D., Bazar, L.S., Wallace, B., and Jacobson, R.J., Heterogeneity of B-cell growth factor receptor reactivity in healthy donors and in patients with chronic lymphatic leukemia: relationship to B-cell-derived lymphokines, *Cell. Immunol.*, 103, 394, 1986.

1107. Smeland, E.B., Blomhoff, H.K., Holte, H., Ruud, E., Beiske, K., Funderud, S., Godal, T., and Ohlsson, R., Transforming growth factor type β (TGFβ) inhibits G_1 to S transition, but not activation of human B lymphocytes, *Exp. Cell Res.*, 171, 213, 1987.

1108. Genot, E., Billard, C., Sigaux, F., Mathiot, C., Degos, L., Falcoff, E., and Kolb, J.-P., Proliferative response of hairy cells to B-cell growth factor (BCGF): in vivo inhibition by interferon-α and in vitro effects of interferon-α, -β, and -γ, *Leukemia*, 1, 590, 1987.

1109. Karray, S., Merle-Béral, H., Vazquez, A., Gerard, J.-P., Debre, P., and Galanaud, P., Functional heterogeneity of B-CLL lymphocytes: dissociated responsiveness to growth factors and distinct requirements for a first activation signal, *Blood*, 70, 1105, 1987.

1110. Lacy, J., Sarkar, N., and Summers, W.C., Induction of c-*myc* expression in human B lymphocytes by B-cell growth factor and anti-immunoglobulin, *Proc. Natl. Acad. Sci. U.S.A.*, 83, 1458, 1986.

1111. Smeland, E.B., Beiske, K., Ek, B., Watt, R., Pfeifer-Ohlsson, S., Blomhoff, H.K., Godal, T., and Ohlsson, R., Regulation of c-*myc* transcription and protein expression during activation of normal human B cells, *Exp. Cell Res.*, 172, 101, 1987.

1112. Suzuki, H., Nakanishi, K., Steinberg, A., and Green, I., Induction of c-myc expression early in the course of B-cell activation: studies in normal humans and patients with systemic lupus erythematosus, *Int. Arch. Allergy Appl. Immunol.*, 79, 380, 1986.

1113. Lemoine, F.M., Krystal, G., Humphries, R.K., and Eaves, C.J., Autocrine production of pre-B-cell stimulating activity by a variety of transformed murine pre-B-cell lines, *Cancer Res.*, 48, 6438, 1988.

1114. Kanowith-Klein, S., Saxon, A., and Uittenbogaart, C.H., Constitutive production of B cell differentiation factor-like activity by human T- and B-cell lines, *Eur. J. Immunol.*, 17, 593, 1987.

1115. Blazar, B.A., Sutton, L.M., and Strome, M., Self-stimulating growth factor production by B-cell lines derived from Burkitt's lymphomas and other lines transformed *in vitro* by Epstein-Barr virus, *Cancer Res.*, 43, 4562, 1983.

1116. Gordon, J., Ley, S.C., Melamed, M.D., English, L.S., and Hughes-Jones, N.C., Immortalized B lymphocytes produce B-cell growth factor, *Nature*, 310, 145, 1984.

1117. Buck, J., Hämmerling, U., Hoffmann, M.K., Levi, E., and Welte, K., Purification and biochemical characterization of a human autocrine growth factor produced by Epstein-Barr virus-transformed B cells, *J. Immunol.*, 138, 2923, 1987.

1118. Ambrus, J.L., Jr., Jurgensen, C.H., Brown, E.J., and Fauci, A.S., Purification to homogeneity of a high molecular weight human B cell growth factor: demonstration of specific binding to activated B cells; and development of a monoclonal antibody to the factor, *J. Exp. Med.*, 162, 1319, 1985.

1119. Uckun, F.M., Fauci, A.S., Heerema, N.A., Song, C.W., Mehta, S.R., Gajl-Peczalska, K., Chandan, M., and Ambrus, J.L., B-cell growth factor receptor expression and B-cell growth factor response of leukemic B-cell precursors and B lineage lymphoid progenitor cells, *Blood*, 70, 1020, 1987.

1120. Perri, R.T., Impaired expression of cell surface receptors for B cell growth factor by chronic lymphocytic leukemia B cells, *Blood*, 67, 943, 1986.

1121. Uckun, F.M., Fauci, A.S., Chandan-Langlie, M., Myers, D.E., and Ambrus, J.L., Detection and characterization of human high molecular weight B-cell growth factor receptors (HMW-BCGF R) on leukemic B-cells in chronic lymphocytic leukemia, *J. Clin. Invest.*, 84, 1595, 1989.

1122. Paganelli, K.A., Evans, S.S., Han, T., and Ozer, H., B cell growth factor-induced proliferation of hairy cell lymphocytes and inhibition by type I interferon in vitro, *Blood*, 67, 937, 1986.

1123. Ford, R.J., Kwok, D., Quesada, J., and Sahasrabuddhe, C.G., Production of B cell growth factor(s) by neoplastic B cells from hairy cell leukemia patients, *Blood*, 67, 573, 1986.

1124. Tosato, G., Seamon, K.B., Goldman, N.D., Sehgal, P.B., May, L.T., Washington, G.C., Jones, K.D., and Pike, S.E., Monocyte-derived human B-cell growth factor identified as interferon-β2 (BSF-2, IL-6), *Science*, 239, 502, 1988.

1125. Gurney, M.E., Heinrich, S.P., Lee, M.R., and Yin, H., Molecular cloning and expression of neuroleukin, a neurotrophic factor for spinal and sensory neurons, *Science*, 234, 566, 1986.

1126. Gurney, M.E., Apatoff, B.R., Spear, G.T., Baumel, M.J., Antel, J.P., Brown Bania, M., and Reder, A.T., Neuroleukin: a lymphokine product of lectin-stimulated T cells, *Science*, 234, 574, 1986.

1127. **Howard, M., Farrar, J., Hilfiker, M., Johnson, B., Takatsu, K., Hamaoka, T., and Paul, W.E.,** Identification of a T-cell-derived B-cell growth factor distinct from interleukin 2, *J. Exp. Med.,* 155, 914, 1982.

1128. **Oliver, K., Noelle, R.J., Uhr, J.W., Krammer, P.H., and Vitetta, E.S.,** B-cell growth factor (B-cell growth factor I or B-cell-stimulating factor, provisional 1) is a differentiation factor for resting B cells and may not induce cell growth, *Proc. Natl. Acad. Sci. U.S.A.,* 82, 2465, 1985.

1129. **Rabin, E.M., Ohara, J., and Paul, W.E.,** B-cell stimulatory factor 1 activates resting B cells, *Proc. Natl. Acad. Sci. U.S.A.,* 82, 2935, 1985.

1130. **Alderson, M.R., Pike, B.L., and Nossal, G.J.V.,** Single cell studies on the role of B-cell stimulatory factor 1 in B-cell activation, *Proc. Natl. Acad. Sci. U.S.A.,* 84, 1389, 1987.

1131. **Finkelman, F.D., Ohara, J., Goroff, D.K., Smith, J., Villacreses, N., Mond, J.J., and Paul, W.E.,** Production of BSF-1 during an in vivo, T-dependent immune response, *J. Immunol.,* 137, 2878, 1986.

1132. **Brown, M.A., Pierce, J.H., Watson, C.J., Falco, J., Ihle, J.N., and Paul, W.E.,** B cell stimulatory factor-1/interleukin-4 mRNA is expressed by normal and transformed mast cells, *Cell,* 50, 809, 1987.

1133. **Ohara, J. and Paul, W.E.,** Production of a monoclonal antibody to and molecular characterization of B-cell stimulatory factor-1, *Nature,* 315, 333, 1985.

1134. **Vitetta, E.S., Ohara, J., Myers, C.D., Layton, J.F., Krammer, P.H., and Paul, W.E.,** Serological, biochemical, and functional identity of B-cell-stimulatory factor 1 and B-cell differentiation factor for IgG1, *J. Exp. Med.,* 162, 1726, 1985.

1135. **Paul, W.E.,** Interleukin 4/B cell stimulatory factor 1: one lymphokine, many functions, *FASEB J.,* 1, 456, 1987.

1136. **Paul, W.E. and Ohara, J.,** B-cell stimulatory factor-1/interleukin 4, *Annu. Rev. Immunol.,* 5, 429, 1987.

1137. **Grabstein, K., Eisenman, J., Mochizuki, D., Shanebeck, K., Conlon, P., Hopp, T., March, C., and Gillis, S.,** Purification to homogeneity of B-cell stimulating factor. A molecule that stimulates proliferation of multiple lymphokine-dependent cell lines, *J. Exp. Med.,* 163, 1405, 1986.

1138. **Ohara, J., Coligan, J.E., Zoon, K., Maloy, W.L., and Paul, W.E.,** High-efficiency purification and chemical characterization of B cell stimulatory factor-1/interleukin 4, *J. Immunol.,* 139, 1127, 1987.

1139. **Ohara, J. and Paul, W.E.,** Up-regulation of interleukin 4/B-cell stimulatory factor 1 receptor expression, *Proc. Natl. Acad. Sci. U.S.A.,* 85, 8221, 1988.

1140. **Takahashi, M., Yoshida, M.C., Satoh, H., Hilgers, J., Yaoita, Y., and Honjo, T.,** Chromosomal mapping of the mouse IL-4 and human IL-5 genes, *Genomics,* 4, 47, 1989.

1141. **Otsuka, T., Villaret, D., Yokota, T., Takebe, Y., Lee, F., Arai, N., and Arai, K.,** Structural analysis of the mouse chromosomal gene encoding interleukin 4 which expresses B-cell, T-cell and mast cell stimulating activities, *Nucleic Acids Res.,* 15, 333, 1987.

1142. **Yokota, T., Otsuka, T., Mosmann, T., Banchereau, J., DeFrance, T., Blanchard, D., De Vries, J.E., Lee, F., and Arai, K.,** Isolation and characterization of a human interleukin cDNA clone homologous to mouse B-cell stimulatory factor 1 that expresses B-cell- and T-cell-stimulating activities, *Proc. Natl. Acad. Sci. U.S.A.,* 83, 5894, 1986.

1143. **Arai, N., Nomora, D., Villaret, D., DeWaal Malefijt, R., Seiki, M., Yoshida, M., Minoshima, S., Fukujama, R., Maekawa, M., Kudoh, J., Shimizu, N., Yokota, K., Abe, E., Yokota, T., Takebe, Y., and Arai, K.,** Complete nucleotide sequence of the chromosomal gene for human IL-4 and its expression, *J. Immunol.,* 142, 274, 1989.

1144. **Lee, J.S., Campbell, H.D., Kozak, C.A., and Young, I.G.,** The *IL-4* and *IL-5* genes are closely linked and are part of a cytokine gene cluster on mouse chromosome 11, *Somat. Cell Mol. Genet.,* 15, 143, 1989.

1145. **Le Beau, M.M., Lemons, R.S., Espinosa, R., III, Larson, R.A., Arai, N., and Rowley, J.D.,** Interleukin-4 and interleukin-5 map to human chromosome 5 in a region encoding growth factors and receptors and are deleted in myeloid leukemias with a del(5q), *Blood,* 73, 647, 1989.

1146. **van Leeuwen, B.H., Martinson, M.E., Webb, G.C., and Young, I.G.,** Molecular organization of the cytokine gene cluster, involving the human IL-3, IL-4, IL-5, and GM-CSF genes, on human chromosome 5, *Blood,* 73, 1142, 1989.

1147. **Powers, R., Garrett, D.S., March, C.J., Frieden, E.A., Gronenborn, A.M., and Clore, G.M.,** Three-dimensional solution structure of human interleukin-4 by multidimensional heteronuclear magnetic resonance spectroscopy, *Science,* 256, 1673, 1992.

1148. **Defrance, T., Vanbervliet, B., Aubry, J.-P., Takebe, Y., Arai, N., Miyajima, A., Yokota, T., Lee, F., Arai, K., de Vries, J.E., and Banchereau, J.,** B cell growth-promoting activity of recombinant human interleukin 4, *J. Immunol.,* 139, 1135, 1987.

1149. **Mosmann, T.R., Yokota, T., Kastelein, R., Zurawski, S.M., Arai, N., and Takebe, T.,** Species-specificity of T cell stimulating activities of IL 2 and BSF-1 (Il-4): comparison of normal and recombinant mouse and human IL 2 and BSF-1 (IL 4), *J. Immunol.,* 138, 1813, 1987.

1150. **Rabin, E.M., Mond, J.J., Ohara, J., and Paul, W.E.,** Interferon-γ inhibits the action of B cell stimulatory factor (BSF)-1 on resting B cells, *J. Immunol.,* 137, 1573, 1986.

1151. **Karray, S., DeFrance, T., Merle-Béral, H., Banchereau, J., Debré, P., and Galanaud, P.,** Interleukin 4 counteracts the interleukin 2-induced proliferation of monoclonal B cells, *J. Exp. Med.,* 168, 85, 1988.

1152. **Han, X., Itoh, K., Balch, C.M., and Pellis, N.R.,** Recombinant interleukin 4 (RIL4) inhibits interleukin 2-induced activation of peripheral blood lymphocytes, *Lymphokine Res.,* 7, 227, 1988.

1153. **Lee, H.-K., Xia, X., and Choi, Y.S.,** IL-4 blocks the upregulation of IL-2 receptors induced by IL-2 in normal human B cells, *J. Immunol.,* 144, 3431, 1990.

1154. **Defrance, T., Vanbervliet, B., Aubry, J.-P., and Banchereau, J.,** Interleukin 4 inhibits the proliferation but not the differentiation of activated human B cells in response to interleukin 2, *J. Exp. Med.,* 168, 1321, 1988.

1155. **Simons, A. and Zharhary, D.,** The role of IL-4 in the generation of B lymphocytes in the bone marrow, *J. Immunol.,* 143, 2540, 1989.

1156. **Snapper, C.M. and Paul, W.E.,** B cell stimulatory factor-1 (interleukin 4) prepares resting murine B cells to secrete IgG1 upon subsequent stimulation with bacterial lipopolysaccharide, *J. Immunol.,* 139, 10, 1987.

1157. **Pène, J., Rousset, Brière, F., Chrétien, I., Bonnefoy, J.-Y., Spits, H., Yokota, T., Arai, N., Arai, K., Banchereau, J., and de Vries, J.E.,** IgE production by normal human lymphocytes is induced by interleukin 4 and suppressed by interferons γ and α and prostaglandin E$_2$, *Proc. Natl. Acad. Sci. U.S.A.,* 85, 6880, 1988.

1158. **Defrance, T., Vanbervliet, B., Pène, J., and Banchereau, J.,** Human recombinant IL-4 induces activated B lymphocytes to produce IgG and IgM, *J. Immunol.,* 141, 2000, 1988.

1159. **Kunimoto, D.Y., Harriman, G.R., and Strober, W.,** Regulation of IgA differentiation in CH12LX B cells by lymphokines. IL-4 induces membrane IgM-positive CH12LX cells to express membrane IgA and IL-5 induces membrane IgA-positive CH12LX cells to secrete IgA, *J. Immunol.,* 141, 713, 1988.

1160. **Finkelman, F.D., Katona, I.M., Urban, J.F., Jr., Snapper, C.M., Ohara, J., and Paul, W.E.,** Suppression of *in vivo* polyclonal IgE responses by monoclonal antibody to the lymphokine B-cell stimulatory factor 1, *Proc. Natl. Acad. Sci. U.S.A.,* 83, 9675, 1986.

1161. **Defrance, T., Aubry, J.P., Rousset, F., Vanbervliet, B., Bonnefoy, J.Y., Arai, N., Takebe, Y., Yokota, T., Lee, F., Arai, K., de Vries, J., and Banchereau, J.,** Human recombinant interleukin 4 induces Fc epsilon receptors (CD23) on normal human B lymphocytes, *J. Exp. Med.,* 165, 1459, 1987.

1162. **Hudak, S.A., Gollnick, S.O., Conrad, D.H., and Kehry, M.R.,** Murine B-cell stimulatory factor 1 (interleukin 4) increases expression of the Fc receptor for IgE on mouse B cells, *Proc. Natl. Acad. Sci. U.S.A.,* 84, 4606, 1987.

1163. **Smeland, E.B., Blomhoff, H.K., Funderud, S., Shalaby, M.F., and Espevik, T.,** Interleukin 4 induces selective production of interleukin 6 from normal human B lymphocytes, *J. Exp. Med.,* 170, 1463, 1989.

1164. **Lee, J.D., Swisher, S.G., Minehart, E.H., McBride, W.H., and Economou, J.S.,** Interleukin-4 downregulates interleukin-6 production in human peripheral blood mononuclear cells, *J. Leukocyte Biol.,* 47, 475, 1990.

1165. **Noelle, R.J., Kuziel, W.A., Maliszewski, C.R., McAdams, E., Vitetta, E.S., and Tucker, P.W.,** Regulation of the expression of multiple class II genes in murine B cells by B cell stimulatory factor-1 (BSF-1), *J. Immunol.,* 137, 1718, 1986.

1166. **Mond, J.J., Carman, J., Sarma, C., Ohara, J., and Finkelman, F.D.,** Interferon-γ suppresses B-cell stimulation factor (BSF-1) induction of class II MHC determinants on B cells, *J. Immunol.,* 137, 3534, 1986.

1167. **Snapper, C.M., Hornbeck, P.V., Atasoy, U., Pereira, G.M.B., and Paul, W.E.,** Interleukin 4 induces membrane Thy-1 expression on normal murine B cells, *Proc. Natl. Acad. Sci. U.S.A.,* 85, 6107, 1988.

1168. **Mosmann, T.R., Bond, M.W., Coffman, R.L., Ohara, J., and Paul, W.E.,** T-cell and mast cell lines response to B-cell stimulatory factor 1, *Proc. Natl. Acad. Sci. U.S.A.,* 83, 5654, 1986.

1169. **Fernandez-Botran, R., Krammer, P.H., Diamantstein, T., Uhr, J.W., and Vitetta, E.S.,** B cell-stimulatory factor 1 (BSF-1) promotes growth of helper T cell lines, *J. Exp. Med.,* 164, 580, 1986.

1170. **Palacios, R., Sideras, P., and von Boehmer, H.,** Recombinant interleukin 4/BSF-1 promotes growth and differentiation of intrathymic T-cell precursors from fetal mice *in vitro, EMBO J.,* 6, 91, 1987.
1171. **Hu-Li, J., Shevach, E.M., Mizuguchi, J., Ohara, J., Mosmann, T., and Paul, W.E.,** B cell stimulatory factor 1 (interleukin 4) is a potent costimulant for normal resting T lymphocytes, *J. Exp. Med.,* 165, 157, 1987.
1172. **Habetswallner, D., Pelosi, E., Bulgarini, D., Camagna, A., Samoggia, P., Montesoro, E., Giannella, G., Lazzaro, D., Isacchi, G., Testa, U., and Peschle, C.,** Activation and proliferation of normal resting human T lymphocytes in serum-free culture: role of IL-4 and IL-6, *Immunology,* 65, 357, 1988.
1173. **Kern, D.E., Peace, D.J., Klarnet, J.P., Cheever, M.A., and Greenberg, P.D.,** IL-4 is an endogenous T-cell growth factor during the immune response to a syngeneic retrovirus-induced tumor, *J. Immunol.,* 141, 2824, 1988.
1174. **Trenn, G., Tkayama, H., Hu-Li, J., Paul, W.E., and Sitkovsky, M.V.,** B cell stimulatory factor 1 (IL-4) enhances the development of cytotoxic T cells from Lyt-2^+ resting murine T lymphocytes, *J. Immunol.,* 140, 1101, 1988.
1175. **Miller, C.L., Hooton, J.W.L., Gillis, S., and Paetkau, V.,** IL-4 potentiates the IL-2-dependent proliferation of mouse cytotoxic T cells, *J. Immunol.,* 144, 1331, 1990.
1176. **Reason, D.C., Ebisawa, M., Saito, H., Nagakura, T., and Ikura, Y.,** Interleukin 4 induces CD4+/CD8– to CD8+/CD4– transformation of human neonatal T cells by way of a double positive intermediate, *Biochem. Biophys. Res. Commun.,* 168, 830, 1990.
1177. **Widmer, M.B. and Grabstein, K.H.,** Regulation of cytolytic T-lymphocyte generation by B-cell stimulatory factor, *Nature,* 326, 795, 1987.
1178. **Fernandez-Botran, R., Sanders, V.M., Oliver, K.G., Chen, Y.-W., Krammer, P.H., Uhr, J.W., and Vitetta, E.S.,** Interleukin 4 mediates autocrine growth of helper T cells after antigenic stimulation, *Proc. Natl. Acad. Sci. U.S.A.,* 83, 9689, 1986.
1179. **Evavold, B.D. and Allen, P.M.,** Separation of IL-4 production from Th cell proliferation by an altered T-cell receptor ligand, *Science,* 252, 1308, 1991.
1180. **Kühn, R., Rajewsky, K., and Müller, W.,** Generation and analysis of interleukin-4 deficient mice, *Science,* 254, 707, 1991.
1181. **Golumbek, P.T., Lazenby, A.J., Levitsky, H.I., Jaffee, L.M., Karasuyama, H., Baker, M., and Pardoll, D.M.,** Treatment of established renal cancer by tumor cells engineered to secrete interleukin-4, *Science,* 254, 713, 1991.
1182. **Wong, H.L., Costa, G.L., Lotze, M.T., and Wahl, S.M.,** Interleukin (IL) 4 differentially regulates monocyte IL-1 family gene expression and synthesis in vitro and in vivo, *J. Exp. Med.,* 177, 775, 1993.
1183. **te Velde, A.A., Klomp, J.P.G., Yard, B.A., de Vries, J.E., and Figdor, C.G.,** Modulation of phenotypic and functional properties of human peripheral blood monocytes by IL-4, *J. Immunol.,* 140, 1548, 1988.
1184. **Standiford, T.J., Strieter, R.M., Chensue, S.W., Westwick, J., Kasahara, K., and Kunkel, S.L.,** IL-4 inhibits the expression of IL-8 from stimulated human monocytes, *J. Immunol.,* 145, 1435, 1990.
1185. **Standiford, T.J., Strieter, R.M., Kasahara, K., and Kunkel, S.L.,** Disparate regulation of interleukin 8 gene expression from blood monocytes, endothelial cells, and fibroblasts by interleukin 4, *Biochem. Biophys. Res. Commun.,* 171, 531, 1990.
1186. **Hamaguchi, Y., Kanakura, Y., Fujita, J., Takeda, S., Nakano, T., Tarui, S., Honjo, T., and Kitamura, Y.,** Interleukin 4 as an essential factor for in vitro clonal growth of murine connective tissue-type mast cells, *J. Exp. Med.,* 165, 268, 1987.
1187. **Sonoda, Y., Okuda, T., Yokota, S., Maekawa, T., Shizumi, Y., Nishigaki, H., Misawa, S., Fujii, H., and Abe, T.,** Actions of human interleukin-4/B-cell stimulatory factor-1 on proliferation and differentiation of enriched hematopoietic progenitor cells in culture, *Blood,* 75, 1615, 1990.
1188. **Favre, C., Saeland, S., Caux, C., Duvert, V., and De Vries, J.E.,** Interleukin-4 has basophilic and eosinophilic cell growth-promoting activity on cord blood cells, *Blood,* 75, 67, 1990.
1189. **Valent, P., Besemer, J., Kishi, K., DiPadova, F., Geissler, K., Lechner, K., and Bettelheim, B.,** Human basophils express interleukin-4 receptors, *Blood,* 76, 1734, 1990.
1190. **Tepper, R.I., Coffman, R.L., and Leder, P.,** An eosinophil-dependent mechanism for the antitumor effect of interleukin 4, *Science,* 257, 548, 1992.
1191. **Zlotnik, A., Fischer, M., Roehm, N., and Zipori, D.,** Evidence for effects of interleukin 4 (B-cell stimulatory factor 1) on macrophages: enhancement of antigen presenting ability of bone marrow-derived macrophages, *Proc. Natl. Acad. Sci. U.S.A.,* 138, 4275, 1987.

1192. **Crawford, R.M., Finbloom, D.S., Ohara, J., Paul, W.E., and Meltzer, M.S.,** B cell stimulatory factor-1 (interleukin 4) activates macrophages for increased tumoricidal activity and expression of Ia antigens, *J. Immunol.,* 139, 135, 1987.
1193. **McInnes, A. and Rennick, D.M.,** Interleukin 4 induces cultured monocytes/macrophages to form giant multinucleated cells, *J. Exp. Med.,* 167, 598, 1988.
1194. **Hart, P.H., Cooper, R.L., and Finlay-Jones, J.J.,** IL-4 suppresses IL-1β, TNF-α and PGE_2 production by human peritoneal macrophages, *Immunology,* 72, 344, 1991.
1195. **Newcom, S.R., Ansari, A.A., and Gu, L.B.,** Interleukin 4 is an autocrine growth factor secreted by the L-428 Reed-Sternberg cell, *Blood,* 79, 191, 1992.
1196. **Peschel, C., Paul, W.E., Ohara, J., and Green, I.,** Effects of B cell stimulatory factor-1/interleukin 4 on hematopoietic progenitor cells, *Blood,* 70, 254, 1987.
1197. **Rennick, D., Yang, G., Muller-Sieburg, C., Smith, C., Arai, N., Takabe, Y., and Gemmell, L.,** Interleukin 4 (B-cell stimulatory factor 1) can enhance or antagonize the factor-dependent growth of hematopoietic progenitor cells, *Proc. Natl. Acad. Sci. U.S.A.,* 84, 6889, 1987.
1198. **Sonoda, Y., Kuzuyama, Y., Tanaka, S., Yokota, S., Maekawa, T., Clark, S.C., and Abe, T.,** Human interleukin-4 inhibits proliferation of megakaryocyte progenitor cells in culture, *Blood,* 81, 624, 1993.
1199. **Kishi, K., Ihle, J.N., Urdal, D.L., and Ogawa, M.,** Murine B-cell stimulatory factor-1 (BSF-1)/interleukin-4 (IL-4) is a multilineage colony-stimulating factor that acts directly on primitive hemopoietic progenitors, *J. Cell. Physiol.,* 139, 463, 1989.
1200. **Peschel, C., Green, I., and Paul, W.E.,** Interleukin-4 induces a substance in bone marrow stromal cells that reversibly inhibits factor-dependent and factor-independent cell proliferation, *Blood,* 73, 1130, 1989.
1201. **Toi, M., Harris, A.L., and Bicknell, R.,** Interleukin-4 is a potent mitogen for capillary endothelium, *Biochem. Biophys. Res. Commun.,* 174, 1287, 1991.
1202. **Watanabe, K., Tanaka, Y., Morimoto, I., Yahata, K., Zeki, K., Fujihara, T., Yamashita, U., and Eto, S.,** Interleukin-4 as a potent inhibitor of bone resorption, *Biochem. Biophys. Res. Commun.,* 172, 1035, 1990.
1203. **Ohara, J. and Paul, W.E.,** Receptors for B-cell stimulatory factor-1 expressed on cells of hematopoietic lineage, *Nature,* 325, 537, 1987.
1204. **Park, L.S., Friend, D., Grabstein, K., and Urdal, D.L.,** Characterization of the high-affinity cell-surface receptor for murine B-cell-stimulatory factor 1, *Proc. Natl. Acad. Sci. U.S.A.,* 84, 1669, 1987.
1205. **Lowenthal, J.W., Castle, B.E., Christiansen, J., Schreurs, J., Rennick, D., Arai, N., Hoy, P., Takebe, Y., and Howard, M.,** Expression of high affinity receptors for murine interleukin 4 (BSF-1) on hemopoietic and nonhemopoietic cells, *J. Immunol.,* 140, 456, 1988.
1206. **Park, L.S., Friend, D., Sassenfeld, H.M., and Urdal, D.L.,** Characterization of the human B-cell stimulatory factor 1 receptor, *J. Exp. Med.,* 166, 476, 1987.
1207. **Cabrillat, H., Galizzi, J.-P., Djossou, O., Arai, N., Yokota, T., Arai, K., and Banchereau, J.,** High affinity binding of human interleukin 4 to cell lines, *Biochem. Biophys. Res. Commun.,* 149, 995, 1987.
1208. **Wagteveld, A.J., Zanten, A.K.V., Esselink, M.T., Halie, M.R., and Vellenga, E.,** Expression and regulation of IL-4 receptors on human monocytes and acute myeloblastic leukemic cells, *Leukemia,* 5, 782, 1991.
1209. **Feldman, G.M. and Finbloom, D.S.,** Induction and regulation of IL-4 receptor expression on murine macrophage cell lines and bone-marrow-derived macrophages by IFN-γ, *J. Immunol.,* 145, 854, 1990.
1210. **Mosley, B., Beckmann, P., March, C.J., Idzerda, R.L., Gimpel, S.D., Vanden Bos, T., Friend, D., Alpert, A., Anderson, D., Jackson, J., Wignall, J.M., Smith, C., Gallis, B., Sims, J.E., Urdal, D., Widmer, M.B., Cosman, D., and Park, L.S.,** The murine interleukin-4 receptor: molecular cloning and characterization of secreted and membrane bound forms, *Cell,* 59, 335, 1989.
1211. **Keegan, A.D., Beckmann, M.P., Park, L.S., and Paul, W.E.,** The IL-4 receptor: biochemical characterization of IL-4-binding molecules in a T-cell line expressing large numbers of receptors, *J. Immunol.,* 146, 2272, 1991.
1212. **Harada, N., Yang, G., Miyajima, A., and Howard, M.,** Identification of an essential region for growth signal transduction in the cytoplasmic domain of the human interleukin-4 receptor, *J. Biol. Chem.,* 267, 22752, 1992.
1213. **Karray, S., Dautry-Varsat, A., Tsudo, M., Merle-Beral, H., Debre, P., and Galanaud, P.,** IL-4 inhibits the expression of high-affinity IL-4 receptors of monoclonal human B cells, *J. Immunol.,* 145, 1152, 1990.

1214. **Galizzi, J.-P., Zuber, C.E., Cabrillat, H., Djossou, O., and Banchereau, J.**, Internalization of human interleukin 4 and transient down-regulation of its receptor in the CD23-inducible Jijoye cells, *J. Biol. Chem.*, 264, 6984, 1989.

1215. **Mizuguchi, J., Beaven, M.A., Ohara, J., and Paul, W.E.**, BSF-1 action on resting B cells does not require elevation of inositol phospholipid metabolism or increased [Ca^{2+}], *J. Immunol.*, 137, 2215, 1986.

1216. **McCann, F.V., McCarthy, D.C., and Noelle, R.J.**, Interleukin-4 activates ion channels in B lymphocytes, *Cell. Signal.*, 3, 483, 1991.

1217. **Justement, L., Chen, Z., Harris, L., Ransom, J., Sandoval, V., Smith, C., Rennick, D., Roehm, N., and Cambier, J.**, BSF1 induces membrane protein phosphorylation but not phosphoinositide metabolism, Ca^{2+} mobilization, protein kinase C translocation, or membrane depolarization in resting murine B lymphocytes, *J. Immunol.*, 137, 3664, 1986.

1218. **Arruda, S. and Ho, J.L.**, IL-4 receptor signal transduction in human monocytes is associated with protein kinase C translocation, *J. Immunol.*, 149, 1258, 1992.

1219. **Izuhara, K. and Harada, N.**, Interleukin-4 (IL-4) induces protein tyrosine phosphorylation of the IL-4 receptor and association of phosphatidylinositol 3-kinase to the IL-4 receptor in a mouse T-cell line, HT2, *J. Biol. Chem.*, 268, 13097, 1993.

1220. **Grusby, M.J., Nabavi, N., Wong, H., Dick, R.F., Bluestone, J.A., Schotz, M.C., and Glimcher, L.H.**, Cloning of an interleukin-4 inducible gene from cytotoxic T lymphocytes and its identification as a lipase, *Cell*, 60, 451, 1990.

1221. **Phillips, N.E., Gravel, K.A., Tumas, K., and Parker, D.C.**, IL-4 (B cell stimulatory factor 1) overcomes Fcγ receptor-mediated inhibition of mouse B lymphocyte proliferation without affecting inhibition of c-*myc* mRNA induction, *J. Immunol.*, 141, 4243, 1988.

1222. **Dokter, W.H.A., Esselink, M.T., Halie, M.R., and Vellenga, E.**, Interleukin-4 inhibits the lipopolysaccharide-induced expression of c-*jun* and c-*fos* messenger RNA and activator protein-1 binding activity in human monocytes, *Blood*, 81, 337, 1993.

1223. **Hoon, D.S.B., Edward, O., Banez, M., Irie, F.R., and Morton, D.L.**, Interleukin 4 alone and with γ-interferon or tumor necrosis factor modulates cell surface antigens on human renal cell carcinoma, *Cancer Res.*, 51, 5687, 1991.

1224. **Obiri, N.I., Hillman, G.G., Haas, G.P., Sud, S., and Puri, R.K.**, Expression of high affinity interleukin-4 receptors on human renal carcinoma cells and inhibition of tumor cell growth in vitro by interleukin-4, *J. Clin. Invest.*, 91, 88, 1993.

1225. **Morisaki, T., Yuzuki, D.H., Lin, R.T., Foshag, L.J., Morton, D.L., and Hoon, D.S.B.**, Interleukin 4 receptor expression and growth inhibition of gastric carcinoma cells by interleukin 4, *Cancer Res.*, 52, 6059, 1992.

1226. **Debinski, W., Puri, R.K., Kreitman, R.J., and Pastan, I.**, A wide range of human cancers express interleukin 4 (IL4) receptors that can be targeted with chimeric toxin composed of IL4 and Pseudomonas exotoxin, *J. Biol. Chem.*, 268, 14065, 1993.

1227. **Harriman, G.R. and Strober, W.**, The immunobiology of interleukin-5, *Yearb. Immunol.*, 5, 160, 1989.

1228. **Banchereau, J.**, Interleukine 5, MS Med. Sci., 6, 954, 1990.

1229. **Sanderson, C.J., O'Garra, A., Warren, D.J., and Klaus, G.G.B.**, Eosinophil differentiation factor also has B-cell growth factor activity: proposed name interleukin 4, *Proc. Natl. Acad. Sci. U.S.A.*, 83, 437, 1986.

1230. **O'Garra, A., Warren, D.J., Holman, M., Popham, A.M., Sanderson, C.J., and Klaus, G.G.B.**, Interleukin 4 (B-cell growth factor II/eosinophil differentiation factor is a mitogen and differentiation factor for preactivated murine B lymphocytes, *Proc. Natl. Acad. Sci. U.S.A.*, 83, 5228, 1986.

1231. **Matsumoto, M., Tominaga, A., Harada, N., and Takatsu, K.**, Role of T cell-replacing factor (TRF) in the murine B-cell differentiation: induction of increased levels of expression of secreted type IgM mRNA, *J. Immunol.*, 138, 1826, 1987.

1232. **Rasmussen, R., Takatsu, K., Harada, N., Takahashi, T., and Bottomly, K.**, T cell-dependent hapten-specific and polyclonal B-cell responses require release of interleukin 5, *J. Immunol.*, 140, 705, 1988.

1233. **Beagley, K.W., Eldridge, J.H., Kiyono, H., Everson, M.P., Koopman, W.J., Honjo, T., and McGhee, J.R.**, Recombinant murine IL-5 induces high rate IgA synthesis in cycling IgA-positive Peyer's patch B cells, *J. Immunol.*, 141, 2035, 1988.

1234. **Lebman, D.A. and Coffman, R.L.,** The effects of IL-4 and IL-5 on the IgA response by murine Peyer's patch B cell subpopulations, *J. Immunol.,* 141, 2050, 1988.
1235. **Takatsu, K., Kikuchi, Y., Takahashi, T., Honjo, T., Matsumoto, M., Harada, N., and Tominaga, A.,** Interleukin 5, a T-cell-derived B-cell differentiation factor also induces cytotoxic T lymphocytes, *Proc. Natl. Acad. Sci. U.S.A.,* 84, 4234, 1987.
1236. **Kawano, M., Matsushima, K., Masuda, A., and Oppenheim, J.J.,** A major 50-kDa human B-cell growth factor-II induces both Tac antigen expression and proliferation by several types of lymphocytes, *Cell. Immunol.,* 111, 273, 1988.
1237. **Clutterbuck, E.J., Hirst, E.M.A., and Sanderson, C.J.,** Human interleukin-5 (IL-5) regulates the production of eosinophils in human bone marrow cultures: comparison and interaction with IL-1, IL-3, IL-6, and GMCSF, *Blood,* 73, 1504, 1989.
1238. **Yamaguchi, Y., Suda, T., Suda, J., Eguchi, M., Miura, Y., Harada, N., Tominaga, A., and Takatsu, K.,** Purified interleukin 5 supports the terminal differentiation and proliferation of murine eosinophilic precursors, *J. Exp. Med.,* 167, 43, 1988.
1239. **Yamaguchi, Y., Hayashi, Y., Sugama, Y., Miura, Y., Kasahara, T., Kitamura, S., Torisu, M., Mita, S., Tominaga, A., Takatsu, K., and Suda, T.,** Highly purified murine interleukin 5 (IL-5) stimulates eosinophil function and prolongs in vitro survival. IL-5 as an eosinophil chemotactic factor, *J. Exp. Med.,* 167, 1737, 1988.
1240. **Enokihara, H., Nagashima, S., Noma, T., Kajitani, H., Hamaguchi, H., Saito, K., Furusawa, S., Shishido, H., and Honjo, T.,** Effect of human recombinant interleukin 5 and G-CSF on eosinophil colony formation, *Immunol. Lett.,* 18, 73, 1988.
1241. **Dent, L.A., Strath, M., Mellor, A.L., and Sanderson, C.J.,** Eosinophilia in transgenic mice expressing interleukin 5, *J. Exp. Med.,* 172, 1425, 1990.
1242. **Denburg, J.A., Silver, J.E., and Abrams, J.S.,** Interleukin-5 is a human basophilopoietin: induction of histamine content and basophilic differentiation of HL-60 cells and of peripheral blood basophil-eosinophil progenitors, *Blood,* 77, 1462, 1991.
1243. **Sutherland, G.R., Baker, E., Callen, D.F., Campbell, H.D., Young, I.G., Sanderson, C.J., Garson, O.M., Lopez, A.F., and Vadas, M.A.,** Interleukin-5 is at 5q31 and is deleted in the 5q- syndrome, *Blood,* 71, 1150, 1988.
1244. **Azuma, C., Tanabe, T., Konishi, M., Kinashi, T., Noma, T., Matsuda, F., Yaoita, Y., Takatsu, K., Hammarström, L., Smith, C.I.E., Severnson, E., and Honjo, T.,** Cloning of cDNA for human T-cell replacing factor (interleukin-5) and comparison with the murine homologue, *Nucleic Acids Res.,* 14, 9149, 1986.
1245. **Yokota, T., Coffman, R.L., Hagiwara, H., Rennick, D.M., Takebe, Y., Yokota, K., Gemmell, L., Shrader, B., Yang, G., Meyerson, P., Luh, J., Hoy, P., Pène, J., Brière, F., Spits, H., Banchereau, J., de Vries, J., Lee, F.D., Arai, N., and Arai, K.,** Isolation and characterization of lymphokine cDNA clones encoding mouse and human IgA-enhancing factor and eosinophil colony-stimulating factor activities: relationship to interleukin 5, *Proc. Natl. Acad. Sci. U.S.A.,* 84, 7388, 1987.
1246. **Tavernier, J., Devos, R., van der Heyden, J., Hauquier, G., Bauden, R., Fache, I., Kawashima, E., Vandekerckhove, J., Contreras, R., and Fiers, W.,** Expression of human and murine interleukin-5 in eukaryotic systems, *DNA,* 8, 491, 1989.
1247. **Kinashi, T., Harada, N., Severinson, E., Tanabe, T., Sideras, T., Konishi, M., Azuma, C., Tominaga, A., Bergstedt-Lindqvist, S., Takahashi, M., Matsuda, F., Yaoita, Y., Takatsu, K., and Honjo, T.,** Cloning of complementary DNA encoding T-cell replacing factor and identity with B-cell growth factor II, *Nature,* 324, 70, 1986.
1248. **Tominaga, A., Matsumoto, M., Harada, N., Takahashi, T., Kikuchi, Y., and Takatsu, K.,** Molecular properties and regulation of mRNA expression for murine T cell-replacing factor/IL-5, *J. Immunol.,* 140, 1175, 1988.
1249. **Chihara, J., Plumas, J., Gruart, V., Tavernier, J., Prin, L., Capron, A., and Capron, M.,** Characterization of a receptor for interleukin 5 on human eosinophils: variable expression and induction by granulocyte/macrophage colony-stimulating factor, *J. Exp. Med.,* 172, 1347, 1990.
1250. **Lopez, A.F., Vadas, M.A., Woodcock, J.M., Milton, S.E., Lewis, A., Elliott, M.J., Gillis, D., Ireland, R., Olwell, E., and Park, L.S.,** Interleukin-5, interleukin-3, and granulocyte-macrophage colony-stimulating factor cross-compete for binding to cell surface receptors on human eosinophils, *J. Biol. Chem.,* 266, 24741, 1991.

1251. Devos, R., Tavernier, J., Plaetinck, G., van der Heyden, J., Rolinck, A., and Fiers, W., Expression of the murine interleukin-5 receptor on Xenopus laevis oocytes, *Biochem. Biophys. Res. Commun.*, 172, 570, 1990.
1252. Mita, S., Harada, N., Naomi, S., Hitoshi, Y., Sakamoto, K., Akagi, M., Tominaga, A., and Takatsu, K., Receptors for T-cell-replacing factor/interleukin 5. Specificity, quantitation, and its implication, *J. Exp. Med.*, 168, 863, 1988.
1253. Mita, S., Tominaga, A., Hitoshi, Y., Sakamoto, K., Honjo, T., Akagi, M., Kikuchi, Y., Yamaguchi, N., and Takatsu, K., Characterization of high-affinity receptors for interleukin 5 on interleukin 5-dependent cell lines, *Proc. Natl. Acad. Sci. U.S.A.*, 86, 2311, 1989.
1254. Yamaguchi, N., Hitoshi, Y., Mita, S., Hosoya, Y., Murata, Y., Kikuchi, Y., Tominaga, A., and Takatsu, K., Characterization of the murine interleukin 5 receptor by using a monoclonal antibody, *Int. Immunol.*, 2, 181, 1990.
1255. Takaki, S., Tominaga, A., Hitoshi, Y., Mita, S., Sonoda, E., Yamaguchi, N., and Takatsu, K., Molecular cloning and expression of the murine interleukin-5 receptor, *EMBO J.*, 9, 4367, 1990.
1256. Migita, M., Yamaguchi, N., Mita, S., Higuchi, S., Hitoshi, Y., Yoshida, Y., Tomonaga, M., Matsuda, I., Tominaga, A., and Takatsu, K., Characterization of the human IL-5 receptors on eosinophils, *Cell. Immunol.*, 133, 487, 1991.
1257. Murata, Y., Takaki, S., Migita, M., Kikuchi, Y., Tominaga, A., and Takatsu, K., Molecular cloning and expression of the human interleukin 5 receptor, *J. Exp. Med.*, 175, 341, 1992.
1258. Tavernier, J., Devos, R., Cornelis, S., Tuypens, T., Van der Heyden, J., Fiers, W., and Plaetinck, G., A human high affinity interleukin-5 receptor (IL5R) is composed of an IL-5-specific α chain and a β chain shared with the receptor for GM-CSF, *Cell*, 66, 1175, 1991.
1259. Isobe, M., Kumura, Y., Murata, Y., Takaki, S., Tominaga, A., Takatsu, K., and Ogita, Z., Localization of the gene encoding the α-subunit of human interleukin-5 receptor *(IL5RA)* to chromosome region 3p24-3p26, *Genomics*, 14, 755, 1992.
1260. Renard, D., Petit-Koskas, E., Génot, E., Dugas, B., Poggioli, J., and Kolb, J.-P., Activation of phoshatidylinositol metabolic pathway by low molecular weight B cell growth factor, *Eur. J. Immunol.*, 18, 1705, 1988.
1261. Yamaguchi, N., Takahashi, T., Harada, N., and Takatsu, K., Mechanisms of the interleukin 5-induced differentiation of B cells, *J. Biochem.*, 106, 837, 1989.
1262. Murata, Y., Yamaguchi, N., Hitoshi, Y., Tominaga, A., and Takatsu, K., Interleukin 5 and interleukin 3 induce serine and tyrosine phosphorylations of several cellular proteins in an interleukin 5-dependent cell line, *Biochem. Biophys. Res. Commun.*, 173, 1102, 1990.
1263. Migita, M., Yamaguchi, N., Katoh, S., Mita, S., Matsumoto, R., Sonoda, E., Tsuchiya, H., Matsuda, I., Tominaga, A., and Takatsu, K., Elevated expression of proto-oncogenes during interleukin-5-induced growth and differentiation of murine B lineage cells, *Microbiol. Immunol.*, 34, 937, 1990.
1264. Le, J. and Vilcek, J., Interleukin 6: a multifunctional cytokine regulating immune reactions and the acute phase protein response, *Lab. Invest.*, 61, 588, 1989.
1265. Sehgal, P.B., Interleukin-6: molecular pathophysiology, *J. Invest. Dermatol.*, 94, 2S, 1990.
1266. Sehgal, P.B., Interleukin 6 in infection and cancer, *Proc. Soc. Exp. Biol. Med.*, 195, 183, 1990.
1267. Hirano, T., Akira, S., Taga, T., and Kishimoto, T., Biological and clinical aspects of interleukin 6, *Immunol. Today*, 11, 443, 1990.
1268. Van Snick, J., Interleukin-6: an overview, *Annu. Rev. Immunol.*, 8, 253, 1990.
1269. Brach, M.A. and Herrmann, F., Interleukin 6 — present and future, *Int. J. Clin. Lab. Res.*, 22, 143, 1992.
1270. Kishimoto, T., Akira, S., and Taga, T., Interleukin-6 and its receptor — a paradigm for cytokines, *Science*, 258, 593, 1992.
1271. Lee, F.D., The role of interleukin-6 in development, *Develop. Biol.*, 151, 331, 1992.
1272. Hirano, T., Interleukin-6 (IL-6) and its receptor — their role in plasma cell neoplasias, *Int. J. Cell Cloning*, 9, 166, 1991.
1273. Sehgal, P.B., May, L.T., Tamm, I., and Vilcek, J., Human β_2 interferon and B-cell differentiation factor BSF-2 are identical, *Science*, 235, 731, 1987.
1274. Poupart, P., Vandenabeele, P., Cayphas, S., Van Snick, J., Haegeman, G., Kruys, V., Fiers, W., and Content, J., B cell growth modulating and differentiating activity of recombinant human 26-kda protein (BSF-2, HuIFN-β_2, HPGF), *EMBO J.*, 6, 1219, 1987.

1275. **Gauldie, J., Richards, C., Harnish, D., Lansdorp, P., and Baumann, H.**, Interferon β_2/B-cell stimulatory factor type 2 shares identity with monocyte-derived hepatocyte-stimulating factor and regulates the major acute phase protein response in liver cells, *Proc. Natl. Acad. Sci. U.S.A.*, 84, 7251, 1987.

1276. **Van Damme, J., Van Beeumen, J., Decock, B., Van Snick, J., de Ley, M., and Billiau, A.**, Separation and comparison of two monokines with lymphocyte-activating factor activity: IL-1β and hybridoma growth factor (HGF). Identification of leukocyte-derived HGF as IL-6, *J. Immunol.*, 140, 1534, 1988.

1277. **Geiger, T., Andus, T., Bauer, J., Northoff, H., Ganter, U., Hirano, T., Kishimoto, T., and Heinrich, P.C.**, Cell-free-synthesized interleukin-6 (BSF-2/IFN-β2) exhibits hepatocyte-stimulating activity, *Eur. J. Biochem.*, 175, 181, 1988.

1278. **Van Damme, J., Cayphas, S., Opdenakker, G., Billiau, A., and Van Snick, J.**, Interleukin 1 and poly(rI).poly(rC) induce production of a hybridoma growth factor by human fibroblasts, *Eur. J. Immunol.*, 17, 1, 1987.

1279. **Houssiau, F.A., Coulie, P.G., and Van Snick, J.**, Distinct roles of IL-1 and IL-6 in human T cell activation, *J. Immunol.*, 143, 2520, 1989.

1280. **Garman, R.D., Jacobs, K.A., Clark, S.C., and Raulet, D.H.**, B-cell-stimulatory factor 2 (β_2 interferon) functions as a second signal for interleukin 2 production by mature murine T cells, *Proc. Natl. Acad. Sci. U.S.A.*, 84, 7629, 1987.

1281. **Uyttenhove, C., Coulie, P.G., and Van Snick, J.**, T cell growth and differentiation induced by interleukin-HP1/IL-6, the murine hybridoma/plasmacytoma growth factor, *J. Exp. Med.*, 167, 1417, 1988.

1282. **Le, J., Fredrickson, G., Reis, L.F.L., Diamantstein, T., Hirano, T., Kishimoto, T., and Vilcek, J.**, Interleukin 2-dependent and interleukin 2-independent pathways of regulation of thymocyte function by interleukin 6, *Proc. Natl. Acad. Sci. U.S.A.*, 85, 8643, 1988.

1283. **Hodgkin, P.D., Bond, M.W., O'Garra, A., Frank, G., Lee, F., Coffman, R.L., Zlotnik, A., and Howard, M.**, Identification of IL-6 as a T cell-derived factor that enhances the proliferative response of thymocytes to IL-4 and phorbol myristate acetate, *J. Immunol.*, 141, 151, 1988.

1284. **Luger, T.A., Krutmann, J., Kirnbauer, R., Urbanski, A., Schwarz, T., Klappacher, G., Köck, A., Micksche, M., Malejczyk, J., Schauer, E., May, L.T., and Sehgal, P.B.**, IFN-β$_2$/IL-6 augments the activity of human natural killer cells, *J. Immunol.*, 143, 1206, 1989.

1285. **Schaafsma, M.R., Fibbe, W.E., Van Damme, J., Duinkerken, N., Ralph, P., Kaushansky, K., Altrock, B.W., Willemze, R., and Falkenburg, J.H.F.**, Interleukin-6 is not involved in the interleukin-1-induced production of colony-stimulating factors by human bone marrow stromal cells and fibroblasts, *Blood*, 74, 2619, 1989.

1286. **Rennick, D., Jackson, J., Yang, G., Wideman, J., Lee, F., and Hudak, S.**, Interleukin-6 interacts with interleukin-4 and other hematopoietic growth factors to selectively enhance the growth of megakaryocytic, erythroid, myeloid, and multipotential progenitor cells, *Blood*, 73, 1828, 1989.

1287. **Ishibashi, T., Kimura, H., Uchida, T., Kariyone, S., Friese, P., and Burstein, S.A.**, Human interleukin 6 is a direct promoter of maturation of megakaryocytes *in vitro*, *Proc. Natl. Acad. Sci. U.S.A.*, 86, 5953, 1989.

1288. **Lotem, J., Shabo, Y., and Sachs, L.**, Regulation of megakaryocyte development by interleukin-6, *Blood*, 74, 1545, 1989.

1289. **Bruno, E. and Hoffman, R.**, Effect of interleukin 6 on in vitro human megakaryocytopoiesis: its interaction with other cytokines, *Exp. Hematol.*, 17, 1038, 1989.

1290. **Hill, R.J., Warren, M.K., and Levin, J.**, Stimulation of thrombopoiesis in mice by recombinant interleukin-6, *J. Clin. Invest.*, 85, 1242, 1990.

1291. **Koike, K., Nakahata, T., Kubo, T., Kikuchi, T., Takagi, M., Ishiguro, A., Tsuji, K., Nagahuma, K., Okano, A., and Akiyama, Y.**, Interleukin-6 enhances murine megakaryocytopoiesis in serum-free culture, *Blood*, 75, 2286, 1990.

1292. **Carrington, P.A., Hill, R.J., Stenberg, P.E., Levin, J., Corash, L., Schreurs, J., Baker, G., and Levin, F.C.**, Multiple in vivo effects of interleukin-3 and interleukin-6 on murine megakaryopoiesis, *Blood*, 77, 34, 1991.

1293. **Navarro, S., Debili, N., Le Couedic, J.-P., Klein, B., Breton-Gorius, J., Doly, J., and Vainchenker, W.**, Interleukin-6 and its receptor are expressed in human megakaryocytes: in vitro effects on proliferation and endoreplication, *Blood*, 77, 461, 1991.

1294. Asano, S., Okano, A., Ozawa, K., Nakahata, T., Ishibashi, T., Koike, K., Kimura, H., Tanioka, Y., Shibuya, A., Hirano, T., Kishimoto, T., Takaku, F., and Akiyama, Y., In vivo effects of recombinant human interleukin-6 in primates: stimulated production of platelets, *Blood,* 75, 1602, 1990.

1295. Hill, R.J., Warren, M.K., Stenberg, P., Levin, J., Corash, L., Drummond, R., Baker, G., Levin, F., and Mok, Y., Stimulation of megakaryocytopoiesis in mice by human recombinant interleukin-6, *Blood,* 77, 42, 1991.

1296. Suda, T., Yamaguchi, Y., Suda, J., Miura, Y., Okano, A., and Akiyama, Y., Effect of interleukin 6 (IL-6) on the differentiation and proliferation of murine and human hemopoietic progenitors, *Exp. Hematol.,* 16, 891, 1988.

1297. Pojda, Z. and Tsuboi, A., In vivo effects of human recombinant interleukin 6 on hemopoietic stem and progenitor cells and circulating blood cells in normal mice, *Exp. Hematol.,* 18, 1034, 1990.

1298. Suzuki, C., Okano, A., Takatsuki, F., Miyasaka, Y., Hirano, T., Kishimoto, T., Ejima, D., and Akiyama, Y., Continuous perfusion with interleukin 6 (IL-6) enhances production of hematopoietic stem cells (CFU-S), *Biochem. Biophys. Res. Commun.,* 159, 933, 1989.

1299. Ulich, T.R., del Castillo, J., and Guo, K., In vivo hematologic effects of recombinant interleukin-6 on hematopoiesis and circulating numbers of RBCs and WBCs, *Blood,* 73, 108, 1989.

1300. Ikebuchi, K., Wong, G.G., Clark, S.C., Ihle, J.N., Hirai, Y., and Ogawa, M., Interleukin 6 enhancement of interleukin 3-dependent proliferation of multipotential hemopoietic progenitors, *Proc. Natl. Acad. Sci. U.S.A.,* 84, 9035, 1987.

1301. Koike, K., Nakahata, T., Takagi, M., Kobayashi, T., Ishiguro, A., Tsuji, K., Naganuma, K., Okano, A., Akiyama, Y., and Akabane, T., Synergism of BSF-2/interleukin 6 and interleukin 3 on development of multipotential hemopoietic progenitors in serum-free culture, *J. Exp. Med.,* 168, 879, 1988.

1302. Wong, G.G., Witek-Giannotti, J.S., Temple, P.A., Kriz, R., Ferenz, C., Hewick, R.M., Clark, S.C., Ikebuchi, K., and Ogawa, M., Stimulation of murine hemopoietic colony formation by human IL-6, *J. Immunol.,* 140, 3040, 1988.

1303. Bot, F.J., van Eijk, L., Broeders, L., Aarden, L.A., and Löwenberg, B., Interleukin-6 synergizes with M-CSF in the formation of macrophage colonies from purified human marrow progenitor cells, *Blood,* 73, 435, 1989.

1304. Caracciolo, D., Clark, S.C., and Rovera, G., Human interleukin-6 supports granulocytic differentiation of hematopoietic progenitor cells and acts synergistically with GM-CSF, *Blood,* 73, 666, 1989.

1305. Borish, L., Rosenbaum, R., Albury, L., and Clark, S., Activation of neutrophils by recombinant interleukin 6, *Cell. Immunol.,* 121, 280, 1989.

1306. May, L.T., Helfgott, D.C., and Sehgal, P.B., Anti-β-interferon antibodies inhibit the increased expression of HLA-B7 mRNA in tumor necrosis factor-treated human fibroblasts: structural studies of the β_2 interferon involved, *Proc. Natl. Acad. Sci. U.S.A.,* 83, 8957, 1986.

1307. Marinkovic, S., Jahreis, G.P., Wong, G.G., and Baumann, H., IL-6 modulates the synthesis of a specific set of acute phase plasma proteins in vivo, *J. Immunol.,* 142, 808, 1989.

1308. Castell, J.V., Gómez-Lechón, M.J., David, M., Hirano, T., Kishimoto, T., and Heinrich, P.C., Recombinant human interleukin-6 (IL-6/BSF-2/HSF) regulates the synthesis of acute phase proteins in human hepatocytes, *FEBS Lett.,* 232, 347, 1988.

1309. Heinrich, P.C., Castell, J.V., and Andus, T., Interleukin-6 and the acute phase response, *Biochem. J.,* 265, 621, 1990.

1310. Castell, J.V., Gómez-Lechón, M.J., David, M., Andus, T., Geiger, T., Trullenque, R., Fabra, R., and Heinrich, P.C., Interleukin-6 is the major regulator of acute phase protein synthesis in adult human hepatocytes, *FEBS Lett.,* 242, 237, 1989.

1311. Grunfeld, C., Adi, S., Soued, M., Moser, A., Fiers, W., and Feingold, K.R., Search for mediators of the lipogenic effects of tumor necrosis factor: potential role for interleukin 6, *Cancer Res.,* 50, 4233, 1990.

1312. Bereta, J., Szuba, K., Fiers, W., Gauldie, J., and Koj, A., Transforming growth factor-β and epidermal growth factor modulate basal and interleukin-6-induced amino acid uptake and acute phase protein synthesis in cultured rat hepatocytes, *FEBS Lett.,* 266, 48, 1990.

1313. **Yamaguchi, M., Matsuzaki, N., Hirota, K., Miyake, A., and Tanizawa, O.,** Interleukin-6 possibly induced by interleukin-1β in the pituitary gland stimulates the release of gonadotropins and prolactin, *Acta Endocrinol.,* 122, 201, 1990.

1314. **Naitoh, Y., Fukata, J., Tominaga, T., Nakai, Y., Tamai, S., Mori, K., and Imura, H.,** Interleukin-6 stimulates the secretion of adrenocorticotropic hormone in conscious, freely-moving rats, *Biochem. Biophys. Res. Commun.,* 155, 1459, 1988.

1315. **Syed, V., Gérard, N., Kaipia, A., Bardin, C.W., Parvinen, M., and Jégou, B.,** Identification ontogeny, and regulation of an interleukin-6-like factor in the rat seminiferous tubule, *Endocrinology,* 132, 293, 1993.

1316. **Sandler, S., Bendtzen, K., Eizirik, D.L., and Welsh, M.,** Interleukin-6 affects insulin secretion and glucose metabolism of rat pancreatic islets *in vitro, Endocrinology,* 126, 1288, 1990.

1317. **Southern, C., Schulster, D., and Green, I.C.,** Inhibition of insulin secretion from rat islets of Langerhans by interleukin-6. An effect distinct from that of interleukin-1, *Biochem. J.,* 272, 243, 1990.

1318. **Campbell, I.L., Cutri, A., Wilson, A., and Harrison, L.C.,** Evidence for IL-6 production by and effects on the pancreatic β cell, *J. Immunol.,* 143, 1188, 1989.

1319. **Jilka, R.L., Hangoc, G., Girasole, G., Passeri, G., Williams, D.C., Abrams, J.S., Boyce, B., Broxmeyer, H., and Manolagas, S.C.,** Increased osteoclast development after estrogen loss: mediation by interleukin 6, *Science,* 257, 88, 1992.

1320. **Satoh, T., Nakamura, S., Taga, T., Matsuda, T., Hirano, T., Kishimoto, T., and Kaziro, Y.,** Induction of neuronal differentiation in PC12 cells by B-cell stimulatory factor 2/interleukin 6, *Mol. Cell. Biol.,* 8, 3546, 1988.

1321. **Sehgal, P.B., Zilberstein, A., Ruggieri, A.-M., May, L.T., Ferguson-Smith, A., Slate, D.L., Revel, M., and Ruddle, F.H.,** Human chromosome 7 carries the β$_2$ interferon gene, *Proc. Natl. Acad. Sci. U.S.A.,* 83, 5219, 1986.

1322. **Zilberstein, A., Ruggieri, R., Korn, J.H., and Revel, M.,** Structure and expression of cDNA and genes for human interferon-β$_2$, a distinct species inducible by growth-stimulatory cytokines, *EMBO J.,* 5, 2529, 1986.

1323. **Hirano, T., Yasukawa, K., Harada, H., Taga, T., Watanabe, Y., Matsuda, T., Kashiwamura, S., Nakajima, K., Koyama, K., Iwamatsu, A., Tsunasawa, S., Sakiyama, F., Matsui, H., Yakahara, Y., Taniguchi, T., and Kishimoto, T.,** Complementary DNA for a novel human interleukin (BSF-2) that induces B lymphocytes to produce immunoglobulin, *Nature,* 324, 73, 1986.

1324. **Van Damme, J., Cayphas, S., Van Snick, J., Conings, R., Put, W., Lenaerts, J.-P., Simpson, R.J., and Billiau, A.,** Purification and characterization of human fibroblast-derived hybridoma growth factor identical to T-cell-derived B-cell-stimulatory factor-2 (interleukin 6), *Eur. J. Biochem.,* 168, 543, 1987.

1325. **Asagoe, Y., Yakusawa, K., Saito, T., Maruo, N., Miyata, K., Kono, T., Miyake, T., Kato, T., Kakidani, H., and Mitani, M.,** Human B-cell stimulatory factor-2 expressed in *Escherichia coli, Biotechnology,* 6, 806, 1988.

1326. **Santhanam, U., Ghrayeb, J., Sehgal, P.B., and May, L.T.,** Post-translational modifications of human interleukin 6, *Arch. Biochem. Biophys.,* 274, 161, 1989.

1327. **May, L.T., Santhanam, U., Tatter, S.B., Bhardwaj, N., Ghrayeb, J., and Sehgal, P.B.,** Phosphorylation of secreted forms of human β$_2$-interferon/hepatocyte stimulating factor/interleukin-6, *Biochem. Biophys. Res. Commun.,* 152, 1144, 1988.

1328. **May, L.T. and Sehgal, P.B.,** Phosphorylation of interleukin-6 at serine-54: an early event in the secretory pathway in human fibroblasts, *Biochem. Biophys. Res. Commun.,* 185, 524, 1992.

1329. **Santhanam, U., Ray, A., and Sehgal, P.B.,** Repression of the interleukin 6 gene promoter by p53 and the retinoblastoma susceptibility gene product, *Proc. Natl. Acad. Sci. U.S.A.,* 88, 7605, 1991.

1330. **Mock, B.A., Nordan, R.P., Justice, M.J., Kozak, C., Jenkins, N.A., Copeland, N.G., Clark, S.C., Wong, G.G., and Rudikoff, S.,** The murine *Il-6* gene maps to proximal region of chromosome 5, *J. Immunol.,* 142, 1372, 1989.

1331. **Van Snick, J., Cayphas, S., Szikora, J.-P., Renauld, J.-C., Van Roost, E., Boon, T., and Simpson, R.J.,** cDNA cloning of murine interleukin-HP1: homology with human interleukin 6, *Eur. J. Immunol.,* 18, 193, 1988.

1332. **Chiu, C.-P., Moulds, C., Coffman, R.L., Rennick, D., and Lee, F.,** Multiple biological activities are expressed by a mouse interleukin 6 cDNA isolated from bone marrow stromal cells, *Proc. Natl. Acad. Sci. U.S.A.,* 85, 7099, 1988.

1333. **Northemann, W., Braciak, T.A., Hattori, M., Lee, F., and Fey, G.H.,** Structure of the rat interleukin 6 gene and its expression in macrophage-derived cells, *J. Biol. Chem.,* 264, 16072, 1989.
1334. **Bauer, J., Ganter, U., Geiger, T., Jacobshagen, U., Hirano, T., Matsuda, T., Kishimoto, T., Andus, T., Acs, G., Gerok, W., and Ciliberto, G.,** Regulation of interleukin-6 expression in cultured human blood monocytes and monocyte-derived macrophages, *Blood,* 72, 1134, 1988.
1335. **Musso, T., Espinoza-Delgado, I., Pulkki, K., Gusella, G.L., Longo, D.L., and Varesio, L.,** IL-2 induces IL-6 production in human monocytes, *J. Immunol.,* 148, 795, 1992.
1336. **Rieckmann, P., D'Alessandro, F., Nordan, R.P., Fauci, A.S., and Kehrl, J.H.,** IL-6 and tumor necrosis factor-α. Autocrine and paracrine cytokines involved in B cell function, *J. Immunol.,* 146, 3462, 1991.
1337. **Navarro, S., Debili, N., Bernaudin, J.-F., Vainchenker, W., and Doly, J.,** Regulation of the expression of IL-6 in human monocytes, *J. Immunol.,* 142, 4339, 1989.
1338. **Miyaura, C., Jin, C.H., Yamaguchi, Y., Tomida, M., Hozumi, M., Matsuda, T., Hirano, T., Kishimoto, T., and Suda, T.,** Production of interleukin 6 and its relation to the macrophage differentiation of mouse myeloid leukemia cells (M1) treated with differentiation-inducing factor and $1\alpha,25$-dihydroxyvitamin D_3, *Biochem. Biophys. Res. Commun.,* 158, 660, 1989.
1339. **Kameda, T., Matsuzaki, N., Sawai, K., Okada, T., Saji, F., Matsuda, T., Hirano, T., Kishimoto, T., and Tanizawa, O.,** Production of interleukin-6 by normal human trophoblasts, *Placenta,* 11, 205, 1990.
1340. **Loppnow, H. and Libby, P.,** Proliferating or interleukin-1-activated human vascular smooth muscle cells secrete copious interleukin-6, *J. Clin. Invest.,* 85, 731, 1990.
1341. **Scotte, M., Daveau, M., Hiron, M., Teniere, P., and Lebreton, J.P.,** Absence of expression of interleukin-6 (IL-6) messenger RNA in regenerating rat liver, *FEBS Lett.,* 315, 159, 1993.
1342. **Kohase, M., May, L.T., Tamm, I., Vilcek, J., and Sehgal, P.B.,** A cytokine network in human diploid fibroblasts: interactions of β-interferons, tumor necrosis factor, platelet-derived growth factor, and interleukin-1, *Mol. Cell. Biol.,* 7, 273, 1987.
1343. **Defilippi, P., Poupart, P., Tavernier, J., Fiers, W., and Content, J.,** Induction and regulation of mRNA encoding 26-kDa protein in human cell lines treated with recombinant human tumor necrosis factor, *Proc. Natl. Acad. Sci. U.S.A.,* 84, 4557, 1987.
1344. **Tabibzadeh, S.S., Santhanam, U., Sehgal, P.B., and May, L.T.,** Cytokine-induced production of IFN-β_2/IL-6 by freshly explanted human endometrial stromal cells. Modulation by estradiol-17β, *J. Immunol.,* 142, 3134, 1989.
1345. **May, L.T., Torcia, G., Cozzolino, F., Ray, A., Tatter, S.B., Santhanam, U., Sehgal, P.B., and Stern, D.,** Interleukin-6 gene expression in human endothelial cells: RNA start sites, multiple IL-6 proteins and inhibition of proliferation, *Biochem. Biophys. Res. Commun.,* 159, 991, 1989.
1346. **Shalaby, M.F., Waage, A., and Espevik, T.,** Cytokine regulation of interleukin 6 production by human endothelial cells, *Cell. Immunol.,* 121, 372, 1989.
1347. **Jablons, D.M., Mulé, J.J., McIntosh, J.K., Sehgal, P.B., May, L.T., Huang, C.M., Rosenberg, S.A., and Lotze, M.T.,** IL-6/IFN-β2 as a circulating hormone. Induction by cytokine administration in humans, *J. Immunol.,* 142, 1542, 1989.
1348. **Yang, Y.-C., Tsai, S., Wong, G.G., and Clark, S.C.,** Interleukin-1 regulation of hematopoietic growth factor production by human stromal fibroblasts, *J. Cell. Physiol.,* 134, 292, 1988.
1349. **Elias, J.A., Lentz, V., and Cummings, P.J.,** Transforming growth factor-β regulation of IL-6 production by unstimulated and IL-1-stimulated human fibroblasts, *J. Immunol.,* 146, 3437, 1991.
1350. **McGee, D.W., Beagley, K.W., Aicher, W.K., and McGhee, J.R.,** Transforming growth factor-β enhances interleukin-6 secretion by intestinal epithelial cells, *Immunology,* 77, 7, 1992.
1351. **Walther, Z., May, L.T., and Sehgal, P.B.,** Transcriptional regulation of the interferon-β_2/hepatocyte-stimulating factor gene in human fibroblasts by other cytokines, *J. Immunol.,* 140, 974, 1988.
1352. **Sehgal, P.B., Walther, Z., and Tamm, I.,** Rapid enhancement of β_2-interferon/B-cell differentiation factor BSF-2 gene expression in human fibroblasts by diacylglycerols and the calcium ionophore A23187, *Proc. Natl. Acad. Sci. U.S.A.,* 84, 3663, 1987.
1533. **Ray, A., Tatter, S.B., May, L.T., and Sehgal, P.B.,** Activation of the human "β_2-interferon/hepatocyte-stimulating factor/interleukin 6" promoter by cytokines, viruses, and second messenger agonists, *Proc. Natl. Acad. Sci. U.S.A.,* 85, 6701, 1988.
1354. **Zhang, Y., Lin, J.-X., and Vilcek, J.,** Interleukin-6 induction by tumor necrosis factor and interleukin-1 in human fibroblasts involves activation of a nuclear factor binding to a kappa B-like sequence, *Mol. Cell. Biol.,* 10, 3818, 1990.

1355. **Poli, V. and Cortese, R.,** Interleukin 6 induces a liver-specific nuclear protein that binds to the promoter of acute-phase genes, *Proc. Natl. Acad. Sci. U.S.A.,* 86, 8202, 1989.
1356. **Baumann, M., Baumann, H., and Fey, G.H.,** Molecular cloning, characterization and functional expression of the rat liver interleukin-6 receptor, *J. Biol. Chem.,* 265, 19853, 1990.
1357. **Kluck, P.M.C., Wiegant, J., Jansen, R.P.M., Bolk, M.W.J., Raap, A.K., Willemze, R., and Ladegent, J.E.,** The human interleukin-6 receptor α-chain gene is localized on chromosome 1 band q21, *Hum. Genet.,* 90, 542, 1993.
1358. **Coulie, P.G., Vanhecke, A., Van Damme, J., Cayphas, S., Poupart, P., De Wit, L., and Content, J.,** High-affinity binding sites for human 26-kDa protein (interleukin 6, B cell stimulatory factor-2, human hybridoma plasmacytoma growth factor, interferon-$β_2$), different from those of type I interferon (α, β), on lymphoblastoid cells, *Eur. J. Immunol.,* 17, 1435, 1987.
1359. **Snyers, L. and Content, J.,** Enhancement of IL-6 receptor β chain (gp130) expression by IL-6, IL-1 and TNF in human epithelial cells, *Biochem. Biophys. Res. Commun.,* 185, 902, 1992.
1360. **Snyers, L., De Wit, L., and Content, J.,** Glucocorticoid upregulation of high-affinity interleukin 6 receptors on human epithelial cells, *Proc. Natl. Acad. Sci. U.S.A.,* 87, 2838, 1990.
1361. **Yamaguchi, M., Michishita, M., Hirayoshi, K., Yasukawa, K., Okuma, M., and Nagata, K.,** Down-regulation of interleukin-6 receptors of mouse myelomonocytic leukemia cells by leukemia inhibitory factor, *J. Biol. Chem.,* 267, 22035, 1992.
1362. **Schroeder, E.J. and Cousins, R.J.,** Interleukin 6 regulates metallothionein gene expression and zinc metabolism in hepatocyte monolayer cultures, *Proc. Natl. Acad. Sci. U.S.A.,* 87, 3137, 1990.
1363. **Calderon, T.M., Sherman, J., Wilkerson, H., Hatcher, V.B., and Berman, J.W.,** Interleukin-6 modulates c-*sis* gene expression in cultured human endothelial cells, *Cell. Immunol.,* 142, 118, 1992.
1364. **Nabata, T., Morimoto, S., Koh, E., Shiraishi, T., and Ogihara, T.,** Interleukin-6 stimulates c-myc expression and proliferation of cultured vascular smooth muscle cells, *Biochem. Int.,* 20, 445, 1990.
1365. **Tabibzadeh, S.S., Poubouridis, D., May, L.T., and Segal, P.B.,** Interleukin-6 immunoreactivity in human tumors, *Am. J. Pathol.,* 135, 427, 1989.
1366. **Takizawa, H., Ohtoshi, T., Ohta, K., Hirohata, S., Yamaguchi, M., Suzuki, N., Ueda, T., Ishii, A., Shindoh, G., Oka, T., Hiramatsu, K., and Ito, K.,** Interleukin 6/B cell stimulatory factor II is expressed and released by normal and transformed human bronchial epithelial cells, *Biochem. Biophys. Res. Commun.,* 187, 596, 1992.
1367. **Van Meir, E., Sawamura, Y., Diserens, A.-C., Hamou, M.E., and de Tribolet, N.,** Human glioblastoma cells release interleukin-6 *in vivo* and *in vitro, Cancer Res.,* 50, 6683, 1990.
1368. **Siegall, C.B., Schwab, G., Nordan, R.P., FitzGerald, D.J., and Pastan, I.,** Expression of the interleukin 6 receptor and interleukin 6 in prostate carcinoma cells, *Cancer Res.,* 50, 7786, 1990.
1369. **Berek, J.S., Chung, C.S., Kaldi, K., Watson, J.M., Knox, R.M., and Martinez-Maza, O.,** Serum interleukin-6 levels correlate with disease status in patients with epithelial ovarian cancer, *Am. J. Obstet. Gynecol.,* 164, 1991.
1370. **Herold, M., Schmalzl, F., and Zwierzina, H.,** Increased serum interleukin-6 levels in patients with myelodysplastic syndromes, *Leukemia Res.,* 16, 585, 1992.
1371. **Miles, S.A., Rezai, A.R., Salazar-González, J.F., Vander Meyden, M., Stevens, R.H., Logan, D.M., Mitsuyasu, R.T., Taga, T., Hirano, T., Kishimoto, T., and Martínez-Maza, O.,** AIDS Kaposi sarcoma-derived cells produce and respond to interleukin 6, *Proc. Natl. Acad. Sci. U.S.A.,* 87, 4068, 1990.
1372. **Hoang, T., Haman, A., Goncalves, O., Wong, G.G., and Clark, S.C.,** Interleukin-6 enhances growth factor-dependent proliferation of the blast cells of acute myeloblastic leukemia, *Blood,* 72, 823, 1988.
1373. **Kurzrock, R., Redman, J., Cabanillas, F., Jones, D., Rothberg, J., and Talpaz, M.,** Serum interleukin-6 levels are elevated in lymphoma patients and correlate with survival in advanced Hodgkin's disease and with B-symptoms, *Cancer Res.,* 53, 2118, 1993.
1374. **Sugiyama, H., Wiener, F., Babonits, M., Silva, S., Hirano, T., Kishimoto, T., and Klein, G.,** v-*abl* Does not abolish IL-6 requirement by murine plasmacytoma cells, *Int. J. Cancer,* 48, 234, 1991.
1375. **Takeda, K., Hosoi, T., Noda, M., Arimura, H., and Konno, K.,** Effect of fibroblast-derived differentiation inducing factor on the differentiation of human monocytoid and myeloid leukemia cell lines, *Biochem. Biophys. Res. Commun.,* 155, 24, 1988.
1376. **Miyaura, C., Onozaki, K., Akiyama, Y., Taniyama, T., Hirano, T., Kishimoto, T., and Suda, T.,** Recombinant human interleukin 6 (B-cell stimulatory factor 2) is a potent inducer of differentiation of mouse myeloid leukemia cells (M1), *FEBS Lett.,* 234, 17, 1988.

1377. Navarro, S., Louache, F., Debili, N., Vainchenker, W., and Doly, J., Autocrine regulation of terminal differentiation by interleukin-6 in the pluripotent KU812 cell line, *Biochem. Biophys. Res. Commun.*, 169, 184, 1990.
1378. Lu, C., Vickers, M.F., and Kerbel, R.S., Interleukin 6: a fibroblast-derived growth inhibitor of human melanoma cells from early but not advanced stages of tumor progression, *Proc. Natl. Acad. Sci. U.S.A.*, 89, 9215, 1992.
1379. Widmer, M.B., Morrisey, P.J., Goodwin, R.G., Grabstein, K.H., Park, L.S., Watson, J.D., Kincade, P.W., Conlon, P.J., and Namen, A.E., Lymphopoiesis and IL-7, *Int. J. Cell Cloning*, 8, 168, 1990.
1380. Namen, A.E., Schmierer, A.E., March, C.J., Overell, R.W., Park, L.S., Urdal, D.L., and Mochizuki, D.Y., B cell precursor growth promoting activity. Purification and characterization of a growth factor active on lymphocyte precursors, *J. Exp. Med.*, 167, 988, 1988.
1381. Namen, A.E., Lupton, S., Hjerrild, K., Wignall, J., Mochizuki, D.Y., Schmierer, A., Mosley, B., March, C.J., Urdal, D., Gillis, S., Cosman, D., and Goodwin, R.G., Stimulation of B-cell progenitors by cloned interleukin-7, *Nature*, 333, 571, 1988.
1382. Goodwin, R.G., Lupton, S., Schmierer, A., Hjerrild, K.J., Jerzy, R., Clevenger, W., Gillis, S., Cosman, D., and Namen, A.E., Human interleukin 7: molecular cloning and growth factor activity on human and murine B-lineage cells, *Proc. Natl. Acad. Sci. U.S.A.*, 86, 302, 1989.
1383. Sutherland, G.R., Baker, E., Fernandez, K.E.W., Callen, D.F., Goodwin, R.G., Lupton, S., Namen, A.E., Shannon, M.F., and Vadas, M.A., The gene for human interleukin 7 *(IL7)* is at 8q12-13, *Hum. Genet.*, 82, 371, 1989.
1384. Lee, G., Namen, A.E., Gillis, S., Ellingsworth, L.R., and Kincade, P.W., Normal B cell precursors responsive to recombinant murine IL-7 and inhibition of IL-7 activity by transforming growth factor-β, *J. Immunol.*, 142, 3875, 1989.
1385. Suda, T., Okada, S., Miura, Y., Ito, M., Sudo, T., Hayashi, S., Nishikawa, S., and Nakauchi, H., A stimulatory effect of recombinant murine interleukin-7 (IL-7) on B-cell colony formation and an inhibitory effect of IL-1α, *Blood*, 74, 1936, 1989.
1386. Billips, L.G., Petitte, D., Dorshkind, K., Narayanan, R., Chiu, C.-P., and Ladreth, K.S., Differential roles of stromal cells, interleukin-7, and *kit*-ligand in the regulation of B lymphopoiesis, *Blood*, 79, 1185, 1992.
1387. Morrissey, P.J., Goodwin, R.G., Nordan, R.P., Anderson, D., Grabstein, K.H., Cosman, D., Sims, J., Lupton, S., Acres, B., Reed, S.G., Mochizuki, D., Eisenman, J., Conlon, P.J., and Namen, A.E., Recombinant interleukin 7, pre-B cell growth factor, has costimulatory activity on purified mature T cells, *J. Exp. Med.*, 169, 707, 1989.
1388. Okazaki, H., Ito, M., Sudo, T., Hattori, M., Kano, S., Katsura, Y., and Minato, N., IL-7 promotes thymocyte proliferation and maintains immunocompetent thymocytes bearing αβ or γδ T-cell receptors in vitro: synergism with IL-2, *J. Immunol.*, 143, 2917, 1989.
1389. Welch, P.A., Namen, A.E., Goodwin, R.G., Armitage, R., and Cooper, M.D., Human IL-7: a novel T-cell growth factor, *J. Immunol.*, 143, 3562, 1989.
1390. Armitage, R.J., Namen, A.E., Sassenfeld, H.M., and Grabstein, K.H., Regulation of human T-cell proliferation by IL-7, *J. Immunol.*, 144, 938, 1990.
1391. Grabstein, K.H., Namen, A.E., Shanebeck, K., Voice, R.F., Reed, S.G., and Widmer, M.B., Regulation of T-cell proliferation by IL-7, *J. Immunol.*, 144, 3015, 1990.
1392. Bertagnolli, M. and Herrmann, S., IL-7 supports the generation of cytotoxic T lymphocytes from thymocytes. Multiple lymphokines required for proliferation and cytotoxicity, *J. Immunol.*, 145, 1706, 1990.
1393. Armitage, R.J., Macduff, B.M., Ziegler, S.F., and Grabstein, K.H., Multiple cytokine secretion by IL-7-stimulated human T cells, *Cytokine*, 4, 461, 1992.
1394. Alderson, M.R., Tough, T.W., Ziegler, S.F., and Grabstein, K.H., Interleukin 7 induces cytokine secretion and tumoricidal activity by human peripheral blood monocytes, *J. Exp. Med.*, 173, 923, 1991.
1395. Damia, G., Komschlies, K.L., Faltynek, C.R., Ruscetti, F.W., and Wiltrout, R.H., Administration of recombinant human interleukin-7 alters the frequency and number of myeloid progenitor cells in the bone marrow and spleen of mice, *Blood*, 79, 1121, 1992.
1396. Park, L.S., Friend, D.J., Schmierer, A.E., Dower, S.K., and Namen, A.E., Murine interleukin 7 (IL-7) receptor. Characterization on an IL-7-dependent cell line, *J. Exp. Med.*, 171, 1073, 1990.

1397. **Goodwin, R.G., Friend, D., Ziegler, S.F., Jerzy, R., Falk, B.A., Gimpel, S., Cosman, D., Dower, S.K., March, C.J., Namen, A.E., and Park, L.S.,** Cloning of the human and murine interleukin-7 receptors: demonstration of a soluble form and homology to a new receptor superfamily, *Cell,* 60, 941, 1990.

1398. **Pleiman, C.M., Gimpel, S.D., Park, L.S., Harada, H., Taniguchi, T., and Ziegler, S.F.,** Organization of the murine and human interleukin-7 receptor genes: two mRNAs generated by differential splicing and presence of a type I-interferon-inducible promoter, *Mol. Cell. Biol.,* 11, 3052, 1991.

1399. **Lynch, M., Baker, E., Park, L.S., Sutherland, G.R., and Goodwin, R.G.,** the interleukin 7 receptor gene is at 5p13, *Hum. Genet.,* 89, 566, 1992.

1400. **Uckun, F.M., Dibirdik, I., Smith, R., Tuel-Ahlgren, L., Langlie, M.-C., Schieven, G.L., Waddick, K.G., Hanson, M., and Ledbetter, J.A.,** Interleukin-7 receptor ligation stimulates tyrosine phosphorylation, inositol phospholipid turnover, and clonal proliferation of human B-cell precursors, *Proc. Natl. Acad. Sci. U.S.A.,* 88, 3589, 1991.

1401. **Uckun, F.M., Tuel-Ahlgren, L., Obuz, V., Smith, R., Dibirdik, I., Hanson, M., Langlie, M.-C., and Ledbetter, J.A.,** Interleukin 7 receptor engagement stimulates tyrosine phosphorylation, inositol phospholipid turnover, proliferation, and selective differentiation of the CD4 lineage by human fetal thymocytes, *Proc. Natl. Acad. Sci. U.S.A.,* 88, 6323, 1991.

1402. **Dadi, H.K., Ke, S., and Roifman, C.M.,** Interleukin 7 receptor mediates the activation of phosphatidylinositol 3-kinase in human B-cell precursors, *Biochem. Biophys. Res. Commun.,* 192, 459, 1993.

1403. **Venkitaraman, A.R. and Cowling, R.J.,** Interleukin-7 receptor functions by recruiting the tyrosine kinase p59^{fyn} through a segment of its cytoplasmic tail, *Proc. Natl. Acad. Sci. U.S.A.,* 89, 12083, 1992.

1404. **Morrow, M.A., Lee, G., Gillis, S., Yancopoulos, G.D., and Alt, F.W.,** Interleukin-7 induces N-*myc* and c-*myc* expression in normal precursor lymphocytes B, *Genes Develop.,* 6, 61, 1992.

1405. **Sica, D., Rayman, P., Stanley, J., Edinger, M., Tubbs, R.R., Klein, E., Bukowski, R., and Finke, J.H.,** Interleukin-7 enhances the proliferation and effector function of tumor-infiltrating lymphocytes from renal-cell carcinoma, *Int. J. Cancer,* 53, 941, 1993.

1406. **Frishman, J., Long, B., Knospe, W., Gregory, S., and Plate, J.,** Genes for interleukin-7 are transcribed in leukemic cell subsets of individuals with chronic lymphocytic leukemia, *J. Exp. Med.,* 177, 955, 1993.

1407. **Touw, I., Pouwels, K., van Gurp, R., Budel, L., Hoogerbrugge, H., Dehwel, R., Goodwin, R., Namen, A., and Löwenberg, B.,** Interleukin-7 is a growth factor of precursor B and T acute lymphoblastic leukemia, *Blood,* 75, 2097, 1990.

1408. **Masuda, M., Motoji, T., Oshimi, K., and Mizoguchi, H.,** Effects of interleukin-7 on proliferation of hematopoietic malignant cells, *Exp. Hematol.,* 18, 965, 1990.

1409. **Digel, W., Schmid, M., Heil, K., Conrad, P., Gillis, S., and Porzsolt, F.,** Human interleukin-7 induces proliferation of neoplastic cells from chronic lymphocytic leukemia and acute leukemias, *Blood,* 78, 753, 1991.

1410. **Young, J.C., Gishizky, M.L., and Witte, O.N.,** Hyperexpression of interleukin-7 is not necessary or sufficient for transformation of a pre-B lymphoid cell line, *Mol. Cell. Biol.,* 11, 854, 1991.

1411. **Overell, R.W., Clark, L., Lynch, D., Jerzy, R., Schmierer, A., Weisser, K.E., Namen, A.E., and Goodwin, R.G.,** Interleukin-7 retroviruses transform pre-B cells by an autocrine mechanism not evident in Abelson murine leukemia virus transformants, *Mol. Cell. Biol.,* 11, 1590, 1991.

1412. **Yoshimura, T., Matsushima, K., Oppenheim, J.J., and Leonard, E.J.,** Neutrophil chemotactic factor produced by lipopolysaccharide (LPS)-stimulated human blood mononuclear leukocytes: partial characterization and separation from interleukin-1 (IL-1), *J. Immunol.,* 139, 788, 1987.

1413. **Baggiolini, M., Walz, A., and Kunkel, S.L.,** Neutrophil-activating peptide-1/interleukin 8, a novel cytokine that activates neutrophils, *J. Clin. Invest.,* 84, 1045, 1989.

1414. **Larsen, C.G., Andersen, A.O., Appella, E., Oppenheim, J.J., and Matsushima, K.,** The neutrophil-activating protein (NAP-1) is also a chemotactic for lymphocytes, *Science,* 243, 1464, 1989.

1415. **Gimbrone, M.A., Jr., Obin, M.S., Brock, A.F., Luis, E.A., Hass, P.E., Hébert, C.A., Yip, Y.K., Leung, D.W., Lowe, D.G., Kohr, W.J., Darbonne, W.C., Bechtol, K.B., and Baker, J.B.,** Endothelial interleukin-8: a novel inhibitor of leukocyte-endothelial interactions, *Science,* 246, 1601, 1989.

1416. **Smyth, M.J., Zachariae, C.O.C., Norihisa, Y., Ortaldo, J.R., Hishinuma, A., and Matsushima, K.,** IL-8 gene expression and production in human peripheral blood lymphocyte subsets, *J. Immunol.,* 146, 3815, 1991.
1417. **Fujishima, S., Hoffman, A.R., Vu, T., Kim, J., Zheng, H., Daniel, D., Kim, Y., Wallace, E.F., Larrick, J.W., and Raffin, T.A.,** Regulation of neutrophil interleukin 8 gene expression and protein secretion by LPS, TNF-α, and IL-1β, *J. Cell. Physiol.,* 154, 478, 1993.
1418. **Rampart, M., Van Damme, J., Zonnekeyn, L., and Herman, A.G.,** Granulocyte chemotactic protein/interleukin-8 induces plasma leakage and neutrophil accumulation in rabbit skin, *Am. J. Pathol.,* 135, 21, 1989.
1419. **Huber, A.R., Kunkel, S.L., Todd, R.F., III, and Weiss, S.J.,** Regulation of transendothelial neutrophil migration by endogenous interleukin-8, *Science,* 254, 99, 1991.
1420. **Schröder, J.-M., Mrowietz, U., and Chrostophers, E.,** Purification and partial biological characterization of a human lymphocyte derived peptide with potent neutrophil stimulating activity, *J. Immunol.,* 140, 3534, 1988.
1421. **Koch, A.E., Polverini, P.J., Kunkel, S.L., Harlow, L.A., DiPietro, L.A., Elner, V.M., Elner, S.G., and Strieter, R.M.,** Interleukin-8 as a macrophage-derived mediator of angiogenesis, *Science,* 258, 1798, 1992.
1422. **Matsushima, K., Morishita, K., Yoshimura, T., Lavu, S., Kobayashi, Y., Lew, W., Appella, E., Kung, H.F., Leonard, E.J., and Oppenheim, J.J.,** Molecular cloning of a human monocyte-derived neutrophil chemotactic factor (MDNCF) and the induction of MDNCF mRNA by interleukin-1 and tumor necrosis factor, *J. Exp. Med.,* 167, 1863, 1988.
1423. **Modi, W.S., Dean, M., Seuanez, H.N., Mukaida, N., Matsushima, K., and O'Brien, S.J.,** Monocyte-derived neutrophil chemotactic factor (MDNCF/IL-8) resides in a gene cluster along with several other members of the platelet factor 4 gene superfamily, *Hum. Genet.,* 84, 185, 1990.
1424. **Thomas, K.M., Taylor, L., and Navarro, J.,** The interleukin-8 receptor is encoded by a neutrophil-specific cDNA clone, F3R, *J. Biol. Chem.,* 266, 14839, 1991.
1425. **Beckmann, M.P., Munger, W.E., Kozlosky, C., VandenBos, T., Price, V., Lyman, S., Gerard, N.P., Gerard, C., and Cerretti, D.P.,** Molecular characterization of the interleukin-8 receptor, *Biochem. Biophys. Res. Commun.,* 179, 784, 1991.
1426. **Holmes, W.E., Lee, J., Kuang, W.-J., Rice, G., and Wood, W.I.,** Structure and functional expression of a human interleukin-8 receptor, *Science,* 253, 1278, 1991.
1427. **Murphy, P.M. and Tiffany, H.L.,** Cloning of complementary DNA encoding a functional human interleukin-8 receptor, *Science,* 253, 1280, 1991.
1428. **Lee, J., Horuk, R., Rice, G.C., Bennett, G.L., Camerato, T., and Wood, W.I.,** Characterization of two high affinity interleukin-8 receptors, *J. Biol. Chem.,* 267, 16283, 1992.
1429. **Morris, S.W., Nelson, N., Valentine, M.B., Shapiro, D.N., Look, A.T., Kozlosky, C.J., Beckmann, M.P., and Cerreti, D.P.,** Assignment of the genes encoding human interleukin-8 receptor type 1 and type 2 and an interleukin-8 receptor pseudogene to chromosome 2q35, *Genomics,* 14, 685, 1992.
1430. **Lloyd, A., Modi, W., Sprenger, H., Cevario, S., Oppenheim, J., and Kelvin, D.,** Assignment of genes for interleukin-8 receptors to (IL8R)-A and IL8R-B to human chromosome band 2q35, *Cytogenet. Cell Genet.,* 63, 238, 1993.
1431. **Samanta, A.K., Oppenheim, J.J., and Matsuchima, K.,** Interleukin 8 (monocyte-derived neutrophil chemotactic factor) dynamically regulates its own receptor expression on human neutrophils, *J. Biol. Chem.,* 265, 183, 1990.
1432. **Wu, Q.D., LaRosa, G.J., and Simon, M.I.,** G-protein-coupled signal transduction pathways for interleukin-8, *Science,* 261, 101, 1993.
1433. **Bacon, K.B. and Camp, R.D.R.,** Interleukin (IL)-8-induced *in vitro* human lymphocyte migration is inhibited by cholera and pertussis toxins and inhibitors of protein kinase C, *Biochem. Biophys. Res. Commun.,* 169, 1099, 1990.
1434. **Pike, M.C., Costello, K.M., and Lamb, K.A.,** IL-8 stimulates phosphatidylinositol 4-phosphate kinase in human polymorphonuclear leukocytes, *J. Immunol.,* 148, 3158, 1992.
1435. **Van Meir, E., Ceska, M., Effenberger, F., Walz, A., Grouzmann, E., Desbaillets, I., Frei, K., Fontana, A., and de Tribolet, N.,** Interleukin-8 is produced in neoplastic and infectious diseases of the human central nervous system, *Cancer Res.,* 52, 4297, 1992.

1436. Uyttenhove, C., Simpson, R.J., and Van Snick, J., Functional and structural characterization of P40, a mouse glycoprotein with T-cell growth factor activity, *Proc. Natl. Acad. Sci. U.S.A.,* 85, 6934, 1988.
1437. Van Snick, J., Goethals, A., Renauld, J.C., Van Roost, E., Uyttenhove, C., Rubira, M.R., Moritz, R.L., and Simpson, R.J., Cloning and characterization of a cDNA for a new mouse T-cell growth factor (P40), *J. Exp. Med.,* 169, 363, 1989.
1438. Simpson, R.J., Moritz, R.L., Gorman, J.J., and Van Snick, J., Complete amino acid sequence of a new murine T-cell growth factor P40, *Eur. J. Biochem.,* 183, 715, 1989.
1439. Yang, Y.-C., Ricciardi, S., Ciarletta, A., Calvetti, J., Kelleher, K., and Clark, S.C., Expression cloning of a cDNA encoding a novel human hematopoietic growth factor: human homologue of murine T-cell growth factor P40, *Blood,* 74, 1880, 1989.
1440. Renauld, J.-C., Goethals, A., Houssiau, F., Merz, H., Van Roost, E., and Van Snick, J., Human P40/IL-9. Expression in activated CD4+ T cells, genomic organization, and comparison with the mouse gene, *J. Immunol.,* 144, 4235, 1990.
1441. Kelleher, K., Bean, K., Clark, S.C., Leung, W.-Y., Yang-Feng, T.L., Chen, J.W., Lin, P.-F., Luo, W., and Yang, Y.-C., Human interleukin-9: genomic sequence, chromosomal location, and sequences essential for its expression in human T-cell leukemia virus (HTLV)-I-transformed human T cells, *Blood,* 77, 1436, 1991.
1442. Houssiau, F.A., Renauld, J.C., Fibbe, W.E., and Van Snick, J., IL-2 dependence of IL-9 expression in human lymphocytes T, *J. Immunol.,* 148, 3147, 1992.
1443. Holbrook, S.T., Ohis, R.K., Schibler, K.R., Yang, Y.-C., and Christensen, R.D., Effect of interleukin-9 on clonogenic maturation and cell-cycle status of fetal and adult hematopoietic progenitors, *Blood,* 77, 2129, 1991.
1444. Schaafsma, M.R., Falkenburg, J.H.F., Duinkerken, N., Van Snick, J., Landegent, J.E., Willemze, R., and Fibbe, W.E., Interleukin-9 stimulates the proliferation of enriched human erythroid progenitor cells: additive effect with GM-CSF, *Ann. Hematol.,* 66, 45, 1993.
1445. Druez, C., Coulie, P., Uyttenhove, C., and Van Snick, J., Functional and biochemical characterization of mouse P40/IL-9 receptors, *J. Immunol.,* 145, 2494, 1990.
1446. Renauld, J.-C., Druez, C., Kermouni, A., Houssiau, F., Uyttenhove, C., Van Roost, E., and Van Snick, J., Expression cloning of the murine and human interleukin 9 receptor cDNAs, *Proc. Natl. Acad. Sci. U.S.A.,* 89, 5690, 1992.
1447. Gruss, H.J., Brach, M.A., Drexler, H.G., Bross, K.J., and Herrmann, F., Interleukin-9 is expressed by primary and cultured Hodgkin and Reed-Sternberg cells, *Cancer Res.,* 52, 1026, 1992.
1448. Merz, H., Houssiau, F.A., Orscheschek, K., Renauld, J.C., Fliedner, A., Herin, M., Noel, H., Kadin, M., Mueller-Hermelink, H.K., Van Snick, J., and Feller, A.C., Interleukin-9 expression in human malignant lymphomas: unique association with Hodgkin's disease and large cell anaplastic lymphoma, *Blood,* 78, 1311, 1991.
1449. Uyttenhove, C., Druez, D., Renauld, J.C., Hérin, M., Noël, H., and Van Snick, J., Autonomous growth and tumorigenicity induced by p40 interleukin-9 cDNA transfection of a mouse p40-dependent T-cell line, *J. Exp. Med.,* 173, 519, 1991.
1450. Moore, K.W., Vieira, P., Fiorentino, D.F., Trounstine, M.L., Khan, T.A., and Mosmann, T.R., Homology of cytokine synthesis inhibitory factor (IL-10) to the Epstein-Barr virus gene BCRF1, *Science,* 248, 1230, 1990.
1451. Hsu, D.-H., de Waal Malefyt, R., Fiorentino, D.F., Dang, M.-N., Vieira, P., de Vries, J., Spits, H., Mosmann, T.R., and Moore, K.W., Expression of interleukin-10 activity by Epstein-Barr virus protein BCRF1, *Science,* 250, 830, 1990.
1452. Zlotnik, A. and Moore, K.W., Interleukin-10, *Cytokine,* 3, 366, 1991.
1453. Spits, H. and Malefyt, R.D., Functional characterization of human IL-10, *Int. Arch. Allergy Immunol.,* 99, 8, 1992.
1454. Moore, K.W., O'Garra, A., Malefyt, R.D., Vieira, P., and Mosmann, T.R., Interleukin-10, *Annu. Rev. Immunol.,* 11, 165, 1993.
1455. MacNeil, I.A., Suda, T., Moore, K.W., Mosmann, T.R., and Zlotnik, A., IL-10, a novel growth cofactor for mature and immature T cells, *J. Immunol.,* 145, 4167, 1990.
1456. Taga, K. and Tosato, G., IL-10 inhibits human T-cell proliferation and IL-2 production, *J. Immunol.,* 148, 1143, 1992.

1457. **Ding, L. and Shevach, E.M.,** IL-10 inhibits mitogen-induced T-cell proliferation by selectively inhibiting macrophage costimulatory function, *J. Immunol.,* 148, 3133, 1992.
1458. **Ralph, P., Nakoinz, I., Sampson-Johannes, A., Fong, S., Lowe, D., Min, H.-Y., and Lin, L.,** IL-10, T-lymphocyte inhibitor of human blood cell production of IL-1 and tumor necrosis factor, *J. Immunol.,* 148, 808, 1992.
1459. **Chomarat, P., Rissoan, M.C., Bancherau, J., and Miossec, P.,** Interferon-γ inhibits interleukin-10 production by monocytes, *J. Exp. Med.,* 177, 523, 1993.
1460. **Go, N.F., Castle, B.E., Barrett, R., Kastelein, R., Dang, W., Mosmann, T.R., Moore, K.W., and Howard, M.,** Interleukin 10, a novel B cell stimulatory factor: unresponsiveness of X chromosome-linked immunodeficiency B cells, *J. Exp. Med.,* 172, 1625, 1990.
1461. **Rousset, F., Garcia, E., Defrance, T., Peronne, C., Vezzio, N., Hsu, D.H., Kastelein, R., Moore, K.W., and Banchereau, J.,** Interleukin-10 is a potent growth and differentiation factor for activated human lymphocytes B, *Proc. Natl. Acad. Sci. U.S.A.,* 89, 1924, 1992.
1462. **Thompson-Snipes, L., Dhar, V., Bond, M.W., Mosmann, T.R., Moore, K.W., and Rennick, D.M.,** Interleukin 10: a novel stimulatory factor for mast cells and their progenitors, *J. Exp. Med.,* 173, 507, 1991.
1463. **Burdin, N., Peronne, C., Banchereau, J., and Rousset, F.,** Epstein-Barr virus transformation induces lymphocytes-B to produce human interleukin-10, *J. Exp. Med.,* 177, 295, 1993.
1464. **Enk, A.H. and Katz, S.I.,** Identification and induction of keratinocyte-derived IL-10, *J. Immunol.,* 149, 92, 1992.
1465. **Howard, M., Muchamuel, T., Andrade, S., and Menon, S.,** Interleukin-10 protects mice from lethal endotoxemia, *J. Exp. Med.,* 177, 1205, 1993.
1466. **Goodman, R.E., Oblak, J., and Bell, R.G.,** Synthesis and characterization of rat interleukin-10 (IL-10) cDNA clones from RNA of cultured OX8-OX22 thoracid duct T cells, *Biochem. Biophys. Res. Commun.,* 189, 1, 1992.
1467. **Vieira, P., de Waal-Malefyt, R., Dang, M.-N., Johnson, K.E., Kastelein, R., Fiorentino, D.F., de Vries, J.E., Ronarola, M.-G., Mosmann, T.R., and Moore, K.W.,** Isolation and expression of human cytokine synthesis inhibitory factor cDNA clones: homology to Epstein-Barr virus open reading frame BCRFI, *Proc. Natl. Acad. Sci. U.S.A.,* 88, 1172, 1991.
1468. **Benjamin, D., Knobloch, T.J., and Dayton, M.A.,** Human B-cell interleukin-10. B cell lines derived from patients with acquired immunodeficiency syndrome and Burkitt's lymphoma constitutively secrete large quantities of interleukin-10, *Blood,* 80, 1289, 1992.
1469. **Emilie, D., Touitou, R., Raphael, M., Peuchmaur, M., Devergnee, O., Rea, D., Coumbraras, J., Crevon, M.C., Edelman, L., Joab, I., et al.,** In vivo production of interleukin-10 by malignant cells in AIDS lymphomas, *Eur. J. Immunol.,* 22, 2937, 1992.
1470. **Paul, S.R. and Schendel, P.,** The cloning and biological characterization of recombinant human interleukin 11, *Int. J. Cell Cloning,* 10, 135, 1992.
1471. **Yang, Y.C. and Ying, T.G.,** Interleukin-11 and its receptor, *Biofactors,* 4, 15, 1992.
1472. **Paul, S.R., Bennett, F., Calvetti, J.A., Kelleher, K., Wood, C.R., O'Hara, R.M., Jr., Leary, A.C., Sibley, B., Clark, S.C., Williams, D.A., and Yang, Y.-C.,** Molecular cloning of a cDNA encoding interleukin 11, a stromal cell-derived lymphopoietic and hematopoietic cytokine, *Proc. Natl. Acad. Sci. U.S.A.,* 87, 7512, 1990.
1473. **McKinley, D., Wu, Q.M., Yang-Feng, T., and Yang, Y.C.,** Genomic sequence and chromosomal location of human interleukin-11 gene *(IL11), Genomics,* 13, 814, 1992.
1474. **Anderson, K.C., Morimoto, C., Paul, S.R., Chauhan, D., Williams, D., Cochran, M., and Barut, B.A.,** Interleukin-11 promotes accessory cell-dependent B-cell differentiation in humans, *Blood,* 80, 2797, 1992.
1475. **Musashi, M., Clark, S.C., Sudo, T., Urdal, D.L., and Ogawa, M.,** Synergistic interactions between interleukin-11 and interleukin-4 in support of proliferation of primitive hematopoietic progenitors of mice, *Blood,* 78, 1448, 1991.
1476. **Hangoc, C., Yin, T.G., Cooper, S., Schendel, P., Yang, Y.C., and Broxmeyer, H.E.,** *In vivo* effects of recombinant interleukin-11 on myelopoiesis in mice, *Blood,* 81, 965, 1993.
1477. **Quesniaux, V.F.J., Clark, S.C., Turner, K., and Fagg, B.,** Interleukin-11 stimulates multiple phases of erythropoiesis *in vitro, Blood,* 80, 1218, 1992.
1478. **Teramura, M., Kobayashi, S., Hoshino, S., Oshimi, K., and Mizoguchi, H.,** Interleukin-11 enhances human megakaryocytopoiesis in vitro, *Blood,* 79, 327, 1992.

1479. **Kobayashi, S., Teramura, M., Sugawara, I., Oshimi, K., and Mizoguchi, H.,** Interleukin-11 acts as an autocrine growth factor for human megakaryoblastic cell lines, *Blood,* 81, 889, 1993.
1480. **Neben, T.Y., Loebelenz, J., Hayes, L., McCarthy, K., Stoudemire, J., Schaub, R., and Goldman, S.J.,** Recombinant human interleukin-11 stimulates megakaryocytopoiesis and increases peripheral platelets in normal and splenectomized mice, *Blood,* 8, 901, 1993.
1481. **Baumann, H. and Schendel, P.,** Interleukin 11 regulates the hepatic expression of the same plasma protein genes as interleukin 6, *J. Biol. Chem.,* 266, 20424, 1991.
1482. **Kawashima, I., Ohsumi, J., Mita-Honjo, K., Shimoda-Takano, K., Ishikawa, H., Sakakibara, S., Miyadai, K., and Taniguchi, Y.,** Molecular cloning of a cDNA encoding adipogenesis inhibitory factor and identity with interleukin 11, *FEBS Lett.,* 283, 199, 1991.
1483. **Yin, T., Miyazawa, K., and Yang, Y.-C.,** Characterization of interleukin-11 receptor and protein tyrosine phosphorylation induced by interleukin-11 in mouse 3T3-L1 cells, *J. Biol. Chem.,* 267, 8347, 1992.
1484. **Hu, J.P., Casano, A., Santoli, D., Clark, S.C., and Hoang, T.,** Effects of interleukin-11 on the proliferation and cell cycle status of myeloid leukemic cells, *Blood,* 81, 1586, 1993.
1485. **Kobayashi, M.L., Fitz, L., Ryan, M., Hewick, R.M., Chan, S., Loudon, R., Sherman, B., Perussia, B., and Trinchieri, G.,** Identification and purification of a natural killer cell stimulatory factor (NKSF), a cytokine with multiple biological effects on human lymphocytes, *J. Exp. Med.,* 170, 827, 1989.
1486. **Stern, A.S., Podlaski, F.J., Hulmes, J.D., Pan, Y.E., Quinn, P.M., Wolitzky, A.G., Familletti, P.C., Stremlo, D.L., Truitt, T., Chizzonite, R., and Gately, M.K.,** Purification to homogeneity and partial characterization of cytotoxic lymphocyte maturation factor from human B-lymphoblastoid cells, *Proc. Natl. Acad. Sci. U.S.A.,* 87, 6808, 1990.
1487. **Gately, M.K., Desai, B.B., Wolitzky, A.G., Quinn, P.M., Dwyer, C.M., Podlaski, F.J., Familletti, P.C., Sinigaglia, F., Chizzonite, R., Gubler, U., and Stern, A.S.,** Regulation of human lymphocyte proliferation by a heterodimeric cytokine, interleukin 12 (cytotoxic lymphocyte maturation factor), *J. Immunol.,* 147, 874, 1991.
1488. **Naume, B., Gately, M.K., Desai, B.B., Sundan, A., and Espevik, T.,** Synergistic effects of interleukin-4 and interleukin-12 on NK cell proliferation, *Cytokine,* 5, 38, 1993.
1489. **Sieburth, D., Jabs, E.W., Warrington, J.A., Li, X., Lasota, U., LaForgia, S., Kelleher, K., Huebner, K., Wasmuth, J.J., and Wolf, S.F.,** Assignment of genes encoding a unique cytokine (IL-12) composed of two unrelated subunits to chromosomes 3 and 5, *Genomics,* 14, 59, 1992.
1490. **Chizzonite, R., Truitt, T., Desai, B.B., Nunes, P., Podlaski, F.J., Stern, A.S., and Gately, M.K.,** IL-12 receptor. I. Characterization of the receptor on phytohemagglutinin-activated human lymphoblasts, *J. Immunol.,* 148, 3117, 1992.
1491. **Desai, B.B., Quinn, P.M., Wolitzky, A.G., Mongini, P.K.A., Chizzonite, R., and Gately, M.K.,** IL-12 receptor. II. Distribution and regulation of receptor expression, *J. Immunol.,* 148, 3125, 1992.
1492. **Chizzonite, R., Truitt, T., Podlaski, F.J., Wolitzky, A.G., Quinn, P.M., Nunes, P., Stern, A.S., and Gately, M.K.,** IL-12: monoclonal antibodies specific for the 40-kDa subunit block receptor binding and biologic activity of activated human lymphoblasts, *J. Immunol.,* 147, 1548, 1991.
1493. **Minty, A., Chalon, P., Derocq, J.-M., Dumont, X., Guillemot, J.-C., Kaghad, M., Labit, C., Leplatois, P., Liauzun, P., Miloux, B., Minty, C., Casellas, P., Loison, G., Lupker, J., Shire, D., Ferrara, P., and Caput, D.,** Interleukin-13 is a new human lymphokine regulating inflammatory and immune responses, *Nature,* 362, 248, 1993.
1494. **Punnonen, J., Aversa, G., Cocks, B.G., McKenzie, A.N.J., Menon, S., Zurawski, G., Malefyt, R.D., and de Vries, J.E.,** Interleukin-13 induces interleukin-4-independent IgG4 and IgE synthesis and CD23 expression by human B cells, *Proc. Natl. Acad. Sci. U.S.A.,* 90, 3730, 1993.
1495. **McKenzie, A.N.J., Culpepper, J.D., Malefyt, R.D., Punnonen, J., Aversa, G., Sato, A., Dang, W., Cocks, B.G., Menon, S., and Zurawski, G.,** Interleukin-13, a T-cell-derived cytokine that regulates human monocyte and B-cell function, *Proc. Natl. Acad. Sci. U.S.A.,* 90, 3735, 1993.
1496. **Smith, A.G., Heath, J.R., Donaldson, D.D., Wong, G.G., Moreau, J., Stahl, M., and Roger, D.,** Inhibition of pluripotential embryonic stem cells differentiation by purified polypeptides, *Nature,* 336, 688, 1988.

1497. **Hilton, D.J., Nicola, N.A., and Metcalf, D.,** Specific binding of murine leukemia inhibitory factor to normal and leukemic monocytic cells, *Proc. Natl. Acad. Sci. U.S.A.,* 85, 5971, 1988.
1498. **Miyaura, C., Jin, C.H., Yamaguchi, Y., Tomida, M., Hozumi, M., Matsuda, T., Hirano, T., Kishimoto, T., and Suda, T.,** Production of interleukin 6 and its relation to the macrophage differentiation of mouse myeloid leukemia cells (M1) treated with differentiation-inducing factor and 1α,25-dihydroxyvitamin D_3, *Biochem. Biophys. Res. Commun.,* 158, 660, 1989.
1499. **Abe, T., Murakami, M., Sato, T., Kajiki, M., Ohno, M., and Kodaira, R.,** Macrophage differentiation inducing factor from human monocytic cells is equivalent to murine leukemia inhibitory factor, *J. Biol. Chem.,* 264, 8941, 1989.
1500. **Okabe-Kado, J., Honma, Y., Hayashi, M., Hozumi, M., Sampi, K., Sakurai, M., Hino, K., and Tsuruoka, N.,** Induction of differentiation of mouse myeloid leukemia M1 cells by serum of patients with chronic myeloid leukemia, *Jpn. J. Cancer Res.,* 79, 1318, 1988.
1501. **Moreau, J.-F., Donaldson, D.D., Bennett, F., Witek-Giannotti, J., Clark, S.C., and Wong, G.G.,** Leukemia inhibitory factor is identical to the myeloid growth factor human interleukin for DA cells, *Nature,* 336, 690, 1988.
1502. **Baumann, H. and Wong, G.G.,** Hepatocyte-stimulating factor III shares structural and functional identity with leukemia-inhibitory factor, *J. Immunol.,* 143, 1163, 1989.
1503. **Yamamori, T., Fukada, K., Aebersold, R., Korsching, S., Fann, M.-J., and Patterson, P.H.,** The cholinergic neuronal differentiation factor from heart cells is identical to leukemia inhibitory factor, *Science,* 246, 1412, 1989.
1504. **Gearing, D.P., Gough, N.M., King, J.A., Hilton, P.J., Nicola, N.A., Simpson, R.J., Nice, E.C., Kelson, A., and Metcalf, D.,** Molecular cloning and expression of cDNA encoding a murine myeloid leukemia inhibitory factor (LIF), *EMBO J.,* 6, 3995, 1987.
1505. **Gough, N.M., Gearing, D.P., King, J.A., Willson, T.A., Hilton, D.J., Nicola, N.A., and Metcalf, D.,** Molecular cloning and expression of the human homolog of the murine gene encoding myeloid leukemia inhibitory factor, *Proc. Natl. Acad. Sci. U.S.A.,* 85, 2623, 1988.
1506. **Lowe, D.G., Nunes, W., Bombara, M., McCabe, S., Ranges, G.E., Henzel, W., Tomida, M., Yamamoto-Yamaguchi, Y., Hozumi, M., and Goeddel, D.V.,** Genomic cloning and heterologous expression of human differentiation-stimulating factor, *DNA,* 8, 351, 1989.
1507. **Sutherland, G.R., Baker, E., Hyland, V.J., Callen, D.F., Stahl, J., and Gough, N.M.,** The gene for human leukemia inhibitory factor *(LIF)* maps to 22q12, *Leukemia,* 3, 9, 1989.
1508. **Jeffery, E., Price, V., and Gearing, D.P.,** Close proximity of the genes for leukemia inhibitory factor and oncostatin M, *Cytokine,* 5, 107, 1993.
1509. **Layton, M.J., Cross, B.A., Metcalf, D., Ward, L.D., Simpson, R.J., and Nicola, N.A.,** A major binding protein for leukemia inhibitory factor in normal mouse serum: identification as a soluble form of the cellular receptor, *Proc. Natl. Acad. Sci. U.S.A.,* 89, 8616, 1992.
1510. **Metcalf, D.,** The leukemia inhibitory factor (LIF), *Int. J. Cell Cloning,* 9, 95, 1991.
1511. **Kurzrock, R., Estrov, Z., Wetzler, M., Gutterman, J.U., and Talpaz, M.,** LIF: not just a leukemia inhibitory factor, *Endocrine Rev.,* 12, 208, 1991.
1512. **Villiger, P.M., Geng, Y., and Lotz, M.,** Induction of cytokine expression by leukemia inhibitory factor, *J. Clin. Invest.,* 91, 1575, 1993.
1513. **Escary, J.L., Perreau, J., Dumenil, D., Enzine, S., and Brulet, P.,** Leukemia inhibitory factor is necessary for maintenance of hematopoietic stem cells and thymocyte stimulation, *Nature,* 363, 361, 1993.
1514. **Leary, A.G., Wong, G.G., Clark, S.C., Smith, A.G., and Ogawa, M.,** Leukemia inhibitory factor differentiation-inhibiting activity/human interleukin for DA cells augments proliferation of human hematopoietic stem cells, *Blood,* 75, 1960, 1990.
1515. **Wetzler, M., Talpaz, M., Lowe, D.G., Baiocchi, G., Gutterman, J.U., and Kurzrock, R.,** Constitutive expression of leukemia inhibitory factor RNA by human bone marrow stromal cells and modulation by IL-1, TNF-α, and TGF-β, *Exp. Hematol.,* 19, 347, 1991.
1516. **Burstein, S.A., Meik R.-L., Henthorn, J., Friese, P., and Turner, K.,** Leukemia inhibitory factor and interleukin-11 promote maturation of murine and human megakaryocytes in vitro, *J. Cell. Physiol.,* 153, 305, 1992.
1517. **Metcalf, D., Nicola, N.A., and Gearing, D.P.,** Effects of injected leukemia inhibitory factor on hematopoietic and other tissues in mice, *Blood,* 76, 50, 1990.

1518. **Abe, E., Tanaka, H., Ishimi, Y., Miyaura, C., Hayashi, T., Nagasawa, H., Tomida, M., Yamaguchi, Y., Hozumi, M., and Suda, T.,** Differentiation-inducing factor purified from conditioned medium of mitogen-treated spleen cell cultures stimulates bone resorption, *Proc. Natl. Acad. Sci. U.S.A.,* 83, 5958, 1986.

1519. **Metcalf, D. and Gearing, D.P.,** Fatal syndrome in mice engrafted with cells producing high levels of the leukemia inhibitory factor, *Proc. Natl. Acad. Sci. U.S.A.,* 86, 5948, 1989.

1520. **Reid, I.R., Lowe, C., Cornish, J., Skinner, S.J.M., Hilton, D.J., Willson, T.A., Gearing, D.P., and Martin, T.J.,** Leukemia inhibitory factor: a novel bone-active cytokine, *Endocrinology,* 126, 1416, 1990.

1521. **Noda, M., Vogel, R.L., Hasson, D.M., and Rodan, G.A.,** Leukemia inhibitory factor suppresses proliferation, alkaline phosphatase activity, and type I collagen messenger ribonucleic acid level and enhances osteopontin mRNA level in murine osteoblast-like (MC3T3E1) cells, *Endocrinology,* 127, 185, 1990.

1522. **Ishimi, Y., Abe, E., Jin, C.H., Miyaura, C., Hong, M.H., Oshida, M., Kurosawa, H., Yamaguchi, Y., Tomida, M., Hozumi, M., and Suda, T.,** Leukemia inhibitory factor/differentiation-stimulating factor (LIF/D-factor): regulation of its production and possible roles in bone metabolism, *J. Cell. Physiol.,* 152, 71, 1992.

1523. **Murray, R., Lee, F., and Chiu, C.-P.,** The genes for leukemia inhibitory factor and interleukin-6 are expressed in mouse blastocyst prior to the onset of hemopoiesis, *Mol. Cell. Biol.,* 10, 4953, 1990.

1524. **Conquet, F. and Brûlet, P.,** Developmental expression of myeloid leukemia inhibitory factor gene in preimplantation blastocysts and in extraembryonic tissue of mouse embryos, *Mol. Cell. Biol.,* 10, 3801, 1990.

Chapter 3

Colony-Stimulating Factors

I. INTRODUCTION

The colony-stimulating factors (CSFs), also called myeloid growth factors, are HGFs crucially involved in controlling the formation from bone marrow progenitors of nonlymphoid cells which include neutrophils, eosinophils, basophils, and monocytes. The CSFs were discovered on the basis of their specific biological activities as assessed in colony assays *in vitro*.[1-4] They are represented by glycoproteins which have recently been purified to homogeneity, and their amino acid sequences have been deduced from the respective cloned genes.[5-18] In addition to the macrophage CSF (M-CSF or CSF-1), the granulocyte-macrophage CSF (GM-CSF or CSF-2), and the granulocyte CSF (G-CSF or CSF-3), IL-3 can also be considered as a CSF. The CSFs are expressed by various bone marrow components, including fibroblasts, preadipose cells, and adipocytes,[19] which are important for normal hematopoiesis. The mechanisms by which CSFs regulate the proliferation and differentiation of marrow cell populations with different lineage specificities include as an important component the activation of the N^+/H^+ antiporter and intracellular alkalinization.[20]

II. COLONY-STIMULATING FACTOR 1

Colony-stimulating factor 1 (CSF-1), also called macrophage colony-stimulating factor (M-CSF), is a lineage-specific HGF that supports the proliferation, differentiation, and survival of mononuclear phagocytes and their precursors.[21] Signals mediated by the interaction of CSF-1 with its receptor on the cell surface may play a deterministic role in the differentiation of macrophage cells.[22] The mononuclear phagocyte system, which consists of monocytes and tissue macrophages, is the major component of the reticuloendothelial system. This system participates in various physiological and pathological events.[23] Phagocytosis by macrophages is essential to metazoan life, and macrophages are involved in the secretion of important biological products.[24] Macrophages are highly active cells that readily respond to hormonal and cellular signals, exhibiting noteworthy interactions with lymphocytes, and participating in immunological responses.

A. BIOLOGICAL EFFECTS OF CSF-1

CSF-1 can elicit a variety of effects on blood cells, both *in vivo* and *in vitro*. Administration of CSF-1 to intact rats induces, in a dose-dependent manner, peripheral monocytosis, neutrophilia, and lymphopenia.[25] *In vitro*, both CSF-1 and IL-3 support macrophage and neutrophil-macrophage colony formation from bone marrow cells of normal mice, but there is evidence that some of the macrophage colony-forming cells that respond to IL-3 are more primitive than those that are sensitive to CSF-1.[26] In addition to its action on progenitor marrow cells, CSF-1 has also certain effects on mature cells. Highly purified CSF-1 induces thromboplastin activity in murine macrophages and human monocytes *in vitro*.[27] Thromboplastin (tissue factor) is the most potent physiological trigger of blood coagulation presently known. It consists of the integral membrane glycoprotein, apoprotein III. CSF-1 also stimulates platelet-activating factor (PAF) and superoxide anion generation by human neutrophils.[28]

Production of IFN and TNF by human blood monocytes is increased by CSF-1.[29] Macrophages stimulated by CSF-1 have inhibitory activity for proliferating lymphocytes, suggesting that CSF-1 may play a role in immunoregulatory mechanisms.[30] Pretreatment of peritoneal macrophages with CSF-1 can increase their tumoricidal capacity.[31] Human monocytes cultured in the presence of CSF-1 can ingest up to 100% of melanoma and neuroblastoma cells in the presence of antitumor monoclonal antibody.[32] Human CSF-1 can augment the tumoricidal activity of human peripheral blood monocytes induced by other agents.[33] CSF-1-induced activation of human macrophages includes the induction of TNF-α, which may result in enhancement of their cytolytic activity against tumor cells.

B. CSF-1 STRUCTURE AND THE CSF-1 GENE

Murine CSF-1 is a heterogeneous glycoprotein of 65 to 70 kDa and the active molecule appears to consist of two subunits of equal molecular weights, linked by disulfide bonds. Mild reduction results in subunit dissociation and the loss of all biological activity. The amino acid composition, the amino-terminal sequence, and the tryptic map of murine L-cell CSF-1 have been determined.[34] CSF-1 contains four or five cysteine residues per subunit, with the unusual configuration of three contiguous cysteine residues (Cys-Cys-Cys) located in the amino-terminal sequence. The murine CSF-1 molecule contains 30 to 40% carbohydrate by weight and exhibits limited homology to CSF-2 or IL-3. The protein undergoes autophosphorylation *in vitro* and *in vivo* following CSF-1 binding. The murine CSF-1 receptor protein expressed in myeloid and fibroblastic cells contains two major sites of tyrosine phosphorylation (Tyr-697 and Tyr-706), and phosphorylation at these sites is stimulated by CSF-1.[35] The gene encoding CSF-1 was cloned from a mouse L-cell cDNA library.[36] CSF-1 transcripts are expressed in several murine tissues in the form of four distinct mRNA species, ranging from 4.5 to 1.4 kb in size. Large qualitative and quantitative differences in the pattern of CSF-1 transcripts are observed between tissues, with liver exhibiting a single 1.4-kb CSF-1 transcript, although no CSF-1 bioactivity is detected in this organ. The CSF-1 gene is located on mouse chromosome 3.[37,38]

CSF-1 has been isolated in microgram amounts and has been purified from murine L cells and human urine.[39,40] Native human urinary CSF-1 is a glycosylated homodimer of approximate 45 kDa. Various amounts of CSF-1 are produced by human cell lines and the pancreatic carcinoma lines, MIA PaCa and PANC, have been found to secrete high levels of CSF-1.[41] These two cell lines stopped secreting CSF-1 when transferred to serum-free medium, but serum-free production of CSF-1 was reinitiated by treatment with phorbol ester (PMA). The human CSF-1 glycoprotein purified from the medium conditioned by cultured human pancreatic carcinoma cells was found to have a subunit molecular weight corresponding to the smallest of four molecular species whose molecular weights range from 40,000 to 23,000 Da.[42] The human CSF-1 protein has been purified in milligram amounts from culture supernatants of SV40-infected CV-1 monkey cells that were transformed with a plasmid containing a human CSF-1 cDNA sequence.[43] A polyclonal antibody to recombinant CSF-1 produced in rabbits was shown to specifically neutralize the biological activity of both recombinant and native CSF-1.

The CSF-1 gene was initially localized to human chromosome band 5q33.1,[44] but was reassigned to region 1p13-p21.[45,46] The complete nucleotide sequences of the human CSF-1 gene were determined from cDNA probes.[47,48] The gene is 18 kb in length and codes for a 224-residue CSF-1 polypeptide. Native human CSF-1 is a glycosylated dimer protein of 45 kDa.[40] Differential posttranslational processing may reflect diverse physiological roles for the products of CSF-1 precursors.[49] A 4-kb mRNA from the human CSF-1 gene encodes a larger (61 kDa) precursor protein which is very similar in its properties to those of CSF-1 isolated from the human urine.[50] The 61-kDa prepro-CSF-1 polypeptide is processed at the amino terminus by removal of the 31-residue signal peptide and at the carboxyl terminus by removal of about 333 residues, to yield a subunit of 189 amino acids with a predicted molecular weight of 21 kDa. Thus, the human CSF-1 gene can be expressed to yield at least two different mRNA species that encode distinct but related forms of CSF-1. The diverse sequences detected in CSF-1 mRNAs arise from differential splicing of a large primary transcript. Two major CSF-1 mRNA species expressed in human endometrial glands during the menstrual cycle predict different forms (soluble or membrane-bound) of the growth factor.[51] These results suggest that different molecular forms of CSF-1 may have distinct roles as mediators of sex steroid hormone action in the endometrium, depending on their mode of presentation to the target cells.

Molecular heterogeneity of the human CSF-1 protein results from both pre- and posttranslational processing, including alternative mRNA splicing, differential glycosylation, and proteolytic processing.[52] The several distinct but related species of CSF-1 could mediate the different biological activities reported for CSF-1. However, studies with a truncated CSF-1 cDNA have shown that CSF-1 amino acid residues 1 to 158 are sufficient for biological activity, including the formation of bone marrow-derived mouse macrophage colonies in semisolid medium.[53] Molecular cloning and expression of human CSF-1 gene deletion mutants indicate that at least 377 carboxy-terminal amino acid residues of the molecule are dispensable for human CSF-1 to exhibit its *in vitro* biological activity on murine marrow cells.[54]

C. PRODUCTION OF CSF-1

CSF-1 gene transcripts are expressed in normal fibroblasts and other mesenchymal cells as well as in some hematopoietic cells such as monocytes. Whereas normal human cells express only CSF-1 transcripts of 4.0 kb, multiple myeloma cells may express 3.5-kb CSF-1 transcripts.[55] CSF-1 activity is produced by a wide variety of mammalian tissues, including brain, heart, and lung.[36] Blood cells may also produce CSF-1 mRNA and protein. CSF-1 transcripts are undetectable in unstimulated human monocytes, but activation of monocytes with IFN-γ or PMA induces CSF-1 expression.[56] CSF-1 mRNA is not detectable in normal human T lymphocytes, either unstimulated or stimulated. In contrast, activated or

EBV-infected B lymphocytes from healthy donors release CSF-1.[57] Increased levels of circulating CSF-1 may be found in patients with preleukemia, leukemia, and lymphoid malignant diseases.[58]

1. Regulation of CSF-1 Production

The production of CSF-1 is controlled at both the transcriptional and posttranscriptional levels in stimulated human monocytes.[59] Different physiological factors are involved in controlling the production of CSF-1. Production of CSF-1 by human bone marrow stroma cell layers in long-term culture is stimulated by IL-1.[60] CSF-2 induces transcriptional and translational expression of the CSF-1 gene in human peripheral blood monocytes.[61] This induction occurs during the continued expression of CSF-1 receptor gene transcripts. Bacterial endotoxin, IL-1, and TNF-α stimulate the transcriptional expression of the CSF-1 gene in cultures of human umbilical vein endothelial (HUVE) cells.[62] EGF stimulates CSF-1 mRNA expression and CSF-1 release in cultured murine stromal cells.[63] PDGF, basic FGF, and TNF-α regulate hematopoiesis indirectly through the production and release of CSF-1 by bone marrow stromal cells.[64] The mouse marrow-derived stromal cell line H-1/A, which undergoes adipocytic differentiation after confluence, produces CSF-1 activity. The production of CSF-1 by H-1/A cells exhibits an early downregulation when the cells differentiate into adipocytes.[65] This decrease in CSF-1 production is due, at least in part, to a posttranscriptional mechanism and is blocked by TNF-α at a transcriptional level.

Pregnancy induces a 1000-fold increase in the concentration of CSF-1 in the mouse uterus, which is under the control of chorionic gonadotropin.[66] Pregnancy is also associated with a twofold elevation of the CSF-1 concentrations in serum and most other tissues, as well as with increases in the number of splenic macrophage precursor cells. Uterine CSF-1 may have a role in regulating both macrophage accumulation and the formation and differentiation of the placenta.[67,68] In situ hybridization and Northern blotting studies localized CSF-1 gene transcription to the uterine endometrium at 11 days of pregnancy. Concentration of CSF-1 in the mouse placenta is regulated by the synergistic action of estradiol and progesterone. IL-1β stimulates CSF-1 production in human term placenta.[69] CSF-1 expression in the placenta is confined mainly to trophoblast cells.[70] Since the placenta expresses high levels of c-Fms/CSF-1 receptor protein, these findings suggest a functional role for interactions between CSF-1 and its receptor in trophoblast development and differentiation.

2. Genetic Deficiency of CSF-1

Mice homozygous for the recessive mutation osteopetrosis *(op)* on chromosome 3 have a restricted capacity for bone remodeling and are severely deficient in mature macrophages and osteoclasts. Both types of cells derive from a common hematopoietic progenitor. The osteopetrotic mice are smaller and stubbier in appearance than their normal littermates, have extensive skeletal deformities, and their life span is reduced. These mice are characterized by a total absence of CSF-1, which is due to a mutation in the coding region of the CSF-1 gene.[71,72] In one of the osteopetrotic mice the mutation was characterized as a single bp insertion 262 bp downstream from the ATG initiation codon, with generation of a stop codon 21 bp downstream of this site, resulting in the production of a nonfunctional CSF-1 protein.

D. THE CSF-1 RECEPTOR

The physiologic actions of CSF-1 are exerted at the cellular level through its binding to a specific receptor located on the cell surface.[73] The factor binds specifically to mononuclear phagocytes and their precursors as well as to macrophages and myelomonocytic cell lines in culture. The CSF-1 receptor was purified from the human choriocarcinoma cell line, BeWo, as well as from normal human peripheral blood monocytes by means of a specific monoclonal antibody to phosphotyrosine.[74] The purified CSF-1 receptor is a protein with an associated tyrosine kinase activity.[75] In addition, the CSF-1 receptor, immunoprecipitated by either antiphosphotyrosine or antireceptor antibodies, is associated with a phosphatidylinositol (PI) 3-kinase activity.[76] This activity requires the receptor tyrosine kinase activity, is triggered by receptor phosphorylation on tyrosine, and correlates with its mitogenic potential.

Binding of CSF-1 to its receptor stimulates dimerization of the receptor.[77] The formation of noncovalent dimers of the CSF-1 receptor is temporally correlated with cellular protein tyrosine phosphorylation. The noncovalent receptor dimers become covalently linked via disulfide bonds and are modified and subsequently internalized. Internalized CSF-1 receptors, in contrast to the receptors for other growth factors such as EGF and NGF, are rapidly destroyed in the lysosomal compartment without segregation into more slowly degrading intracellular compartments.[78] All CSF-1 that does not initially dissociate from the cells is ultimately degraded. Ligand-induced internalization and degradation of the CSF-1 receptor may require phosphorylation on tyrosine residues of a protein other than the receptor itself.[79]

1. The CSF-1 Receptor and the v-Fms and c-Fms Proteins

The murine cellular receptor for CSF-1 is a glycoprotein composed of a single polypeptide chain of 165 kDa which has an associated tyrosine kinase activity.[80] The McDonough strain of feline sarcoma virus (SM-FeSV) transduces the oncogene v-*fms* whose product is a glycoprotein, termed gp140$^{v\text{-}fms}$ or v-Fms, whose structure and topology resembles that of known surface receptors.[81,82] Like the v-Erb-B oncoprotein, the v-Fms protein has an amino-terminal portion orientated to the cell surface, a membrane-spanning sequence, and a carboxy-terminal signal transducing function corresponding to the kinase domain. Infection of long-term mouse bone marrow cultures with SM-FeSV results in effects which recapitulate those of the v-*abl* oncogene on immature B-lineage cells, leading to the clonal high-density outgrowth of early pre-B cells which eventually evolve to a tumorigenic phenotype.[83] Infection of the IL-3-dependent murine myeloid cell line FDC-P1 with a retrovirus vector containing the v-*fms* oncogene results in transformation and IL-3 independence.[84] However, an autocrine mechanism is not involved in this transformation since the factor-independent cells do not synthesize growth factors capable of stimulating either parental FDC-P1 cells or CSF-1-dependent macrophages.

Neoplastic transformation by the v-Fms oncoprotein depends on glycosylational processing and cell surface expression.[85] Treatment of SM-FeSV-transformed REF cells with the glycosylation-processing inhibitor, castanospermine, decreases the association of v-Fms with the plasma membrane, which results in reversion to the nontransformed phenotype in spite of the fact that the tyrosine kinase activity of the oncoprotein is not affected by the treatment.[86] Growth of v-*fms*-transformed cells becomes serum-dependent when the N-linked carbohydrates of the oncoprotein are modified by the presence of specific trimming inhibitors in the culture fluid.[87] Specific binding occurs between CSF-1 and the v-Fms oncoprotein.[88] It is thus most interesting that the CSF-1 receptor is closely related to the *fms* oncogene product.[89-94]

The product of the cat c-*fms* gene is a 170-kDa protein with tyrosine kinase activity.[95] The primary structure of the c-Fms and v-Fms proteins differ mainly at their carboxyl-terminal ends. The v-Fms oncoprotein contains at this end a residue (Thr-939) that is phosphorylated *in vivo* by a serine/threonine protein kinase.[96] The mature form of the human c-Fms product is a 150-kDa glycoprotein which is composed of an amino-terminal extracellular CSF-1-binding domain, a central membrane-spanning region, and a carboxy-terminal cytoplasmic tyrosine kinase domain. Comparison of the sequences of the feline v-*fms* oncogene and the human c-*fms* proto-oncogene indicates a high degree of evolutionary conservation, but the two proteins have markedly different carboxyl termini.[97] Antibodies to distal carboxyl-terminal epitopes present in the v-Fms glycoprotein do not cross react with the c-Fms protein.[98]

A cDNA clone corresponding to the murine c-*fms* gene has been isolated, sequenced, and expressed in mammalian cells.[99] The murine c-Fms protein, as deduced from the cDNA clone, is composed of 976 amino acids and has 75% general homology with the human c-Fms protein. The homology between the human and murine proteins is strongest (95%) in the cytoplasmic kinase domain and weakest (63%) in the external domain. The murine c-Fms protein can specifically bind human CSF-1.

Replacement of carboxy-terminal truncation of v-*fms* with c-*fms* proto-oncogene sequences markedly reduces transformation potential of the protein.[100] An alteration of the v-Fms oncoprotein at its extreme carboxyl terminus represents the major structural difference between the viral protein and the normal c-Fms protein, and this difference may affect the tyrosine kinase activity of the v-Fms oncoprotein.[90] While the tyrosine kinase activity of the normal CSF-1 receptor is stimulated by CSF-1, the v-Fms kinase appears to act constitutively and is refractory to the ligand.[101] Tyrosine phosphorylation of the v-Fms oncoprotein in membranes occurs in the absence of CSF-1 and is not enhanced by addition of CSF-1. Although the mechanism of v-*fms*-induced transformation is unknown, v-*fms*-transformed cells have a constitutively elevated activity of guanine nucleotide-dependent, phosphatidylinositol-4,5-bisphosphate-specific phospholipase C.

Site-directed mutagenesis analysis may contribute to a better definition of the functional domains of the v-Fms oncoprotein and their relationship to the domains of the c-Fms protein.[102] Different insertion mutations can affect the capacity of the oncogene to transform cells *in vitro,* as well as the processing, intracellular distribution, and tyrosine kinase activity of the v-Fms protein. Substitution of serine for leucine at position 301 in the extracellular domain of the human CSF-1 receptor protein is sufficient to activate its oncogenic potential.[103] The mutated protein can induce morphologic transformation, anchorage-independent growth, and tumorigenicity in NIH/3T3 cells. The mechanism of *fms*-induced transformation is unknown, but NIH/3T3 cells transformed by the v-*fms* oncogene or an activated c-*fms* gene exhibit higher levels of phosphorylation of a 57-kDa protein than untransformed NIH/3T3 cells expressing the normal c-*fms* proto-oncogene.[104] A 60- to 100-amino acid insert present in the v-Fms and c-Fms proteins, as well as in the c-Kit/SCGF receptor tyrosine kinase, with no counterpart in other protein tyrosine kinases, is not required for enzymatic and transforming activities, but may play a specific function in cells such as monocytes and trophoblasts that normally express the CSF-1 receptor.[105]

Tyr-809 is a site of ligand-dependent phosphorylation of the human CSF-1 receptor *in vivo*. A point mutation at this position impairs its ability to induce mitogenic effects, but does not abrogate tyrosine kinase activity, association with PI 3-kinase, or induction of c-*fos* and *jun*-B proto-oncogenes.[106] The mutant receptor is likely to be impaired in its ability to interact with critical cellular effectors whose activity is required for mitogenesis.

2. The Human c-*fms*/CSF-1 Receptor Gene

The human c-*fms* proto-oncogene spans over a DNA region of 32 kbp and its nucleotide sequences have been determined. A RFLP of the c-*fms* gene was detected in a patient with ALL and congenital hypothyroidism.[107] The abnormal allele of the c-*fms* gene present in the patient contained a deletion 426 bp in size located in close proximity to a putative c-*fms* exon. The patient was homozygous for the abnormal allele, which was inherited from each of his parents.[108] The possible relationship between the genetic finding and the clinical condition of the patient remained undetermined. RFLP of the c-*fms* locus may be common in the human population, with the existence of apparent selective pressure in favor of heterozygotes.[109]

The c-*fms* gene has been assigned to human chromosome 5, at either region 5q34 or 5q33.2-q33.3.[110,111] This gene is deleted in the 5q- syndrome, an acquired cytogenetic abnormality associated with refractory macrocytic or aplastic anemia or with polycytemia vera. It has been postulated that hemizygosity at the c-*fms* locus as a consequence of the 5q- deletion may lead to abnormalities in the maturation of hematopoietic cells.[112] However, c-*fms* is just one of several different genes involved in deletions observed in the 5q- syndrome and its role in the development of this syndrome is not understood. The c-*fms*/CSF-1 receptor gene and the PDGF receptor gene are physically linked in a head-to-tail array and are separated by less than 500 bp on human chromosome 5q.[113] Other genes contained in the same human chromosome region are those coding for IL-3, CSF-2, IL-5, and CSF-1.

3. Expression of the c-*fms*/CSF-1 Receptor Gene

The human c-*fms* gene product has been characterized as a 140-kDa protein which is expressed in cells of the monocyte-macrophage lineage.[114] The c-Fms/CSF-1 receptor protein is expressed by less mature bone marrow progenitors, but the number of receptors per cell increases as the cells become committed to the mononuclear phagocytic lineage, and circulating peripheral blood monocytes express relatively high numbers of the receptors.[115] CSF-1 receptors are also expressed by normal and malignant human B lymphocytes.[116]

Various cytokines are involved in the regulation of CSF-1 receptor expression in normal and transformed cells. IL-2, but not IFN-γ, augments c-Fms/CSF-1 receptor expression in human monocytes.[117] TNF-α increases c-*fms*/CSF-1 receptor mRNA in HL-60 cells, which is due to mechanisms operating at both the transcriptional and posttranscriptional levels.[118] The murine macrophage cell line ANA-1 constitutively express c-Fms/CSF-1 receptor mRNA, and treatment of ANA-1 cells with LPS, but not IFN-γ, downregulates this expression.[119] Introduction of the murine c-*fms*/CSF-1 receptor gene into the factor-dependent blast cell line FDC-P1 results in growth and differentiation in the presence of exogenous CSF-1.[120] Expression of the human c-Fms/CSF-1 receptor in IL-3-dependent murine myeloid leukemia cell line 32CD13 induces CSF-1 responsiveness, but inhibits its granulocytic differentiation.[121]

In addition to mononuclear phagocytes and their precursors, expression of c-*fms* gene transcripts has been detected in a diversity of mammalian organs including spleen, brain, and liver.[95] Transcripts of the c-*fms* gene have been detected in murine osteoclasts.[122] Intimal smooth muscle cells derived from the aorta of a rabbit model of arteriosclerotic lesion express the c-*fms* proto-oncogene.[123] Expression of c-Fms/CSF-1 receptor in smooth muscle cells coincides with the phenotypic conversion of these cells to the phagocytic phenotype found in atherosclerotic lesions. These cells coexpress the PDGF receptor, suggesting that both CSF-1 and PDGF may function in an autocrine or paracrine manner in the proliferation and migration of vascular smooth muscle cells associated with the process of atherogenesis. The c-*fms* gene is expressed at high levels in the normal human placenta as well as in choriocarcinoma cell lines.[124,125] The c-Fms/CSF-1 receptor is also expressed in different types of human tumors.[126] CSF-1 receptors expressed by human choriocarcinoma cell lines are similar or identical to the c-Fms protein expressed on the surface of normal human peripheral blood mononuclear cells.[124]

4. Phosphorylation and Internalization of the CSF-1 Receptor

The binding of CSF-3 to the extracellular segment of the CSF-1 receptor triggers phosphorylation of the receptor on tyrosine, which subsequently leads to the phosphorylation of cellular substrates and the eventual transmission of mitogenic signals to the nucleus. This is followed by a rapid internalization and degradation of the CSF-1 receptor. Studies with a kinase-defective mutant of the CSF-1 receptor indicated that phosphorylation of the receptor occurs via a bimolecular interaction between receptor monomers.[127] Two functionally important autophosphorylation sites of the murine CSF-1 receptor are represented by Tyr-706, located in the kinase insert, and by Tyr-807, a residue conserved in all tyrosine kinases. Phosphorylation of Tyr-807 may be required for full activation of the CSF-1 receptor.[128] Mutational analysis indicates that Gly-807 mutant receptors lack tyrosine kinase activity, fail to respond to CSF-1, and are defective in biosynthetic processing.

5. Expression of c-fms Transcripts in Neoplastic Cells

Human leukemic cells may express c-fms mRNA. Expression of the c-fms gene is a constant finding in the leukemic cells of AML patients, regardless of the degree of differentiation of the leukemic clone.[129] The high levels of c-fms gene expression present in AML cells are not associated with amplification or rearrangement of the gene. In contrast, the c-fms gene is not expressed in ALL, whether of T- or B-cell origin. Thus, c-fms gene expression has been considered to represent a specific marker for leukemogenesis occurring in the myeloid lineage.

Neoplastic cells of nonhematopoietic origin may express the c-fms gene. All of five cell lines derived from primary rat tracheal epithelial (RTE) cells transformed by treatment with N-methyl-N'-nitro-N-nitrosoguanidine (MNNG) *in vitro* expressed elevated levels of 9.5-kb transcripts from a c-fms-related gene.[130] The gene expressed in the transformed RTE cells may be distinct from the gene encoding the CSF-1 receptor, whose transcripts in the rat are 3.8 kb long. No amplification or rearrangement of the c-fms gene was detected in the cell lines expressing high levels of c-fms-related transcripts.

6. Growth Factor Independence of v-fms-Transformed Cells

Transformation induced by the v-fms oncogene does not depend on an exogenous source of CSF-1, and neutralizing antibodies to CSF-1 do not affect the transformed phenotype.[90] SV40-immortalized macrophages infected with SM-FeSV do not produce CSF-1 or show constitutive down-modulation of their CSF-1 receptors, indicating that their conversion to factor independence is directly mediated by the v-Fms kinase rather than an autocrine mechanism.[131] Thus, although the v-Fms oncoprotein includes the ligand-binding domain of the CSF-1 receptor, it can function as an unregulated enzyme without the growth factor ligand. NIH/3T3 mouse cells transformed by either the feline v-fms oncogene or a mutated human c-fms gene are able to proliferate in the complete absence of exogenous growth factors.[132] A monoclonal antibody that prevents signal transduction by the human CSF-1 receptor inhibited the proliferation of cells transformed by the activated c-fms gene, indicating that CSF-1 receptor function is required to abrogate growth factor requirements and to maintain the transformed state.

7. Tumor Promoters, Differentiation Inducers, and c-fms/CSF-1 Receptor Expression

Phorbol ester (TPA) can stimulate mouse bone marrow cells to form myeloid colonies in agar cultures without the addition of exogenous CSFs, suggesting that it can mimic the action of CSFs.[133] Phorbol ester causes a rapid but transient decrease in the expression of its own receptor, protein kinase C, (homologous downregulation) as well as in the expression of CSF-1 receptors (heterologous downregulation) on the membrane of murine peritoneal exudate macrophages.[134] Contrarily, CSF-1, which causes homologous downregulation of its own receptor, fails to induce heterologous downregulation of phorbol ester receptors in the same cells. Whether TPA induces phosphorylation of the CSF-1 receptor through activation of protein kinase C is not yet clear. Protein kinase C does not appear to trigger down-modulation by directly phosphorylating the CSF-1 receptor, but rather by activation of a protease which recognizes the receptor as a substrate.[135]

Cells from the human HL-60 promyelocytic leukemia cell line mature morphologically and functionally towards granulocytes after induction with DMSO or hexamethylene bisacetamide, and can be induced to differentiate along a monocyte/macrophage pathway when treated with TPA or calcitriol. Although no c-fms gene transcripts are detected in uninduced HL-60 cells, these transcripts are detectable after treatment with either TPA or calcitriol.[136] Both CSF-1 and c-fms transcripts are expressed during TPA-induced monocytic differentiation of HL-60 cells.[137,138] In contrast, c-fms mRNA was not detected following induction of HL-60 cells with DMSO or HMBA. Thus, c-fms expression is induced when the

HL-60 cells mature along the monocyte/macrophage, but not the granulocyte, pathway. The c-*fms* transcripts appear 6 h after TPA addition, and the maximum levels of c-*fms* mRNA are present 24 to 48 h after induction initiation.[136] In contrast, c-*fos* mRNA is detectable within 1 h of treating HL-60 cells with TPA, and c-*myc* expression is not detected before 24 h after TPA induction. However, the relation between monocytic differentiation of HL-60 cells and c-*fms* gene expression is not clear. Both IFN-γ and TNF-α can induce this differentiation, which is accompanied by the appearance of membrane-bound tyrosine protein kinase activity, but it is not related to expression of the c-*fms* proto-oncogene.[139]

E. POSTRECEPTOR MECHANISMS OF ACTION OF CSF-1

Little is known about the events responsible for signal transduction after the binding of CSF-1 to its receptor. The c-Fms/CSF-1 receptor kinase is phosphorylated on tyrosine *in vivo* and is rapidly degraded after CSF-1 binding.[140] Stimulation of the CSF-1 receptor induces phosphorylation of other cellular proteins on tyrosine, which would mediate biochemical and functional changes that occur in the target cells. A 56-kDa protein of unknown function is phosphorylated on tyrosine by the action of CSF-1 on the human BeWo choriocarcinoma cell line as well as in peripheral blood mononuclear leukocytes.[74] In addition to tyrosine phosphorylation, several cellular proteins (61 to 260 kDa) are phosphorylated on serine upon incubation of murine macrophages with CSF-1.[141] The phosphorylated proteins are predominantly located on the cytoplasm, but their identity is unknown.

Glucose uptake is stimulated by CSF-1 in cells such as the mouse bone marrow-derived macrophages.[142] It is known that quiescent cells stimulated to proliferation increase their uptake of glucose through a specific transport system, so that more glucose is rendered available to meet the additional energy requirements associated with growth. Changes in ion fluxes may be involved in the transmission of the signal initiated by CSF-1 binding to its receptor. CSF-1 rapidly stimulates a Na^+/K^+-ATPase-mediated K^+ influx in quiescent mouse marrow-derived macrophages.[143] This effect is transient and the degree of stimulation is dependent on the dose of CSF-1. The biological relevance of this change is unknown, but the intracellular K^+ levels may be involved in the regulation of the protein biosynthetic machinery, which eventually exerts a control on the processes related to DNA synthesis and cell proliferation.

CSF-1-induced stimulation of proliferation in cells such as murine marrow-derived macrophages is apparently independent of increased phosphoinositide turnover.[144] However, stimulation of diglyceride production by phosphatidylcholine-specific phospholipase C may be a component of CSF-1 signal transduction through a pathway leading to c-*fos* and *jun*-B proto-oncogene expression, and formation of AP-1 transcription factors which may collaborate with c-*myc*, but is independent of protein kinase C-δ and Ras protein activation.[145] CSF-1 stimulates the generation of 1,2-diacylglycerol in murine marrow-derived macrophages, but not in resident peritoneal macrophages, which also respond to the factor.[146] In NIH/3T3 cells expressing the CSF-1 receptor, the phospholipase C form PLC-II/PLC-γ is not phosphorylated on tyrosine during the mitogenic response to CSF-1.[147] The receptor for CSF-1 associates with PI 3-kinase in various types of cells.[148,149] Activation of the CSF-1 receptor may result in the accumulation of phosphoinositide metabolites phosphorylated at the D-3 position of the inositol ring. However, the precise physiological significance of the PI-3 kinase remains unknown since none of the products of this enzyme are in the metabolic pathway for generating the Ca^{2+}-regulating second messenger, inositol 1,4,5-trisphosphate. PI 3-kinase contains a binding site for the CSF-1 receptor, but only a minority of ligand-activated CSF-1 receptors form a stable complex with the enzyme *in vivo* and the biological significance of this binding, if any, is unknown.[150]

F. REGULATION OF GENE EXPRESSION BY CSF-1

Some of the physiological effects of CSF-1 may depend on the regulation of gene expression. Two of three cyclin-related genes (*CYL* genes) are regulated by CSF-1 during the G_1 phase of the macrophage cell cycle.[151] Deprivation of CSF-1 during G_1 leads to rapid degradation of *CYL*-encoded 36-kDa proteins (p36^{CYL}) and correlates with failure to initiate DNA synthesis. However, after entering S phase, macrophages no longer require CSF-1 and can complete cell division without expressing *CYL* genes. During G_1, the p36^{CYL} protein is phosphorylated and associates with cdc2 protein.

G. CSF-1 AND PROTO-ONCOGENE EXPRESSION

CSF-1 stimulates macrophage proliferation, and this effect is associated with changes in the level of expression of several proto-oncogenes, including c-*myc*, c-*fos*, and c-*jun*. Expression of c-*myc* may have a central role in CSF-1-induced mitogenesis.[152] Reduced levels of c-*fos* and c-*myc* gene expression and absence of cell proliferation occurs in primary cultures of bone marrow-derived mouse macrophages deprived of CSF-1, and the addition of CSF-1 results in transient induction of the expression of both proto-oncogenes and reinitiation of cell proliferation.[153] CSF-1-induced expression of c-*fos* gene in macrophages is associated with phospholipid breakdown and the ensuing activation of protein kinase C and release of Ca^{2+}.[154] Similar results were obtained with stimulation of rat alveolar macrophages with CSF-1.[155] In addition to c-*fos* and c-*myc*, the expression of the c-*fgr* gene, but not the c-*src*, c-*yes*, or c-*fms* genes, is stimulated by the action of CSF-1 on mouse monocytic cells.[156] The kinetics of these inductions were different for each proto-oncogene. The c-*fgr* gene is induced in bone marrow-derived monocytic cells, not only by CSF-1 but also by CSF-2, LPS, and IFN-γ, suggesting that the c-Fgr kinase may be essential for mediating the effects of different monocytic stimuli.[157] High levels of c-*myb* expression are observed during the normal processes of macrophage differentiation,[158] but their relation to CSF-1 action mechanism is not understood.

Oncoproteins with protein kinase activity may be involved in CSF-1 signal transduction mechanisms. Members of the Src protein family, including the Src, Fyn, and Yes proteins, are activated in NIH/3T3 cells expressing high levels of human CSF-1 receptor and become associated with the receptor.[159] The Raf-1 serine/threonine kinase is a downstream second messenger involved in CSF-1-mediated signal transduction.[160,161] The c-Raf-1 protein is not a substrate for the c-Fms/CSF-1 receptor kinase *in vivo* and its activation may represent a step in a phosphorylation cascade initiated by the interaction of the ligand-stimulated CSF-1 receptor at the cell surface that may eventually lead to cell proliferation.

The mechanisms involved in the regulation of gene expression by CSF-1 are unknown, but the activity of Ras proteins is required for the proliferative response to CSF-1. Signals transduced by both the CSF-1 receptor and Ras stimulate transcription from promoter elements containing overlapping binding sites for Fos-Jun/AP-1 and Ets transcription factors.[162] The Ets family of transcription factors may play a central role in integrating both CSF-1 receptor and Ras-induced mitogenic signals and in modulating the *myc* gene response to CSF-1 stimulation.

H. ROLE OF CSF-1 IN NEOPLASTIC PROCESSES

The role of CSF-1 and its receptor in oncogenic processes is not understood. Transformation of mouse marrow cells by transfection with R-*myc*, a human proto-oncogene related to c-*myc*, is associated with endogenous production of CSF-1.[163] R-*myc* has homology to the 5' and 3' coding exons of c-*myc*, but its restriction map is different. A murine monocyte tumor induced by a helper-free c-*myc* retrovirus was found to contain a DNA rearrangement at the CSF-1 locus, resulting in high levels of CSF-1 production and autocrine growth.[164] The CSF-1 gene rearrangement was associated with integration of a murine BALB/c ecotropic retrovirus.

Constitutive expression of the c-*fms*/CSF-1 receptor gene, either by mutation or gene rearrangement, may contribute to leukemogenesis.[165] Cotransfection of a human c-*fms*/CSF-1 receptor gene and a cDNA clone encoding a precursor of the human CSF-1 polypeptide results in transformation of NIH/3T3 fibroblasts by an autocrine mechanism.[166] Introduction of a cloned human CSF-1 gene into the immortalized mouse macrophage cell line BAC1.2F5 abrogates the specific growth factor dependence, but does not render the cells tumorigenic in nude mice.[167] Certain point mutations can activate the oncogenic potential of the c-Fms/CSF-1 receptor protein. Replacement of Leu-301 in the human CSF-1 receptor by serine, threonine, glutamic acid, or proline induces ligand-independent transforming activity of the protein in mouse NIH/3T3 cells.[168] Probably, any mutation that activates a ligand-independent protein kinase activity of the human CSF-1 receptor, without completely inhibiting its transport to the cell surface or decreasing its stability, might induce transformation potential.

The role of CSF-1 and its receptor in human leukemia is not clear. In 24 patients with AML, CSF-1 mRNA expression was found to be the exception in the neoplastic cells, whereas normal tissue macrophages from the lung and monocytes matured *in vitro* regularly showed coexpression of the mRNAs for CSF-1 and its receptor.[169] The c-Fms/CSF-1 receptor mRNA was only weakly expressed in AML cells, as compared with monocytes, and in about half of the cases is was completely missing. CSF-1 receptor mRNA was detected in the leukemic blasts from 15 of 50 children with AML, compared with 4 of 26 adults with the disease.[170] By contrast, CSF-1 receptors were uniformly absent on blast cells from 19 children with ALL. No rearrangements of the CSF-1 receptor gene were detected by Southern blotting analyses of DNA from 47 cases of AML. The study of fresh human AML cells with Northern blotting hybridization analysis, using specific cDNA probes, allowed the detection of CSF-1 transcripts in 10 of 17 cases and c-*fms* mRNA in 7 of 15 cases; coexpression of CSF-1 and c-*fms* transcripts was observed in 5 cases, and in 5 other cases neither gene was expressed.[171] These clinical studies suggest that CSF-1 does not play a significant role in the development of acute leukemias. However, coexpression of CSF-1 and its receptor in the blast cells from a subset of AMLs suggests the operation of an autocrine mechanism of tumor cell growth in such cases.

CSF-1 may have a role in nonhematopoietic human neoplasms. Ovarian and endometrial epithelial cancers may express high levels of CSF-1/c-*fms* transcripts, correlating strongly with high-grade, high-stage presentations, and prognostic of poor outcome.[172] In a study of 14 tissue specimens of human ovarian adenocarcinomas, it was found that all tumors expressed c-*fms* transcripts and that about half of the invasive carcinoma specimens coexpressed CSF-1 and its receptor, suggesting the operation of an autocrine or paracrine mechanism of growth in these tumors involving CSF-1.[173]

CSF-1 has an apparently limited capacity for the induction of differentiation of leukemic cells *in vitro*. Exposure of human leukemic blast progenitors to CSF-1 *in vitro* results in weak stimulation of terminal cell divisions, but not in stimulation of self-renewal of leukemic blast progenitors.[174] CSF-1 is not able to induce the differentiation of leukemic blast progenitors into normal macrophage-monocytes.

III. COLONY-STIMULATING FACTOR 2

Granulocyte-macrophage colony-stimulating factor (GM-CSF), also called colony-stimulating factor-2 (CSF-2), was first identified in crude preparations of conditioned media that stimulate immature hematopoietic cells to proliferate and differentiate *in vitro* into mature granulocytes and macrophages.[1] However, there are several factors capable of controlling the formation and function of granulocytes and macrophages. Available evidence indicates that the factor originally defined as GM-CSF/CSF-2 may have important effects on a diversity of hematopoietic and nonhematopoietic cells.[175-179]

A. BIOLOGICAL EFFECTS OF CSF-2

The production and functional activities of different types of blood cells, including leukocytes and lymphocytes, may be regulated by CSF-2. The neutrophil is usually the first line of defense against bacterial infections, and an important factor involved in neutrophil development and function is CSF-2. The factor is required for the formation of colonies of neutrophil granulocyte/macrophage progenitor cells (CFU-GM) in culture.[180] CSF-2 would act predominantly to prevent monocyte/macrophage development, probably through alteration of CSF-1 receptor mRNA.[181] Granulocyte development may require both the activation of the program associated with granulocytic differentiation and the suppression of the program associated with monocyte/macrophage differentiation. The tumor cells from patients with myelogenous leukemia are absolutely dependent on CSF-2 for proliferation *in vitro*.[182] The stimulating activity of CSF-2 on progenitor cells of the granulocyte/macrophage lineage would be counteracted by an inhibitor factor which is released by mature granulocytes.[183]

CSF-2 may have important actions on mature blood cells. Human CSF-2 stimulates the function of mature granulocytes (neutrophils and eosinophils), enhances the expression of certain functional surface antigens on these cells, and prolongs their survival *in vitro*.[184] CSF-2 behaves as a factor inhibiting the migration of human peripheral blood neutrophils under agarose, and as a potent activator of phagocytosis. CSF-2 supports long-term growth *in vitro* of mouse tissue macrophages, including bone-derived macrophages, and enhances the responsiveness of macrophages to CSF-1.[185] CSF-2 is involved in regulating the growth of macrophage precursors, and concentrations of CSF-2 at the picogram level can enhance the responsiveness of bone marrow progenitors to CSF-1, resulting in an increased number of macrophage colonies.[186] Growth of murine pulmonary alveolar macrophage colonies *in vitro* is directly stimulated by CSF-2 and the response of these cells to CSF-1 is enhanced, thereby favoring the production of more mature and functionally competent macrophages.[187] Polymorphonuclear leukocytes stimulated by CSF-2 accumulate transcripts for cytokines including TNF-α, CSF-1, and CSF-3.[188]

CSF-2 can act on B lymphocytes and displays plasmacytoma growth factor activity similar to that of IL-6.[189] CSF-2 stimulates the production of antibody by B cells.[190] In addition, it functions as a growth factor for T lymphocytes. The growth of HT-2 cells can be maintained for up to 2 months in the presence of CSF-2 as the sole TCGF.[191] Both CSF-2 and IL-3 exert a marked potentiating effect on the IL-2-stimulated growth of freshly isolated human peripheral blood T lymphocytes and *in vitro*-stimulated T cells.[192] Recombinant human CSF-2 enhances the ability of human peripheral blood monocytes to serve as accessory cells for mitogen- and antigen-stimulated T-cell proliferation.[193] It enhances monocyte surface HLA-DR expression and stimulate IL-1 secretion, both critical requirements for antigen presentation to T lymphocytes. CSF-2 stimulates peripheral blood monocytes *in vitro* to become cytotoxic for tumor cells, such as the malignant melanoma cell line A375.[194] CSF-2 may stimulate the antibody-independent cytotoxicity of monocytes against tumor cells indirectly, through an enhancement of the production of TNF-α.[195] The effects of CSF-2 and IL-3 on monocytes are very similar, suggesting that they may be mediated through some common mechanisms.[196]

CSF-2 is a multilineage HGF. In addition to its well characterized granulocyte-monocyte CFU activity, CSF-2 stimulates the formation of colonies derived from multipotential progenitors.[197] The progenitor target cell spectrum of CSF-2 is strikingly similar to that of IL-3. However, IL-3 supports a larger number of erythroid and megakaryocyte progenitors than CSF-2, while CSF-2 supports more myeloid progenitors.[198] Studies on normal human cord blood cells expressing the CD34 antigen, which is present on hematopoietic progenitors and early precursors, indicate that a sequential action of IL-3 followed by CSF-2 is important for myeloid expansion, in spite of the existence of a wide overlap of CD34$^+$ cells responsive to either IL-3 or CSF-2.[199] Studies with primates *in vivo* suggest that IL-3 expands an early hematopoietic cell population that subsequently requires the action of CSF-2 to complete its development.[200] However, the activity of CSF-2 on hematopoietic progenitors is exerted through cooperation with accessory cells.[201,202] CSF-2 alone may be ineffective in supporting colony formation and may be unable, by itself, to support the terminal maturation of human granulocyte/macrophage progenitors.[203]

CSF-2 works synergistically with CSF-3 and erythropoietin in supporting human neutrophil and erythroid progenitor proliferation in culture. Blast-cell colonies that respond to CSF-2 may be represented by a subpopulation of multipotential progenitors responding to IL-3.[204] Human CSF-2 does not stimulate erythroid colony formation, but in combination with erythropoietin it increases erythroid and multipotential colony formation in cultures of peripheral blood cells.[205] Recombinant human CSF-2 stimulates antibody-dependent cytolysis of tumor cells by both human neutrophils and eosinophils, and increases eosinophil autofluorescence and phagocytosis by neutrophils. CSF-2 has a direct action on megakaryocyte progenitor cells, favoring the development of megakaryocyte colonies (CFU-Meg) *in vitro*.[206,207] However, an effective stimulation of megakaryocytopoiesis *in vivo*, bringing about an increase in the levels of blood platelets, may require interaction of CSF-2 with other cytokines. IL-3 and CSF-2 have additive effects in stimulating the formation of CFU-Meg colonies.

Murine, but not human, CSF-2 is active both *in vitro* and *in vivo* in the rat.[208] The hematologic effects of a single i.v. injection of murine CSF-2 in the rat consist in peripheral neutropenia and monocytopenia, which is followed by induction of neutrophilia and monocytosis. At 6 h after injection the marrow exhibits a myeloproliferative effect. Once-daily injection of CSF-2 to rats for 1 week results in a repetitive daily neutrophilia of the same magnitude. After 1 week of daily injections the marrow does not exhibit a generalized myeloid hyperplasia, but shows an increase in eosinophils and a decrease in lymphocytes. The hematologic effects of CSF-2 have been confirmed in kinetic studies performed on human subjects *in vivo*.[209]

CSF-2 may exert important effects on nonhematopoietic cells. It is able to stimulate the proliferation of normal human marrow fibroblast precursors as well as that of some neoplastically transformed cells, including human osteogenic sarcoma and breast carcinoma cell lines.[210] Human CSF-2 stimulates *in vitro* the growth of osteoblast-like cells derived from human trabacular bone.[211] In addition, CSF-2 antagonizes the induction by calcitriol of osteocalcin synthesis and alkaline phosphatase activity, two characteristic products of osteoblasts. Thus, CSF-2 may have a broad role as a normal regulator of the growth of normal and transformed cells of both hematopoietic and nonhematopoietic origin, although it is not a general growth factor for all transformed cells.

B. CSF-2 STRUCTURE AND THE CSF-2 GENE

The gene encoding CSF-2 is located on mouse chromosome 11, near the IL-3 gene, and cDNAs corresponding to this gene have been constructed.[212,213] These cDNAs are capable of directing CSF-2 synthesis in *Escherichia coli* and in *Xenopus laevis* oocytes. The primary structure of murine CSF-2, as deduced from the cDNA clones, is composed of a single-chain polypeptide of 13,500 Da containing 118 amino acids. The higher molecular weight forms of CSF-2 detected in mouse tissues would correspond to posttranslational modifications of the polypeptide. The biological activities of native CSF-2 and recombinant CSF-2 are similar despite the fact that the latter is nonglycosylated.[214] Both recombinant murine CSF-2 and native CSF-2 stimulate the growth of granulocyte and macrophage colonies in serum-free cultures of mouse bone marrow cells.[215] Antibodies raised against recombinant murine CSF-2 neutralize the biological activity of both native and recombinant CSF-2. Recombinant CSF-2 obtained from a murine T-cell line acts preferentially and directly on committed granulocyte-macrophage progenitor cells, without affecting either pluripotent stem cells or progenitors of cells other than neutrophils and macrophages.[214] Four regions critical to the biological activity of the murine CSF-2 protein have been delineated by generating a series of small deletions scanning the entire length of the molecule.[216]

The human CSF-2 gene has been cloned, sequenced, and expressed in heterologous systems.[217-221] The predicted human CSF-2 polypeptide weighs 16,293 Da, contains 144 amino acids, and has 54% homology with mouse CSF-2. The naturally occurring human CSF-2 is a 22-kDa glycoprotein which contains up to 34% carbohydrate by weight.[219] Human CSF-2 produced in *Escherichia coli* is deglycosylated and displays higher immunoreactivity and bioactivity than native human CSF-2.[222] Removal of N-linked oligosaccharides from recombinant human CSF-2 proteins produced in yeast or animal cells (COS cells) results in significant increases in their immunological and biological properties.

The general structures of the mouse and human CSF-2 genes are highly homologous, both being composed of three introns and four exons.[223] The gene contains two promoters that give rise to alternative mRNAs which encode CSF-2 precursor polypeptides with different amino terminal sequences.[224] The human CSF-2 gene is approximately 2.5 kbp in length and contains at least three introns. Expression of the human CSF-2 gene is *cis*-regulated by 5′-flanking DNA sequences, and depends on the interaction of cell-specific and inducible proteins with a specific region of the CSF-2 gene promoter.[225,226] A complex pattern of regulation of CSF-2 expression exists in T cells, and both positive and negative regulatory sequences may play critical roles in controlling the expression of the gene in the marrow microenvironment and in localized inflammatory responses.[227]

The CSF-2 gene has been mapped to human chromosome region 5q23-q31,[111,228] most probably being located at 5q23.[229] This region is involved in interstitial deletions occurring in the 5q- syndrome associated with refractory anemia.[230] Total or partial monosomy of human chromosome 5 has been described in ANLL.

C. PRODUCTION OF CSF-2

CSF-2 is produced and secreted by various types of cells under the regulation of a diversity of stimuli. Normal and neoplastic human B lymphocytes produce CSF-2 but not IL-3.[231] Phagocytosis and inflammatory stimuli induce the accumulation of CSF-2 mRNA in macrophages through posttranscriptional regulatory mechanisms.[232] Lymphokines are involved in the regulation of CSF-2 synthesis. IL-1 induces CSF-2 release from human mononuclear phagocytes.[233] Purified T cells stimulated by IL-1 secrete CSF-2, and this effect of IL-1 takes place at the level of gene transcription.[234] The prostaglandin PGE_2 may function in synergy with IL-2 to elicit CSF-2 production by T cells.[235]

Substantial amounts of CSF-2 are produced by unstimulated rat microvascular endothelial cells.[236] IL-1 and TNF-α induce human endothelial cells to produce the CSF-2.[237-239] The immortalized human endothelial cell line, HEC KSV, constitutively produces CSF-2. The immunosuppressive agent, cyclosporine A, inhibits the production of IL-2 and IL-3 at the transcriptional level, but is ineffective in blocking CSF-2 production.[240] Other types of cells such as keratinocytes can produce CSF-2.[241] Keratinocyte-derived CSF-2 may play an important role in regulating cutaneous macrophage responses occurring in infections and noninfectious cutaneous diseases. IL-2 stimulates the production of CSF-2 by stroma cells *in vitro* and probably also *in vivo*.[242] Production of CSF-2 by some fibroblastic cell lines is greatly increased by infection with murine retroviruses *in vitro*.[243] Dexamethasone and calcitriol, but not cyclosporine A, inhibit the production of CSF-2 by human fibroblasts.[244] Astrocytes, which may play a central role in the regulation of immune-mediated processes in the central nervous system, express transcripts for CSF-2 and CSF-3 and synthesize CSF-2.[245,246] An IL-3-like factor previously identified in astrocytes may rather correspond to CSF-2 and CSF-3 secreted by these cells.

Tumor cells may be able to produce CSF-2. A factor secreted by the human bladder carcinoma cell line HTB9, and capable of contributing to the proliferation of clonogenic blast cells, was identified as CSF-2.[247] The clonal rat osteosarcoma cell line ROS secretes CSF-2 under the stimulus of bone-resorbing agents such as parathyroid hormone and LPS.[248] In some tumor cell-host systems, CSF-2-like factors produced constitutively by the tumor cells may play a role in the development of tumor metastasis, mediated through functional suppression of host lymphoid tissues.[249]

D. THE CSF-2 RECEPTOR

High-affinity CSF-2 receptors are present in normal and leukemic human myeloid cells.[250-252] Whereas one single class of CSF-2 receptor was identified in human peripheral neutrophils, two classes of these receptors exist in human peripheral monocytes and CSF-2-responsive myeloid cell lines.[253,254] Cross-linking studies suggested the existence of at least three distinct species of molecules with affinity for human CSF-2, with molecular weights of 135, 100, and 80 kDa, respectively. The biological significance and relationships between these forms of the CSF-2 receptor are unknown, but recent evidence indicates that the CSF-2 receptor consists of two subunits, termed α and β, and that the β subunit is shared with the IL-3 and IL-5 receptors.[255-257] The β subunit of the CSF-2 receptor is phosphorylated on tyrosine residues, and the CSF-2 and IL-3 receptors induce tyrosine phosphorylation of an almost identical set of proteins.[258] The human gene encoding the CSF-2 receptor β chain is located on chromosome region 22q12.2-q13.1, which also contains the gene for IL-2Rβ.[259] The low-affinity human CSF-2 receptor α subunit can be converted to a high-affinity CSF binding complex in the presence of the β subunit. A homologue of the human CSF-2 receptor α subunit with low affinity for the ligand has been isolated.[260]

CSF-2 receptors are present in mouse cells of myelomonocytic origin as well as in the tumor cell lines LSTRA and LBRM-33, which are of T-cell origin.[261] However, no binding sites for CSF-2 were detected in other T-cell lines, including two subclones of LBRM-33, which would indicate that expression of CSF-2 receptors on T cells might be limited to discrete, perhaps aberrant, cell populations. Human nonhematopoietic cell lines, including cell lines derived from non-small-cell lung cancer, stomach cancer, colon cancer, and osteosarcoma, frequently express low-affinity CSF-2 receptor proteins of 65 to 85 kDa.[262] High-affinity receptors for CSF-2 were not detected in human nonhematopoietic tumor cells.

E. POSTRECEPTOR MECHANISM OF ACTION OF CSF-2

The postreceptor mechanisms of CSF-2 action are poorly understood. Addition of CSF-2 to human granulocytes does not result in alteration of the resting transmembrane potential, the pH_i, or the $[Ca^{2+}]_i$.[263] However, the $[Ca^{2+}]_i$ is increased by CSF-2, as well as by erythropoietin in immature precursors derived from human cord blood erythroid progenitor cells whose proliferation and differentiation is regulated, at least in part, by CSF-2.[264] The role of phosphoinositide metabolism in the mechanism of CSF-2 action is not known. In K562 cells, both CSF-2 and IL-3 induce the expression of the inositol trisphosphate receptor.[265] The action of CSF-2 in suspensions of human neutrophils is associated with upregulation of phospholipase D activity, which gives rise to the generation of choline-linked phosphoglyceride breakdown products, including phosphatidic acid.[266]

CSF-2 can induce the release of arachidonic acid from plasma membrane within minutes of addition to the cell culture, which suggests that direct activation of phospholipase C and/or protein kinase C is part of the cellular response to CSF-2. Stimulation of macrophage proliferation by CSF-2 is associated with a persistent activation of the Na^+/H^+ antiporter.[267] The participation of G proteins in the mechanism of CSF-2 action is suggested by the fact that CSF-2-associated proliferative pathways are sensitive to both pertussis and cholera toxins.[268] There are synergistic mitogenic effects between CSF-2 and the insulin family of hormones in the insulin-dependent human acute myeloid leukemic cell line AML-193, indicating that CSF-2 and insulin receptors may be linked to different signaling mechanisms in addition to sharing some G protein-coupled pathways.

Phosphorylation of cellular proteins on tyrosine residues may be an important mechanism of CSF-2 action. Treatment of both murine hematopoietic cell lines and human peripheral blood neutrophils with CSF-2 results in phosphorylation on tyrosine of cellular proteins with molecular weights ranging from 40 to 150 kDa.[269,270] In human U-937 and HL-60 cells, CSF-2 rapidly stimulates phosphorylation on tyrosine residues of several proteins.[271] CSF-2 induces in human neutrophils the phosphorylation on tyrosine of microtubule-associated protein (MAP) kinase.[272] Treatment of MO7E cells, derived from an infant with acute megakaryocytic leukemia, with either CSF-2 or IL-3 results in increased phosphorylation of a similar or identical set of cytoplasmic proteins on tyrosine residues.[273] Phosphorylation of the Raf-1 kinase by CSF-2 in human myeloid cells may be part of the transductional mechanism of CSF-2 action.[274] Since the CSF-2 and IL-3 receptors do not possess tyrosine kinase activity, the phosphorylation of cellular proteins on tyrosine stimulated by CSF-2 and IL-3 must depend on the secondary activation of intracellular tyrosine kinases, which could include products of the Src family. Internalization of CSF-2 receptors after ligand binding is not required for activation of tyrosine kinase, which suggests that CSF-2 receptor internalization may be a consequence of signal transduction.[275] Ras proteins may have been an important role in the transductional mechanism of CSF-2 action.

F. ROLE OF CSF-2 IN NEOPLASTIC PROCESSES

CSF-2 is capable of inducing tumoricidal activity in human alveolar macrophages and monocytes.[276] The mechanisms by which activated macrophages destroy susceptible tumor cells may include both direct and indirect actions. The direct process consists in the binding of activated macrophages to the target cells, whereas the indirect mechanism may involve the release of diffusible cytotoxic molecules. CSF-2-induced activation of tumoricidal properties in alveolar macrophages does not seem to involve alterations in oxidative metabolism or secretion of cytokines such as IL-1β or TNF-α.

Formation of leukemic cell colonies *in vitro* generally requires the addition of growth factors, but the exact factors required remain incompletely defined. CSF-2 alone or in combination with other HGFs may be required for the growth of transformed cells *in vitro*. Specific receptors for CSF-2 are present in human AML blast cells,[277] and CSF-2 is frequently required for the establishment and continuous proliferation of human AML cells *in vitro*.[278,279] CSF-2, and to a slightly lesser extent CSF-3, can support the growth of AML cell colonies.[280,281] For many cases of AML, CSF-2 can completely replace standard conditioned media, but in other cases growth with CSF-2 alone is suboptimal, and in some cases no growth of AML colony-forming cells is observed at all. In some cases the effects of CSF-2 and CSF-3 are additive in promoting maximum AML colony size. CSF-2 appears to be a primary endogenous regulator of the growth of juvenile chronic myelogenous leukemia cells through an autocrine/paracrine stimulation.[282]

CSF-2 may contribute to regulate the growth of HL-60 human leukemia cells. Purified CSF-2 can induce differentiation of HL-60 cells with suppression of clonogenicity.[283] The growth of these cells can be inhibited by DMSO at the G_1 phase of the cycle and this effect is reversed by CSF-2, which partially restores HL-60 cell growth.[284,285] Differentiation of the human monoblast-like cell line U-937 is synergistically stimulated by CSF-2 and calcitriol.[286] Apparently, this effect is mediated by the calcitriol-induced expression of CSF-2 receptors in U-937 cells.

Most frequently, AML patients do not express CSF-2 and CSF-3 transcripts in their blast cells, but in some cases abnormally large CSF-2 transcripts can be detected.[287] Constitutive expression of CSF-2 mRNA and protein occurs in some human tumors. Using a full-length CSF-2 cDNA as a probe, expression of the CSF-2 gene was detected in 3 of 24 human solid tumors and tumor-cell lines and in 1 of 12 human leukemia-cell lines.[288] No rearrangement of the tumor-cell DNA was detected by the CSF-2 cDNA probe. The mechanism and biological significance of CSF-2 gene expression by tumor cells are unknown.

The acute retrovirus A-MuLV is capable, by action of its v-*abl* oncogene, of inducing transformation of CSF-2-dependent, nontumorigenic myeloid cell lines into CSF-2-independent, tumorigenic cell lines, but this transformation is not associated with the production of the specific growth factor by a kind of autocrine type of stimulation.[289] CSF-2 is able to stimulate differentiation in promonocytic leukemia-cell lines derived from A-MuLV-infected mice,[290] which shows that malignant cells expressing the v-*abl* oncogene are not irreversibly blocked in their capacity to differentiate.

G. CSF-2 AND PROTO-ONCOGENE EXPRESSION

The physiological actions of CSF-2 are partially exerted at the level of gene expression. Expression of some proto-oncogenes may be influenced by CSF-2. Treatment of rat alveolar macrophages with CSF-2 causes induction of c-*fos* and c-*myc* mRNA.[156] The mechanism of this induction is unknown. Myelomonocytic leukemia WEHI-3B cells are induced by CSF-2 to differentiate into monocytes-macrophages and granulocytes in the presence of actinomycin D. This differentiation is accompanied by decreased expression of c-*myc* and c-*myb* and markedly increased expression of c-*fos*, whereas the expression of other proto-oncogenes is unaltered (c-*abl*, c-K-*ras*, and c-*fes*) or not detectable (c-*src*, c-*sis*, c-*mos*, c-*erb*-A, and c-*erb*-B).[291] Expression of c-*fos* is tightly correlated with monocyte differentiation in both normal and leukemic cells and may also be required for the expression of some macrophage-specific functions. CSF-2 can stimulate the proliferation and clonogenicity of HL-60 human promyelocytic leukemia cells and under certain conditions can induce the differentiation of these cells; these effects are associated with increased transcriptional expression of the c-*myc* gene.[292]

Expression of the c-*fes* proto-oncogene is confined mainly to hematopoietic cells, in particular myeloid cells. The 93-kDa c-Fes tyrosine kinase may be involved in the mechanisms of action of CSF-2.[293,294] The human myeloblastoid cell line, KG-1, expresses the c-Fes protein and can be induced to differentiate in response to CSF-2, while the KG-1a variant of the same cell line does not express the c-Fes protein and, concomitantly, has lost the capacity to differentiate and respond to CSF-2. Two other hematopoietic cell lines, LTBM and IO-3, have an absolute dependence on CSF-2, IL-3, or both for their growth, and the c-*fes* gene is expressed by both cell lines. Such correlations suggest that the c-Fes protein may be involved in the cellular response of myeloid cells to CSF-2 and other HGFs.

CSF-2 rapidly and markedly induces *egr*-1 mRNA expression in murine peritoneal macrophages through a mechanism that does not require *de novo* protein synthesis or protein kinase C activation.[295] The *egr*-1 gene is a member of the early growth response family and its product is a nuclear protein that binds, in the presence of zinc, to a DNA consensus sequence. Expression of another gene, c-*fgr*, is transiently induced in normal murine bone marrow-derived monocytic cells by activating signals, including LPS,

CSF-1, CSF-2, LPS, and IFN-γ.[158] These results suggest that the c-Fgr tyrosine kinase may be essential for the mediation of the intracellular effects of many monocytic stimuli.

H. INFLUENCE OF VIRAL ONCOGENES ON CSF-2 EXPRESSION

During the first 3 h of stimulation of bone marrow cells by CSF-2 there is both creation of DNA breaks and closure of preexisting DNA breaks, as demonstrated with inhibitors of ADP-ribosyl transferase activity.[296] DNA rearrangements may occur not only during B-lymphocyte differentiation, but also in other cell lineages like the monocyte-macrophage lineage. Such rearrangements might provide a molecular basis for differentiation of the different cell lineages. The possible relationship between DNA rearrangements and proto-oncogene activation in different cell lineages during the respective differentiation processes remains uncharacterized. Infection of long-term murine bone marrow cultures with a recombinant murine amphotropic virus carrying the v-*src* oncogene results in an alteration of the normal differentiation program of the stem cells, which is accompanied by a 25- to 50-fold increase in the level of CSF-2.[297]

Infection of individual multilineage hematopoietic colonies with the acute retrovirus A-MuLV, which carries the v-*abl* oncogene, results in the production of mast cell lines which exhibits transcriptional activation of the CSF-2 gene and production of CSF-2 protein.[298] However, these results were not confirmed by other investigators, who did not detect production of HGFs after infection of a growth factor-dependent myeloid cell line (FDC-P1 cells) by A-MuLV.[288] The reason for such discrepant results is unknown.

I. PRODUCTION OF CSF-2 BY TUMOR CELLS

CSF-2 is produced by the malignant cells in some human leukemias. Constitutive expression of the CSF-2 gene was detected in the leukemic cells of 11 of 22 cases of AML, whereas no expression of the gene was found in 11 cases of common (pre-B) ALL and 4 cases of CML.[299] Biologically active CSF-2 was detected in 6 of 11 cases of AML which were positive for the presence of CSF-2 transcripts. The results suggest that expression of the CSF-2 gene may contribute to the abnormal growth properties of some human AMLs.

The fibroblastoid cell line BMA-1, established from mouse marrow cells transfected with Ad5 DNA, produces CSF-2. Transplantation of these cells into splenectomized mice induces granulocytosis.[300] The factor produced by BMA-1 cells stimulated the formation of spleen colony-forming cells and granulocyte-macrophage colony-forming cells in the tumor bearing animals, which were associated with a granulopoietic response. Production of CSF-2 by human glioblastoma cells *in vitro* can be stimulated by IL-1 or TNF-α, but CSF-2 is not expressed by human glioblastomas *in vivo*.[301]

J. ONCOGENIC POTENTIAL OF THE CLONED CSF-2 GENE

Expression of a retroviral vector carrying a cDNA coding for CSF-2 in the factor-dependent murine cell line FDC-P1 (FD cells), results in proliferation of the cells in the absence of exogenous CSF-2, and the transfected cells, unlike the parental cells, exhibit tumorigenic properties and produce transplanted leukemias in recipient syngeneic mice.[302] The only change relevant to the tumorigenic properties of the transfected FD cells is the synthesis of CSF-2, which is thus sufficient to convert the cells to a tumorigenic phenotype. Although the cloned CSF-2 gene behaves in these experiments in a way which is similar to that of active oncogenes, capable of inducing oncogenic transformation, the recipient FD cells are not normal cells but are immortalized cells that may have a block in terminal differentiation. Thus, FD cells may have already undergone at least one step in the transformation process. The constructed retroviral vector carrying the CSF-2 gene is not capable of transforming hematopoietic cells from normal fetal liver or bone marrow. An intriguing observation is that the CSF-2 protein secreted by the cells transfected with the vector carrying the CSF-2 gene is apparently not responsible for the independence of these cells of exogenous CSF-2.[302] An antiserum against CSF-2 failed to inhibit the growth of the transfected cells. Rather, the growth factor produced in the transfected cells could bind to its receptor in an intracellular compartment before the receptor reaches the cell surface, which would lead to autonomous growth. Another possible explanation is production in the transfected cells of a secreted growth factor distinct from CSF-2, but dependent on its action at an intracellular level.

Other cell lines may be susceptible to CSF-2-induced neoplastic transformation. Transfection of cDNAs encoding the α and β subunits of the CSF-2 receptor into NIH/3T3 cells, which normally do not express CSF-2 receptors, results in the expression of a transformed phenotype, as assessed by the appearance of foci of altered cells.[303] This alteration is conditioned by the presence of CSF-2 in the culture medium, suggesting the operation of an autocrine or paracrine mechanism.

K. CSF-2 AS AN AGENT FOR THE TREATMENT OF CANCER AND AIDS

The biological activity of CSF-2 has been verified *in vivo*. Injection of normal mice from different strains with recombinant CSF-2 results in increases in the numbers of circulating granulocytes and macrophages as well as in enhanced macrophage phagocytic activity.[304] Administration of human CSF-2 to rhesus monkeys *in vivo* results in the induction of leukocytosis and the stimulation of phagocytic function of mature neutrophils.[305-308]

Administration of recombinant human CSF-2 accelerated myeloid recovery in cancer patients treated with high-dose chemotherapy and autologous bone marrow transplantation.[309] Administration of CSF-2 to sarcoma patients during the leukocyte recovery period following chemotherapy resulted in a marked increase in the number of granulocyte-macrophage colony-forming units (CFU-GM) and erythroid-burst-forming units (BFU-E) in the peripheral blood.[310] CFU-GM and BFU-E correspond to hematopoietic stem cells, and are normally found in small amounts in the peripheral blood of mammals, including man. Treatment of patients with refractory carcinoma with human CSF-2 resulted in enhancement of the oxidative metabolism (superoxide release) from polymorphonuclear leukocytes while chemotaxis was not changed.[311] CSF-2 infusion to cancer patients increased the number of monocytes and neutrophils in peripheral blood and activated the antitumor potential of peripheral blood monocytes, with secretion of TNF-α and interferon by these cells.[312] These results suggest that CSF-2 could be a useful adjunct in the therapy of patients with cancer.

Neutrophils from AIDS patients respond normally to CSF-2 *in vitro*, and administration of CSF-2 to AIDS patients is well tolerated and may correct neutrophil functional defects in phagocytosis and intracellular killing of germs such as *Staphylococcus aureus*.[313,314] The number of circulating neutrophils increases in AIDS patients treated with CSF-2 in a dose-dependent manner.

IV. COLONY-STIMULATING FACTOR 3

The granulocyte colony-stimulating factor (G-CSF) was first identified as a glycoprotein that can induce differentiation in murine myeloid and myelomonocytic leukemia cell lines.[315] The structure and function of human and murine G-CSF and their receptors have been reviewed.[316-318] Studies performed in healthy volunteers and patients with various hematologic disorders indicate that G-CSF plays an important physiologic role as a circulating neutrophilopoietin.[319] The designation of G-CSF as colony-stimulating factor-3 (CSF-3) was proposed by the author.[12]

A. BIOLOGICAL EFFECTS OF CSF-3

CSF-3 specifically stimulates the growth of committed bone marrow precursor cells to form granulocyte colonies.[320,321] Purified CSF-3 protein promotes the formation in serum-free cultures of human granulocyte colonies.[322] In addition, CSF-3 promotes the terminal differentiation of granulocytes and exerts a strong stimulus for the activity of mature neutrophils, including the production of alkaline phosphatase.[323-325] The striking effects of CSF-3 on granulopoiesis *in vitro* have been verified in patients with metastatic breast cancer *in vivo*.[326] CSF-3 can cross the placenta and stimulates fetal rat granulopoiesis.[327]

In addition to granulopoietic cells, other types of cells may also respond to CSF-3. In appropriate assay systems, human CSF-3 can stimulate neutrophils to transcription of IFN-α mRNA.[328] Since IFN-α is known to suppress myelopoiesis, including neutrophil production, the evidence suggests that the IFN-α/CSF-3 system may participate in the feedback inhibitory regulation of neutropoiesis. CSF-3 can also contribute to stimulate the formation of macrophage colonies and may support early erythroid colonies and mixed colony formation.[329]

In certain systems *in vitro*, CSF-3 may stimulate the growth of multipotential hematopoietic precursors.[330] However, CSF-3 as a single agent is unable to support the formation of multilineage colonies, erythroid burst, and megakaryocyte colonies.[331] It may act synergistically with IL-3 to shorten the G_0 period of hematopoietic stem cells, resulting in an earlier appearance of multilineage colonies.[332] Human CSF-3 can support the survival and proliferation of the IL-3-dependent diploid murine progenitor cell line, 32D C13.[333] In this system, IL-3 supports the proliferation of the stem-cell population and CSF-3 stimulates the terminal differentiation of the cells into neutrophilic granulocytes. Concurrent administration of IL-3 and CSF-3 to intact rats results in additive effects for the production of neutrophilia.[334] IL-3 and CSF-3 act synergistically on human AML cells whether measured by blast colony assay or thymidine incorporation into DNA.[335] The initial exposure to IL-3 or CSF-2 may prime the leukemic cells for a subsequent response to the second stimulus represented by CSF-3. The synergistic interaction between CSF-2 and CSF-3 is via a direct effect on progenitor cells that are not stimulated by CSF-2 or CSF-3 alone, and it is not mediated by growth factor production by accessory cells.[336] CSF-3 and erythropoietin may act synergistically with IL-3 or CSF-2 in supporting human neutrophil colony and BFU-E formation, respectively.[203] Administration of CSF-3 either *in vivo* or *in vitro* may induce an up-modulation of IL-1 receptor expression on murine bone marrow cells, and this effect is synergistically enhanced by glucocorticoids.[337]

The possibility that CSF-3 may exert some effects on nonhematopoietic cells is suggested by the expression of CSF-3 receptors in these cells. In fact, there is evidence that CSF-3 may have mitogenic effects on cultured mouse fibroblasts.[338] The designation of G-CSF as a CSF-3 may be justified on the basis of these properties.

Certain derivatives of CSF-3 may exhibit enhanced biological properties. A CSF-3 derivative termed KW-2228, in which amino acids were replaced at five positions of the amino-terminal region of human CSF-3 by gene mutagenic techniques, showed two to four times higher specific activity to mouse marrow progenitor cells by colony-forming units in soft agar and by cell-proliferation assay in liquid culture, as compared to intact human recombinant CSF-3.[339] The mechanism for the high specific activity of KW-2228 remains to be elucidated.

B. CSF-3 STRUCTURE AND THE CSF-3 GENE

Human CSF-3 is a hydrophobic glycoprotein of 19.6 kDa composed of 174 amino acids.[329,340] The chromosomal gene structure and two mRNAs coding for human CSF-3 were characterized.[341] cDNA coding for human CSF-3 was cloned from a human squamous carcinoma cell line (CHU-2) which constitutively produces CSF-3. Expression of this cDNA in monkey COS cells gave rise to a protein showing authentic CSF-3 activity.[342] The human CSF-3 gene was also cloned from the bladder carcinoma cell line 5637 and was expressed in *Escherichia coli*, and the native human CSF-3 protein was purified from this cell line.[329] This protein is O-glycosylated and has a molecular weight of approximately 19 kDa. The CSF-3 gene was also cloned, using a synthetic oligonucleotide probe, from a cDNA library of LPS-stimulated human peripheral blood macrophages.[343] A study of human CSF-3 by site-directed *in vitro* mutagenesis indicated that most mutations located on the internal and carboxy-terminal regions of the CSF-3 molecule abolished its biological activity, whereas mutants without some terminal amino acids retain the activity.[344] Moreover, some substitutions at the amino-terminal amino acid sequences resulted in enhanced specific activity. Analysis of the three-dimensional structure of recombinant human CSF-3 by X-ray crystallography showed that CSF-3 belongs to a distinct class of growth factors which includes CSF-2, IL-2, IL-4, and IFN-β, as well as growth hormone, and which is characterized by the presence of a common motif of a four-α-helix bundle with two long crossover connections.[345] This structure exists despite little amino acid sequence similarity. Differences between the members of this class of growth factors include the number and position of disulfide bonds and the local conformation of their loops. The extracellular portion of the cell surface receptors for growth factors includes a conserved "cytokine-binding" domain of about 210 residues, suggesting that these signaling ligands may all bind to their respective receptors with equivalent geometries.

Molecular hybridization analysis of DNA from normal human leukocytes and CHU-2 cells showed that the human genome contains only one gene coding for CSF-3 and that some rearrangement occurred within one of the alleles of the CSF-3 gene in CHU-2 cells. No structural homology was detected between the human CSF-3 protein and other proteins, including CSF-2 and IL-3.[342] The gene for CSF-3 is located on human chromosome region 17q, at a region involved in translocations frequently associated with acute promyelocytic leukemia (APML).[346] More precisely, the CSF-3 gene is located on human chromosome 17q11, proximal to the breakpoint of the t(15;17) translocation associated with APML.[347] No rearrangement of the CSF-3 gene occurs in APML cells.[348] The proto-oncogenes c-*erb*-A and c-*neu*/*erb*-B2, as well as the NGF receptor gene, are located on human chromosome region 17q21-q22, but these genes are not involved in the development of APML.

cDNA clones coding for murine CSF-3 were isolated from the murine fibrosarcoma cell line NFSA, which synthesizes CSF-3 mRNA constitutively.[349] This cDNA encodes a polypeptide consisting of a 30-amino acid signal sequence, followed by a mature CSF-3 sequence of 178 amino acids with a calculated molecular weight of approximately 19,000 Da. The murine cDNA can direct the synthesis in COS cells of a protein with authentic CSF-3 activity. The overall homology of the mature human and murine CSF-3 polypeptides is about 73%. Another cDNA clone, derived from chromosomal DNA extracted from mouse spleen, showed that the murine CSF-3 gene, like the human gene, is interrupted by four introns, but the nucleotide sequences of the human and murine CSF-3 genes exhibit little sequence homology, except for the intron-exon junction parts which are necessary for RNA splicing.[350] In contrast, the 5′ flanking sequences of the human and murine CSF-3 genes are highly conserved. These sequences are probably involved in the control of CSF-3 gene expression.

A factor with CSF-3-like activity, called neutrophil CSF, is a sialoglycoprotein obtained from the medium conditioned by RSP-2.P3 cells, a line of rat spleen cells maintained for several years in medium without either lipids or proteins.[351] The addition of sodium butyrate and LPS results in an increased production of neutrophil CSF by RSP-2.P3 cells, but it is not known whether this factor is similar or identical to CSF-3 derived from mouse peritoneal cells.

C. PRODUCTION OF CSF-3

CSF-3 is produced and secreted by different types of cells. Mouse peritoneal cells can be used to obtain CSF-3.[320] Cultured human umbilical vein endothelial cells express CSF-3 mRNA when they are stimulated with LPS, IL-1, or TNF-α.[237] Human vascular smooth muscle cells also synthesize CSF-3, and stimulation of these cells with IL-1α and TNF-α results in a marked increase in CSF-3 synthesis.[352] These results suggest that CSF-3 may contribute to the development of vasculitis lesions. The production of CSF-3 by human marrow stromal layers in long-term culture is stimulated by IL-1.[60] This factor also stimulates the production of CSF-3 by the human stromal fibroblast cell line, ST-1.[353] CSF-3 is produced by a diversity of cell lines.[354] Astrocytes, which may play a central role in the regulation of immune-mediated processes, express transcripts for both CSF-2 and CSF-3.[355] An IL-3-like factor identified in astrocytes may be represented by CSF-2 and CSF-3 secreted by these cells.

Using an enzyme immunoassay specific for CSF-3, the factor could not be detected in the serum of most healthy persons, but elevated levels were present in patients with abnormal absolute neutrophil count.[356] Serum levels ranging from 46 to >2000 pg/ml were found in patients with idiopathic aplastic anemia, Fanconi's anemia, myelodysplastic syndrome, chronic lymphoid leukemia, as well as in cases of acute leukemia without any blast cells in the blood. In addition, some patients with lung cancer, cyclic neutropenia, malignant lymphoma, and acute infection had high levels of circulating CSF-3. Interestingly, a reverse correlation was found between blood neutrophil count and serum CSF-3 level in patients with aplastic anemia. Patients with severe congenital neutropenia have increased serum levels of CSF-3.[357] These results support the concept that CSF-3 is a circulating hormone specific for neutrophilopoiesis.

D. THE CSF-3 RECEPTOR

The physiologic action of CSF-3 is initiated by its binding to specific high-affinity receptors expressed on the surface of responsive cells present in the bone marrow.[358] cDNAs encoding the human CSF-3 receptor have been cloned from HL-60 cells and the gene was mapped to human chromosome region 1p32-p34.[359] The human CSF-3 receptor is a protein of 150 kDa which is expressed on circulating neutrophils.[360] The receptor is composed of a single subunit of 813 amino acids and shows high homology to its murine counterpart.[361] It contains extracellular, transmembrane, and cytoplasmic domains. At least three different mRNA species, probably originating from alternative splicing mechanisms, code for the human CSF-3 receptor. Two variants of the CSF-3 receptors are present in the human placenta.

In the murine myelomonocytic leukemia cell line WEHI-3B D+, the CSF-3 receptor is also represented by a 150-kDa protein.[362] The receptor, purified to apparent homogeneity from the solubilized membrane fraction of mouse myeloid leukemia NFS-60 cells, is represented under reducing conditions by a single polypeptide of 100 to 130 kDa, which may show aggregation in the form of oligomers.[363] The murine CSF-3 receptor, as deduced from cDNA clones, is a polypeptide composed of 812 amino acids residues with a single transmembrane domain.[364] The extracellular domain, which consists of 601 amino acids, contains a region of 220 amino acids that exhibits a high degree of similarity to the growth hormone and prolactin receptors. Chimeric molecules containing CSF-3 receptor and growth hormone receptor sequences are capable of transducing signals by similar mechanisms.[365] The cytoplasmic domain of the murine CSF-3 receptor exhibits similarity with parts of the cytoplasmic domain of the murine IL-4 receptor. Analysis of various mouse tissues indicated that transcripts of the CSF-3 receptor gene are present only in marrow cells that contain the progenitor for neutrophilic granulocytes. No difference exists in CSF-3 binding capacity between normal blast cells and cells of the myelomonocytic leukemia cell line WEHI-3B D+. Murine and human CSF-3 exhibit almost complete biological and receptor-binding cross reactivities to normal and leukemic mouse or human cells.[366]

Expression of human and mouse CSF-3 receptor cDNA in various cell lines demonstrated that the extracellular domain of the receptor molecule has a composite structure consisting of an Ig-like domain, a cytokine receptor homologous (CRH) domain, and three fibronectin type II (FNIII) domains.[367] The cytoplasmic domain of the receptor has a limited similarity to that of the IL-4 receptor and does not contain a domain with kinase or other enzymatic activity. Mutational analysis of the CSF-3 receptor expressed in the IL-3-dependent murine myeoloid cell line, FDC-P1, indicated that the amino-terminal half of the CRH domain is essential for the recognition of CSF-3, but the Ig-like FNIII and cytoplasmic domains were not. The CRH domain and a portion of the cytoplasmic domain of about 100 amino acids are indispensable for transduction of the CSF-3-triggered signal. Expression in a human myeloid leukemia cell line (FDC-P1) of a hybrid molecule containing the extracellular binding domain of the human growth hormone receptor linked to the transmembrane and intracellular domains of the murine CSF-3 receptor is capable of inducing proliferation of the cells after addition of growth hormone.[368] Distinct regions of the human CSF-3 receptor cytoplasmic domain may be required for proliferation and gene induction.[369]

Functional high-affinity CSF-3 receptors have been detected in platelets[370] and in nonhematopoietic cells such as normal human endothelial cells, as well as in human choriocarcinoma and small-cell lung carcinoma cell lines.[371-373] CSF-3 receptors are also present in human placental membranes and trophoblastic cells.[374] These results suggest that CSF-3 plays some role in the feto-placental unit during human development. Contrary to studies suggesting the restriction of biological activities of CSF-3 to hematopoietic cells, nonhematopoietic cells may also respond to CSF-3. However, the exact role of CSF-3 in nonhematopoietic cells is not unknown.

Multiple endogenous and exogenous factors, including other CSFs, may be involved in the regulation of CSF-3 receptor expression. TNF-α modulates the expression of CSF-3 receptors on murine peritoneal exudate macrophages.[375] Modulation of CSF-3 receptor expression in macrophages and other types of cells by HGFs and cytokines may be important for the diverse physiological actions of CSF-3, including inflammatory responses.

E. POSTRECEPTOR MECHANISM OF ACTION OF CSF-3

Little is known about the postreceptor mechanism of action of CSF-3. Addition of human CSF-3 to isolated human granulocytes in concentrations sufficient to induce maximal stimulation of the proliferation and differentiation of granulocyte-macrophage progenitor cells does not result in alteration of the resting membrane electric potential, the pH_i, or the $[Ca^{2+}]_i$.[263] However, CSF-3 induces release of arachidonic acid from the plasma membrane within minutes of addition to the culture, suggesting that activation of phospholipase C and/or protein kinase C is part of the cellular response to CSF-3. Binding of human CSF-3 to the CSF-3 receptor on the surface of murine myeloblastic NFS-60 cells induces proliferation of the cells, and this effect is associated with activation of the G protein/adenylate cyclase system.[376] The possible role of proto-oncogene expression in the action mechanism of CSF-3 is unknown, but in the established human myeloid leukemia cell line, NKM-1, both CSF-3 and CSF-1 induce c-*fos* and *jun*-B, but not c-*jun*, gene expression.[377]

F. EFFECTS OF *IN VIVO* ADMINISTRATION OF CSF-3

The efficacy and specificity of CSF-3 has been demonstrated in intact animals. Continuous i.v. administration of human CSF-3 to golden Syrian hamsters induced an elevation (five- to sixfold) in peripheral blood neutrophils, whereas other types of blood cells (monocytes, lymphocytes, and eosinophils) remained stable.[378] Similar observations were made in mice receiving i.p. injections of human CSF-3 every day for 14 d.[379] In these mice, the number of circulating leukocytes began to increase on 4th day and reached more than 10 times the control on the 14th day, with neutrophilic granulocytes representing 88.5% of total leukocytes. A dose-dependent increase in the number of blood neutrophils was also observed in mice receiving s.c. injections of human CSF-3 twice daily for a period of 4 to 5 d.[380] However, a puzzling feature observed in the CSF-3-treated mice was a decrease in marrow cellularity, with a strong inhibition of erythropoiesis.

Injection of a single dose of CSF-3 in mice resulted in a 2.5-fold increase of neutrophil counts within 2 h, and these high levels were maintained for at least 8 h.[381] Compared with single injections, repeated injection of CSF-3 induced a progressive and marked rise in neutrophile counts, reaching a level 8 times above the preinjection level after 15 days of injections. Progressive elevation of splenic progenitor cell levels was observed in the CSF-3-treated mice. Moreover, neutropenia induced in mice by injection of cyclophosphamide was not only obviated by CSF-3 treatment, but the blood neutrophil levels increased, rather than decreased, in the treated animals. Daily administration of purified human CSF-3 can accelerate the recovery from neutropenia induced by total-body irradiation in mice.[382] Similar results were obtained with s.c. injections of recombinant human CSF-3 into Golden Syrian hamsters and *Cynomolgus* monkeys.[383,384]

A single i.v. injection of human CSF-3 in rats caused an initial peripheral neutropenia between 3 and 15 min and a subsequent neutrophilia beginning at 0.5 h, peaking between 12 and 24 h, and subsiding to normal between 30 to 36 h.[385] Simultaneous observations made in bone marrow and peripheral blood of the treated rats indicated that CSF-3 acts not only as a mitogen and growth factor for early cells in the myeloid series, but also as a factor that induces the release of mature neutrophils from the bone marrow. Dexamethasone and IFN-γ inhibited the magnitude of the CSF-3-induced neutrophilia, suggesting that endogenous glucocorticoids and IFN-γ may play a negative feedback role in the endogenous regulation of hematopoiesis. Continuous infusion of recombinant human CSF-3 in patients with small-cell lung carcinoma resulted in an early fall in the number of peripheral neutrophils within the first hour, followed by a rapid influx of mature neutrophils into the circulatory pool.[386] These effects were accompanied by stimulation of the proliferation and differentiation of neutrophil precursors in the bone marrow.

Administration of human CSF-3 to patients with myelodysplastic syndromes (which may represent preleukemic diseases) resulted in repair of neutrophil anomalies with enhanced activity of neutrophil alkaline phosphatase, an enzyme that is considered to be a marker of neutrophil maturity.[387] Moreover, the production of superoxide anion (O_2^-) by neutrophils is frequently decreased in patients with myelodysplastic syndromes, and treatment with CSF-3 may induce a significant increase of this anion in most of the treated patients. The results suggest that CSF-3 may be clinically useful for the treatment of neutropenic and preleukemic patients.

Treatment with recombinant human CSF-3 has been assayed with good results in patients with congenital agranulocytosis (Kostmann's syndrome).[388] Children with this lethal disease have severe, persistent absolute neutropenia and bone marrow morphological alterations which suggest a maturational arrest of neutrophil precursors at the promyelocytic stage. The patients have a propensity to local bacterial infections which easily progress to severe septicemia, meningitis, peritonitis, or enteritis, which accounts for the high mortality seen in this disease in early childhood. The difficulty of finding an HLA-compatible sibling donor limits the possibility of a successful bone marrow transplantation in these children. Treatment with CSF-3 can lead to an increase in the numbers of functional neutrophils in patients with congenital agranulocytosis. The mechanisms involved in this disease have not been elucidated, but may include a deleted or mutated CSF-3 gene or altered cellular mechanisms of action of CSF-3 at the receptor or postreceptor levels.

G. ROLE OF CSF-3 IN NEOPLASTIC PROCESSES

Although CSF-3 has been shown to stimulate the proliferation of human leukemic blast cells, the precise role of CSF-3 in neoplasia is little understood. Examination of human leukemia cell lines and blast cells from patients with leukemia demonstrated the presence of high-affinity binding sites for CSF-3 in myeloid cell lines and in the blasts obtained from AML patients.[389,390] In contrast, no specific binding of CSF-3 was observed in lymphoblastic cell lines or the blast cells of ALL or lymphoma. Relatively few CSF-3 receptors may be required to allow activation of AML cell growth by CSF-3, but the presence of the specific high-affinity receptors may not be a strict indicator of the proliferative responsiveness of the blast cells to CSF-3. However, a proliferative response of AML blasts to CSF-3 may be predicted when the blasts express a large number of CSF-3 receptors.[391] A subline established from an AML patient responded with exponential growth to CSF-3, although the morphology and phenotype of this subline were similar to those of the original cell line, which did not respond to CSF-3.[392] The molecular basis of this difference was not established.

CSF-3 can suppress leukemic stem-cell self-regeneration and can induce the differentiation in some murine myeloid leukemia cell lines.[315] Human CSF-3 can induce the terminal differentiation of cultured murine and human leukemia cells into macrophages and granulocytes.[329,393,394] Purified CSF-3 can induce differentiation of human HL-60 cells with suppression of clonogenicity.[283] Human CSF-3 stimulates the proliferation of human APL cells and does not induce, by itself, the differentiation of these cells *in vitro*, but can enhance retinoic acid-induced differentiation of the cells.[395] Differentiation of human leukemic cells *in vitro* by CSF-3 and other inducers, such as retinoic acid or DMSO, is associated with the phosphorylation on serine of a 22-kDa cytosolic protein.[396]

The possible use of CSF-3 for the treatment of hematologic malignancies remains to be evaluated. Administration of CSF-3 to patients with AML may stimulate the self-renewal and terminal differentiation of the blast progenitor cells, but the effects are heterogeneous among different patients.[397] The differentiation-inducing properties of CSF-3 may be restricted to certain types of tumor cells. In a study on the *in vitro* response of human AML cells to CSF-2 and CSF-3, it was observed that a number of leukemic cells become morphologically differentiated in suspension culture, but this occurred both with and without the addition of the CSFs.[398] Thus, there was no evidence of differentiation-induction by either CSF-2 or CSF-3. Even under optimum conditions of exposure to CSF-3, 30 to 40% of the blastic cell population from M1 mouse myeloid leukemia remains unaltered.[399] The growth-promoting effects of CSF-3 may limit its potential as a differentiation-inducing agent.[400] Not a reduced, but an increased growth of i.d.-inoculated tumors was observed in mice after i.p. administration of CSF-3.[401] Further studies are required for a proper evaluation of the possible use of CSFs in the treatment of leukemias.

V. MEGAKARYOCYTE COLONY-STIMULATING FACTORS

Megakaryocytopoiesis is one of the differentiation pathways of pluripotent hematopoietic stem cells.[402] It is related to the production of blood platelets (thrombocytopoiesis) and is regulated through specific humoral factors by both the platelet demand and the megakaryocyte mass.[403,404] The terminal differentiation of megakaryocytes is characterized by the appearance of specific organelles, the synthesis of platelet proteins, and the increase of DNA content by an endomitotic process, which results in a marked increase in megakaryocyte ploidy and size. Platelets arise from the fragmentation of megakaryocyte cytoplasm.

Normal megakaryocytopoiesis implicates various progenitor cells, which include the burst-forming unit megakaryocyte (BFU-MK) and the colony-forming unit megakaryocyte (CFU-MK). The BFU-MK (megakaryoblast) is the most primitive progenitor committed to the megakaryocyte lineage. The megakaryoblasts cannot be identified by morphological criteria, but are recognized by their ability to divide and give rise to colonies of mature megakaryocytes. The megakaryoblast is a precursor of transitional immature megakaryocytes, which are small mononuclear cells that express platelet markers and represent a bridge between progenitors and morphologically identifiable megakaryocytes. The mature megakaryocytes are readily recognized in the bone marrow due to their large size and multilobulated nuclei. The mature megakaryocyte gives origin to platelets circulating in the blood.

The study of megakaryocytopoiesis has been hampered by the rarity of megakaryocytes in normal bone marrow (0.03 to 0.06% of all nucleated cells present in human marrow) and by the difficulty in growing megakaryocyte progenitor cells in culture. These methodologic pitfalls have been circumvented, in part, by the establishment of a number of continuous cell lines originating from normal or leukemic human bone marrow that express a range of megakaryocytic phenotypic properties. The process of megakaryocytopoiesis initially involves a phase characterized by mitotic division of a progenitor cell, followed by a wave of nuclear endoreplications that occur in a nonproliferating cell, which results in megakaryocytes possessing different polyploidy values. The morphologically identifiable mature megakaryocytes are characterized by the presence of cytoplasmic organelles, the expression of membrane antigens and glycoproteins, and the release of mature platelets.[404]

Studies in animal models indicate that normal megakaryocytopoiesis depends, at least in part, on the action of humoral factors, and this is supported by the analysis of megakaryocytopoietic systems *in vitro*.[405] Well-characterized growth factors and cytokines are implicated in megakaryocytopoiesis, including TGF-β, IL-3, IL-6, CSF-2, and erythropoietin.[406] Two HGFs more specifically involved in regulating megakaryocyte maturation and platelet production are the megakaryocyte colony-stimulating factor and the thrombocytopoiesis-stimulating factor, or thrombopoietin. In addition to these stimulating factors, normal megakaryocytopoiesis may also involve the action of a factor with inhibitory properties. The regulation of megakaryocytopoiesis by a growth factor may involve changes in the expression of proto-oncogenes such as c-*fos* and c-*jun*, which encode the AP-1 transcription factor and are expressed by human megakaryocytes.[407]

A. MEGAKARYOCYTE COLONY-STIMULATING FACTOR

The megakaryocyte colony-stimulating factor (MK-CSF), also called megakaryocyte colony-stimulating activity (MK-CSA), would be specifically involved in stimulating the proliferation of megakaryoblasts.[408,409] This factor is necessary for the formation of megakaryocyte colonies (CFU-MK) in cultures of cells from bone marrow and other hematopoietic organs. The *in vivo* significance of MK-CSF is not clear.

The structure and function of MK-CSF is a subject of much controversy. The partial purification of human urinary MK-CSF has been reported.[410] A factor with MK-CSF activity was isolated from the human T lymphoblast cell line Mo.[411] MK-CSF isolated from the conditioned medium of WEHI-3 cells is identical with IL-3.[412,413] The megakaryocyte-stimulating properties of IL-3 have been confirmed in human cells with IL-3 cloned from a gibbon ape cell line.[414] The stimulation of megakaryocytopoiesis by IL-3 is limited to the early stages of the process.[415] IL-3 promotes predominantly the mitotic component of megakaryocyte colony development and early megakaryocytic differentiation, but has no stimulatory effect on later events such as megakaryocyte nuclear endoreduplication. Another factor involved in the control of megakaryocytopoiesis is IL-6. This factor may act in concert with other interleukins and HGFs, including IL-3, IL-11, CSF-2, and erythropoietin for promoting CFU-MK and the maturation of megakaryocytes.[416-420] In contrast, the IFNs usually have inhibitory effects on megakaryocyte growth *in vitro*.[421] However, the precise role of IL-3, IL-6, CSF-2, IFNs, erythropoietin, and other cytokines and HGFs on megakaryocyte growth and platelet production *in vivo* remains to be evaluated. Recent evidence suggests that the MK-CSF present in the sera from patients with megakaryocyte aplasia in the bone marrow is distinct from both IL-3 and CSF-2, as well as from other defined cytokines and HGFs.[422]

In addition to the positive control represented by MK-CSF, megakaryocytopoiesis may be subjected to negative regulation by an inhibitory factor which is stored in the platelets α-granules.[423] This inhibitor may be identical to TGF-β.

B. THROMBOCYTOPOIESIS-STIMULATING FACTOR

The thrombocytopoiesis-stimulating factor (TSF), also called thrombopoietin, is a putative growth factor involved in the control of megakaryocytopoiesis, i.e., in the proliferation and maturation of megakaryoblasts.[424,425] TSF is present in the blood and urine of some thrombocytopenic patients as well as in the medium from cultured human embryonic kidney cells. The exact structure, origin, and function of TSF have not been elucidated. The major role of TSF may be to promote the cytoplasmic maturation of megakaryocytes rather than influencing the proliferative capacity of CFU-MK.[426] The relationship between TSF and a factor, termed megakaryocyte potentiator,[427] that accelerates cytoplasmic maturation of morphologically recognizable megakaryocytes, remains to be elucidated.

VI. MACROPHAGE-DERIVED GROWTH FACTORS

Monocytes and macrophages are the blood and tissue phases, respectively, of the same cell lineage that has its origin in the bone marrow. Monocytes give origin to macrophages *in vivo* and *in vitro*, and the macrophage can be considered as more highly differentiated and functionally more active than its less mature precursor.[428] Macrophages are cells directly involved in inflammatory processes, host defense mechanisms, and injury repair. At least in *in vitro* systems, activated macrophages are capable of destroying neoplastic cells, while they leave nonneoplastic cells unharmed even under conditions of cocultivation.[429]

A. MACROPHAGE COLONY-STIMULATING ACTIVITY

Multiple secretory products have been identified in macrophages, including different types of growth factors. Unfortunately, many of the putative growth factors present in macrophages remain poorly characterized. A factor, named macrophage colony-stimulating activity, may be synergistically involved in potentiating the resorption of bone tissue induced by IL-1.[430]

B. MACROPHAGE-DERIVED GROWTH FACTOR

The action of some of the growth factors associated with macrophages may not be limited to these cells, but may be involved in stimulating a broad spectrum of cells. One of these factors is IL-1. Another factor, the macrophage-derived growth factor (MDGF), is a potent mitogen for nonlymphoid mesenchymal cells, including fibroblasts, smooth-muscle cells, and endothelial cells. MDGF may be identical with FGF.[431] However, a significant part of MDGF activity secreted by human alveolar or peritoneal macrophages consists of at least two forms of PDGF-like products.[432]

C. MACROPHAGE-ACTIVATING FACTORS

Activation of macrophages *in vivo* results from their interaction with a specific lymphokine, the macrophage-activating factor (MAF). This substance is constitutively produced by an HTLV-positive human T-cell line (C10/MJ-2).[433] MAF is a 50- to 67-kDa protein which induces protein synthesis in macrophages and enhances cytolytic activity towards tumor cells.[434] MAF is capable of activating human monocytes to lyse tumor cells. In the presence of MAF some virgin marrow cells rapidly mature and acquire the capacity to kill a wide array of syngeneic, allogeneic, and xenogeneic tumor cells, as shown in a cytotoxicity assay.[435] However, decay of this tumoricidal activity takes place even in the continued presence of MAF, indicating that the effector cells lose responsiveness to the stimulatory signal. Recent evidence indicates that MAF activity released by stimulated lymphocytes may be identical with IFN-γ.[436] However, IFN-γ is not the only cytokine with MAF activity. Macrophages possess receptors for BSF-1/IL-4, and this factor is a potent activator of the tumoricidal properties of peritoneal macrophages against malignant cells such as fibrosarcoma cells.[437] MAF activity is constitutively produced by the HTLV-I-infected human T-cell line DGA-1, but not by the parent cell line C91 PL.[438] This MAF is distinct from IFN-γ and CSF-2.

D. MACROPHAGE MIGRATION FACTORS

Stimulation of human mononuclear cells with concanavalin A may result in the production of either macrophage migration inhibition factor (MIF) or macrophage migration stimulation factor (MSF).[439] In contrast, stimulation with PHA almost invariably results in production of MIF. Soluble factors from OKT8+ cells would be involved in determining MIF or MSF response to concanavalin A stimulation.

E. MACROPHAGE PROINFLAMMATORY PROTEINS

The macrophage inflammatory proteins (MIPs), also called monocyte chemoattractant proteins (MCPs), are monokines that cause localized inflammatory reactions characterized by a rapid influx of polymorphonuclear cells.[440] The MIPs have the ability to activate human polymorphonuclear cells *in vitro* and synergize with some HGFs to enhance CSF-3 colony formation.

Two members of the MIP family have been termed MIP-1 (MCP-1) and MIP-2 (MCP-2).[440] MIP-1/MCP-1 is composed of two distinct gene products, MIP-1α and MIP-1β. The genes coding for MIP-1α and MIP-1β have been cloned and sequenced, allowing the deduction of the complete amino acid sequence of their protein products. The cDNA for MIP-1α predicts a mature polypeptide of 69 amino acids with a molecular weight of 7889 Da, which contains no sites for N-glycosylation. The cDNA for MIP-1β predicts a mature polypeptide also of 69 amino acids, with a molecular weight of 7832 Da and containing one potential N-glycosylation site. The two MIP-1 subtypes exhibit a high degree of amino acid identities. MIP-2/MCP-2 is a heparin binding protein secreted by endotoxin-stimulated macrophages. It is a potent chemotactic agent for human polymorphonuclear cells and can synergize with CSF-1 and CSF-2 in stimulating colony growth.

Amino acid sequence analysis has demonstrated that MIPs are members of a superfamily of proinflammatory peptides which consists of no less than 20 different peptides.[441] The first member to be described in this family was the platelet factor-4 (PF-4), a chemotactic factor for neutrophils and monocytes.[442] Another member of this family is β-thromboglobulin, a protein contained in platelet α granules that functions as a chemotactic agent for fibroblasts. β-Thromboglobulin is synthesized as a 15-kDa precursor called platelet basic protein (PBP). IL-8 is also a member of the same superfamily. The most salient structural feature of the proteins of this superfamily is the presence in the mature proteins of four cysteine (C) residues. The relative order of the first two C residues in these proteins serves to subdivide the superfamily into the C-C family, in which they are adjacent to each other, and the C-X-C family, in which the first two cysteines are separated by one amino acid. The members of the C-C family, such as MIP-1/MCP-1, target monocytes, whereas the members of the C-X-C family, such as IL-8, activate neutrophils.

A recently identified additional member of the superfamily of proinflammatory peptides is the FIC protein, which is a member of the C-C family.[443] The *fic* gene behaves as an immediate-early gene in serum-stimulated cells (quiescent NIH/3T3 cells). The *fic* gene is located, along with genes coding for other cytokines, on human chromosome 11, and encodes a 97-amino acid polypeptide with a predicted molecular weight of 11,084 Da. The secreted FIC protein has a predicted molecular weight of 8597 Da and binds to a subpopulation of MIP-1/MCP-1, but not MIP-2/MCP-2, receptors in monocytes and endothelial cells. The FIC protein transduces its intracellular signal through a pertussis toxin-sensitive G protein, as do other members of the superfamily of proinflammatory cytokines. Fic induces changes in the $[Ca^{2+}]_i$ in human monocytes, but not in platelets, neutrophils, or lymphocytes. The precise role of the FIC protein remains to be elucidated, but it may be involved in the processes associated with wound healing and tissue repair.

REFERENCES

1. **Bradley, T.R. and Metcalf, D.,** The growth of mouse bone marrow cells in vitro, *Aust. J. Exp. Biol. Med. Sci.,* 44, 287, 1966.
2. **Ichikawa, Y., Pluznik, D.H., and Sachs, L.,** In vitro control of the development of macrophage and granulocyte colonies, *Proc. Natl. Acad. Sci. U.S.A.,* 56, 488, 1966.
3. **Golde, D.W., Finley, T.N., and Cline, M.J.,** Production of colony-stimulating factor by human macrophages, *Lancet,* 2, 1397, 1972.

4. **Stanley, E.R., Hansen, G., Woodcock, J., and Metcalf, D.,** Colony stimulating factor and the regulation of granulopoiesis and macrophage production, *Fed. Proc.,* 34, 2272, 1975.
5. **Metcalf, D.,** The granulocyte-macrophage colony-stimulating factors, *Science,* 229, 16, 1985.
6. **Metcalf, D.,** The molecular biology and functions of the granulocyte-macrophage colony-stimulating factors, *Blood,* 67, 257, 1986.
7. **Clark, S.C. and Kamen, R.,** The human hematopoietic colony-stimulating factors, *Science,* 236, 1229, 1987.
8. **Ralph, P. and Warren, M.K.,** Molecular biology, cell biology and clinical future of myeloid growth factors, *Yearb. Immunol.,* 5, 103, 1989.
9. **Weisbart, R.H., Gasson, J.C., and Golde, D.W.,** Colony-stimulating factors and host defense, *Ann. Intern. Med.,* 110, 297, 1989.
10. **Andreeff, M. and Welte, K.,** Hematopoietic colony-stimulating factors, *Semin. Oncol.,* 16, 211, 1989.
11. **Whetton, A.D. and Dexter, T.M.,** Myeloid haematopoietic growth factors, *Biochim. Biophys. Acta,* 989, 111, 1989.
12. **Pimentel, E.,** Colony-stimulating factors, *Ann. Clin. Lab. Sci.,* 20, 36, 1990.
13. **Metcalf, D.,** The colony-stimulating factors: discovery, development, and clinical applications, *Cancer,* 65, 2185, 1990.
14. **Golde, D.W.,** Overview of myeloid growth factors, *Semin. Hematol.,* 27 (Suppl. 3), 1, 1990.
15. **Heyworth, C.M., Vallance, S.J., Whetton, A.D., and Dexter, T.M.,** The biochemistry and biology of the myeloid haemopoietic cell growth factors, *J. Cell Sci.,* Suppl. 13, 57, 1990.
16. **Gregory, S.H., Magee, D.M., and Wing, E.J.,** The role of colony-stimulating factors in host defenses, *Proc. Soc. Exp. Biol. Med.,* 197, 349, 1991.
17. **Metcalf, D.,** Control of granulocytes and macrophages: molecular, cellular, and clinical aspects, *Science,* 254, 529, 1991.
18. **Rapoport, A.P., Abboud, C.N., and DiPersio, J.F.,** Granulocyte-macrophage colony-stimulating factor (GM-CSF) and granulocyte colony-stimulating factor (G-CSF): receptor biology, signal transduction, and neutrophil activation, *Blood Rev.,* 6, 43, 1992.
19. **Harrington, M.A., Falkenburg, J.H.F., Daub, R., and Broxmeyer, H.E.,** Effect of myogenic and adipogenic differentiation on expression of colony-stimulating factor genes, *Mol. Cell. Biol.,* 10, 4948, 1990.
20. **Cook, N., Dexter, T.M., Lord, B.I., Cragoe, E.J., Jr., and Whetton, A.D.,** Identification of a common signal associated with cellular proliferation stimulated by four haemopoietic growth factors in a highly enriched population of granulocyte/macrophage colony-forming cells, *EMBO J.,* 8, 2967, 1989.
21. **Stanley, E.R., Guilbert, L.J., Tushinski, R.J., and Bartelmez, S.H.,** CSF-1 — a mononuclear phagocyte lineage-specific hemopoietic growth factor, *J. Cell. Biochem.,* 21, 151, 1983.
22. **Borzillo, G.V., Ashmun, R.A., and Sherr, C.J.,** Macrophage lineage switching of murine early pre-B lymphoid cells expressing transduced *fms* genes, *Mol. Cell. Biol.,* 10, 2703, 1990.
23. **Unanue, E.R. and Allen, P.M.,** The basis for the immunoregulatory role of macrophages and other accessory cells, *Science,* 236, 551, 1987.
24. **Nathan, C.F.,** Secretory products of macrophages, *J. Clin. Invest.,* 79, 319, 1987.
25. **Ulich, T.R., del Castillo, J., Watson, L.R., Yin, S., and Garnick, M.B.,** In vivo hematologic effects of recombinant human macrophage colony-stimulating factor, *Blood,* 75, 846, 1990.
26. **Koike, K., Stanley, E.R., Ihle, J.N., and Ogawa, M.,** Macrophage colony formation supported by purified CSF-1 and/or interleukin 3 in serum-free culture: evidence for hierarchical difference in macrophage colony-forming cells, *Blood,* 67, 859, 1986.
27. **Lyberg, T., Stanley, E.R., and Prydz, H.,** Colony-stimulating factor-1 induces thromboplastin activity in murine macrophages and human monocytes, *J. Cell. Physiol.,* 132, 367, 1987.
28. **DeNichilo, M.O., Stewart, A.G., Vadas, M.A., and Lopez, A.F.,** Granulocyte-macrophage colony-stimulating factor is a stimulant of platelet-activating factor and superoxide anion generation by human neutrophils, *J. Biol. Chem.,* 266, 4896, 1991.
29. **Warren, M.K. and Ralph, P.,** Macrophage growth factor CSF-1 stimulates human monocyte production of interferon, tumor necrosis factor, and colony stimulating activity, *J. Immunol.,* 137, 2281, 1986.
30. **Wing, E.J., Magee, D.M., Pearson, A.C., Waheed, A., and Shadduck, R.K.,** Peritoneal macrophages exposed to purified macrophage colony-stimulating factor (M-CSF) suppress mitogen-and antigen-stimulated lymphocyte proliferation, *J. Immunol.,* 137, 2768, 1986.

31. **Ralph, P. and Nakoinz, I.,** Stimulation of macrophage tumoricidal activity by the growth and differentiation factor CSF-1, *Cell. Immunol.,* 105, 270, 1987.
32. **Munn, D.H. and Cheung, N.-K.V.,** Phagocytosis of tumor cells by human monocytes cultured in recombinant macrophage colony-stimulating factor, *J. Exp. Med.,* 172, 231, 1990.
33. **Sampson-Johannes, A. and Carlino, J.A.,** Enhancement of human monocyte tumoricidal activity by recombinant M-CSF, *J. Immunol.,* 141, 3680, 1988.
34. **Ben-Avram, C.M., Shively, J.E., Shadduck, R.K., Waheed, A., Rajavashisth, T., and Lusis, A.J.,** Amino-terminal amino acid sequence of murine colony-stimulating factor 1, *Proc. Natl. Acad. Sci. U.S.A.,* 82, 4486, 1985.
35. **Tapley, P., Kazlauskas, A., Cooper, J.A., and Rohrschneider, L.R.,** Macrophage colony-stimulating factor-induced tyrosine phosphorylation of c-*fms* proteins expressed in FDC-P1 and BALB/c 3T3 cells, *Mol. Cell. Biol.,* 10, 2528, 1990.
36. **Rajavashisth, T.B., Eng, R., Shadduck, R.K., Waheed, A., Ben-Avram, C.M., Shively, J.E., and Lusis, A.J.,** Cloning and tissue-specific expression of mouse macrophage colony-stimulating factor mRNA, *Proc. Natl. Acad. Sci. U.S.A.,* 84, 1157, 1987.
37. **Gisselbrecht, S., Sola, B., Fichelson, S., Bordereaux, D., Tambourin, P., Mattei, M.-G., Simon, D., and Guenet, J.-L.,** The murine M-CSF gene is localized on chromosome 3, *Blood,* 73, 1742, 1989.
38. **Buchberg, A.M., Jenkins, N.A., and Copeland, N.G.,** Localization of the murine macrophage colony-stimulating factor gene to chromosome 3 using interspecific backcross analysis, *Genomics,* 5, 363, 1989.
39. **Waheed, A. and Shadduck, R.K.,** Purification of colony-stimulating factor by affinity chromatography, *Blood,* 60, 238, 1982.
40. **Das, S.K. and Stanley, E.R.,** Structure-function studies of a colony-stimulating factor (CSF-1), *J. Biol. Chem.,* 257, 13679, 1982.
41. **Ralph, P., Warren, M.K., Lee, M.T., Csejtey, J., Weaver, J.F., Broxmeyer, H.E., Williams, D.E., Stanley, E.R., and Kawasaki, E.S.,** Inducible production of human macrophage growth factor, CSF-1, *Blood,* 68, 633, 1986.
42. **Csejtey, J. and Boosman, A.,** Purification of human macrophage colony-stimulating factor (CSF-1) from medium conditioned by pancreatic carcinoma cells, *Biochem. Biophys. Res. Commun.,* 138, 238, 1986.
43. **Halenbeck, R., Shadle, P.J., Lee, P.-J., Lee, M.-T., and Koths, K.,** Purification and characterization of recombinant human macrophage colony-stimulating factor and generation of a neutralizing antibody useful for Western analysis, *J. Biotechnol.,* 8, 45, 1988.
44. **Pettenati, M.J., Le Beau, M.M., Lemons, R.S., Shima, E.A., Kawasaki, E.S., Larson, R.A., Sherr, C.J., Diaz, M.O., and Rowley, J.D.,** Assignment of *CSF-1* to 5q33.1: evidence for clustering of genes regulating hematopoiesis and for their involvement in the deletion of the long arm of chromosome 5 in myeloid disorders, *Proc. Natl. Acad. Sci. U.S.A.,* 84, 2970, 1987.
45. **Morris, S.W., Valentine, M.B., Shapiro, D.N., Sublett, J.E., Deaven, L.L., Foust, J.T., Roberts, W.M., Cerretti, D.P., and Look, A.T.,** Reassignment of the human *CSF1* gene to chromosome 1p13-p21, *Blood,* 78, 2013, 1991.
46. **Saltman, D.L., Dolganov, G.M., Hinton, L.M., and Lovett, M.,** Reassignment of the human macrophage colony-stimulating factor gene to chromosome 1p13-21, *Biochem. Biophys. Res. Commun.,* 182, 1139, 1992.
47. **Ralph, P., Warren, M.K., Nakoinz, I., Lee, M.-T., Brindley, L., Sampson-Johannes, A., Kawasaki, E.S., Ladner, M.B., Strickler, J.E., Boosman, A., Csejtey, J., and White, T.J.,** Biological properties and molecular biology of the human macrophage growth factor, CSF-1, *Immunobiology,* 172, 194, 1986.
48. **Ladner, M.B., Martin, G.A., Noble, J.A., Nikoloff, D.M., Tal, R., Kawasaki, E.S., and White, T.J.,** Human CSF-1: gene structure and alternative splicing of mRNA precursors, *EMBO J.,* 6, 2693, 1987.
49. **Rettenmier, C.W. and Roussel, M.F.,** Differential processing of colony-stimulating factor 1 precursors encoded by two human cDNAs, *Mol. Cell. Biol.,* 8, 5026, 1988.
50. **Wong, G.G., Temple, P.A., Leary, A.C., Witek-Giannotti, J.S., Yang, Y.-C., Ciarletta, A.B., Chung, M., Murtha, P., Kriz, R., Kaufman, R.J., Ferenz, C.R., Sibley, B.S., Turner, K.J., Hewick, R.M., Clark, S.C., Yanai, N., Yokota, H., Yamada, M., Saito, M., Motoyoshi, K., and Takaku, F.,** Human CSF-1: molecular cloning and expression of 4-kb cDNA encoding the human urinary protein, *Science,* 235, 1504, 1987.

51. **Pampfer, S., Tabibzadeh, S., Chuan, F.-C., and Pollard, J.W.,** Expression of colony-stimulating factor (CSF-1) messenger RNA in human endometrial glands during the menstrual cycle: molecular cloning of a novel transcript that predicts a cell surface form of CSF-1, *Mol. Endocrinol.,* 5, 1931, 1991.
52. **Shadle, P.J., Aldwin, L., Nitecki, D.E., and Koths, K.,** Human macrophage colony-stimulating factor heterogeneity results from alternative mRNA splicing, differential glycosylation, and proteolytic processing, *J. Cell. Biochem.,* 40, 91, 1989.
53. **Heard, J.M., Roussel, M.F., Rettenmier, C.W., and Sherr, C.J.,** Synthesis, post-translational processing, and autocrine transforming activity of a carboxylterminal truncated form of colony stimulating factor-1, *Oncogene Res.,* 1, 423, 1987.
54. **Takahashi, M., Hirato, T., Takano, M., Nishida, T., Nagamura, K., Kamogashira, T., Nakai, S., and Hirai, Y.,** Amino-terminal region of human macrophage colony-stimulating factor (M-CSF) is sufficient for its *in vitro* biological activity: molecular cloning and expression of carboxyl-terminal deletion mutants of human M-CSF, *Biochem. Biophys. Res. Commun.,* 161, 892, 1989.
55. **Nakamura, M., Merchav, S., Carter, A., Ernst, T.J., Demetri, G.D., Furukawa, Y., Anderson, K., Freedman, A.S., and Griffin, J.D.,** Expression of a novel 3.5-kb macrophage colony-stimulating factor transcript in human myeloma cells, *J. Immunol.,* 143, 3543, 1989.
56. **Rambaldi, A., Young, D.C., and Griffin, J.D.,** Expression of the M-CSF (CSF-1) gene by human monocytes, *Blood,* 69, 1409, 1987.
57. **Reisbach, G., Sindermann, J., Kremer, J.P., Hültner, L., Wolf, H., and Dörner, P.,** Macrophage colony-stimulating factor (CSF-1) is expressed by spontaneously outgrown EBV-B cell lines and activated normal B lymphocytes, *Blood,* 74, 959, 1989.
58. **Janowska-Wieczorek, A., Belch, A.R., Jacobs, A., Bowen, D., Padua, R.A., Paietta, E., and Stanley, E.R.,** *Blood,* 77, 1796, 1991.
59. **Horiguchi, J., Sariban, E., and Kufe, D.,** Transcriptional and posttranscriptional regulation of *CSF-1* gene expression in human monocytes, *Mol. Cell. Biol.,* 8, 3951, 1988.
60. **Fibbe, W.E., van Damme, J., Billiau, A., Goselink, H.M., Voogt, P.J., van Eeden, G., Ralph, P., Altrock, B.W., and Falkenburg, J.H.,** Interleukin 1 induces human marrow stromal cells in long-term culture to produce granulocyte colony-stimulating factor and macrophage colony-stimulating factor, *Blood,* 71, 430, 1988.
61. **Horiguchi, J., Warren, M.K., and Kufe, D.,** Expression of the macrophage-specific colony-stimulating factor in human monocytes treated with granulocyte-macrophage colony-stimulating factor, *Blood,* 69, 1259, 1987.
62. **Seelentag, W.K., Mermod, J.-J., Montesano, R., and Vassalli, P.,** Additive effects of interleukin 1 and tumour necrosis factor-α on the accumulation of the three granulocyte and macrophage colony-stimulating factor mRNAs in human endothelial cells, *EMBO J.,* 6, 2261, 1987.
63. **Abboud, S.L.,** Epidermal growth factor stimulates macrophage colony-stimulating factor (M-CSF) messenger RNA expression and M-CSF release in cultured murine stromal cells, *Br. J. Haematol.,* 80, 452, 1992.
64. **Abboud, S.L. and Pinzani, M.,** Peptide growth factors stimulate macrophage colony-stimulating factor in murine stromal cells, *Blood,* 78, 103, 1991.
65. **Umezawa, A., Tachibana, K., Harigaya, K., Kusakari, S., Kato, S., Watanabe, Y., and Takano, T.,** Colony-stimulating factor 1 expression is down-regulated during the adipocyte differentiation of H-1/A marrow stromal cells and induced by cachectin/tumor necrosis factor, *Mol. Cell. Biol.,* 11, 920, 1991.
66. **Bartocci, A., Pollard, J.W., and Stanley, E.R.,** Regulation of colony-stimulating factor 1 during pregnancy, *J. Exp. Med.,* 164, 956, 1986.
67. **Pollard, J.W., Bartocci, A., Arceci, R., Orlofsky, A., Ladner, M.B., and Stanley, E.R.,** Apparent role of the macrophage growth factor, CSF-1, in placental development, *Nature,* 330, 484, 1987.
68. **Arceci, R.J., Shanahan, F., Stanley, E.R., and Pollard, J.W.,** Temporal expression and location of colony-stimulating factor 1 (CSF-1) and its receptor in the female reproductive tract are consistent with CSF-1-regulated placental development, *Proc. Natl. Acad. Sci. U.S.A.,* 86, 8818, 1989.
69. **Kauma, S.W.,** Interleukin-1β stimulates colony-stimulating factor 1 production in human term placenta, *J. Clin. Endocrinol. Metab.,* 76, 701, 1993.
70. **Regenstreif, L.J. and Rossant, J.,** Expression of the c-*fms* proto-oncogene and of the cytokine, CSF-1, during mouse embryogenesis, *Develop. Biol.,* 133, 284, 1989.

71. Yoshida, H., Hayashi, S.-I., Kunisada, T., Ogawa, M., Nishikawa, S., Okamura, H., Sudo, T., Shultz, L.D., and Nishikawa, S.-I., The murine mutation osteopetrosis is in the coding region of the macrophage colony stimulating factor gene, *Nature,* 345, 442, 1990.
72. Wiktor-Jedrzejczak, W., Bartocci, A., Ferrante, A.W., Jr., Ahmed-Ansari, A., Sell, K.W., Pollard, J.W., and Stanley, E.R., Total absence of colony-stimulating factor 1 in the macrophage-deficient osteopetrotic *(op/op)* mouse, *Proc. Natl. Acad. Sci. U.S.A.,* 87, 4828, 1990.
73. Sherr, C.J., Colony-stimulating factor-1 receptor, *Blood,* 75, 1, 1990.
74. Huhn, R.D., Cicione, M.E., and Frackelton, A.R., Jr., Identification of tyrosine-phosphorylated colony-stimulating factor 1 (CSF-1) receptor and a 56-kilodalton protein phosphorylated in intact human cells in response to CSF-1, *J. Cell. Physiol.,* 39, 129, 1989.
75. Yeung, Y.G., Jubinsky, P.T., Sengupta, A., Yeung, D.C.Y., and Stanley, L.R., Purification of the colony-stimulating factor 1 receptor and demonstration of its tyrosine kinase activity, *Proc. Natl. Acad. Sci. U.S.A.,* 84, 1268, 1987.
76. Shurtleff, S.A., Downing, J.R., Rock, C.O., Hawkins, S.A., Roussel, M.F., and Sherr, C.J., Structural features of the colony-stimulating factor 1 receptor that affect its association with phosphatidylinositol 3-kinase, *EMBO J.,* 9, 2415, 1990.
77. Li, W. and Stanley, E.R., Role of dimerization and modification of the CSF-1 receptor in its activation and internalization during the CSF-1 response, *EMBO J.,* 10, 277, 1991.
78. Guilbert, L.J., Tynan, P.W., and Stanley, E.R., Uptake and destruction of ^{125}I-CSF-1 by peritoneal exudate macrophages, *J. Cell. Biochem.,* 31, 203, 1986.
79. Carlberg, K., Tapley, P., Haystead, C., and Rohrschneider, L., The role of kinase activity and the kinase insert region in ligand-induced internalization and degradation of the c-*fms* protein, *EMBO J.,* 10, 877, 1991.
80. Sherr, C.J., Rettenmier, C.W., Sacca, R., Roussel, M.F., Look, A.T., and Stanley, E.R., The c-*fms* proto-oncogene product is related to the receptor for the mononuclear phagocyte growth factor, CSF-1, *Cell,* 41, 665, 1985.
81. Manger, R., Najita, L., Nichols, E.J., Hakomori, S., and Rohrschneider, L., Cell surface expression of the McDonough strain of feline sarcoma virus *fms* gene product (gp140^{fms}), *Cell,* 39, 327, 1984.
82. Rettenmier, C.W., Roussel, M.F., Quinn, C.O., Kitchingman, G.R., Look, A.T., and Sherr, C.J., Transmembrane orientation of glycoproteins encoded by the v-*fms* oncogene, *Cell,* 40, 971, 1985.
83. Borzillo, G.V. and Sherr, C.J., Early pre-B-cell transformation induced by the v-*fms* oncogene in long-term mouse bone marrow cultures, *Mol. Cell. Biol.,* 9, 3973, 1989.
84. Wheeler, E.F., Askew, D., May, S., Ihle, J.N., and Sherr, C.J., The v-*fms* oncogene induces factor-independent growth and transformation of the interleukin-3-dependent myeloid cell line FDC-P1, *Mol. Cell. Biol.,* 7, 1673, 1987.
85. Nichols, E.J., Manger, R., Hakomori, S., Herscovics, A., and Rohrschneider, L.R., Transformation by the v-*fms* oncogene product: role of glycosylational processing and cell surface expression, *Mol. Cell. Biol.,* 5, 3467, 1985.
86. Nichols, E.J., Manger, R., Hakomori, S.-I., and Rohrschneider, L.R., Transformation by the oncogene v-*fms:* the effects of castanospermine on transformation-related parameters, *Exp. Cell Res.,* 173, 486, 1987.
87. Hadwiger, A., Niemann, H., Käbisch, A., Bauer, H., and Tamura, T., Appropriate glycosylation of the *fms* gene product is a prerequisite for its transforming potency, *EMBO J.,* 5, 689, 1986.
88. Sacca, R., Stanley, E.R., Sherr, C.J., and Rettenmier, C.W., Specific binding of the mononuclear phagocyte colony-stimulating factor CSF-1 to the product of the v-*fms* oncogene, *Proc. Natl. Acad. Sci. U.S.A.,* 83, 3331, 1986.
89. Sherr, C.J. and Rettenmier, C.W., The *fms* gene and the CSF-1 receptor, *Cancer Surv.,* 5, 221, 1986.
90. Rettenmier, C.W., Jackowski, S., Rock, C.O., Roussel, M.F., and Sherr, C.J., Transformation by the v-*fms* oncogene product: an analog of the CSF-1 receptor, *J. Cell. Biochem.,* 33, 109, 1987.
91. Sherr, C.J., Roussel, M.F., and Rettenmier, C.W., Colony-stimulating factor-1 receptor (c-*fms*), *J. Cell. Biochem.,* 38, 179, 1988.
92. Sherr, C.J., The *fms* oncogene, *Biochim. Biophys. Acta,* 948, 225, 1988.
93. Rettenmier, C.W., Roussel, M.F., and Sherr, C.J., The colony stimulating factor 1 (CSF-1) receptor (c-*fms* proto-oncogene product) and its ligand, *J. Cell Sci.,* Suppl. 9, 27, 1988.
94. Sherr, C.J., Rettenmier, C.W., and Roussel, M.F., Macrophage colony-stimulating factor, CSF-1, and its proto-oncogene-encoded receptor, *Cold Spring Harbor Symp. Quant. Biol.,* 53, 521, 1988.

95. **Rettenmier, C.W., Chen, J.H., Roussel, M.F., and Sherr, C.J.,** The product of the c-*fms* proto-oncogene: a glycoprotein with associated tyrosine kinase activity, *Science,* 228, 320, 1985.
96. **Smola, U., Hennig, D., Hadwiger-Fangmeier, A., Schütz, B., Pfaff, E., Niemann, H., and Tamura, T.,** Reassessment of the v-*fms* sequence: threonine phosphorylation of the COOH-terminal domain, *J. Virol.,* 65, 6181, 1991.
97. **Coussens, L., Van Beveren, C., Smith, D., Chen, E., Mitchell, R.L., Isacke, C.M., Verma, I.M., and Ullrich, A.,** Structural alteration of viral homologue of receptor proto-oncogene *fms* at carboxyl terminus, *Nature,* 320, 277, 1986.
98. **Furman, W.L., Rettenmier, C.W., Chen, J.H., Roussel, M.F., Quinn, C.O., and Sherr, C.J.,** Antibodies to distal carboxyl terminal epitopes in the v-*fms*-coded glycoprotein do not cross-react with the c-*fms* gene product, *Virology,* 152, 432, 1986.
99. **Rothwell, V.M. and Rohrschneider, L.R.,** Murine c-*fms* cDNA: cloning, sequence analysis and retroviral expression, *Oncogene Res.,* 1, 311, 1987.
100. **Browning, P.J., Bunn, H.F., Cline, A., Shuman, M., and Nienhuis, A.W.,** "Replacement" of COOH-terminal truncation of v-*fms* with c-*fms* sequences markedly reduces transformation potential, *Proc. Natl. Acad. Sci. U.S.A.,* 83, 7800, 1986.
101. **Sherr, C.J.,** Fibroblast and hematopoietic cell transformation by the *fms* oncogene (CSF-1 receptor), *J. Cell. Physiol.,* Suppl. 5, 83, 1987.
102. **Lyman, S.D. and Rohrschneider, L.R.,** Analysis of functional domains of the v-*fms*-encoded protein of Susan McDonough strain feline sarcoma virus by linker insertion mutagenesis, *Mol. Cell. Biol.,* 7, 3287, 1987.
103. **Roussel, M.F., Downing, J.R., Rettenmier, C.W., and Sherr, C.J.,** A point mutation in the extracellular domain of the human CSF-1 receptor (c-*fms* proto-oncogene product) activates its transforming potential, *Cell,* 55, 979, 1988.
104. **Li, W., Yeung, Y.G., and Stanley, E.R.,** Tyrosine phosphorylation of a common 57-kDa protein in growth factor-stimulated and -transformed cells, *J. Biol. Chem.,* 266, 6808, 1991.
105. **Taylor, G.R., Reedijk, M., Rothwell, V., Rohrschneider, L, and Pawson, T.,** The unique insert of cellular and viral *fms* protein tyrosine kinase domains is dispensable for enzymatic and transforming activities, *EMBO J.,* 8, 2029, 1989.
106. **Roussel, M.F., Shurtleff, S.A., Downing, J.R., and Sherr, C.J.,** A point mutation at tyrosine-809 in the human colony-stimulating factor 1 receptor impairs mitogenesis without abrogating tyrosine kinase activity, association with phosphatidylinositol 3-kinase, or induction of c-*fos* and *junB* genes, *Proc. Natl. Acad. Sci. U.S.A.,* 87, 6738, 1990.
107. **Verbeek, J.S., Roebroek, A.J.M., van den Ouwenland, A.M.W., Bloemers, H.P.J., and Van de Ven, W.J.M.,** Human c-*fms* proto-oncogene: comparative analysis with an abnormal allele, *Mol. Cell. Biol.,* 5, 422, 1985.
108. **Verbeek, J.S., van Heerikhuizen, H., de Pauw, B.E., Haanen, C., Bloemers, H.P.J., and Van de Ven, W.J.M.,** A hereditary abnormal c-*fms* proto-oncogene in a patient with acute lymphocytic leukaemia and congenital hypothyroidism, *Br. J. Haematol.,* 61, 135, 1985.
109. **Xu, D.Q., Guilhot, S., and Galibert, F.,** Restriction fragment length polymorphism of the human c-*fms* gene, *Proc. Natl. Acad. Sci. U.S.A.,* 82, 2862, 1985.
110. **Groffen, J., Heisterkamp, N., Spurr, N., Dana, S., Wasmuth, J.J., and Stephenson, J.R.,** Chromosomal localization of the human c-*fms* oncogene, *Nucleic Acids Res.,* 11, 6331, 1983.
111. **Le Beau, M.M., Westbrook, C.A., Diaz, M.O., Larson, R.A., Rowley, J.D., Gasson, J.C., Golde, D.W., and Sherr, C.J.,** Evidence for the involvement of *GM-CSF* and *FMS* in the deletion (5q) in myeloid disorders, *Science,* 231, 984, 1986.
112. **Nienhuis, A.W., Bunn, H.F., Turner, P.H., Gopal, T.V., Nash, W.G., O'Brien, S.J., and Sherr, C.J.,** Expression of the human c-*fms* proto-oncogene in hematopoietic cells and its deletion in the 5q-syndrome, *Cell,* 42, 421, 1985.
113. **Roberts, W.M., Look, A.T., Roussel, M.F., and Sherr, C.J.,** Tandem linkage of human CSF-1 receptor (c-*fms*) and PDGF receptor genes, *Cell,* 55, 655, 1988.
114. **Woolford, J., Rothwell, V., and Rohrschneider, L.,** Characterization of the human c-*fms* gene product and its expression in cells of the monocyte-macrophage lineage, *Mol. Cell. Biol.,* 5, 3458, 1985.
115. **Bartelmez, S.H. and Stanley, E.R.,** Synergism between hemopoietic growth factors (HGFs) detected by their effects on cells bearing receptors for a lineage specific HGF: assay of hemopoietin-1, *J. Cell. Physiol.,* 122, 370, 1985.

116. **Baker, A.H., Ridge, S.A., Hoy, T., Cachia, P.G., Culligan, D., Baines, P., Whittaker, J.A., Jacobs, A., and Padua, R.A.,** Expression of the colony-stimulating factor 1 receptor in B lymphocytes, *Oncogene,* 3, 371, 1993.
117. **Espinoza-Delgado, I., Longo, D.L., Gusella, G.O., and Varesio, L.,** IL-2 enhances c-fms expression in human monocytes, *J. Immunol.,* 145, 1137, 1990.
118. **Sherman, M.L., Weber, B.L., Datta, R., and Kufe, D.W.,** Transcriptional and posttranscriptional regulation of macrophage-specific colony stimulating factor gene expression by tumor necrosis factor. Involvement of arachidonic acid metabolism, *J. Clin. Invest.,* 85, 442, 1990.
119. **Gusella, G.L., Ayroldi, E., Espinoza-Delgado, I., and Varesio, L.,** Lipopolysaccharide, but not IFN-γ, down-regulates c-fms mRNA proto-oncogene expression in murine macrophages, *J. Immunol.,* 144, 3574, 1990.
120. **Rohrschneider, L.R. and Metcalf, D.,** Induction of macrophage colony-stimulating factor-dependent growth and differentiation after introduction of the murine c-*fms* gene into FDC-P1 cells, *Mol. Cell. Biol.,* 9, 5081, 1989.
121. **Kato, J. and Sherr, C.J.,** Human colony-stimulating factor 1 (CSF-1) receptor confers CSF-1 responsiveness to interleukin-3-dependent 32DCL3 mouse myeloid cells and abrogates differentiation in response to granulocyte CSF, *Blood,* 75, 1780, 1990.
122. **Hofstetter, W., Wetterwald, A., Cecchini, M.C., Felix, R., Fleisch, H., and Mueller, C.,** Detection of transcripts for the receptor for macrophage colony-stimulating factor, c-*fms,* in murine osteoclasts, *Proc. Natl. Acad. Sci. U.S.A.,* 89, 9637, 1992.
123. **Inaba, T., Yamada, N., Gotoda, T., Shimano, H., Shimada, M., Momomura, K., Kadowaki, T., Motoyoshi, K., Tsukada, T., Morisaki, N., Saito, Y., Yoshida, S., Takaku, F., and Yazaki, Y.,** Expression of M-CSF receptor encoded by c-*fms* on smooth muscle cells derived from arteriosclerotic lesion, *J. Biol. Chem.,* 267, 5693, 1992.
124. **Müller, R., Slamon, D.J., Adamson, E.D., Tremblay, J.M., Müller, D., Cline, M.J., and Verma, I.M.,** Transcription of c-*onc* genes c-*ras*^{Ki} and c-*fms* during mouse development, *Mol. Cell. Biol.,* 3, 1062, 1983.
125. **Rettenmier, C.W., Sacca, R., Furman, W.L., Roussel, M.F., Holt, J.T., Nienhuis, A.W., Stanley, E.R., and Sherr, C.J.,** Expression of the human c-*fms* proto-oncogene product (colony-stimulating factor-1 receptor) on peripheral blood mononuclear cells and choriocarcinoma cell lines, *J. Clin. Invest.,* 77, 1740, 1986.
126. **Slamon, D.J., de Kernion, J.B., Verma, I.M., and Cline, M.J.,** Expression of cellular oncogenes in human malignancies, *Science,* 224, 256, 1984.
127. **Ohtsuka, M., Roussel, M.F., Sherr, C.J., and Downing, J.R.,** Ligand-induced phosphorylation of the colony-stimulating factor 1 receptor can occur through an intermolecular reaction that triggers receptor down modulation, *Mol. Cell. Biol.,* 10, 1664, 1990.
128. **van der Geer, P. and Hunter, T.,** Tyrosine 706 and 807 phosphorylation site mutants in the murine colony-stimulating factor-1 receptor are unaffected in their ability to bind or phosphorylate phosphatidylinositol-3 kinase but show differential defects in their ability to induce early response gene transcription, *Mol. Cell. Biol.,* 11, 4698, 1991.
129. **Dubreuil, P., Torrès, H., Courcoul, M.-A., Birg, F., and Mannoni, P.,** c-*fms* Expression is a molecular marker of human acute myeloid leukemias, *Blood,* 72, 1081, 1988.
130. **Walker, C., Nettesheim, P., Barrett, J.C., and Gilmer, T.M.,** Expression of a *fms*-related oncogene in carcinogen-induced neoplastic epithelial cells, *Proc. Natl. Acad. Sci. U.S.A.,* 84, 1804, 1987.
131. **Wheeler, E.F., Rettenmier, C.W., Look, A.T., and Sherr, C.J.,** The v-*fms* oncogene induces factor independence and tumorigenicity in CSF-1 dependent macrophage cell line, *Nature,* 324, 377, 1986.
132. **Roussel, M.F. and Sherr, C.J.,** Mouse NIH 3T3 cells expressing human colony-stimulating factor 1 (CSF-1) receptors overgrow in serum-free medium containing human CSF-1 as their only growth factor, *Proc. Natl. Acad. Sci. U.S.A.,* 86, 7924, 1989.
133. **Stuart, R.K. and Hamilton, J.A.,** Tumor-promoting esters stimulate hematopoietic colony formation in vitro, *Science,* 208, 402, 1980.
134. **Chen, B.D.-M. and Wilkins, K.L.,** Role of phorbol ester receptors in the 12-O-tetradecanoyl-phorbol-13-acetate (TPA)-induced down-regulation of colony-stimulating factor (CSF-1) binding to murine peritoneal exudate macrophates, *J. Cell. Physiol.,* 124, 305, 1985.
135. **Downing, J.R., Roussel, M.F., and Sherr, C.J.,** Ligand and protein kinase C downmodulate the colony-stimulating factor 1 receptor by independent mechanisms, *Mol. Cell. Biol.,* 9, 2890, 1989.

136. Sariban, E., Mitchell, T., and Kufe, D., Expression of the c-*fms* proto-oncogene during human monocytic differentiation, *Nature,* 316, 64, 1985.
137. Horiguchi, J., Warren, M.K., Ralph, P., and Kufe, D., Expression of the macrophage specific colony-stimulating factor (CSF-1) during human monocytic differentiation, *Biochem. Biophys. Res. Commun.,* 141, 924, 1986.
138. Wakamiya, N., Horiguchi, J., and Kufe, D., Detection of c-fms and CSF-1 RNA by in situ hybridization, *Leukemia,* 1, 518, 1987.
139. Glazer, R.I., Chapekar, M.S., Hartman, K.D., and Knode, M.C., Appearance of membrane-bound tyrosine kinase during differentiation of HL-60 leukemia cells by immune interferon and tumor necrosis factor, *Biochem. Biophys. Res. Commun.,* 140, 908, 1986.
140. Downing, J.R., Rettenmier, C.W., and Sherr, C.J., Ligand-induced tyrosine kinase activity of the colony-stimulating factor 1 receptor in a murine macrophage cell line, *Mol. Cell. Biol.,* 8, 1795, 1988.
141. Sengupta, A., Liu, W.-K., Yeung, Y.G., Yeung, D.C.Y., Frackelton, A.R., Jr., and Stanley, E.R., Identification and subcellular localization of proteins that are rapidly phosphorylated in tyrosine in response to colony-stimulating factor 1, *Proc. Natl. Acad. Sci. U.S.A.,* 85, 8062, 1988.
142. Hamilton, J.A., Vairo, G., and Lingelbach, S.R., CSF-1 stimulates glucose uptake in murine bone marrow-derived macrophages, *Biochem. Biophys. Res. Commun.,* 138, 445, 1986.
143. Vairo, G. and Hamilton, J.A., CSF-1 stimulates Na$^+$K$^+$-ATPase mediated ^{86}Rb$^+$ uptake in mouse bone marrow-derived macrophages, *Biochem. Biophys. Res. Commun.,* 132, 430, 1985.
144. Whetton, A.D., Monk, P.N., Consalvey, S.D., and Downes, C.P., The haemopoietic growth factors interleukin 3 and colony-stimulating factor-1 stimulate proliferation but do not induce inositol lipid breakdown in murine bone-marrow-derived macrophages, *EMBO J.,* 5, 3281, 1986.
145. Xu, X.X., Tessner, T.G., Rock, C.O., and Jackowski, S., Phosphatidylinositol hydrolysis and c-*myc* expression are in collaborating mitogenic pathways activated by colony-stimulating factor 1, *Mol. Cell. Biol.,* 13, 1522, 1993.
146. Veis, N. and Hamilton, J.A., Colony-stimulating factor 1 stimulates diacylglycerol generation in murine bone marrow-derived macrophages, but not in resident peritoneal macrophages, *J. Cell Physiol.,* 147, 298, 1991.
147. Downing, J.R., Margolis, B.L., Zilberstein, A., Ashmun, A., Ullrich, A., Sherr, C.J., and Schlessinger, J., Phospholipase Cγ, a substrate for PDGF receptor kinase, is not phosphorylated on tyrosine during the mitogenic response to CSF-1, *EMBO J.,* 8, 3345, 1989.
148. Varticovski, L., Druker, B., Morrison, D., Cantley, L., and Roberts, T., The colony-stimulating factor-1 receptor associates with an activates phosphatidylinositol-3 kinase, *Nature,* 342, 699, 1989.
149. Reedijk, M., Liu, X., and Pawson, T., Interactions of phosphatidylinositol kinase, GTPase-activating protein (GAP), and GAP-associated proteins with colony-stimulating factor 1 receptor, *Mol. Cell. Biol.,* 10, 5601, 1990.
150. Downing, J.R., Shurtleff, S.A., and Sherr, C.J., Peptide antisera to human colony-stimulating factor 1 receptor detect ligand-induced conformational changes and a binding site for phosphatidylinositol 3-kinase, *Mol. Cell. Biol.,* 11, 2489, 1991.
151. Matsushime, H., Roussel, M.F., Ashmun, R.A., and Sherr, C.J., Colony-stimulating factor 1 regulates novel cyclins during the G1 phase of the cell cycle, *Cell,* 65, 701, 1991.
152. Roussel, M.F., Cleveland, J.L., Shurtleff, S.A., and Sherr, C.J., *Myc* rescue of a mutant CSF-1 receptor impaired in mitogenic signaling, *Nature,* 353, 361, 1991.
153. Müller, R., Curran, T., Müller, D., and Guilbert, L., Induction of c-*fos* during myelomonocytic differentiation and macrophage proliferation, *Nature,* 314, 546, 1985.
154. Bravo, R., Neuberg, M., Burckhardt, J., Almendral, J., Wallich, R., and Müller, R., Involvement of common and cell type-specific pathways in c-*fos* gene control: stable induction by cAMP in macrophages, *Cell,* 48, 251, 1987.
155. Schaberg, T. and Filderman, A.E., Colony-stimulating factor induction of protooncogene expression in rat alveolar macrophages, *Am. J. Physiol.,* 159, L144, 1990.
156. Willman, C.L., Stewart, C.C., Griffith, J.K., Stewart, S.J., and Tomasi, T.B., Differential expression and regulation of the c-*src* and c-*fgr* protooncogenes in myelomonocytic cells, *Proc. Natl. Acad. Sci. U.S.A.,* 84, 4480, 1987.
157. Yi, T.-L. and Willman, C.L., Cloning of the murine c-*fgr* proto-oncogene cDNA and induction of c-*fgr* expression by proliferation and activation factors in normal bone marrow-derived monocytic cells, *Oncogene,* 4, 1081, 1989.

158. **Duprey, S.P. and Boettiger, D.,** Developmental regulation of c-*myb* in normal myeloid progenitor cells, *Proc. Natl. Acad. Sci. U.S.A.,* 82, 6937, 1985.
159. **Courtneidge, S.A., Dhand, R., Pilat, D., Twamley, G.M., Waterfield, M.D., and Roussel, M.F.,** Activation of Src family kinases by colony stimulating factor-1, and their association with its receptor, *EMBO J.,* 12, 943, 1993.
160. **Choudhury, G.G., Sylvia, V.L., Pfeifer, A., Wang, L.-M., Smith, A.E., and Sakaguchi, A.Y.,** Human colony stimulating factor-1 receptor activates the c-*raf*-1 proto-oncogene kinase, *Biochem. Biophys. Res. Commun.,* 172, 154, 1990.
161. **Baccarini, M., Sabatini, D.M., App, H., Rapp, U.R., and Stanley, E.R.,** Colony stimulating factor-1 (CSF-1) stimulates temperature dependent phosphorylation and activation of the RAF-1 proto-oncogene product, *EMBO J.,* 9, 3649, 1990.
162. **Langer, S.J., Bortner, D.M., Roussel, M.F., Sherr, C.J., and Ostrowski, M.C.,** Mitogenic signaling by colony-stimulating factor 1 and *ras* is suppressed by the *ets*-2 DNA-binding domain and restored by *myc* overexpression, *Mol. Cell. Biol.,* 12, 5355, 1992.
163. **Sklar, M.D., Tereba, A., Chen, B.D.-M., and Walker, W.S.,** Transformation of mouse bone marrow cells by transfection with a human oncogene related to c-myc is associated with the endogenous production of macrophage colony stimulating factor 1, *J. Cell. Physiol.,* 125, 403, 1985.
164. **Baumbach, W.R., Colston, E.M., and Cole, M.D.,** Integration of the BALB/c ecotropic provirus into the colony-stimulating factor-1 growth factor locus in a myc retrovirus-induced murine monocyte tumor, *J. Virol.,* 62, 3151, 1988.
165. **Sherr, C.J.,** The role of the CSF-1 receptor gene (c-*fms*) in cell transformation, *Leukemia,* 2, 132S, 1988.
166. **Rettenmier, C.W., Roussel, M.F., Ashmun, R.A., Ralph, P., Price, K., and Sherr, C.J.,** Synthesis of membrane-bound colony-stimulating factor 1 (CSF-1) and downmodulation of CSF-1 receptors in NIH 3T3 cells transformed by cotransfection of the human CSF-1 and c-*fms* (CSF-1 receptor) genes, *Mol. Cell. Biol.,* 7, 2378, 1987.
167. **Roussel, M.F., Rettenmier, C.W., and Sherr, C.J.,** Introduction of a human colony stimulating factor-1 gene into a mouse macrophage cell line induces CSF-1 independence but not tumorigenicity, *Blood,* 71, 1218, 1988.
168. **Roussel, M.F., Downing, J.R., and Sherr, C.J.,** Transforming activities of human CSF-1 receptors with different point mutations at codon 301 in their extracellular domains, *Oncogene,* 5, 25, 1990.
169. **Parwaresch, M.R., Kreipe, H., Felgner, J., Heidorn, K., Jaquet, K., Bödewadt-Radzun, S., and Radzun, H.J.,** M-CSF and M-CSF-receptor gene expression in acute myelomonocytic leukemias, *Leukemia Res.,* 14, 27, 1990.
170. **Ashmun, R.A., Look, A.T., Roberts, W.M., Roussel, M.F., Seremetis, S., Ohtsuka, M., and Sherr, C.J.,** Monoclonal antibodies to the human CSF-1 receptor (c-*fms* proto-oncogene product) detect epitopes on normal mononuclear phagocytes and on human myeloid leukemic blast cells, *Blood,* 73, 827, 1989.
171. **Rambaldi, A., Wakamiya, N., Vellenga, E., Horiguchi, J., Warren, M.K., Kufe, D., and Griffin, J.D.,** Expression of the macrophage colony-stimulating factor and c-*fms* genes in human acute myeloblastic leukemia cells, *J. Clin. Invest.,* 81, 1030, 1988.
172. **Kacinski, B.M., Carter, D., Mittal, K., Kohorn, E.I., Bloodgood, R.S., Donahue, J., Donofrio, L., Edwards, R., Schwartz, P.E., Chambers, J.T., and Chambers, S.K.,** High level expression of fms proto-oncogene mRNA is observed in clinically aggressive human endometrial adenocarcinomas, *Int. J. Radiat. Oncol. Biol. Phys.,* 15, 823, 1988.
173. **Kacinski, B.M., Carter, D., Mittal, K., Yee, L.D., Scata, K.A., Donofrio, L., Chambers, S.K., Wang, K.-I., Yang-Feng, T., Rohrschneider, L.R., and Rothwell, V.M.,** Ovarian adenocarcinomas express *fms*-complementary transcripts and *fms* antigen, often with coexpression of CSF-1, *Am. J. Pathol.,* 137, 135, 1990.
174. **Suzuki, T., Nagata, K., Murohashi, I., and Nara, N.,** Effect of recombinant human M-CSF on the proliferation of leukemic blast progenitors in AML patients, *Leukemia,* 2, 358, 1988.
175. **Bonnem, E.M. and Morstyn, G.,** Granulocyte macrophage colony stimulating factor (GM-CSF). Current status and future development, *Semin. Oncol.,* 15, 46, 1988.
176. **Coffey, R.G.,** Mechanism of GM-CSF stimulation of neutrophils, *Immunol. Res.,* 8, 236, 1989.
177. **Monroy, R.L., Davis, T.A., and MacVittie, T.J.,** Granulocyte-macrophage colony-stimulating factor: more than a hemopoietin, *Clin. Immunol. Immunopathol.,* 54, 333, 1990.

178. Gasson, J.C., Molecular physiology of granulocyte-macrophage colony-stimulating factor, *Blood*, 77, 1131, 1991.
179. Baldwin, G.C., The biology of granulocyte-macrophage colony-stimulating factor. Effects on hematopoietic and nonhematopoietic cells, *Develop. Biol.*, 151, 352, 1992.
180. Pluznik, D.H., Cunningham, R.E., and Noguchi, P.D., Colony-stimulating factor (CSF) controls proliferation of CSF-dependent cells by acting during the G_1 phase of the cell cycle, *Proc. Natl. Acad. Sci. U.S.A.*, 81, 7451, 1984.
181. Gliniak, B.C. and Rohrschneider, L.R., Expression of the M-CSF receptor is controlled posttranscriptionally by the dominant actions of GM-CSF or multi-CSF, *Cell*, 63, 1073, 1990.
182. Griffin, J.D., Young, D., Herrmann, F., Wiper, D., Wagner, K., and Sabbath, K.D., Effects of recombinant human GM-CSF on proliferation of clonogenic cells in acute myeloblastic leukemia, *Blood*, 67, 1448, 1986.
183. Boyum, A., Lovhaug, D., Kolsto, A.B., Helgestad, J., and Melby, T., Colony inhibiting factor in mature granulocytes from normal individuals and patients with chronic myeloid leukemia, *Eur. J. Haematol.*, 38, 318, 1987.
184. Lopez, A.F., Williamson, D.J., Gamble, J.R., Begley, C.G., Harlan, J.M., Klebanoff, S.J., Waltersdorph, A., Wong, G., Clark, S.C., and Vadas, M.A., Recombinant human granulocyte-macrophage colony-stimulating factor stimulates in vitro mature human neutrophil and eosinophil function, surface expression, and survival, *J. Clin. Invest.*, 78, 1220, 1986.
185. Chen, B.D.-M., Clark, C.R., and Chou, T., Granulocyte/macrophage colony-stimulating factor stimulates monocyte and tissue macrophage proliferation and enhances their responsiveness to macrophage colony-stimulating factor, *Blood*, 71, 997, 1988.
186. Caracciolo, D., Shirsat, N., Wong, G.G., Lange, B., Clark, S., and Rovera, G., Recombinant human macrophage colony-stimulating factor (M-CSF) requires subliminal concentrations of granulocyte/macrophage (GM)-CSF for optimal stimulation of human macrophage colony formation in vitro, *J. Exp. Med.*, 166, 1851, 1987.
187. Chen, B.D.M., Mueller, M., and Chou, T., Role of granulocyte/macrophage colony-stimulating factor in the regulation of murine alveolar macrophage proliferation and differentiation, *J. Immunol.*, 141, 139, 1988.
188. Lindemann, A., Riegel, D., Oster, W., Ziegler-Heitbrock, H.W.L., Mertelsmann, R., and Herrmann, F., Granulocyte-macrophage colony-stimulating factor induces cytokine secretion by human polymorphonuclear leukocytes, *J. Clin. Invest.*, 83, 1308, 1989.
189. Vink, A., Vandenabeele, P., Uyttenhove, C., Cayphas, S., and Van Snick, J., Plasmacytoma growth factor activity of murine granulocyte-macrophage colony-stimulating factor, *J. Immunol.*, 141, 1996, 1988.
190. Grabstein, K., Mochizuki, D., Kronheim, S., Price, V., Cosman, D., Urdal, D., Gillis, S., and Conlon, P., Regulation of antibody production *in vitro* by granulocyte-macrophage colony stimulating factor, *J. Mol. Cell. Immunol.*, 2, 199, 1986.
191. Kupper, T., Flood, P., Coleman, D., and Horowitz, M., Growth of an interleukin 2/interleukin 4-dependent T-cell line induced by granulocyte-macrophage colony-stimulating factor (GM-CSF), *J. Immunol.*, 138, 4288, 1987.
192. Santoli, D., Clark, S.C., Kreider, B.L., Maslin, P.A., and Rovera, G., Amplification of IL-2-driven T-cell proliferation by recombinant human IL-3 and granulocyte-macrophage colony-stimulating factor, *J. Immunol.*, 141, 519, 1988.
193. Smith, P.D., Lamerson, C.L., Wong, H.L., Wahl, L.M., and Wahl, S.M., Granulocyte-macrophage colony-stimulating factor stimulates human monocyte accessory cells function, *J. Immunol.*, 144, 3829, 1990.
194. Grabstein, K.H., Urdal, D.L., Tushinski, R.J., Mochizuki, D.Y., Price, V.L., Cantrell, M.A., Gillis, S., and Conlon, P.J., Induction of macrophage tumoricidal activity by granulocyte-macrophage colony-stimulating factor, *Science*, 232, 506, 1986.
195. Cannistra, S.A., Vellenga, E., Groshek, P., Rambaldi, A., and Griffin, J.D., Human granulocyte-monocyte colony-stimulating factor and interleukin 3 stimulate monocyte cytotoxicity through a tumor necrosis factor-dependent mechanism, *Blood*, 71, 672, 1988.
196. Elliott, M.J., Vadas, M.A., Eglinton, J.M., Park, L.S., To, L.B., Cleland, L.G., Clark, S.C., and Lopez, A.F., Recombinant human interleukin-3 and granulocyte-macrophage colony-stimulating factor show common biological effects and binding characteristics on human monocytes, *Blood*, 74, 2349, 1989.

197. **Sieff, C.A., Emerson, S.G., Donahue, R.E., Nathan, D.G., Wang, E.A., Wong, G.G., and Clark, S.C.,** Human recombinant granulocyte-macrophage colony-stimulating factor: a multilineage hematopoietin, *Science,* 230, 1171, 1985.
198. **Emerson, S.G., Yang, Y.-C., Clark, S.C., and Long, M.W.,** Human recombinant granulocyte-macrophage colony stimulating factor and interleukin 3 have overlapping but distinct hematopoietic activities, *J. Clin. Invest.,* 82, 1282, 1988.
199. **Saeland, S., Caux, C., Favre, C., Duvert, V., Pébusque, M.-J., Mannoni, P., and de Vries, J.E.,** Combined and sequential effects of human IL-3 and GM-CSF on the proliferation of CD34+ hematopoietic cells from cord blood, *Blood,* 73, 1195, 1989.
200. **Donahue, R.E., Seehra, J., Metzger, M., Lefebvre, D., Rock, B., Carbone, S., Nathan, D.G., Garnick, M., Sehgal, P.K., Laston, LaVallie, E., McCoy, J., Schendel, P.F., Norton, C., Turner, K., Yang, Y.-C., and Clark, S.C.,** Human IL-3 and GM-CSF act synergistically in stimulating hematopoiesis in primates, *Science,* 241, 1820, 1988.
201. **Ferrero, D., Tarella, C., Badoni, R., Caracciolo, D., Bellone, G., Pileri, A., and Gallo, E.,** Granulocyte-macrophage colony-stimulating factor requires interaction with accessory cells or granulocyte-colony stimulating factor for full stimulation of human myeloid progenitors, *Blood,* 73, 402, 1989.
202. **Bot, F.J., van Eijk, L., Schipper, P., and Löwenberg, B.,** Human granulocyte-macrophage colony-stimulating factor (GM-CSF) stimulates immature marrow precursors but not CFU-GM, CF-Y-G, or CFU-M, *Exp. Hematol.,* 17, 292, 1989.
203. **Sonoda, Y., Yang, Y.-C., Wong, G.G., Clark, S.C., and Ogawa, M.,** Analysis in serum-free culture of the targets of recombinant human hemopoietic growth factors: interleukin 3 and granulocyte/macrophage-colony-stimulating factor are specific for early developmental stages, *Proc. Natl. Acad. Sci. U.S.A.,* 85, 4360, 1988.
204. **Koike, K., Ogawa, M., Ihle, J.N., Miyake, T., Shimizu, T., Miyajima, A., Yokota, T., and Arai, K.,** Recombinant murine granulocyte-macrophage (GM) colony-stimulating factor supports formation of GM and multipotential blast cell colonies in culture: comparison with the effects of interleukin-3, *J. Cell. Physiol.,* 131, 458, 1987.
205. **Metcalf, D., Begley, C.G., Johnson, G.R., Nicola, N.A., Vadas, M.A., Lopez, A.F., Williamson, D.J., Wong, G.G., Clark, S.C., and Wang, E.A.,** Biologic properties in vitro of a recombinant human granulocyte-macrophage colony-stimulating factor, *Blood,* 67, 37, 1986.
206. **Robinson, B.E., McGrath, H.E., and Quesenberry, P.J.,** Recombinant murine granulocyte macrophage colony-stimulating factor has megakaryocyte colony-stimulating activity and augments megakaryocyte colony stimulation by interleukin 3, *J. Clin. Invest.,* 79, 1648, 1987.
207. **Vannucchi, A.M., Grossi, A., Rafanelli, D., and Ferrini, P.L.,** In vivo stimulation of megakaryocytopoiesis by recombinant murine granulocyte-macrophage colony-stimulating factor, *Blood,* 76, 1473, 1990.
208. **Ulich, T.R., del Castillo, J., McNiece, I., Watson, L., Yin, S., and Andresen, J.,** Hematologic effects of recombinant murine granulocyte-macrophage colony-stimulating factor on the peripheral blood and bone marrow, *Am. J. Pathol.,* 137, 369, 1990.
209. **Aglietta, M., Piacibello, W., Sanavio, F., Stacchini, A., Aprá, F., Schena, M., Mossetti, C., Carnino, F., Caligaris-Cappio, F., and Gavosto, F.,** Kinetics of human hemopoietic cells after in vivo administration of granulocyte-macrophage colony-stimulating factor, *J. Clin. Invest.,* 83, 551, 1989.
210. **Dedhar, S., Gaboury, L., Galloway, P., and Eaves, C.,** Human granulocyte-macrophage colony-stimulating factor is a growth factor active on a variety of cell types of nonhemopoietic origin, *Proc. Natl. Acad. Sci. U.S.A.,* 85, 9253, 1988.
211. **Evans, D.B., Bunning, R.A.D., and Russell, R.G.G.,** The effects of recombinant human granulocyte-macrophage colony-stimulating factor (rhGM-CSF) on human osteoblast-like cells, *Biochem. Biophys. Res. Commun.,* 160, 588, 1989.
212. **Gough, N.M., Gough, J., Metcalf, D., Kelso, A., Grail, D., Nicola, N.A., Burgess, A.W., and Dunn, A.R.,** Molecular cloning of cDNA encoding a murine haematopoietic growth regulator, granulocyte-macrophage colony-stimulating factor, *Nature,* 309, 763, 1984.
213. **Kajigaya, S., Suda, T., Suda, J., Saito, M., Miura, Y., Iizuka, M., Kobayashi, S., Minato, N., and Sudo, T.,** A recombinant murine granulocyte/macrophage (GM) colony-stimulating factor derived from an inducer T cell line (IH5.5), *J. Exp. Med.,* 164, 1102, 1986.

214. **Metcalf, D., Burgess, A.W., Johnson, G.R., Nicola, N.A., Nice, E.C., DeLamarter, J., Thatcher, D.R., and Mermod, J.-J.,** In vitro actions on hemopoietic cells of recombinant murine GM-CSF purified after production in *Escherichia coli:* comparison with purified native GM-CSF, *J. Cell. Physiol.,* 128, 421, 1986.
215. **DeLarmarter, J.F., Mermod, J.-J., Liang, C.-M., Eliason, J.F., and Thatcher, D.R.,** Recombinant murine GM-CSF from *E. coli* has biological activity and is neutralized by a specific antiserum, *EMBO J.,* 4, 2575, 1985.
216. **Shanafelt, A.B. and Kastelein, R.A.,** Identification of critical regions in mouse granulocyte-macrophage colony-stimulating factor by scanning-deletion analysis, *Proc. Natl. Acad. Sci. U.S.A.,* 86, 4872, 1989.
217. **Wong, G.G., Witek, J.S., Temple, P.A., Wilkens, K.M., Leary, A.C., Luxenberg, D.P., Jones, S.S., Brown, E.L., Kay, R.M., Orr, E.C., Shoemaker, C., Golde, D.W., Kaufman, R.J., Hewick, R.M., Wang, E.A., and Clark, S.C.,** Human GM-CSF: molecular cloning of the complementary DNA and purification of the natural and recombinant proteins, *Science,* 228, 810, 1985.
218. **Lee, F., Yokota, T., Otsuka, T., Gemmell, L., Larson, N., Luh, J., Arai, K., and Rennick, D.,** Isolation of cDNA for a human granulocyte-macrophage colony-stimulating factor by functional expression in mammalian cells, *Proc. Natl. Acad. Sci. U.S.A.,* 82, 4360, 1985.
219. **Cantrell, M.A., Anderson, D., Cerretti, D.P., Price, V., McKereghan, K., Tushinski, R.J., Mochizuki, D.Y., Larsen, A., Grabstein, K., Gillis, S., and Cosman, D.,** Cloning, sequence, and expression of a human granulocyte/macrophage colony-stimulating factor, *Proc. Natl. Acad. Sci. U.S.A.,* 82, 6250, 1985.
220. **Kaushansky, K., O'Ohara, P.J., Berkner, K., Segal, G.M., Hagen, F.S., and Adamson, J.W.,** Genomic cloning, characterization, and multilineage growth-promoting activity of human granulocyte-macrophage colony-stimulating factor, *Proc. Natl. Acad. Sci. U.S.A.,* 83, 3101, 1986.
221. **Libby, R.T., Braedt, G., Kronheim, S.R., March, C.J., Urdal, D.L., Chiaverotti, T.A., Tushinski, R.J., Mochizuki, D.Y., Hopp, T.P., and Cosman, D.,** Expression and purification of native human granulocyte-macrophage colony-stimulating factor from an *Escherichia coli* secretion vector, *DNA,* 6, 221, 1987.
222. **Moonen, P., Mermod, J.-J., Ernst, J.F., Hirschi, M., and DeLamarter, J.F.,** Increased biological activity of deglycosylated recombinant human granulocyte/macrophage colony-stimulating factor produced by yeast or animal cells, *Proc. Natl. Acad. Sci. U.S.A.,* 84, 4428, 1987.
223. **Miyatake, S., Otsuka, T., Yokota, T., Lee, F., and Arai, K.,** Structure of the chromosomal gene for granulocyte-macrophage colony stimulating factor: comparison of the mouse and human genes, *EMBO J.,* 4, 2561, 1985.
224. **Stanley, E., Metcalf, D., Sobieszczuk, P., Gough, N.M., and Dunn, A.R.,** The structure and expression of the murine gene encoding granulocyte-macrophage colony stimulating factor: evidence for utilisation of alternative promoters, *EMBO J.,* 4, 2569, 1985.
225. **Chan, J.Y., Slamon, D.J., Nimer, S.D., Golde, D.W., and Gasson, J.C.,** Regulation of expression of human granulocyte/macrophage colony-stimulating factor, *Proc. Natl. Acad. Sci. U.S.A.,* 83, 8669, 1986.
226. **Shannon, M.F., Gamble, J.R., and Vadas, M.A.,** Nuclear proteins interacting with the promoter region of the human granulocyte/macrophate colony-stimulating factor gene, *Proc. Natl. Acad. Sci. U.S.A.,* 85, 674, 1988.
227. **Nimer, S.D., Morita, E.A., Martis, M.J., Wachsman, W., and Gasson, J.C.,** Characterization of the human granulocyte-macrophage colony-stimulating factor promoter region by genetic analysis: correlation with DNase I footprinting, *Mol. Cell. Biol.,* 8, 1979, 1988.
228. **Huebner, K., Isobe, M., Croce, C.M., Golde, D.W., Kaufman, S.E., and Gasson, J.C.,** The human gene encoding GM-CSF is at 5q21-q32, the chromosome region deleted in the 5q- anomaly, *Science,* 230, 1282, 1985.
229. **Huebner, K., Nagarajan, L., Besa, E., Angert, E., Lange, B.J., Cannizzaro, L.A., van den Berghe, H., Santoli, D., Finan, J., Croce, C.M., and Nowell, P.C.,** Order of genes on human chromosome 5q with respect to 5q interstitial deletions, *Am. J. Hum. Genet.,* 46, 26, 1990.
230. **van den Berghe, H., Vermaelen, K., Mecucci, C., Barbieri, D., and Tricot, G.,** The 5q- anomaly, *Cancer Genet. Cytogenet.,* 17, 189, 1985.
231. **Zupo, S., Perussia, B., Baldi, L., Corcione, A., Dono, M., Ferrarini, M., and Pistoia, V.,** Production of granulocyte-macrophage colony-stimulating factor but not IL-3 by normal and neoplastic human lymphocytes B, *J. Immunol.,* 148, 1423, 1992.

232. **Thorens, B., Mermod, J.-J., and Vassalli, P.,** Phagocytosis and inflammatory stimuli induce GM-CSF mRNA in macrophage through posttranscriptional regulation, *Cell,* 48, 671, 1987.
233. **Fibbe, W.E., Van Damme, J., Billiau, A., Voogt, P.J., Duinkerken, N., Kluck, P.M.C., and Falkenburg, J.H.F.,** Interleukin-1 (22-K factor) induces release of granulocyte-macrophage colony-stimulating activity from human mononuclear phagocytes, *Blood,* 68, 1316, 1986.
234. **Herrmann, F., Oster, W., Meuer, S.C., Lindemann, A., and Mertelsmann, R.H.,** Interleukin 1 stimulates T lymphocytes to produce granulocyte-monocyte colony-stimulating factor, *J. Clin. Invest.,* 81, 1415, 1988.
235. **Quill, H., Gaur, A., and Phipps, R.P.,** Prostaglandin E_2-dependent induction of granulocyte-macrophage colony-stimulating factor secretion by cloned murine helper T cells, *J. Immunol.,* 142, 813, 1989.
236. **Malone, D.G., Pierce, J.H., Falko, J.P., and Metcalfe, D.D.,** Production of granulocyte-macrophage colony-stimulating factor by primary cultures of unstimulated rat microvascular endothelial cells, *Blood,* 71, 684, 1988.
237. **Seelentag, W.K., Mermod, J.-J., Montesano, R., and Vassalli, P.,** Additive effects of interleukin 1 and tumour necrosis factor-α on the accumulation of the three granulocyte and macrophage colony-stimulating factor mRNAs in human endothelial cells, *EMBO J.,* 6, 2261, 1987.
238. **Broudy, V.C., Kaushansky, K., Segal, G.M., Harlan, J.M., and Adamson, J.W.,** Tumor necrosis factor type α stimulates human endothelial cells to produce granulocyte/macrophage colony-stimulating factor, *Proc. Natl. Acad. Sci. U.S.A.,* 83, 7467, 1986.
239. **Sieff, C.A., Tsai, S., and Faller, D.V.,** Interleukin 1 induces cultured human endothelial cell production of granulocyte-macrophage colony-stimulating factor, *J. Clin. Invest.,* 79, 48, 1987.
240. **Bickel, M., Tsuda, H., Amstad, P., Evequoz, V., Mergenhangen, S.E., Wahl, S.M., and Pluznik, D.H.,** Differential regulation of colony-stimulating factors and interleukin 2 production by cyclosporin A, *Proc. Natl. Acad. Sci. U.S.A.,* 84, 3274, 1987.
241. **Chodakewitz, J.A., Kupper, T.S., and Coleman, D.L.,** Keratinocyte-derived granulocyte/macrophage colony-stimulating factor induces DNA synthesis by peritoneal macrophages, *J. Immunol.,* 140, 832, 1988.
242. **Yang, Y.-C., Tsai, S., Wong, G.G., and Clark, S.C.,** Interleukin-1 regulation of hematopoietic growth factor production by human stromal fibroblasts, *J. Cell. Physiol.,* 134, 292, 1988.
243. **Koury, M.J. and Pragnell, I.B.,** Retroviruses induce granulocyte-macrophage colony stimulating activity in fibroblasts, *Nature,* 299, 638, 1982.
244. **Tobler, A., Marti, H.P., Gimmi, C., Cachelin, A.B., Saurer, S., and Fey, M.F.,** Dexamethasone and 1,25-dihydroxyvitamin-D_3, but not cyclosporine-A, inhibit production of granulocyte-macrophage colony-stimulating factor in human fibroblasts, *Blood,* 77, 1912, 1991.
245. **Malipiero, U.V., Frei, K., and Fontana, A.,** Production of hemopoietic colony-stimulating factors by astrocytes, *J. Immunol.,* 144, 3816, 1990.
246. **Ohno, K., Suzumura, A., Sawada, M., and Marunouchi, T.,** Production of granulocyte/macrophage colony-stimulating factor by cultured astrocytes, *Biochem. Biophys. Res. Commun.,* 169, 719, 1990.
247. **Hayashi, S., Okamura, S., Asano, Y., Ohhara, N., Otsuka, T., Shibuya, T., Otsuka, T., and Niho, Y.,** Human bladder carcinoma cell line HTB9, which secretes a factor to stimulate clonogenic leukemic blast growth, expresses the granulocyte-macrophage colony-stimulating factor gene, *Jpn. J. Cancer Res.,* 78, 1224, 1987.
248. **Weir, E.C., Insogna, K.L., and Horowitz, M.C.,** Osteoblast-like cells secrete granulocyte-macrophage colony-stimulating factor in response to parathyroid hormone and lipopolysaccharide, *Endocrinology,* 124, 899, 1989.
249. **Tsuchiya, Y., Igarashi, M., Suzuki, R., and Kumagai, K.,** Production of colony-stimulating factor by tumor cells and the factor-mediated induction of suppressor cells, *J. Immunol.,* 141, 699, 1988.
250. **Gasson, J.C., Kaufman, S.E., Weisbart, R.H., Tomonaga, M., and Golde, D.W.,** High-affinity binding of granulocyte-macrophage colony-stimulating factor to normal and leukemic human myeloid cells, *Proc. Natl. Acad. Sci. U.S.A.,* 83, 669, 1986.
251. **Park, L.S., Friend, D., Gillis, S., and Urdal, D.L.,** Characterization of the cell surface receptor for human granulocyte/macrophage colony-stimulating factor, *J. Exp. Med.,* 164, 251, 1986.
252. **Kelleher, C.A., Wong, G.G., Clark, S.C., Schendel, P.F., Minden, M.F., and McCulloch, E.A.,** Binding of iodinated recombinant human GM-CSF to the blast cells of acute myeloblastic leukemia, *Leukemia,* 2, 211, 1988.

253. Chiba, S., Tojo, A., Kitamura, T., Urabe, A., Miyazono, K., and Takaku, F., Characterization and molecular features of the cell surface receptor for human granulocyte-macrophage colony-stimulating factor, *Leukemia,* 4, 29, 1990.
254. Cannistra, S.A., Koenigsmann, M., DiCarlo, J., Groshek, P., and Griffin, J.D., Differentiation-associated expression of two functionally distinct classes of granulocyte-macrophage colony-stimulating factor receptors by human myeloid cells, *J. Biol. Chem.,* 265, 12656, 1990.
255. Budel, L.M., Elbaz, O., Hoogerbrugge, H., Delwel, R., Mahmoud, L.A., Löwenberg, B., and Touw, I.P., Common binding structure for granulocyte macrophage colony-stimulating factor and interleukin-3 on human acute myeloid cells and monocytes, *Blood,* 75, 1439, 1990.
256. Hayashida, K., Kitamura, T., Gorman, D.M., Arai, K., Tokota, T., and Miyajima, A., Molecular cloning of a second subunit of the receptor for human granulocyte-macrophage colony-stimulating factor (GM-CSF): reconstitution of a high-affinity GM-CSF receptor, *Proc. Natl. Acad. Sci. U.S.A.,* 87, 9655, 1990.
257. Kitamura, T., Sato, N., Arai, K., and Miyajima, A., Expression cloning of the human IL-3 receptor cDNA reveals a shared β subunit for the human IL-3 and GM-CSF receptors, *Cell,* 66, 1165, 1991.
258. Duronio, V., Clark-Lewis, I., Federsppiel, B., Wieler, J.S., and Schrader, J.W., Tyrosine phosphorylation of receptor β subunits and common substrates in response to interleukin-3 and granulocyte-macrophage colony-stimulating factor, *J. Biol. Chem.,* 267, 21856, 1992.
259. Shen, Y., Baker, E., Callen, D.F., Sutherland, G.R., Willson, T.A., Rakar, S., and Gough, N.M., Localization of the human GM-CSF receptor β-chain gene *(CSF2RB)* to chromosome 22q12.2-q13.1, Cytogenet. Cell Genet., 61, 175, 1992.
260. Park, L.S., Martin, U., Sorensen, R., Luhr, S., Morrissey, P.J., Cosman, D., and Larsen, A., Cloning of the low-affinity murine granulocyte-macrophage colony-stimulating factor receptor and reconstitution of a high-affinity receptor complex, *Proc. Natl. Acad. Sci. U.S.A.,* 89, 4295, 1992.
261. Park, L.S., Friend, D., Gillis, S., and Urdal, D.L., Characterization of the cell surface receptor for granulocyte-macrophage colony-stimulating factor, *J. Biol. Chem.,* 261, 4177, 1986.
262. Miyagawa, K., Chiba, S., Shibuya, K., Piao, Y.-F., Matsuki, S., Yokota, J., Terada, M., Miyazono, K., and Takaku, F., Frequent expression of receptors for granulocyte-macrophage colony-stimulating factor on human nonhematopoietic tumor cell lines, *J. Cell. Physiol.,* 143, 483, 1990.
263. Sullivan, R., Griffin, J.D., Simons, E.R., Schafer, A.I., Meshulam, T., Fredette, J.P., Maas, A.K., Gadenne, A.-S., Leavitt, J.L., and Melnick, D.A., Effects of recombinant human granulocyte and macrophage colony-stimulating factors on signal transduction pathways in human granulocytes, *J. Immunol.,* 139, 3422, 1987.
264. Miller, B.A., Scaduto, R.C., Jr., Tillotson, D.L., Botti, J.J., and Cheung, J.Y., Erythropoietin stimulates a rise in intracellular free calcium concentration in single early human erythroid precursors, *J. Clin. Invest.,* 82, 309, 1988.
265. Bradford, P.G., Jin, Y.Y., Hui, P., and Wang, X.H., IL-3 and GM-CSF induce the expression of the inositol trisphosphate receptor in K562 myeloblast cells, *Biochem. Biophys. Res. Commun.,* 187, 438, 1992.
266. Bourgoin, S., Plante, E., Gaudry, M., Naccache, P.H., Borgeat, P., and Poubelle, P.E., Involvement of a phospholipase D in the mechanism of action of granulocyte-macrophage colony-stimulating factor (GM-CSF): priming of human neutrophils in vitro with GM-CSF is associated with accumulation of phosphatidic acid and diacylglycerol, *J. Exp. Med.,* 172, 767, 1990.
267. Vallance, S.J., Downes, C.P., Cragge, E.J., and Whetton, A.D., Granulocyte-macrophage colony-stimulating factor can stimulate macrophage proliferation via persistent activation of Na^+/H^+ antiport. Evidence for two distinct roles for Na^+/H^+ antiport activation, *Biochem. J.,* 265, 359, 1990.
268. Oksenberg, D., Dieckmann, B.S., and Greenberg, P.L., Functional interactions between colony-stimulating factors and the insulin family hormones for human myeloid leukemic cells, *Cancer Res.,* 50, 6471, 1990.
269. Morla, A.O., Schereurs, J., Miyajima, A., and Wang, J.Y.J., Hematopoietic growth factors activate the tyrosine phosphorylation of distinct sets of proteins in interleukin-3-dependent murine cell lines, *Mol. Cell. Biol.,* 8, 2214, 1988.
270. Gomez-Cambronero, J., Huang, C.-K., Bonak, V.A., Wang, E., Casnellie, J.E., Shiraishi, T., and Sháafi, R.I., Tyrosine phosphorylation in human neutrophil, *Biochem. Biophys. Res. Commun.,* 162, 1478, 1989.

271. **Adunyah, S.E.,** Granulocyte-macrophage colony-stimulating factor stimulates rapid phosphorylation of proteins on tyrosines in human U937 and HL-60 leukemic cells, *Biochem. Biophys. Res. Commun.,* 193, 890, 1993.
272. **Gomez-Cambronero, J., Huang, C.-K., Gomez-Cambronero, T.M., Waterman, W.H., Becker, E.L., and Shaafi, R.I.,** Granulocyte-macrophage colony-stimulating factor-induced protein tyrosine phosphorylation of microtubule-associated protein kinase in human neutrophils, *Proc. Natl. Acad. Sci. U.S.A.,* 89, 7551, 1992.
273. **Yanakura, Y., Druker, B., Cannistra, S.A., Furukawa, Y., Torimoto, Y., and Griffin, J.D.,** Signal transduction of the human granulocyte-macrophage colony-stimulating factor and interleukin-3 receptors involves tyrosine phosphorylation of a common set of cytoplasmic proteins, *Blood,* 76, 706, 1990.
274. **Kanakura, Y., Druker, B., Wood, K.W., Mamon, H.J., Okuda, K., Roberts, T.M., and Griffin, J.D.,** Granulocyte-macrophage colony-stimulating factor and interleukin-3 induce rapid phosphorylation and activation of the proto-oncogene Raf-1 in a human factor-dependent myeloid cell line, *Blood,* 77, 243, 1991.
275. **Okuda, K., Druker, B., Kanakura, Y., Koenigsmann, M., and Griffin, J.D.,** Internalization of the granulocyte-macrophage colony-stimulating factor receptor is not required for induction of protein tyrosine phosphorylation in human myeloid cells, *Blood,* 78, 1928, 1991.
276. **Thomassen, M.J., Barna, B.P., Rankin, D., Wiedemann, H.P., and Ahmad, M.,** Differential effect of recombinant granulocyte macrophage colony-stimulating factor on human monocytes and alveolar macrophages, *Cancer Res.,* 49, 4086, 1989.
277. **Onetto-Pothier, N., Aumont, N., Haman, A., Bigras, C., Wong, G.G., Clark, S.C., De Lean, A., and Hoang, T.,** Characterization of granulocyte-macrophage colony-stimulating factor receptor on the blast cells of acute myeloblastic leukemia, *Blood,* 75, 59, 1990.
278. **Lange, B., Valtieri, M., Santoli, D., Caracciolo, D., Mavllio, F., Gemperlein, I., Griffin, C., Emanuel, B., Finan, J., Nowell, P., and Rovera, G.,** Growth factor requirements of childhood acute leukemia: establishement of GF-CSF-dependent cell lines, *Blood,* 70, 192, 1987.
279. **Motoji, T., Takanashi, M., Fuchinoue, M., Masuda, M., Oshimi, K., and Mizoguchi, H.,** Effect of recombinant GM-CSF and recombinant G-CSF on colony formation of blast progenitors in acute myeloblastic leukemia, *Exp. Hematol.,* 17, 56, 1989.
280. **Vellenga, E., Young, D.C., Wagner, K., Wiper, D., Ostapovicz, D., and Griffin, J.D.,** The effects of GM-CSF in promoting growth of clonogenic cells in acute myeloblastic leukemia, *Blood,* 69, 1771, 1987.
281. **Vellenga, E., Delwel, H.R., Touw, I.P., and Löwenberg, B.,** Patterns of acute myeloid leukemia colony growth in response to recombinant granulocyte-macrophage colony-stimulating factor (FGM-CSF), *Exp. Hematol.,* 15, 652, 1987.
282. **Gualtieri, R.J., Emanuel, P.D., Zuckerman, K.S., Martin, G., Clark, S.C., Shadduck, R.K., Dracker, R.A., Akabutu, J., Nitschke, R., Hetherington, M.L., Dickerman, J.D., Hakami, N., and Castleberry, R.P.,** Granulocyte-macrophage colony-stimulating factor is an endogenous regulator of cell proliferation in juvenile chronic myelogenous leukemia, *Blood,* 74, 2360, 1989.
283. **Begley, C.G., Metcalf, D., and Nicola, N.A.,** Purified colony-stimulating factors (G-CSF and GM-CSF) induce differentiation in human HL60 leukemic cells with suppression of clonogenicity, *Int. J. Cancer,* 39, 99, 1987.
284. **Brennan, J.K., Lee, K.S., Abboud, C.N., Erickson-Miller, C.L., and Keng, P.C.,** Interactions of dimethyl sulfoxide and granulocyte-macrophage colony-stimulating factors on the growth and maturation of HL-60 cells, *J. Cell. Physiol.,* 132, 246, 1987.
285. **Schwartz, E.L. and Maher, A.M.,** Enhanced mitogenic responsiveness to granulocyte-macrophage colony-stimulating factor in HL-60 promyelocytic leukemia cells upon induction of differentiation, *Cancer Res.,* 48, 2863, 1988.
286. **Zuckerman, S.H., Surprenant, Y.M., and Tang, J.,** Synergistic effect of granulocyte-macrophage colony-stimulating factor and 1,25-dihydroxyvitamin D_3 on the differentiation of the human monocytic cell line U937, *Blood,* 71, 619, 1988.
287. **Cheng, G.Y.M., Kelleher, C.A., Miyauchi, J., Wang, C., Wong, G., Clark, S.C., McCulloch, E.A., and Minden, M.D.,** Structure and expression of genes of GM-CSF and G-CSF in blast cells from patients with acute myeloblastic leukemia, *Blood,* 71, 204, 1988.
288. **Mano, H., Nishida, J., Usuki, K., Maru, Y., Kobayashi, Y., Hirai, H., Okabe, T., Urabe, A., and Takaku, F.,** Constitutive expression of the granulocyte-macrophage colony-stimulating factor gene in human solid tumors, *Jpn. J. Cancer Res.,* 78, 1041, 1987.

289. Cook, W.D., Metcalf, D., Nicola, N.A., Burgess, A.W., and Walker, F., Malignant transformation of a growth factor-dependent myeloid cell line by Abelson virus without evidence of an autocrine mechanism, *Cell,* 41, 677, 1985.
290. Hines, D.L., Differentiation of Abelson murine leukemia virus-infected promonocytic leukemia cells, *Int. J. Cancer,* 36, 233, 1985.
291. Gonda, T.J. and Metcalf, D., Expression of *myb, myc* and *fos* proto-oncogenes during the differentiation of a murine myeloid leukaemia, *Nature,* 310, 249, 1984.
292. Schwartz, E.L., Chamberlin, H., and Brechbühl, A.-B., Regulation of c-*myc* expression by granulocyte-macrophage colony-stimulating factor in human leukemia cells, *Blood,* 77, 2716, 1991.
293. Feldman, R.A., Gabrilove, J.L., Tam, J.P., Moore, M.A.S., and Hanafusa, H., Specific expression of the human cellular *fps/fes*-encoded protein NCP92 in normal and leukemic myeloid cells, *Proc. Natl. Acad. Sci. U.S.A.,* 82, 2379, 1985.
294. Smithgall, T.E., Yu, G., and Glazer, R.I., Identification of the differentiation-associated p93 tyrosine protein kinase of HL-60 leukemia cells as the product of the human c-*fes* locus and its expression in myelomonocytic cells, *J. Biol. Chem.,* 263, 15050, 1988.
295. Liu, J., Lacy, J., Sukhatme, V.P., and Coleman, D.L., Granulocyte-macrophage colony-stimulating factor induces transcriptional activation of *Egr-1* in murine peritoneal macrophages, *J. Biol. Chem.,* 266, 5929, 1991.
296. Francis, G.E., Ho, A.D., Gray, D.A., Berney, J.J., Wing, M.A., Yaxley, J.J., Ma, D.D.F., and Hoffbrand, A.V., DNA strand breakage and ADP-ribosyl transferase mediated DNA ligation during stimulation of human bone marrow cells by granulocyte-macrophage colony stimulating activity, *Leukemia Res.,* 8, 407, 1984.
297. Boettiger, D. and Dexter, T.M., Altered stem cell (CFU-S) function following infection of hematopoietic cells with a virus carrying v-*src, Blood,* 67, 398, 1986.
298. Chung, S.W., Wong, P.M.C., Shen-Ong, G., Ruscetti, S., Ishizaka, T., and Eaves, C.J., Production of granulocyte-macrophage colony-stimulating factor by Abelson virus-induced tumorigenic mast cell lines, *Blood,* 68, 1074, 1986.
299. Young, D.C., Wagner, K., and Griffin, J.D., Constitutive expression of the granulocyte-macrophage colony-stimulating factor gene in acute myeloblastic leukemia, *J. Clin. Invest.,* 79, 100, 1987.
300. Sawada, H., Tezuka, H., Sakoda, H., Nishikori, M., Yoshida, Y., Uchino, H., Miyanomae, T., Fujita, J., Inoue, T., and Mori, K.J., Effect of colony-stimulating factor-producing tumor on hemopoiesis in splenectomized mice, *Jpn. J. Cancer Res.,* 77, 1235, 1986.
301. Frei, K., Piani, D., Malipiero, U.V., van Meir, E., de Tribolet, N., and Fontana, A., Granulocyte-macrophage colony-stimulating factor (GM-CSF) production by glioblastoma cells. Despite the presence of inducing signals GM-CSF is not expressed in vivo, *J. Immunol.,* 148, 3140, 1992.
302. Lang, R.A., Metcalf, D., Gough, N.M., Dunn, A.R., and Gonda, T.J., Expression of a hemopoietic growth factor cDNA in a factor-dependent cell line results in autonomous growth and tumorigenicity, *Cell,* 43, 531, 1985.
303. Areces, L.B., Jücker, M., San Miguel, J.A., Mui, A., Miyajima, A., and Feldman, R.A., Ligand-dependent transformation by the receptor for human granulocyte/macrophage colony-stimulating factor and tyrosine phosphorylation of the receptor β subunit, *Proc. Natl. Acad. Sci. U.S.A.,* 90, 3963, 1993.
304. Metcalf, D., Begley, C.G., Williamson, D.J., Nice, E.C., De Lamarter, J., Mermod, J.-J., Thatcher, D., and Schmidt, A., Hemopoietic responses in mice injected with purified recombinant murine GM-CSF, *Exp. Hematol.,* 15, 1, 1987.
305. Gasson, J.C., Weisbart, R.H., Kaufman, S.E., Clark, S.C., Hewick, R.M., Wong, G.G., and Golde, D.W., Purified human granulocyte-macrophage colony-stimulating factor: direct action on neutrophils, *Science,* 226, 1339, 1984.
306. Weisbart, R.H., Golde, D.W., Clark, S.C., Wong, G.G., and Gasson, J.C., Human granulocyte-macrophage colony-stimulating factor is a neutrophil activator, *Nature,* 314, 361, 1985.
307. Fleischmann, J., Golde, D.W., Weisbart, R.H., and Gasson, J.C., Granulocyte-macrophage colony-stimulating factor enhances phagocytosis of bacteria by human neutrophils, *Blood,* 68, 708, 1986.
308. Mayer, P., Lam, C., Obenaus, H., Liehl, E., and Besemer, J., Recombinant human GM-CSF induces leukocytosis and activates peripheral blood polymorphonuclear neutrophils in nonhuman primates, *Blood,* 70, 206, 1987.

309. **Brandt, S.J., Peters, W.P., Atwater, S.K., Kurtzberg, J., Borowitz, M.J., Jones, R.B., Shpall, E.J., Bast, R.C., Jr., Gilbert, C.J., and Oette, D.H.,** Effect of recombinant human granulocyte-macrophage colony-stimulating factor on hematopoietic reconstitution after high-dose chemotherapy and autologous bone marrow transplantation, *N. Engl. J. Med.,* 318, 869, 1988.
310. **Socinski, M.A., Cannistra, S.A., Elias, A., Antman, K.H., Schnipper, L., and Griffin, J.D.,** Granulocyte-macrophage colony-stimulating factor expands the circulating haemopoietic progenitor cell compartment in man, *Lancet,* 1, 1194, 1988.
311. **Kaplan, S.S., Basford, R.E., Wing, E.J., and Shadduck, R.K.,** The effect of recombinant human granulocyte macrophage colony-stimulating factor on neutrophil activation in patients with refractory carcinoma, *Blood,* 73, 636, 1989.
312. **Wing, E.J., Magee, D.M., Whiteside, T.L., Kaplan, S.S., and Shadduck, R.K.,** Recombinant human granulocyte/macrophage colony-stimulating factor enhances monocyte cytotoxicity and secretion of tumor necrosis factor α and interferon in cancer patients, *Blood,* 73, 643, 1989.
313. **Groopman, J.E., Mitsuyasu, R.T., DeLeo, M.J., Oette, D.H., and Golde, D.W.,** Effect of recombinant human granulocyte-macrophage colony-stimulating factor on myelopoiesis in the acquired immunodeficiency syndrome, *N. Engl. J. Med.,* 317, 593, 1987.
314. **Baldwin, G.C., Gasson, J.C., Quan, S.G., Fleischmann, J., Weisbart, R., Oette, D., Mitsuyasu, R.T., and Golde, D.W.,** Granulocyte-macrophage colony-stimulating factor enhances neutrophil function in acquired immunodeficiency syndrome patients, *Proc. Natl. Acad. Sci. U.S.A.,* 85, 2763, 1988.
315. **Nicola, N.A., Metcalf, D., Matsumoto, M., and Johnson, G.R.,** Purification of a factor inducing differentiation in murine myelomonocytic leukemia cells: identification as granulocyte colony-stimulating factor, *J. Biol. Chem.,* 258, 9017, 1983.
316. **Nagata, S.,** Gene structure and function of granulocyte colony-stimulating factor, *Bioessays,* 10, 113, 1989.
317. **Nagata, S.,** Granulocyte colony-stimulating factor, *Handb. Exp. Pharmacol.,* 95, 699, 1990.
318. **Demetri, G.D. and Griffin, J.D.,** Granulocyte colony-stimulating factor and its receptor, *Blood,* 78, 2791, 1991.
319. **Watari, K., Asano, S., Shirafuji, N., Kodo, H., Ozawa, K., Takaku, F., and Kamachi, S.,** Serum granulocyte colony-stimulating factor levels in healthy volunteers and patients with various disorders as estimated by enzyme immunoassay, *Blood,* 73, 117, 1989.
320. **Metcalf, D. and Nicola, N.A.,** Synthesis by mouse peritoneal cells of G-CSF, the differentiation inducer for myeloid leukemia cells: stimulation by endotoxin, M-CSF and multi-CSF, *Leukemia Res.,* 9, 35, 1985.
321. **Metcalf, D. and Nicola, N.A.,** Proliferative effects of purified granulocyte colony-stimulating factor (G-CSF) on normal mouse hemopoietic cells, *J. Cell. Physiol.,* 116, 198, 1983.
322. **Ieki, R., Kudoh, S., Kimura, H., Ozawa, K., Asano, S., and Takaku, F.,** Human granulocyte colony formation in serum-free cultures stimulated with purified recombinant granulocyte colony-stimulating factor, *Exp. Hematol.,* 18, 883, 1990.
323. **Lopez, A.F., Nicola, N.A., Burgess, A.W., Metcalf, D., Battye, F.L., Sewell, W.A., and Vadas, M.,** Activation of granulocyte cytotoxic function by purified mouse colony-stimulating factors, *J. Immunol.,* 131, 2938, 1984.
324. **Kitagawa, S., Yuo, A., Souza, L.M., Saito, M., Miura, Y., and Takaku, F.,** Recombinant human granulocyte colony-stimulating factor enhances superoxide release in human granulocytes stimulated by the chemotactic peptide, *Biochem. Biophys. Res. Commun.,* 144, 1143, 1987.
325. **Sato, N., Asano, S., Koeffler, H.P., Yoshida, S., Takaku, F., and Takatani, O.,** Identification of neutrophil alkaline phosphatase-inducing factor in cystic fluid of a human squamous cell carcinoma as granulocyte colony-stimulating factor, *J. Cell. Physiol.,* 137, 272, 1988.
326. **Lord, B.I., Bronchud, M.H., Owens, S., Chang, J., Howell, A., Souza, L., and Dexter, T.M.,** The kinetics of human granulopoiesis following treatment with granulocyte colony-stimulating factor *in vivo, Proc. Natl. Acad. Sci. U.S.A.,* 86, 9499, 1989.
327. **Medlock, E.E., Kaplan, D.L., Ceccini, M., Ulich, T.R., Del Castillo, J., and Andressen, J.,** Granulocyte colony-stimulating factor crosses the placenta and stimulates fetal rat granulopoiesis, *Blood,* 81, 916, 1993.
328. **Shirafuji, N., Matsuda, S., Ogura, H., Tani, K., Kodo, H., Ozawa, K., Nagata, S., Asano, S., and Takaku, F.,** Granulocyte colony-stimulating factor stimulates human mature neutrophilic granulocytes to produce interferon-α, *Blood,* 75, 17, 1990.

329. Souza, L.M., Boone, T.C., Gabrilove, J., Lai, P.H., Zsebo, K.M., Murdock, D.C., Chazin, V.R., Bruszewski, J., Lu, H., Chen, K.K., Barendt, J., Platzer, E., Moore, M.A.S., Mertelsmann, R., and Welte, K., Recombinant human granulocyte colony-stimulating factor: effects on normal and leukemic myeloid cells, *Science,* 232, 61, 1986.
330. Suda, T., Yamaguchi, Y., Suda, J., Miura, Y., Okano, A., and Akiyama, Y., Effect of interleukin 6 (IL-6) on the differentiation and proliferation of murine and human hemopoietic progenitors, *Exp. Hematol.,* 16, 891, 1988.
331. Messner, H.A., Yamasaki, K., Jamal, N., Minden, M.M., Yang, Y.-C., Wong, G.G., and Clark, S.C., Growth of human hemopoietic colonies in response to recombinant gibbon interleukin 3: comparison with human recombinant granulocyte and granulocyte-macrophage colony-stimulating factor, *Proc. Natl. Acad. Sci. U.S.A.,* 84, 6765, 1987.
332. Ikebuchi, K., Clark, S.C., Ihle, J.N., Souza, L.M., and Ogawa, M., Granulocyte colony-stimulating factor enhances interleukin 3-dependent proliferation of multipotential hemopoietic progenitors, *Proc. Natl. Acad. Sci. U.S.A.,* 85, 3445, 1988.
333. Valtieri, M., Tweardy, D.J., Caracciolo, D., Johnson, K., Mavilio, F., Altmann, S., Santoli, D., and Rovera, G., Cytokine-dependent granulocytic differentiation. Regulation of proliferative and differentiative responses in a murine progenitor cell line, *J. Immunol.,* 138, 3829, 1987.
334. Ulich, T.R., del Castillo, J., McNiece, I.K., Yin, S., Irwin, B., Busser, K., and Guo, K., Acute and subacute hematologic effects of multi-colony stimulating factor in combination with granulocyte colony-stimulating factor in vivo, *Blood,* 75, 48, 1990.
335. Pébusque, M.-J., Fay, C., Lafage, M., Sempéré, C., Seeland, S., Caux, C., and Mannoni, P., Recombinant human IL-3 and G-CSF act synergistically in stimulating the growth of acute myeloid leukemia cells, *Leukemia,* 3, 200, 1989.
336. McNiece, I., Andrews, R., Stewart, M., Clark, S., Boone, T., and Quesenberry, P., Action of interleukin-3, G-CSF, and GM-CSF on highly enriched human hematopoietic progenitor cells: synergistic interaction of GM-CSF plus G-CSF, *Blood,* 74, 110, 1989.
337. Shieh, J.-H., Peterson, R.H.F., and Moore, M.A.S., Granulocyte colony-stimulating factor modulation of cytokine receptors on murine bone marrow cells. In vivo and in vitro studies, *J. Immunol.,* 147, 2984, 1991.
338. Mendoza, J.F., Céceres, J.R., Santiago, E., Mora, L.M., Sénchez, L., Corona, T.M., Machuca, C., Zambrano, I.R., Martínez, R.D., and Weiss-Steider, B., Evidence that G-CSF is a fibroblast growth factor that induces granulocytes to increase phagocytosis and to present a mature morphology, and that macrophages secrete 45-kd molecules with these activities as well as with G-CSF-like activity, *Exp. Hematol.,* 18, 903, 1990.
339. Okabe, M., Asano, M., Kuga, T., Komatsu, Y., Yamasaki, M., Yokoo, Y., Itoh, S., Morimoto, M., and Oka, T., In vitro and in vivo hematopoietic effect of mutant human granulocyte colony-stimulating factor, *Blood,* 75, 1788, 1990.
340. Nomura, H., Imazeki, I., Oheda, M., Kubota, N., Tamura, M., Ono, M., Ueyama, Y., and Asano, S., Purification and characterization of human granulocyte colony-stimulating factor (G-CSF), *EMBO J.,* 5, 871, 1986.
341. Nagata, S., Tsuchiya, M., Asano, S., Yamamoto, O., Hirata, Y., Kubota, N., Oheda, M., Nomura, H., and Yamazaki, T., The chromosomal gene structure and two mRNAs for human granulocyte colony-stimulating factor, *EMBO J.,* 5, 575, 1986.
342. Nagata, S., Tsuchiya, M., Asano, S., Kaziro, Y., Yamazaki, T., Yamamoto, O., Hirata, Y., Kubota, N., Oheda, M., Nomura, H., and Ono, M., Molecular cloning and expression of cDNA for human granulocyte colony-stimulating factor, *Nature,* 319, 415, 1986.
343. Komatsu, Y., Matsumoto, T., Kuga, T., Nishi, T., Sekine, S., Saito, A., Okabe, M., Morimoto, M., Itoh, S., Okabe, T., and Takaku, F., Cloning of granulocyte colony-stimulating factor cDNA from human macrophages and its expression in *Escherichia coli, Jpn. J. Cancer Res.,* 78, 1179, 1987.
344. Kuga, T., Komatsu, Y., Yamasaki, M., Sekine, S., Miyaji, H., Nishi, T., Sato, M., Yokoo, Y., Asano, M., Okabe, M., Morimoto, M., and Itoh, S., Mutagenesis of human granulocyte colony stimulating factor, *Biochem. Biophys. Res. Commun.,* 159, 103, 1989.
345. Hill, C.P., Osslund, T.D., and Eisenberg, D., The structure of granulocyte-colony-stimulating factor and its relationship to other growth factors, *Proc. Natl. Acad. Sci. U.S.A.,* 90, 5167, 1993.
346. Kanda, N., Fukushige, S., Murotsu, T., Yoshida, M.C., Tsuchiya, M., Asano, S., Kaziro, Y., and Nagata, S., Human gene coding for granulocyte-colony stimulating factor is assigned to the q21-q22 region of chromosome 17, *Somat. Cell Mol. Genet.,* 13, 679, 1987.

347. Le Beau, M.M., Lemons, R.S., Carrino, J.J., Pettenati, M.J., Souza, L.M., Diaz, M.O., and Rowley, J.D., Chromosomal localization of the human *G-CSF* gene to 17q11 proximal to the breakpoint of the t(15;17) in acute promyelocytic leukemia, *Leukemia,* 1, 795, 1987.
348. Simmers, R.N., Webber, L.M., Shannon, M.F., Garson, O.M., Wong, G., Vadas, M.A., and Sutherland, G.R., Localization of the G-CSF gene on chromosome 17 proximal to the breakpoint in the t(15;17) in acute promyelocytic leukemia, *Blood,* 70, 330, 1987.
349. Tsuchiya, M., Asano, S., Kaziro, Y., and Nagata, S., Isolation and characterization of the cDNA for murine granulocyte colony-stimulating factor, *Proc. Natl. Acad. Sci. U.S.A.,* 83, 7633, 1986.
350. Tsuchiya, M., Kaziro, Y., and Nagata, S., The chromosomal gene structure for murine granulocyte colony-stimulating factor, *Eur. J. Biochem.,* 165, 7, 1987.
351. Tsuneoka, K. and Shikita, M., A colony-stimulating factor for neutrophil granulocytes: a marked increase of its production by the addition of sodium butyrate and lipopolysaccharide in serum-free culture of RSP-2.P3 cells, *J. Cell. Physiol.,* 125, 436, 1985.
352. Zoellner, H., Filonzi, E.L., Stanton, H.R., Layton, J.E., and Hamilton, J.A., Human arterial smooth muscle cells synthesize granulocyte colony-stimulating factor in response to interleukin-1α and tumor necrosis factor-α, *Blood,* 80, 2805, 1992.
353. Yang, Y.-C., Tsai, S., Wong, G.G., and Clark, S.C., Interleukin-1 regulation of hematopoietic growth factor production by human stromal fibroblasts, *J. Cell. Physiol.,* 134, 292, 1988.
354. Devlin, J.J., Devlin, P.E., Myambo, K., Lilly, M.B., Rado, T.A., and Warren, M.K., Expression of granulocyte colony-stimulating factor by human cell lines, *J. Leukocyte Biol.,* 41, 302, 1987.
355. Malipiero, U.V., Frei, K., and Fontana, A., Production of hemopoietic colony-stimulating factors by astrocytes, *J. Immunol.,* 144, 3816, 1990.
356. Watari, K., Asano, S., Shirafuji, N., Kodo, H., Ozawa, K., Takaku, F., and Kamachi, S., Serum granulocyte colony-stimulating factor levels in healthy volunteers and patients with various disorders as estimated by enzyme immunoassay, *Blood,* 73, 117, 1989.
357. Mempel, K., Pietsch, T., Menzel, T., Zeidler, C., and Welte, K., Increased serum levels of granulocyte colony-stimulating factor in patients with severe congenital neutropenia, *Blood,* 77, 1919, 1991.
358. Nicola, N.A. and Metcalf, D., Binding of ^{125}I-labeled granulocyte colony-stimulating factor to normal murine hemopoietic cells, *J. Cell. Physiol.,* 124, 313, 1985.
359. Tweardy, D.J., Anderson, K., Cannizzaro, L.A., Steinman, R.A., Croce, C.M., and Huebner, K., Molecular cloning of cDNAs for the human granulocyte colony-stimulating factor receptor from HL-60 and mapping of the gene to chromosome region 1p32-34, *Blood,* 79, 1148, 1992.
360. Uzumaki, H., Okabe, T., Sasaki, N., Hagiwara, K., Takaku, F., and Itoh, S., Characterization of receptor for granulocyte colony-stimulating factor on human circulating neutrophils, *Biochem. Biophys. Res. Commun.,* 156, 1026, 1988.
361. Fukunaga, R., Seto, Y., Mizushima, S., and Nagata, S., Three different mRNAs encoding human granulocyte colony-stimulating factor receptor, *Proc. Natl. Acad. Sci. U.S.A.,* 87, 8702, 1990.
362. Nicola, N.A. and Peterson, L., Identification of distinct receptors for two hemopoietic growth factors (granulocyte colony-stimulating factor and multipotential colony-stimulating factor) by chemical cross-linking, *J. Biol. Chem.,* 261, 12384, 1986.
363. Fukunaga, R., Ishizaka-Ikeda, E., and Nagata, S., Purification and characterization of the receptor for murine granulocyte colony-stimulating factor, *J. Biol. Chem.,* 265, 14008, 1990.
364. Fukunaga, R., Ishizaka-Ikeda, E., Seto, Y., and Nagata, S., Expression cloning of a receptor for murine granulocyte colony-stimulating factor, *Cell,* 61, 341, 1990.
365. Ishizaka-Ikeda, E., Fukunaga, R., Wood, W.I., Goeddel, D.V., and Nagata, S., Signal transduction mediated by growth hormone receptor and its chimeric molecules with the granulocyte colony-stimulating factor receptor, *Proc. Natl. Acad. Sci. U.S.A.,* 90, 123, 1993.
366. Nicola, N.A., Begley, C.G., and Metcalf, D., Identification of the human analogue of a regulator that induces differentiation in murine leukaemic cells, *Nature,* 314, 625, 1985.
367. Fukunaga, R., Ishizaka-Ikeda, E., Pan, C.-X., Seto, Y., and Nagata, S., Functional domains of the granulocyte colony-stimulating factor receptor, *EMBO J.,* 10, 2855, 1991.
368. Fuh, G., Cunningham, B.C., Fukunaga, R., Nagata, S., Goeddel, D.V., and Wells, J.A., Rational design of potent antagonists to the human growth hormone receptor, *Science,* 256, 1677, 1992.
369. Ziegler, S.F., Bird, T.A., Morella, K.K., Mosley, B., Gearing, D.P., and Baumann, H., Distinct regions of the human granulocyte colony-stimulating factor receptor cytoplasmic domain are required for proliferation and gene induction, *Mol. Cell. Biol.,* 13, 2384, 1993.

370. Shimoda, K., Okamura, S., Harada, N., Kondo, S., Okamura, T., and Niho, Y., Identification of a functional receptor for granulocyte colony-stimulating factor on platelets, *J. Clin. Invest.,* 91, 1310, 1993.
371. Bussolino, F., Wang, J.M., Defilippi, P., Turrini, F., Sanavio, F., Edgell, C.-J.S., Aglietta, M., Arese, P., and Mantovani, A., Granulocyte- and granulocyte-macrophage-colony-stimulating factors induce human endothelial cells to migrate and proliferate, *Nature,* 337, 471, 1989.
372. Avalos, B.R., Gasson, J.C., Hevat, C., Quan, S.G., Baldwin, G.C., Weisbart, R.H., Williams, R.E., Golde, W.E., and DiPersio, J.F., Human granulocyte colony-stimulating factor: biologic activities and receptor characterization on hematopoietic cells and small cell lung cancer cell lines, *Blood,* 75, 851, 1990.
373. Kuwaki, T., Hosoi, T., Hanazono, Y., Tsumura, H., Ishikawa, F., Miyazono, K., Miyagawa, K., and Takaku, F., Distribution of human granulocyte colony-stimulating factor receptors on hematopoietic and nonhematopoietic tumor cell lines, *Jpn. J. Cancer,* 82, 560, 1990.
374. Uzumaki, H., Okabe, T., Sasaki, N., Hagiwara, K., Takaku, F., Tobita, M., Yasukawa, K., Ito, S., and Umezawa, Y., Identification and characterization of receptors for granulocyte colony-stimulating factor on human placenta and trophoblastic cells, *Proc. Natl. Acad. Sci. U.S.A.,* 86, 9323, 1989.
375. Shieh, J.-H., Peterson, R.H.F., and Moore, M.A.S., Modulation of granulocyte colony-stimulating factor receptors on murine peritoneal exudate macrophages by tumor necrosis factor-α, *J. Immunol.,* 146, 2648, 1991.
376. Matsuda, S., Shirafuji, N., and Asano, S., Human granulocyte colony-stimulating factor specifically binds to murine myeloblastic NFS-60 cells and activates their guanosine triphosphate binding proteins/adenylate cyclase system, *Blood,* 74, 2343, 1989.
377. Adachi, K. and Saito, H., Induction of junB expression, but not c-*jun,* by granulocyte colony-stimulating factor or macrophage colony-stimulating factor in the proliferative response of human myeloid leukemia cells, *J. Clin. Invest.,* 89, 1657, 1992.
378. Zsebo, K.M., Cohen, A.M., Murdock, D.C., Boone, T.C., Inoue, H., Chazin, V.R., Hines, D., and Souza, L.M., Recombinant human granulocyte colony stimulating factor: molecular and biological characterization, *Immunobiology,* 172, 175, 1986.
379. Fujisawa, M., Kobayashi, Y., Okabe, T., Takaku, F., Komatsu, Y., and Itoh, S., Recombinant human granulocyte colony-stimulating factor induces granulocytosis in vivo, *Jpn. J. Cancer Res.,* 77, 866, 1986.
380. Pojda, Z., Molineux, G., and Dexter, T.M., Hemopoietic effects of short-term in vivo treatment of mice with various doses of rhG-CSF, *Exp. Hematol.,* 18, 27, 1990.
381. Tamura, M., Hattori, K., Nomura, H., Oheda, M., Kubota, N., Imazeki, I., Ono, M., Ueyama, Y., Nagata, S., Shirafuji, N., and Asano, S., Induction of neutrophilic granulocytosis in mice by administration of purified human native granulocyte colony-stimulating factor (G-CSF), *Biochem. Biophys. Res. Commun.,* 142, 454, 1987.
382. Kobayashi, Y., Okabe, T., Urabe, A., Suzuki, N., and Takaku, F., Human granulocyte colony-stimulating factor produced by Escherichia coli shortens the period of granulocytopenia induced by irradiation in mice, *Jpn. J. Cancer Res.,* 78, 763, 1987.
383. Cohen, A.M., Zsebo, K.M., Inoue, H., Hines, D., Boone, T.C., Chazin, V.R., Tsai, L., Ritch, T., and Souza, L.M., In vivo stimulation of granulopoiesis by recombinant human granulocyte colony-stimulating factor, *Proc. Natl. Acad. Sci. U.S.A.,* 84, 2484, 1987.
384. Welte, K., Bonilla, M.A., Gillio, A.P., Boone, T.C., Potter, G.K., Gabrilove, J.L., Moore, M.A.S., O'Reilly, R.J., and Souza, L.M., Recombinant human granulocyte colony-stimulating factor: effects on hematopoiesis in normal and cyclophosphamide-treated primates, *J. Exp. Med.,* 165, 941, 1987.
385. Ulich, T.R., del Castillo, J., and Souza, L., Kinetics and mechanisms of recombinant human granulocyte-colony stimulating factor-induced neutrophilia, *Am. J. Pathol.,* 133, 630, 1988.
386. Bronchud, M.H., Potter, M.R., Morgenstern, G., Blasco, M.J., Scarffe, J.H., Thatcher, N., Crowther, D., Souza, L.M., Alton, N.K., Testa, N.G., and Dexter, T.M., *In vitro* and *in vivo* analysis of the effects of recombinant human granulocyte colony-stimulating factor in patients, *Br. J. Cancer,* 58, 64, 1988.
387. Yuo, A., Kitagawa, S., Okabe, T., Urabe, A., Komatsu, Y., Itoh, S., and Takaku, F., Recombinant human granulocyte colony-stimulating factor repairs the abnormalities of neutrophils in patients with myelodysplastic syndromes and chronic myelogenous leukemia, *Blood,* 70, 404, 1987.

388. **Bonilla, M.A., Gillio, A.P., Ruggiero, M., Kernan, N.A., Brochstein, J.A., Abboud, M., Fumagalli, L., Vincent, M., Gabrilove, J.L., Welte, K., Souza, L.M., and O'Reilly, R.J.,** Effects of recombinant human granulocyte colony-stimulating factor on neutropenia in patients with congenital agranulocytosis, *N. Engl. J. Med.,* 320, 1574, 1989.
389. **Budel, L.M., Touw, I.P., Delwel, R., and Löwenberg, B.,** Granulocyte colony-stimulating factor receptors in human acute myelocytic leukemia, *Blood,* 74, 2668, 1989.
390. **Piao, Y.-F. and Okabe, T.,** Receptor binding of human granulocyte colony-stimulating factor to the blast cells of myeloid leukemia, *Cancer Res.,* 50, 1671, 1990.
391. **Motoji, T., Watanabe, M., Uzumaki, H., Kusaka, M., Fukamachi, H., Shimosaka, A., Oshimi, K., and Mizoguchi, H.,** Granulocyte colony-stimulating factor (G-CSF) receptors on acute myeloblastic leukaemia cells and their relationship with the proliferative response to G-CSF in clonogenic assay, *Br. J. Haematol.,* 77, 54, 1991.
392. **Nara, N., Suzuki, T., Nagata, K., Tohda, S., Yamashita, Y., Nakamura, Y., Imai, Y., Morio, T., and Minamisamatsu, M.,** Granulocyte colony-stimulating factor-dependent growth of an acute myeloblastic leukemia cell line, *Jpn. J. Cancer Res.,* 81, 625, 1990.
393. **Tomida, M., Yamamoto-Yamaguchi, Y., Hozumi, M., Okabe, T., and Takaku, F.,** Induction by recombinant human granulocyte colony-stimulating factor of differentiation of mouse myeloid leukemic M1 cells, *FEBS Lett.,* 207, 271, 1986.
394. **Nicola, N.A.,** Granulocyte colony-stimulating factor and differentiation induction in myeloid leukemic cells, *Int. J. Cell Cloning,* 5, 1, 1987.
395. **Nakamaki, T., Sakashita, A., Sano, M., Hino, K., Suzuki, K., Tomoyasu, S., Tsuruoka, N., Honma, Y., and Hozumi, M.,** Granulocyte-colony stimulating factor and retinoic acid cooperatively induce granulocytic differentiation of acute promyelocytic leukemia cells *in vitro, Jpn. J. Cancer Res.,* 80, 1077, 1989.
396. **Yamamoto, M., Nishimura, J., Ideguchi, H., and Ibayashi, H.,** Specific phosphorylation of 22-kD proteins by various inducers for granuloid differentiation in myeloid leukemic cells, *Leukemia Res.,* 12, 71, 1988.
397. **Nara, N., Murohashi, I., Suzuki, T., Yamashita, Y., Maruyama, Y., Aoki, N., Tanikawa, S., and Onozawa, Y.,** Effects of recombinant human granulocyte colony-stimulating factor (G-CSF) on blast progenitors from acute myeloblastic leukaemia patients, *Br. J. Cancer,* 56, 49, 1987.
398. **Jinnai, I.,** *In vitro* growth response to G-CSF and GM-CSF by bone marrow cells of patients with acute myeloid leukemia, *Leukemia Res.,* 14, 227, 1990.
399. **Tsuda, H., Neckers, L.M., and Pluznik, D.H.,** Colony stimulating factor-induced differentiation of murine M1 myeloid leukemia cells is permissive in early G_1 phase, *Proc. Natl. Acad. Sci. U.S.A.,* 83, 4317, 1986.
400. **Irvine, A.E., Berney, J.J., and Francis, G.E.,** Dissociation of the proliferation and differentiation stimuli of granulocyte colony-stimulating factor (G-CSF), *Leukemia,* 4, 203, 1990.
401. **Segawa, K., Ueno, Y., and Kataoka, T.,** *In vivo* tumor growth enhancement by granulocyte colony-stimulating factor, *Jpn. J. Cancer Res.,* 82, 440, 1991.
402. **Kanz, L., Löhr, G.W., and Fauser, A.A.,** Human megakaryocytic progenitor cells, *Klin. Wochenschr.,* 65, 297, 1987.
403. **McDonald, T.P.,** The regulation of megakaryocyte and platelet production, *Int. J. Cell Cloning,* 7, 139, 1989.
404. **Hoffman, R.,** Regulation of megakaryocytopoiesis, *Blood,* 74, 1196, 1989.
405. **Gewirtz, A.M. and Calabretta, B.,** Molecular regulation of human megakaryocyte development, *Int. J. Cell Cloning,* 8, 267, 1990.
406. **Withy, R.M., Rafield, L.F., Beck, A.K., Hoppe, H., Williams, N., and McPherson, J.M.,** Growth factors produced by human embryonic kidney cells that influence megakaryopoiesis include erythropoietin, interleukin-6, and transforming growth factor-β, *J. Cell. Physiol.,* 153, 362, 1992.
407. **Mouthon, M.-A., Navarro, S., Katz, A., Breton-Gorius, J., and Vainchenker, W.,** Both c-*jun* and c-*fos* are expressed by human megakaryocytes, *Exp. Hematol.,* 20, 909, 1992.
408. **Straneva, J.E., Yang, H.H., Hui, S.L., Bruno, E., and Hoffman, R.,** Effects of megakaryocyte colony-stimulating factor on terminal cytoplasmic maturation of human megakaryocytes, *Exp. Hematol.,* 15, 657, 1987.
409. **de Alarcon, P.A.,** Megakaryocyte colony-stimulating factor (Mk-CSF): its physiologic significance, *Blood Cells,* 15, 173, 1989.

410. Ogata, K., Kuriya, S., Dan, K., and Nomura, T., Partial purification of human urinary megakaryocyte colony-stimulating factor, *Exp. Cell Biol.,* 57, 19, 1989
411. Bagnara, G.P., Guarini, A., Gaggioli, L., Zauli, G., Catani, L., Valvassori, L., Zunica, G., Gugliotta, L., and Marini, M., Human T-lymphocyte-derived megakaryocyte colony-stimulating activity, *Exp. Hematol.,* 15, 679, 1987.
412. Quesenberry, P.J., Synergistic hematopoietic growth factors, *Int. J. Cell Cloning,* 4, 3, 1986.
413. Williams, N., Sparrow, R., Gill, K., Yasmeen, D., and McNiece, I., Murine megakaryocyte colony-stimulating factor: its relationship to interleukin 3, *Leukemia Res.,* 9, 1487, 1985.
414. Lopez, A.F., To, L.B., Yang, Y.-C., Ganble, J.R., Shannon, M.F., Burns, G.F., Dyson, P.G., Juttner, C.A., Clark, S., and Vadas, M.A., Stimulation of proliferation, differentiation, and function of human cells by primate interleukin 3, *Proc. Natl. Acad. Sci. U.S.A.,* 84, 2761, 1987.
415. Mazur, E.M., Cohen, J.L., Bogart, L., Mufson, R.A., Gesner, T.G., Yang, Y.-C., and Clark, S.C., Recombinant gibbon interleukin-3 stimulates megakaryocyte colony growth in vitro from human peripheral blood progenitor cells, *J. Cell. Physiol.,* 136, 439, 1988.
416. Ishibashi, T., Kimura, H., Uchida, T., Kariyone, S., Friese, P., and Burstein, S.A., Human interleukin 6 is a direct promoter of maturation of megakaryocytes in vitro, *Proc. Natl. Acad. Sci. U.S.A.,* 86, 5953, 1989.
417. Lotem, J., Shabo, Y., and Sachs, L., Regulation of megakaryocyte development by interleukin-6, *Blood,* 74, 1545, 1989.
418. Teramura, M., Katahira, J., Hoshino, S., Motoji, T., Oshimi, K., and Mizoguchi, H., Effect of recombinant hemopoietic growth factors on human megakaryocyte colony formation in serum-free cultures, *Exp. Hematol.,* 17, 1011, 1989.
419. Bruno, E. and Hoffman, R., Effect of interleukin 6 on in vitro human megakaryocytopoiesis: its interaction with other cytokines, *Exp. Hematol.,* 17, 1038, 1989.
420. Paul, S.R., Bennett, F., Calvetti, J.A., Kelleher, K., Wood, C.R., O'Hara, R.M., Jr., Leary, A.C., Sibley, B., Clark, S.C., Williams, D.A., and Yang, Y.-C., Molecular cloning of a cDNA encoding interleukin 11, a stromal cell-derived lymphopoietic and hematopoietic cytokine, *Proc. Natl. Acad. Sci. U.S.A.,* 87, 7512, 1990.
421. Griffin, C.G. and Grant, B.W., Effects of recombinant interferons on human megakaryocyte growth, *Exp. Hematol.,* 18, 1013, 1990.
422. Mazur, E.M., Cohen, J.L., Newton, J., Sohl, P., Narendran, A., Gesner, T.G., and Mufson, R.A., Human serum megakaryocyte colony-stimulating activity appears to be distinct from interleukin-3, granulocyte-macrophage colony-stimulating factor, and lymphocyte-conditioned medium, *Blood,* 76, 290, 1990.
423. Mitjavila, M.T., Vinci, G., Villeval, J.L., Kieffer, N., Henri, A., Testa, U., Breton-Gorius, J., and Vainchenker, W., Human platelet α granules contain a nonspecific inhibitor of megakaryocyte colony formation: its relationship to type β transforming growth factor (TGF-β), *J. Cell. Physiol.,* 134, 83, 1988.
424. Levin, J. and Evatt, B.L., Humoral control of thrombopoiesis, *Blood Cells,* 5, 105, 1979.
425. McDonald, T.P., Thrombopoietin: its biology, purification, and characterization, *Exp. Hematol.,* 16, 201, 1988.
426. Straneva, J.E., Briddell, R.A., McDonald, T.P., Yang, H.H., and Hoffman, R., Effects of thrombocytopoiesis-stimulating factor on terminal cytoplasmic maturation of human megakaryocytes, *Exp. Hematol.,* 17, 1122, 1989.
427. Williams, N., Eger, R.R., Jackson, H.M., and Nelson, D.J., Two factor requirement for murine megakaryocyte colony formation, *J. Cell. Physiol.,* 110, 101, 1982.
428. Golde, D.W., Finley, T.N., and Cline, M.J., Production of colony-stimulating factor by human macrophages, *Lancet,* 2, 1397, 1972.
429. Fidler, I.J. and Raz, A., The induction of tumoricidal capabilities in mouse and rat macrophages by lymphokines, in *Lymphokines,* Vol. 3, Pick, E., Ed., Academic Press, New York, 1981, 345.
430. Sato, K., Fujii, Y., Kasono, K., Saji, M., Tsushima, T., and Shizume, K., Stimulation of prostaglandin E_2 and bone resorption by recombinant human interleukin 1α in fetal mouse bones, *Biochem. Biophys. Res. Commun.,* 138, 618, 1986.
431. Baird, A., Mormede, P., and Böhlen, P., Immunoreactive fibroblast growth factor in cells of peritoneal exudate suggests its identity with macrophage-derived growth factor, *Biochem. Biophys. Res. Commun.,* 126, 358, 1985.

432. **Shimokado, K., Raines, E.W., Madtes, D.K., Barrett, T.R., Benditt, E.P., and Ross, R.,** A significant part of macrophage-derived growth factor consists of at least two forms of PDGF, *Cell,* 43, 277, 1985.
433. **Kleinerman, E.S., Zicht, R., Sarin, P.S., Gallo, R.C., and Fidler, I.J.,** Constitutive production and release of a lymphokine with macrophage-activating factor activity distinct from γ-interferon by a human T-cell leukemia virus-positive cell line, *Cancer Res.,* 44, 4470, 1984.
434. **Baliga, B.S., Rorher, S.D., Maumenee, A.E., and Peterson, R.D.A.,** Biosynthesis of macrophage activating factor, *Lymphokine Res.,* 5, 141, 1986.
435. **Keller, R. and Kleist, R.,** Induction, maintenance, and reinduction of tumoricidal activity in bone-marrow-derived mononuclear phagocytes by macrophage-activating lymphokines, *Cell. Immunol.,* 101, 659, 1986.
436. **Talmadge, K.W., Gallati, H., Sinigaglia, F., Walz, A., and Garotta, G.,** Identity between human interferon-γ and "macrophage-activating factor" produced by human T lymphocytes, *Eur. J. Immunol.,* 16, 1471, 1986.
437. **Crawford, R.M., Finbloom, D.S., Ohara, J., Paul, W.E., and Meltzer, M.S.,** B cell stimulatory factor-1 (interleukin 4) activates macrophages for increased tumoricidal activity and expression of Ia antigens, *J. Immunol.,* 139, 135, 1987.
438. **Jones, M.P.A., Gunapala, D.E., Matutes, E., Catovsky, D., and Coates, A.R.M.,** A novel human macrophage-activating factor: distinction from interferon-γ (IFN-γ) and granulocyte-macrophage colony-stimulating factor (GMCSF), *Cell. Immunol.,* 113, 361, 1988.
439. **MacSween, J.M., Rajaraman, K., and Rajaraman, R.,** The cellular basis for differential lymphokine responses to mitogen stimulation, *Cell. Immunol.,* 101, 82, 1986.
440. **Wolpe, S.D. and Cerami, A.,** Macrophage inflammatory proteins 1 and 2: members of a novel superfamily of cytokines, *FASEB J.,* 3, 2565, 1989.
441. **Oppenheim, J.J., Zachariae, C.O.C., Mukaida, N., and Matusushima, K.,** Properties of the novel proinflammatory supergene "intercrine" cytokine family, *Annu. Rev. Immunol.,* 9, 617, 1991.
442. **Deuel, T.F., Keim, P.S., Farmer, M., and Heinrikson, R.L.,** Amino acid sequence of human platelet factor 4, *Proc. Natl. Acad. Sci. U.S.A.,* 74, 2256, 1977.
443. **Heinrich, J.N., Ryseck, R.-P., Macdonald-Bravo, H., and Bravo, R.,** The product of a novel growth factor-activated gene, *fic,* is a biologically active "C-C"-type cytokine, *Mol. Cell. Biol.,* 13, 2020, 1993.

Chapter 4

Interferons

I. INTRODUCTION

The interferons (IFNs) are cellular proteins which were first identified by their ability to protect cells against viral infections.[1] The IFNs are also involved in the mechanisms of protection against bacterial and parasitic infections. In addition, IFNs have an important role in the physiologic processes associated with the regulation of cell proliferation and differentiation.[2-10] The effects of IFN on cellular proliferation are mostly inhibitory, but the effects of different IFNs on cell differentiation are much more complicated. The important role of the IFNs in human malignant diseases has been documented by experimental and clinical studies.

IFNs are a family of proteins with molecular weights in the range of 15 to 30 kDa. This family includes three major types of IFNs, designated α, β, and γ. The α and β IFNs are also called leukocyte and fibroblast IFNs, respectively, and are generically known as class I (type I) IFNs. Class I IFNs are synthesized in response to viral infection, and a single cell line can produce mixtures of IFN-α and IFN-β. Production of IFN-β is induced by treatment of fibroblasts with double-stranded RNA (dsRNA) molecules such as polyinosinic acid:polycytidylic acid. IFN-γ is produced in T lymphocytes following mitogenic or antigenic stimulation and is known as immune IFN or class II (type II) IFN. Human B-cell lines may also express the IFN-γ gene.[11]

IFNs are synthesized and secreted by a variety of cell types in response to different substances and factors acting as IFN inducers, and exert their effects *in vivo* as a result of interaction with other cells in distant parts of the body in a way similar to that of hormones. A functional similarity with hormones is further emphasized by the existence in target cells of specific membrane receptors for IFNs and by the multiplicity of biological effects which result from the interaction of IFNs with their cellular receptors. Different types of transformed cells may act as IFN inducers through the interaction of a specific lymphocyte receptor with a glycoprotein inducer on the surface of the transformed cell. Paradoxically, retinoic acid, which is an inhibitor of tumor cell growth, inhibits in a time- and dose-dependent manner the ability of mouse and human tumor cell lines to induce IFN production by nonsensitized lymphocytes.[12]

II. REGULATION OF INTERFERON PRODUCTION

Induction of IFN production by IFN inducers occurs primarily by an increase in the transcriptional expression of IFN genes and does not require protein synthesis. IFN genes are normally not expressed and are probably repressed, but are turned on following induction. The molecular mechanisms involved in the regulation of IFN production are only partially understood.[9] DNA-binding factors may recognize specific DNA sequences that act as promoters or enhancers of IFN gene expression. The first intron of the human IFN-γ gene contains a binding site for the c-Rel proto-oncogene product.[13] The c-Rel protein shares extensive sequence homology with the p50 and p65 subunits of the NF-κB transcription factor, and the nucleotide sequence recognized by c-Rel is partially identical with an IFN-stimulatable response element (ISRE), suggesting that c-Rel may play a role in IFN-γ gene induction. After IFN protein production, transcription of the IFN gene is downregulated, perhaps by the action of specific repressors. The duration of IFN production may be regulated, in part, by mRNA stability.

Complex endogenous and exogenous factors are involved in the regulation of the synthesis and secretion of the different IFNs, which partially depends on the cell type and the nature of the specific stimulus. Stimulation of human lymphocytes with PHA induces the synthesis of mRNAs for both IFN-β and IFN-γ.[14] Lymphocytes appear to be the only cells normally capable of producing IFN-γ, and this production is regulated by growth factors such as PDGF, EGF, and FGF.[15]

IL-1 and IL-2 have important roles in the regulation of IFN-γ production.[16] Bacterial LPS can induce IFN-γ production by human peripheral T lymphocytes in the presence of accessory monocytes, and it has been demonstrated that induction of IFN-γ by LPS depends mainly on the generation of IL-1 by monocytes/macrophages as well as on an enhanced expression of IL-2 receptors on T lymphocytes.[17] Highly purified T cells can be stimulated to produce IFN-γ by a synergistic action of IL-1 and IL-2. IL-2 induces the transcriptional expression of the IFN-γ gene in murine T cells.[18] This effect may be mediated, at least in part, by protein kinase C activation and Ca^{2+} mobilization. Arachidonic acid plays a pivotal role as an intracellular mediator of the IL-2-elicited signal for the stimulation of IFN-γ production.[19] IL-2-induced production of IFN-γ is dependent on the interaction of IL-2 with IL-2 receptors.[20]

Highly purified human T cells from peripheral blood fail to produce IFN-γ *in vitro* in the absence of accessory cells, but their ability to produce IFN-γ upon stimulation with PHA or concanavalin A is restored when the cells are cocultivated in the presence of allogeneic human fibroblasts.[21] Addition of IL-1α or IL-1β to PHA-stimulated T cells cocultured with fibroblasts results in stimulation of IFN production. However, preincubation of fibroblasts with IL-1α, IL-1β, or TNF-α causes a dose-dependent suppression of the ability of fibroblasts to augment PHA- and concanavalin A-induced IFN-γ production by T cells. Thus, fibroblasts can have marked effects on T-cell functions, and IL-1 and TNF-α can exert immunoregulatory activities indirectly by altering the interactions of fibroblasts with T cells and can modify the capacity of T cells to produce interferon in the presence of fibroblasts. The nature of the interactions responsible for the accessory activity of human fibroblasts for mitogen-activated T cells is not understood.

TNF-α may play a role in regulating the production and effects of IFNs. Cultured FS-4 human foreskin fibroblasts produce IFN-β and secrete it into the medium, and TNF-α induces a severalfold increase in the level of IFN-β mRNA and enhances the production of endogenous IFN-β protein in these cells.[22] Unstimulated FS-4 cells produce small amounts of IFN-β transcripts, as demonstrated by the highly sensitive PCR technique. These small concentrations of autocrine IFN-β may be sufficient to produce a strong synergistic action with TNF-α. These results indicate that autocrine secretion of cytokines, at concentrations that may escape detection by conventional assays, can result in potent biological actions.

III. INTERFERON STRUCTURE AND THE INTERFERON GENES

The genes for IFN-α are located on human chromosome region 9p22 (about 15 active genes), and the gene for IFN-β is located on the same chromosome region.[23] The human IFN-α and IFN-β genes are devoid of introns and code for proteins with very similar biological properties. cDNAs for human IFN-α and IFN-β have been constructed and the nucleotide sequences and deduced amino acid sequences determined.[24-27] The human IFN-α gene codes for a polypeptide of 166 amino acids with a molecular weight of 19,360 Da, and the human IFN-β gene codes for a polypeptide of 165 amino acids with a molecular weight of 20,040 Da. The human IFN-β protein contains three cysteine residues which contribute to the maintenance of the configuration and function of the protein through the existence of disulfide bonds. The human IFN-β protein is preceded by a 21-amino acid signal sequence.

Multiple (more than 15) IFN-α genes are present in the human genome and several different, but homologous, proteins are synthesized by human cells.[28-31] In contrast to the majority of mammalian genes, human IFN-α and IFN-β genes are devoid of intron sequences.[32-35] Human IFN-α and IFN-β are structurally related, showing 45% homology at the nucleotide level and 29% at the amino acid level.[36] Human IFN-α and IFN-β genes give rise to mRNA species which are unusually long polyadenylated structures.[37]

There is a single gene for IFN-γ in the human genome. Human IFN-α cDNA, cloned and expressed in *Escherichia coli*, is biologically active, being capable of protecting squirrel monkeys from lethal encephalomyocarditis virus infection.[38,39] A cDNA coding for human IFN-α was also expressed in yeast.[40] Mouse L cells transformed with a cloned IFN-α gene produced IFN-α mRNA under the normal biochemical control mechanisms of the cell.[41] A cDNA sequence coding for human IFN-γ was identified and cloned and was expressed in *E. coli*.[42,43] This sequence codes for a polypeptide of 166 amino acids, 20 of which constitute a signal peptide, and is quite basic in character. Human IFN-γ bears little structural homology to IFN-α or IFN-β.[44] The total chemical synthesis of a human IFN-γ gene and its expression in *E. coli* have been reported.[45] The human IFN-γ gene cloned in recombinant plasmids and transfected into cultured monkey cells directs the synthesis of the human IFN-γ protein. The single IFN-γ gene contained in the human genome has very little polymorphism and gives rise to a single class of mRNA.[46] Transcriptional regulation of IFN-γ synthesis takes place at T-cell-specific, DNase I-hypersensitive DNA sequences located in both the first intron and the distal 5' flanking region of the human IFN-γ gene.[47] Several additional structural domains of the IFN-γ gene, including a proximal, promoter-associated site that appears only after PHA/PMA-mediated IFN-γ induction, may also be involved in the transcriptional activation of the gene.

Several distinct IFN-β genes have been detected in the human genome.[48] Whereas the IFN-$β_1$ gene is situated on chromosome 9p near a region that carries the IFN-$α_1$-related gene cluster, the IFN-$β_2$ gene is located on chromosome 7, and additional IFN-β-related genes may be located on chromosomes 2 and 4.[49] The human IFN-β1 gene has no introns but the human IFN-β2 gene has several introns. IFN-β1 may represent the ultimate mediator of the antiviral effects attributed to IL-1 and TNF-α.[50] The antiviral effects of TNF-α and IL-1 can be neutralized by specific antibodies against IFN-$β_1$.

The structure and expression of a cDNA coding for human IFN-$β_2$ has been reported.[51,52] The sequence encodes a 23.7-kDa polypeptide of 212 amino acids. The amino acid sequence of IFN-$β_2$, as deduced from its mRNA induced by TNF-α in FS-4 human fibroblasts, shares structural similarities with IFN α and β. It has been shown that IFN-$β_2$ and BSF-2/IL6 are identical molecules.[53,54] Moreover, IFN-$β_2$/BSF-2/IL-6 is identical with a protein called hepatocyte-stimulating factor, which plays an essential role in the development of the acute response to inflammation and trauma.[55]

IV. INTERFERON RECEPTORS

The initial event of IFN action consists in its binding to specific high-affinity cell surface receptors.[56-58] IFN-α and IFN-β appear to bind to a common receptor, named the type I receptor, whereas IFN-γ binds to a distinct receptor, the type II receptor. The gene for the type I IFN receptor is located on human chromosome 21q, and the gene for the type II IFN receptor on chromosome 6, although a component contributed by chromosome 21 appears necessary for full expression.[59] Differential expression of two IFN-α-binding complexes (140 to 160 kDa and 60 kDa) occurs in both proliferating and nonproliferating cells.[60] The biological significance of this difference is unknown.

There is a single class of high-affinity IFN-γ receptor expressed in human cells of distinct tissue origin. The gene coding for the IFN-γ receptor is located on the long arm of human chromosome 6, at region 6q16-q22, close to the c-ros proto-oncogene locus.[61,62] A cDNA encoding the human IFN-γ receptor has been isolated and transfected into mouse cells.[63] As inferred from the cDNA sequence, the human IFN-γ receptor shows no similarities to known proteins. The functional IFN-γ receptor appears to be represented by a dimeric molecule composed of two subunits.[64] As deduced from a cDNA clone, the mouse IFN-γ receptor is a transmembrane protein of 477 amino acid residues.[65] The receptor contains a large cytoplasmic domain of 200 amino acids which have a role in signal transduction, but it has no structural homology with the catalytic domains of growth factor receptors with tyrosine kinase activity, nor does it have a sequence suggestive of an ATP-binding domain.

Normal human B lymphocytes and EBV-immortalized B-cell lines constitutively express IFN-γ receptors of 90 kDa.[66] The IFN-γ receptor was found to be expressed in the vast majority of human tumor cells derived from various tissue origins, and large differences in the number of IFN-γ membrane receptors were found on distinct tumor cells of the same cell type, ranging from a few hundred up to 2 × 10^4 for both carcinoma cells and leukemic cells. Corticosteroids enhance the binding of IFN-γ to human monocytes.[67] A fractional occupancy of less than 5% of murine IFN-γ receptors by the physiological ligand is sufficient to produce the biological response.[68] The IFN-γ receptor numbers do not change during cell cycle progression of *in vitro* established human cell lines.[64] Moreover, unlike other inducible receptors for lymphokines, expression of IFN-γ receptors appears to be constitutive in different types of human tumor cells and is not altered by agents inducing differentiation in leukemic cells.

The effects of IFN, especially at the transcriptional level, correlate to the number of IFN receptors occupied. However, it has been difficult to demonstrate significant correlation between IFN binding and the degree of cellular effects or biological effects.[57,58] Several findings do not support the concept that binding of IFN to surface receptors, by itself, induces all subsequent cellular activities. There is evidence suggesting that IFN receptors, alone or in combination with bound IFN, may act as messengers upon their transport into the nucleus by a process of facilitated receptor-mediated endocytosis, and the possibility exists that intracellular IFN molecules can exert physiological activity, bypassing surface receptors.

V. POSTRECEPTOR MECHANISMS OF INTERFERON ACTION

Little is known about the signal molecules involved in transduction of IFN-induced cellular responses. Mechanisms possibly associated with IFN signal transduction include cytoplasmic alkalinization, phosphatidylinositol metabolism, cytoplasmic concentrations of free Ca^{2+}, intracellular levels of cAMP and/or cGMP, and protein kinase activity. Some of the most important changes elicited by IFNs are exerted through specific regulation of gene expression. After IFN α/β binding to its receptor, a signal is generated that leads to the activation of a latent cytoplasmic DNA-binding factor, the IFN-stimulated gene factor (ISGF). Expression of the adenoviral oncogene E1A may interfere with the IFN signal transduction pathway by inhibiting the DNA-binding activity of ISGF3.[69]

Changes in phosphoinositide metabolism may be prominent in the transductional mechanisms of IFN action. Human IFN-α and IFN-β, but not IFN-γ, stimulated a transient increase in the concentration of diacylglycerol and inositol bis- and trisphosphates within seconds in different types of human and murine cells.[70] No changes in $[Ca^{2+}]_i$ were detected in the IFN-stimulated cells. These results suggest that protein kinase C may have a role in the mediation of cellular IFN effects. There is indeed evidence that the effects of IFN-γ on macrophage functions are mediated by an enhancement in the catalytic activity of protein kinase C, which then results in increased phosphorylation of particular cellular proteins.[71] In the murine pre-B-like cell line 70Z/3, IFN-γ induces translocation of protein kinase C to the cell membrane and increases Na^+/H^+ exchange across the cell membrane, but the enhancement in monovalent ion exchange is independent of the activation of protein kinase C.[72] The antiproliferative activity exerted by IFN-β and IFN-γ on human tumor cells (Hep-2 and KHm14 cells) is associated with modulation of protein kinase C activity.[73] IFN-γ induces a phospholipase D-dependent triphasic activation of protein kinase C in endothelial cells.[74] Protein kinase C may be involved in the cellular responses to IFN-α,[75] but the precise role of this kinase in the growth-inhibitory effect of IFNs remains to be evaluated. Signal transduction by IFN-α may include alterations in arachidonic acid metabolism.[76]

Phosphorylation of cellular proteins on tyrosine may have a role in the postreceptor mechanism of action of interferon. Tyrosine phosphorylation is an early and requisite signal induced by IFN-γ in HL-60 human leukemia cells.[77] As the IFN receptor does not contain sequences characteristic of tyrosine kinases, IFN-induced tyrosine phosphorylation of cellular proteins must be induced by accessory enzymes. A tyrosine kinase is involved in the signaling pathway of IFN α/β, and a transcription factor containing SH2 and SH3 domains is directly activated by IFN-α-induced cytoplasmic tyrosine kinase.[78,79]

The antiviral action and other physiological effects of IFN are associated with the induction of new protein syntheses, which may involve regulatory changes at the genomic level. The best-characterized of the IFN-induced proteins is 2′,5′-oligoadenylate synthetase (2′,5′-A synthetase), an enzyme which catalyzes, in the presence of double-stranded RNA and ATP, the synthesis of oligomers of adenylic acid in a 2′,5′ phosphodiester bond. The synthesized oligomers activate then a latent RNase, which may lead to the degradation of RNA molecules. At least four different forms of 2′,5′-A synthetase have been found in human cells.[80] The question of whether this enzyme plays a role in cell proliferation and differentiation is still open, but M-MuSV-transformed NIH/3T3 cells treated with IFN result in a severalfold increase of 2′,5′-A synthetase gene expression.[81] The M-MuSV-transformed cells, which are relatively resistant to cytolytic virus infection, contain elevated basal levels of the synthetase transcripts and protein. A 27-fold increase in 2′,5′-A synthetase activity has been observed in HL-60 human leukemia cells treated with DMSO, a compound capable of inducing the granulocytic differentiation of these cells.[82] In addition to stimulating the synthesis of specific proteins, IFNs may have an inhibitory effect on the synthesis of certain cellular proteins.

VI. EFFECTS OF INTERFERON ON GENE EXPRESSION

Some of the most important physiologic changes induced by IFNs are exerted through the regulation of gene expression, including proto-oncogenes. Specific consensus DNA sequences are involved in the regulation of gene expression by IFN. The sequence GAAANNGAAA may be an element involved in this regulation.[9] This sequence is present in the 5′ promoter region of all the IFN-inducible genes and is called IFN-stimulated response element (ISRE) or IFN-responsive sequence (IRS). Nuclear binding factors may recognize ISREs in IFN-inducible genes. Some IFN-inducible genes can also be induced by viruses or other external stimuli.

The concentrations of mRNAs coding for several proteins may be altered in cells exposed to exogenous IFNs,[6] and the synthesis of various proteins is modulated by IFN in cells such as human fibroblasts.[83] These proteins include enzymes, surface antigens, and other proteins of unknown function. The expression of HLA-DR antigens is enhanced by IFN-γ on a diversity of cells, including human and murine monocytes, fibroblasts, and endothelial cells, and the level of HLA-DR expression is reduced by treatment of the cells with TGF-$β_1$.[84]

Expression of genes encoding cytokines or their receptors may be induced or repressed by the action of different IFN classes. The IL-2 receptor gene is induced by IFN-γ in human peripheral blood monocytes as well as in the monocytic cell line U-937.[85] IFN-γ stimulates the expression of the TNF-α, IL-1, and urokinase-type plasminogen activator genes in mouse peritoneal macrophages.[86] Transcription of these genes is apparently kept under negative control by repressor proteins. Screening of a cDNA library prepared from lymphokine-stimulated RAW 264.7 cells (a mouse monocyte/macrophage cell line) led to the identification of a set of genes that are induced by IFN-γ.[87] One of these genes, m119, is selectively induced by IFN-γ and encodes a 14.5-kDa protein which is a member of a family of cytokines that include platelet factor 4 (PF4), melanoma growth-stimulatory activity, and IL-8. The name *mig* was proposed for this new member of the PF4 gene family. The m119/mig protein may be a cytokine that affects the growth, movement, or activation state of cells that participate in immune and inflammatory responses.

Class I IFNs induce a marked increase in the transcriptional activity of distinct mammalian genes.[88] Human genes that are induced by IFN-α and IFN-β have been identified and later expressed in manipulated murine cells.[89,90] A gene whose expression is increased 20-fold in Ehrlich ascites tumor cells treated with IFN-β was also cloned.[91] This gene encodes a 56-kDa protein whose function is unknown. Another protein of 15 kDa induced by IFN has been characterized, its amino acid sequence was determined, and the gene coding for this protein was cloned.[92]

A gene inducible by IFN encodes a 98-amino acid protein, IP-10, which shows homology to some chemotactic and mitogenic peptides and is secreted in response to IFN by a variety of cells including monocytes, endothelial cells, and fibroblasts. The gene coding for IP-10 has been mapped to human chromosome region 4q21, a locus associated with an acute monocytic/B-lymphocytic lineage leukemia that exhibits the nonrandom translocation t(4;11)(q21;q23).[93] The c-*ets*-1 proto-oncogene is located on human chromosome region 11q23 and may be involved in this translocation. However, the possible role of c-*ets*-1 in human leukemia is unknown.

The mechanisms involved in the regulation of specific genes by IFN remain to be characterized. A set of genes is rapidly induced by treatment of the human glioblastoma cell line T98G with IFN, and this activation is linked to IFN surface receptor occupancy.[94] The regulation of IFN-inducible genes may be exerted primarily at the level of the plasma membrane by the concentration of occupied IFN receptors. The signals that mediate the transcriptional response to IFN remain unknown. No changes in pH_i, Ca^{2+} influx, and phosphoinositide turnover may be detected during early treatment of human cells with IFN. However, protein kinase C activity and intracellular Ca^{2+} mobilization may have a role in the induction of macrophage tumoricidal activity by IFN-γ.[95] The IFNs can activate specific latent cytoplasmic transcription factors and this effect may be associated with IFN-dependent tyrosine phosphorylation.[96,97] A common transcription factor, IRF-1, may have a critical role in the regulation of IFN-inducible genes.[98] IRF-1 is an immediate-early gene in prolactin-stimulated T cells, which suggests that it is a multifunctional molecule.[99] In addition to its role in regulating growth-inhibitory effects of IFN-inducible genes, IRF-1 may play a stimulatory role in the proliferation of certain types of cells.

A. PROTO-ONCOGENE AND TUMOR SUPPRESSOR GENE EXPRESSION

Exposure of cells to IFN may induce alteration in the level of proto-oncogene expression. However, a general correlation between the cytostatic effects of IFNs and changes in the levels of proto-oncogene expression is not readily apparent. The growth-inhibitory effects of IFN-α in various human leukemic cell lines is associated with altered expression of proto-oncogenes encoding nuclear protein products such as Myc and Fos, but inhibition of growth is not obligatorily coupled to inhibition of proto-oncogene expression.[100] IFN-induced inhibition of the proliferation of normal human fibroblasts is not associated with downregulation of c-*fos* or c-*myc* gene expression.[101] The effects of IFN on proto-oncogene expression can also be observed *in vivo*. Treatment of human malignant diseases with IFNs may be associated with altered expression of particular proto-oncogenes. For example, changes in c-*myc* and c-*fos* gene expression are observed during treatment of hairy cell leukemia with IFN-α.[102] The biological significance of changes in proto-oncogene expression during the treatment of malignant or nonmalignant diseases with IFN is unknown.

Conflicting results have been obtained in studies related to the effect of IFN on c-*myc* gene expression. The discrepant results may be attributed, at least in part, to differences in the experimental protocols, including the class of IFN and the type of cell. Treatment of the HL-60 and Daudi human hematopoietic cell lines with IFN-γ may result in an increase of Myc protein levels.[103] However, a selective reduction in the levels of c-*myc* mRNA has been observed in Daudi cells treated with different IFNs, including IFN-β, and this reduction was accompanied by inhibition of cell growth.[104-106] A close link would exist, at least in some cases, between reduction of c-*myc* expression and IFN-induced arrest of cells at the G_0/G_1 phase of the cycle.[107] The cell-cycle responses to IFN and IL-6 of M1 myeloblastic cells are mediated by the negative effects that these cytokines exert on c-*myc* mRNA and protein expression.[108] Downregulation of c-*myc* gene expression by IFN-γ and TNF-α precedes growth arrest in cultured human melanoma cells.[109]

Regulation of c-*myc* gene expression by interferon may occur at either the transcriptional or posttranscriptional level. In Daudi cells, both IFN-α and IFN-β may regulate c-*myc* expression at the posttranscriptional level by reducing the half-life of c-*myc* mRNA.[110-112] Reduction of c-*myc* mRNA is observed in Daudi cells whose protein synthesis is inhibited by more than 95% with cycloheximide or emetine, indicating that neither sustained nor IFN-induced protein synthesis is required for the regulation of c-*myc* mRNA in these cells.[113]

Decreased levels of c-*myc* gene expression are associated with some IFN-treated cells, but in other cases these changes are not observed and their possible physiological significance remains controversial. In the HL-60 and U-937 human leukemia cell lines, IFN-α and IFN-β do not reduce c-*myc* mRNA levels.[107,112] Reduced c-*myc* expression is a late event in IFN-γ-induced differentiation of HL-60 cells, suggesting that it is not required for the commitment of cells to differentiate.[114] The basis of the difference observed between Daudi cells and other leukemic cell lines is unknown. Both HL-60 cells and U-937 cells display normal induction of other IFN-regulated activities and show a decline in c-*myc* gene expression when they become arrested in the G_0/G_1 phase of the cycle as part of their terminal differentiation.[107]

The growth-inhibitory effect of IFN-α on Daudi cells and HL-60 cells does not depend on changes in the expression of the transferrin receptor.[112] IFN and calcitriol may reduce the expression of c-*myc* in HL-60 cells in a cooperative manner related to inhibition of cell proliferation.[115] Human IFN-γ alters c-*myc* gene expression and growth pattern of the U-937 cell line, but not of its subclone 1937.[116] In clones of Daudi cells selected for resistance to the antiproliferative action of IFN the level of c-*myc* mRNA did not change following IFN treatment, but a clone of the IFN-resistant cells, which had reverted to almost complete sensitivity to the antiproliferative action of IFN, remained refractory to IFN modulation of c-*myc* gene expression.[117] In general, these results obtained with IFN-treated hematopoietic cells suggest that a reduced level of c-*myc* mRNA may not be a prerequisite for inhibition of cell proliferation in IFN-treated cells. Thus, the precise relationships between IFN action, c-*myc* expression, and the control mechanisms of cell proliferation are unknown.

Discrepant results of the effects of interferon on c-*myc* gene expression have also been obtained in the study of nonhematopoietic cells. IFN-γ induces a reduction of c-*myc* mRNA levels in HeLa cells, which is associated with a specific arrest in the G_0/G_1 phase of the cell cycle.[118] This effect is dependent on protein synthesis and is enhanced by TNF-α. The mechanism by which IFN-β slows the growth rate of some human lung-cancer cell lines may not directly involve downregulation of c-*myc* gene expression, which is overexpressed in these tumor cells.[119] Amplification of the N-*myc* gene in a rat neuroblastoma cell line was found to be associated with down-modulation of MHC class I antigen expression, and treatment of these cells with IFN-γ resulted in reversion of MHC antigen expression without affecting the steady-state level of N-*myc* mRNA.[120]

The effects of IFN on c-*fos* expression are variable. Treatment of normal peritoneal macrophages with either IFN-β or IFN-γ, which are potent macrophage activators eliciting tumoricidal activity, may alter the levels of c-*fos* transcripts.[121] IFN-γ-induced downregulation of c-*fos* mRNA expression in human macrophages occurs at the posttranscriptional level.[122] IFN induces c-*fos* expression in NIH/3T3 and F9EC cells.[123] However, the inhibitory effect of IFN on the proliferation of 3T3 mouse cells may not be associated with enhanced c-*fos* expression.[124] Regulation of c-*fos* gene expression by IFN-α in murine and human cells depends on the binding of nuclear factors — in particular, a 98-kDa protein to a DNA sequence element located in the 5' upstream region of the c-*fos* gene.[125]

IFN is capable of inhibiting the transformation of mouse cells caused by exogenous cellular or viral genes.[126] The development of transformed foci in NIH/3T3 cells transfected with v-H-*ras*, v-*mos*, or EJ/T24 c-*ras* DNA is inhibited by IFN treatment.[127] IFN also inhibits transformation of established rodent cell lines by mutant human c-H-*ras* and c-K-*ras* genes.[128] Moreover, prolonged treatment with mouse IFN-α/β can induce phenotypic reversion in NIH/3T3 cells transformed by an LTR-activated human c-H-*ras* gene, but not in cells transformed by a mutant c-H-*ras* gene.[127,129,130]

Proto-oncogene expression may have a role in the cytostatic effects of IFN. Treatment of A431 human epidermoid carcinoma cells with IFN-γ, but not IFN-α or IFN-β, results in a rapid appearance of morphological alterations followed by cell death, and these changes are accompanied by elevated expression of the c-H-*ras* and c-*erb*-B mRNA and protein.[131] IFN-γ-induced killing of A431 cells may be the consequence of an acceleration of terminal differentiation. Addition of double-stranded RNA to cultures of NIH/3T3 cells results in the synthesis of IFN, and this effect is followed by the induction of c-H-*ras* gene expression.[132]

Treatment of cells transformed by acute retroviruses with IFN may result in differential regulation of oncogene expression. In BALB/c 3T3 cells transformed by the genomic incorporation of K-MuSV carrying the v-K-*ras* oncogene, IFN-α/β treatment results in phenotypic cellular changes which are accompanied by differential expression of v-K-*ras*, c-*myc*, and IAP genes.[133] Treatment of RSV-transformed rat cells with rat IFN-α causes a 50% reduction in intracellular v-Src kinase activity, which is accompanied by a reduction in the growth rate of the transformed cells.[134] IFN is also capable of lowering the steady-state concentrations of c-H-*ras* and c-*src* mRNAs in human bladder carcinoma cells.[135] The mechanisms responsible for such IFN inhibitory effects are poorly understood.

The inhibitory effect of IFN on the expression of Ras protein in cells transformed by an LTR-activated *ras* gene takes place at the transcriptional level.[136] In contrast to the reversibility of cellular changes seen after exposure to IFN for several days, the phenotypic reversion of RS485 cells established after 1 to 2 months of IFN treatment persists long after treatment is discontinued.[137] The persistent revertants express high levels of Ras protein, yet are not tumorigenic. These cells are resistant to retransformation by a variety of viral and cellular oncogenes, but they can be readily transformed by the oncogenes after exposure to DNA demethylating drugs such as 5-azacytidine. The persistent reversion transformants revert again when they are treated with IFN. These results suggest that DNA methylation is involved in IFN-induced persistent reversion of oncogene-transformed cells. Cellular genes other than proto-oncogenes may be involved in IFN-induced phenotypic changes.[138]

Phenotypic changes induced by IFN in malignant cells are not necessarily associated altered proto-oncogene expression.[139] In some human tumor cell lines (OHA osteosarcoma cells, EJ bladder carcinoma cells, and SHAC gastric carcinoma cells) the transforming ability and the level of expression of activated c-*ras* proto-oncogenes (c-K-*ras*, c-H-*ras*, and N-*ras*) were unaltered with long-term IFN-α treatment. Although this treatment induced a partial reversion of some aspects of the tumor cell phenotype it did not reverse, but even potentiated, other phenotypic characteristics including tumorigenicity. Thus, there is no simple relationship between the results of IFN treatment and the level of expression of c-*ras* genes in human tumor cells.

Different classes of IFN may have different effects in the level of proto-oncogene expression. For example, treatment of A431 human vulval squamous carcinoma cells with IFN-α or IFN-β results in diminished expression of the c-H-*ras* gene, but the expression of the same gene is elevated two- to threefold by treatment with IFN-γ.[139] Expression of the EGF receptor gene, as determined with v-*erb*-B as a probe, also increased three- to sevenfold after a 1-day treatment of A431 cells with IFN-γ. Thus, both the type of cell and the class of IFN may crucially determine the final response in relation to the level of expression of particular proto-oncogenes.

Functional activation of normal murine marrow-derived monocytic cells by IFN-γ, CSF-2, or LPS is accompanied by transient induction of c-*fgr* proto-oncogene expression.[140] Induction of the c-*fgr* gene is also observed when the proliferation of these cells is stimulated by exposure to CSF-1. These results suggest that the function of the c-Fgr tyrosine kinase may be essential for the mediation of the intracellular effects of many monocytic stimuli.

VII. EFFECTS OF INTERFERON ON CELL PROLIFERATION AND CELL DIFFERENTIATION

The IFNs have important effects on the processes of cell proliferation and cell differentiation.[6] These effects are exerted, at least in part, at the transcriptional level, and may include changes in the expression of specific proto-oncogenes.[141] In general, the effects of IFNs on cell proliferation are inhibitory, but in some cellular systems, for example, in the proliferation of human umbilical vein endothelial cells *in vitro*, low concentrations of IFN-γ can induce an increase in cell growth.[142] The effects of IFNs on cellular differentiation are variable — with either inhibition, stimulation, or no effect —according to the cell type and the physiologic conditions.

Modulation of the interactions of growth factors with their receptors and/or the postreceptor actions of growth factors may represent an important mechanism in the mediation of IFN effects on cell proliferation and cell differentiation. Down-modulation of transferrin receptors may be a mechanism of the antiproliferative action of IFNs on lymphoid cells.[143,144] Inhibition of the growth of mouse AKR-2B cells by IFN-α/β is associated with decreased expression of both EGF receptors and EGF-stimulated c-*myc* gene transcription.[145] Human IFN-α_2 inhibits the growth of Madin-Darby bovine kidney cells by a mechanism involving modulation of the expression of the EGF receptor on the cell surface.[146] As demonstrated by the use of double-stranded RNA IFN inducers, IFN-β blocks the mitogenic action of PDGF in serum-free cultures of human foreskin fibroblasts and the IFN-β system may be considered as a very potent autocrine inhibitory pathway.[147] Both IFNs and TNF-α are involved in inhibiting granulocyte-macrophage colony-forming units (GM-CFU).[148] Moreover, IFNs may induce the synthesis and release of TNF-α from bone marrow accessory cells. It has been suggested that IFNs and TNF-α may synergistically exert a cytotoxic action,[149] but dissociation is observed between IFN-induced regulation of TNF-α receptor expression and cytotoxic activity.[150] The effects of IFNs on the growth of human megakaryocytes *in vitro* are mainly inhibitory.[151]

The IFNs have an important role in the activation of cellular and humoral immune responses. IFN-γ can activate monocytes and macrophages as well as NK cells. In addition, IFN-γ directly exerts stimulatory effects on T lymphocytes, with preferential activation of CD8+ cells.[152] IFNs modulate the induction of cytotoxic cell responses to IL-2.[153] IFNs may promote the differentiation of cytotoxic T cells and NK cells and may possibly be involved in the regulation of T-cell growth. However, IFN-γ produced by treatment of human peripheral blood cells with IL-2 does not play an essential role in increasing NK cell activity, which depends on a direct action of IL-2 on large granular lymphocytes.[154]

IFN-γ may exert important physiological effects not only on T cells but also on B cells. IFN-γ may be involved in promoting the proliferation of activated human B lymphocytes and may sensitize these cells to suboptimal mitogenic concentrations of antibody.[155,156] IFN-γ and IL-2 may act synergistically on distinct steps of *in vitro* terminal human B-cell maturation.[157] However, the effects of IFN-γ on B cells are probably indirect and are mediated by non-B cells since IFN-γ does not perturb the physiology of purified B cells.[158] IFN-γ alone may not have a stimulatory effect on B-cell proliferation, but may act synergistically with IL-2 in inducing this proliferation.[159]

IFN-γ induces IL-2 receptor expression on the surface of human peripheral blood monocytes as well as in the human monocytic cell line U-937.[160] IFN-γ-induced expression of IL-2 receptors in these cells is not due to translocation of a cryptic receptor to the cell surface, but is caused by increased transcriptional activity of the IL-2 receptor gene.

Apparently there is no absolute tissue specificity of the different IFN classes, and no single stage of the cell cycle is uniquely sensitive to IFN action. The antiproliferative effect of IFN and the mitogenic action of growth factors are independent cell-cycle events, as demonstrated in studies with G_0/G_1-arrested normal bovine vascular smooth-muscle cells and endothelial cells.[161] In general, IFNs lower the probability of cells to exit from the quiescent G_0 state under adverse growth conditions. The G_1 phase is also prolonged in actively proliferating cells following IFN treatment. In some cell types, particularly in transformed cells, other phases of the cycle may be prolonged.[6] In certain cell types, IFN action may lead to cessation of DNA replication. The mechanism of the antimitogenic activity of IFNs is unknown, but all types of IFNs inhibit the mitogenic response of quiescent human dermal fibroblasts to PDGF, which suggests that IFNs may inhibit cell proliferation by suppressing the biological activity of PDGF, or may act by a signaling pathway onto which the activity pathways of PDGF and other mitogens converge.[162] In BALB/c 3T3 mouse fibroblasts, IFN may inhibit cell proliferation through an indirect mechanism which consists in preventing PDGF-induced changes of intracellular Ca^{2+}, which are necessary for entry of cells into the S phase of the cycle.[163]

Usually, the different IFN types have synergistic effects, but functional antagonism may occur for some of the effects elicited by class I and class II IFNs, for example, on H_2O_2 production by human monocytes and macrophages during the respiratory burst.[164] Thus, the consequences of upsetting the natural physiological balance should be considered when a combined IFN therapy is indicated.

VIII. ROLE OF INTERFERONS IN NEOPLASTIC PROCESSES

The IFNs play an important role in neoplastic processes, but this role is a complex one and many aspects of this topic have not been characterized as yet. Recent evidence suggests that the IFNs may function, at least in some cases, as tumor suppressor genes.[165] The high incidence of chromosome 9 abnormalities involving breakage at 9p22, the region which contains the loci for IFN-α and IFN-β, and the deletions and translocations of 9p seen in association with ALL and non-Hodgkin's lymphoma, support the possibility that a tumor suppressor gene(s) may be located in this chromosome region. However, congenital deletion of chromosome 9 does not always result in increased incidence of leukemia.

A. INTERFERON-INDUCED DIFFERENTIATION OF NEOPLASTIC CELLS

The IFNs can induce the differentiation of some malignant hematopoietic cells. IFN-α and IFN-β, but not IFN-γ, can regulate the *in vitro* differentiation of multilineage lympho-myeloid stem cells from hairy-cell leukemia.[166] Both IFN-γ and TNF-α have the ability to induce monocytic differentiation of HL-60 human promyelocytic leukemia cells, and this induction is accompanied by the appearance of a membrane-bound tyrosine kinase activity.[167] This activity is not related to the product of the c-*fms* proto-oncogene, whose expression is induced in monocytic differentiation of HL-60 cells.[168] TNF-α-induced differentiation of the mouse myeloid leukemia cell line M1 is mediated by IFN-$β_1$.[169] The combination of IFNs with retinoic acid may result in a synergistic induction of HL-60 cell differentiation.[170-172] TNF-α and IFN-γ act synergistically in the induction of differentiation of ML-1 human myeloblastic leukemia cells.[173] In contrast to most inducers of HL-60 cell differentiation, IFN-γ-induced differentiation of HL-60 cells is not associated with downregulation of c-*myc* gene expression.[174] Moreover, the synergistic effect of IFN-γ and TNF-α on HL-60 cell differentiation is not reflected in a synergy in reduction of c-*myc* expression. These results suggest that IFN-γ-induced differentiation of HL-60 cells occurs through a pathway different from that of other differentiation inducers.

B. CYTOSTATIC AND TUMORICIDAL EFFECTS OF INTERFERON

The IFNs can display inhibitory effects on the proliferation of certain types of normal cells. IFN-γ can inhibit the growth of human basal keratinocytes *in vitro* without affecting cell viability.[175] IFNs exert strong cytostatic and cytocidal effects on a wide variety of tumor cells. These effects can be either direct or indirect, and are frequently exerted through complex interactions with other cytokines. IL-1β and TNF-α, alone or in combination, can neither directly lyse TNF-α-insensitive P815 mastocytoma cells nor activate resident peritoneal macrophages to be tumoricidal for this target, but a synergistic induction of tumoricidal activity against P815 cells occurs when either of these monokines is combined with IFN-γ.[176]

Examination of the growth-modulating effects of IFN-γ, either alone or in combination with IL-1, showed that whereas in some human tumor cell lines (lung carcinoma CALU-1 and colon carcinoma SW-48) IL-1 stimulates growth and offsets the growth-inhibitory effects of IFN-γ, in other lines (cervical carcinoma HeLa, transformed milk line HBL-100, and myelogenous leukemia K562) IFN-γ alone has a growth-inhibitory effect and IL-1 has no effect.[177] In other cell lines (mammary carcinomas MCF-7 and MDA-MB-415) the growth-inhibitory effects of IL-1 and IFN-γ are additive. The effects of IFN-γ and IL-1 on cell growth may be mediated by different mechanisms. Different types of IFN may have different effects on particular types of tumor cells. IFN-$α_2$ and IFN-β, but not IFN-γ, inhibit the BCGF-induced proliferation of the hairy-cell type of leukemia cells, which are cells of B-cell origin.[178]

Different types of blood cells may be involved in mediating the antitumor effects of IFN. NK cells may have a role in the initiation of these effects, but studies with cells transformed by the acute retrovirus M-MuSV, which carries the oncogene v-*mos*, indicate that T cells are necessary for maintenance of the tumor-suppressed state and thus for tumor inhibition.[179] Mononuclear cells may function as mediators of the tumoricidal effects of IFN. In order to activate the *in vitro* tumoricidal capacity of monocytes, IFN-γ requires the exogenous addition of LPS.[180] Although the mechanism of action of LPS on mononuclear blood cells is not understood, LPS induces an early change in the synthesis of proteins from 85 to 36 kDa in murine macrophages.[181] Remodelation in the protein composition of macrophages induced by the combined action of IFN-γ and LPS may be required for these cells to acquire tumoricidal properties. Human tumor-associated macrophages may become tumoricidal under the influence of IFN-γ, producing a diffusable substance in agarose culture which causes antiproliferative effects on the tumor cells.[182]

IFN-γ not only stimulates the phagocytic and tumoricidal activity of macrophages, but also induces the expression of class I and class II MHC antigens on the cell surface. The induction of class II antigens is important for antigen presentation by macrophages during the first phase of T-cell activation. In K562 human leukemic cells, IFN-γ induces the expression of genes for class I HLA antigens in the absence of differentiation effects.[183] Accumulation of MHC class I gene transcripts in IFN-treated cells may be due to interaction of IFN with a transcriptional enhancer located within the 5′-flanking region of these genes.[184] Human TNF-α increases mRNA levels and cell surface expression of HLA-A and HLA-B antigens in endothelial cells and dermal fibroblasts *in vitro*.[185]

IFN-γ can act in a synergistic manner with other factors for effecting tumor cell killing. IFN-γ sensitizes tumor cells to the lytic action of TNF-α.[186,187] Some human tumor cell lines, not sensitive to TNF-α alone, may become highly sensitive when IFN-γ is present as well. Combined treatment with suboptimal doses of IFN-γ and TNF-α may be useful for the control of metastatic cancer *in vivo*.[188] The molecular mechanisms of the synergistic effects of IFN-γ and TNF-α in tumor cell killing are not understood, but may involve immunomodulatory changes. IFN-α, but not IFN-γ, induces IL-1 secretion by human monocytes.[189] On the other hand, IFN-γ, but not IFN-α, renders the monocytes more sensitive to certain other IL-1-inducing stimuli.

In certain cellular systems *in vitro*, including human tumor cell lines, exposure to IFN may result not in decreased but in enhanced expression of the malignant phenotype and increased ability of the transformed cells to form tumors *in vivo*.[190] Growth of human osteosarcoma cells is enhanced by exposure to IFN-γ.[191] Thus, great caution should be exerted with the clinical use of IFN for the treatment of cancer patients, because it could cause an exacerbation of the disease.

C. INTERFERON-INDUCED REVERSION OF THE TRANSFORMED PHENOTYPE

Treatment of HL-60 cells with IFN-γ results in induction of their monocytic differentiation, but alterations in proto-oncogene expression may not be a requisite for the commitment of this differentiation.[114] Transcripts of the c-*fos* gene remain undetectable until day 5 of IFN-γ treatment, c-*fms* mRNA is induced only after day 7, and c-*sis* expression at the RNA and protein levels remains undetectable after induction with IFN-γ.

M-MuSV-transformed embryonic mouse fibroblasts revert to an apparently normal phenotype and lose their tumorigenic properties after long-term treatment with low concentrations of mouse IFN-α/β, and the reverted nonmalignant state can remain stable even after 60 to 100 passages in the absence of IFN.[192] This reversion occurs in spite of the continued integrated M-MuSV genome and the expression of v-*mos* transcripts in the IFN-treated cells. The mechanisms involved in the IFN-induced reversion of M-MuSV-transformed cells, and the persistence of this reversion in spite of the continuous expression of the v-*mos* oncogene, even in the absence of IFN, are unknown. IFN-γ is capable of inducing a complete, but reversible, suppression of the neoplastic properties of mouse NIH/3T3 fibroblasts transformed by a retroviral vector containing the v-*mos* oncogene.[193] This suppression is due to a selective downregulation of the expression of v-*mos* transcripts which are under the control of retroviral promoters.

D. EFFECT OF INTERFERON ON ONCOGENE-TRANSFORMED CELLS

The possible role of interferons on the mechanism of action of viral oncogenes is not understood. The v-Myc oncoprotein can inhibit terminal differentiation of U-937 human leukemia cells induced by PMA, calcitriol, or retinoic acid, but the response to IFN-γ is similar in cells expressing v-*myc* and control U-937 cells.[194] Thus, IFN-γ induces a signal(s) that circumvents the biological activity of the v-Myc oncoprotein.

The effect of IFN inducers on the growth of tumors induced *in vivo* by inoculation of acute retroviruses may depend on a diversity of factors. Tumor growth or tumor regression is observed in C57BL/6J mice inoculated with M-MuSV carrying the v-*mos* oncogene and treated with the IFN inducer, avridine.[195] The IFN-inducing agent not only can inhibit tumor growth in these animals, but can also produce a marked enhancement of tumor growth depending on the timing of administration relative to tumor challenge.

E. ONCOSUPPRESSOR ACTIVITY OF INTERFERONS

The antiproliferative effects or interferons on normal and tumor cells may occur, at least in part, through activation of oncosuppressor genes. The retinoblastoma susceptibility gene, *RB1*, encodes a nuclear phosphoprotein, RB, which has growth-suppressive activity, and IFN-γ can directly modulate RB mRNA expression in monocytoid cells.[196] In other types of cells, cotreatment with the protein synthesis inhibitor, cycloheximide, is required for IFN-γ to increase the level of RB mRNA.

The interferons may have an activity similar to that of the products of oncosuppressor genes. Homozygous and hemizygous deletions of IFN genes on human chromosome 9p21-22 have been found in samples of leukemia cells from some patients with acute lymphocytic leukemia.[197,198] Deletions affecting human chromosome 9p are frequently found in primary human gliomas.[199] The gliomas with 9p deletions are hemi- or nullizygous for IFN-$β_1$ and the IFN-α gene cluster. IFN nullizygosity occurs in gliomas of highest histological malignancy (glioblastomas). However, such deletions may comprise not only the IFN genes, but also other neighboring genes which could include an unidentified oncosuppressor gene. The possible role of these deletions in the tumorigenic process remains to be elucidated.

REFERENCES

1. **Isaacs, A. and Lindemann, J.,** Virus interference. I. The interferon, *Proc. R. Soc. London,* B147, 258, 1957.
2. **Lengyel, P.,** Biochemistry of interferons and their actions, *Annu. Rev. Biochem.,* 51, 225, 1982.
3. **Grossberg, S.E. and Taylor, J.L.,** Interferon effects on cell differentiation, *Interferon,* 3, 299, 1984.
4. **Sreevalsan, T.,** Effects of interferons on cell physiology, *Interferon,* 3, 343, 1984.
5. **Fisher, P.B. and Grant, S.,** Effect of interferon on differentiation of normal and tumor cells, *Pharmacol. Ther.,* 27, 143, 1985.
6. **Clemens, M.J. and McNurlan, M.A.,** Regulation of cell proliferation and differentiation by interferon, *Biochem. J.,* 226, 345, 1985.
7. **Moritz, T. and Kirchner, H.,** The effect of interferons on cellular differentiation, *Blut,* 53, 361, 1986.
8. **Romeo, G., Fiourucci, G., and Rossi, G.B.,** Interferons in cell growth and development, *Trends Genet.,* 5, 19, 1989.
9. **Taylor, J.L. and Grossberg, S.E.,** Recent progress in interferon research: molecular mechanisms of regulation, action, and virus circumvention, *Virus Res.,* 15, 1, 1990.
10. **Farrar, M.A. and Schreiber, R.D.,** The molecular biology of interferon-γ and its receptor, *Annu. Rev. Immunol.,* 11, 571, 1993.
11. **Dayton, M.A., Knobloch, T.J., and Benjamin, D.,** Human B-cell lines express the interferon-γ gene, *Cytokine,* 4, 454, 1992.
12. **Hughes, T.K., Russell, J.K., and Blalock, J.E.,** Induction of interferon by transformed cells: inhibition by retinoic acid, *Biochem. Biophys. Res. Commun.,* 138, 47, 1986.
13. **Sica, A., Tan, T.-H., Rice, N., Kretzschmar, M., Ghosh, P., and Young, H.A.,** The c-*rel* protooncogene product c-Rel but not NF-κB binds to the intronic region of the human interferon-γ gene at a site related to an interferon-stimulable response element, *Proc. Natl. Acad. Sci. U.S.A.,* 89, 1740, 1992.
14. **Vaquero, C., Sanceau, J., Weissenbach, J., Beranger, F., and Falcoff, R.,** Regulation of human γ-interferon and β-interferon gene expression in PHA-activated lymphocytes, *J. Interferon Res.,* 6, 161, 1986.
15. **Johnson, H.M. and Torres, B.A.,** Peptide growth factors PDGF, EGF, and FGF regulate interferon-γ production, *J. Immunol.,* 134, 2824, 1985.
16. **Croll, A.D. and Morris, A.G.,** The regulation of γ-interferon production by interleukins 1 and 2, *Cell. Immunol.,* 102, 33, 1986.
17. **Le, J., Lin, J.-X., Henriksen-DeStefano, D., and Vilcek, J.,** Bacterial lipopolysaccharide-induced interferon-γ production: roles of interleukin 1 and interleukin 2, *J. Immunol.,* 136, 4525, 1986.
18. **Farrar, W.L., Birchenall-Sparks, M.C., and Young, H.B.,** Interleukin 2 induction of interferon-γ mRNA synthesis, *J. Immunol.,* 137, 3836, 1986.
19. **Russell, J.K., Torres, B.A., and Johnson, H.M.,** Phospholipase A_2 treatment of lymphocytes provides helper signal for interferon-γ induction. Evidence for second messenger role of endogenous arachidonic acid, *J. Immunol.,* 139, 3442, 1987.
20. **Vilcek, J., Henriksen-DeStefano, D., Siegel, D., Klion, A., Robb, R.J., and Le, J.,** Regulation of IFN-γ induction in human peripheral blood cells by exogenous and endogenously produced interleukin 2, *J. Immunol.,* 135, 1851, 1985.
21. **Le, J. and Vilcek, J.,** Accessory function of human fibroblasts in mitogen-stimulated interferon-γ production by T lymphocytes: inhibition by interleukin 1 and tumor necrosis factor, *J. Immunol.,* 139, 3330, 1987.
22. **Reis, L.F.L., Lee, T.H., and Vilcek, J.,** Tumor necrosis factor acts synergistically with autocrine interferon-β and increases interferon-β mRNA levels in human fibroblasts, *J. Biol. Chem.,* 264, 16351, 1989.
23. **Trent, J.M., Olson, S., and Lawn, R.M.,** Chromosomal localization of human leukocyte, fibroblast, and immune interferon by means of *in situ* hybridization, *Proc. Natl. Acad. Sci. U.S.A.,* 79, 7809, 1982.
24. **Mantei, N., Schwarzstein, M., Streuli, M., Panem, S., Nagata, S., and Weissmann, C.,** The nucleotide sequence of a cloned human leukocyte interferon cDNA, *Gene,* 10, 1, 1980.
25. **Taniguchi, T., Ohno, S., Fujii-Kuriyama, Y., and Muramatsu, M.,** The nucleotide sequence of human fibroblast interferon cDNA, *Gene,* 10, 11, 1980.
26. **Derynck, R., Content, J., DeClercq, E., Volckaert, G., Tavernier, J., Devos, R., and Fiers, W.,** Isolation and structure of a human fibroblast interferon gene, *Nature,* 285, 542, 1980.

27. **Lawn, R.M., Gross, M., Houck, C.M., Franke, A.E., Gray, P.V., and Goeddel, D.V.,** DNA sequence of a major human leukocyte interferon gene, *Proc. Natl. Acad. Sci. U.S.A.,* 78, 5435, 1981.
28. **Nagata, S., Mantei, N., and Weissmann, C.,** The structure of one of the eight or more distinct chromosomal genes for human interferon-α, *Nature,* 287, 401, 1980.
29. **Allen, G. and Fantes, K.H.,** A family of structural genes for human lymphoblastoid (leukocyte-type) interferon, *Nature,* 287, 408, 1980.
30. **Goeddel, D.V., Leung, D.W., Dull, T.J., Gross, M., Lawn, R.M., McCandliss, R., Seeburg, P.H., Ullrich, A., Yelverton, E., and Gray, P.W.,** The structure of eight distinct cloned human leukocyte interferon cDNAs, *Nature,* 290, 20, 1981.
31. **Weissmann, C., Nagata, S., Boll, W., Fountoulakis, M., Fujisawa, A., Fujisawa, J.-I., Haynes, J., Henco, K., Mantei, N., Ragg, H., Schein, C., Schmid, J., Shaw, G., Streuli, M., Taira, H., Todokoro, K., and Weidle, U.,** Structure and expression of human IFN-α genes, *Philos. Trans. R. Soc. London,* B299, 7, 1982.
32. **Houghton, M., Jackson, I.J., Porter, A.G., Doel, S.M., Catlin, G.H., Barber, C., and Carey, N.H.,** The absence of introns within a human fibroblast interferon gene, *Nucleic Acids Res.,* 9, 247, 1981.
33. **Tavernier, J., Derynck, R., and Fiers, W.,** Evidence for a unique human fibroblast interferon (IFN-β_1) chromosomal gene, devoid of intervening sequences, *Nucleic Acids Res.,* 9, 461, 1981.
34. **Lawn, R.M., Adelman, J., Franke, A.E., Houck, C.M., Gross, M., Najarian, R., and Goeddel, D.V.,** Human fibroblast interferon gene lacks introns, *Nucleic Acids Res.,* 9, 1045, 1981.
35. **Ohno, S. and Taniguchi, T.,** Structure of a chromosomal gene for human interferon β, *Proc. Natl. Acad. Sci. U.S.A.,* 78, 5305, 1981.
36. **Taniguchi, T., Mantei, N., Schwarzstein, M., Nagata, S., Muramatsu, M., and Weissmann, C.,** Human leukocyte and fibroblast interferons are structurally related, *Nature,* 285, 547, 1980.
37. **Sehgal, P.B., May, L.T., LaForge, K.S., and Inouye, M.,** Unusually long mRNA species coding for human α and β interferons, *Proc. Natl. Acad. Sci. U.S.A.,* 79, 6932, 1982.
38. **Goeddel, D.V., Yelverton, E., Ullrich, A., Heynecker, H.L., Miozzari, G., Holmes, W., Seeburg, P.H., Dull, T., May, L., Stebbing, N., Crea, R., Maeda, S., McCandliss, R., Sloma, A., Tabor, J.M., Gross, M., Familletti, P.C., and Pestka, S.,** Human leukocyte interferon produced by *E. coli* is biologically active, *Nature,* 287, 411, 1980.
39. **Weissbach, H., Goeddel, D.V., McCandliss, R., Maeda, S., Familletti, P.C., Redfield, B., Staehelin, T., and Pestka, S.,** In vitro synthesis of biologically active human leukocyte interferon directed by recombinant plasmid DNA, *Arch. Biochem. Biophys.,* 210, 417, 1981.
40. **Hitzeman, R.A., Hagie, F.E., Levine, H.L., Goeddel, D.V., Ammerer, G., and Hall, B.D.,** Expression of a human gene for interferon in yeast, *Nature,* 293, 717, 1981.
41. **Mantei, N. and Weissmann, C.,** Controlled transcription of a human α-interferon gene introduced into mouse L cells, *Nature,* 297, 128, 1982.
42. **Gray, P.W., Leung, D.W., Pennica, D., Yelverton, E., Najarian, R., Simonsen, C.C., Derynck, R., Sherwood, P.J., Wallace, D.M., Berger, S.L., Levinson, A.D., and Goeddel, D.V.,** Expression of human immune interferon cDNA in *E. coli* and monkey cells, *Nature,* 295, 503, 1982.
43. **Gray, P.W. and Goeddel, D.V.,** Structure of the human immune interferon gene, *Nature,* 298, 859, 1982.
44. **Devos, R., Cheroutre, H., Taya, Y., Degrave, W., Van Heuverswyn, H., and Fiers, W.,** Molecular cloning of human immune interferon cDNA and its expression in eukaryotic cells, *Nucleic Acids Res.,* 10, 2487, 1982.
45. **Tanaka, S., Oshima, T., Ohsuye, K., Ono, T., Mizono, A., Ueno, A., Nakazato, H., Tsujimoto, M., Higashi, N., and Noguchi, T.,** Expression in *Escherichia coli* or chemically synthesized gene for the human immune interferon, *Nucleic Acids Res.,* 11, 1707, 1983.
46. **Derynck, R., Leung, D.W., Gray, P.W., and Goeddel, D.V.,** Human interferon γ is encoded by a single class of mRNA, *Nucleic Acids Res.,* 10, 3605, 1982.
47. **Hardy, K.J., Manger, B., Newton, M., and Stobo, J.D.,** Molecular events involved in regulating human interferon-γ gene expression during T cell activation, *J. Immunol.,* 138, 2353, 1987.
48. **Sagar, A.D., Sehgal, P.B., Slate, D.L., and Ruddle, F.H.,** Multiple human β interferon genes, *J. Exp. Med.,* 156, 744, 1982.
49. **Sehgal, P.B., Zilberstein, A., Ruggieri, A.-M., May, L.T., Ferguson-Smith, A., Slate, D.L., Revel, M., and Ruddle, F.H.,** Human chromosome 7 carries the β_2 interferon gene, *Proc. Natl. Acad. Sci. U.S.A.,* 83, 5219, 1986.

50. Van Damme, J., De Ley, M., Van Snick, J., Dinarello, C.A., and Billiau, A., The role of interferon-β_1 and the 26-kDa protein (interferon-β_2) as mediators of the antiviral effect of interleukin 1 and tumor necrosis factor, *J. Immunol.*, 139, 1867, 1987.
51. May, L.T., Helfgott, D.C., and Sehgal, P.B., Anti-β-interferon antibodies inhibit the increased expression of HLA-B7 mRNA in tumor necrosis factor-treated human fibroblasts: structural studies of the β_2 interferon involved, *Proc. Natl. Acad. Sci. U.S.A.*, 83, 8957, 1986.
52. Zilberstein, A., Ruggieri, R., Korn, J.H., and Revel, M., Structure and expression of cDNA and genes for human interferon-β_2, a distinct species inducible by growth-stimulatory cytokines, *EMBO J.*, 5, 2529, 1986.
53. Sehgal, P.B., May, L.T., Tamm, I., and Vilcek, J., Human β_2 interferon and B-cell differentiation factor BSF-2 are identical, *Science*, 235, 731, 1987.
54. Poupart, P., Vandenabeele, P., Cayphas, S., Van Snick, J., Haegeman, G., Kruys, V., Fiers, W., and Content, J., B cell growth modulating and differentiating activity of recombinant human 26-kda protein (BSF-2, HuIFN-β_2, HPGF), *EMBO J.*, 6, 1219, 1987.
55. Gauldie, J., Richards, C., Harnish, D., Lansdorp, P., and Baumann, H., Interferon β_2/B-cell stimulatory factor type 2 shares identity with monocyte-derived hepatocyte-stimulating factor and regulates the major acute phase protein response in liver cells, *Proc. Natl. Acad. Sci. U.S.A.*, 84, 7251, 1987.
56. Rubinstein, M. and Orchansky, P., The interferon receptors, *Crit. Rev. Biochem.*, 21, 249, 1986.
57. Branca, A.A., Interferon receptors, *In Vitro Cell. Dev. Biol.*, 24, 155, 1988.
58. Langer, J. and Pestka, S., Interferon receptors, *Immunol. Today*, 9, 393, 1988.
59. Langer, J.A., Rashidbaigi, A., Lai, L.-W., Patterson, D., and Jones, C., Sublocalization on chromosome 21 of human interferon-α receptor gene and the gene for an interferon-γ response protein, *Somat. Cell Mol. Genet.*, 16, 231, 1990.
60. Hannigan, G.E., Lau, A.S., and Williams, B.R.G., Differential human interferon α receptor expression on proliferating and nonproliferating cells, *Eur. J. Biochem.*, 157, 187, 1986.
61. Rashidbaigi, A., Langer, J.A., Jung, V., Jones, C., Morse, H.G., Tischfield, J.A., Trill, J.J., Kung, H., and Pestka, S., The gene for the human immune interferon receptor is located on chromosome 6, *Proc. Natl. Acad. Sci. U.S.A.*, 83, 384, 1986.
62. Pfizenmaier, K., Wiegmann, K., Scheurich, P., Krönke, M., Merlin, G., Aguet, M., Knowles, B.B., and Ücer, U., High affinity human IFN-γ-binding capacity is encoded by a single receptor gene located in proximity to c-*ros* on human chromosome region 6q16 to 6q22, *J. Immunol.*, 141, 856, 1988.
63. Aguet, M., Dembic, Z., and Merlin, G., Molecular cloning and expression of the human interferon-γ receptor, *Cell*, 55, 273, 1988.
64. Ücer, U., Bartsch, H., Scheurich, P., Berkovic, D., Ertel, C., and Pfizenmaier, K., Quantitation and characterization of γ-interferon receptors on human tumor cells, *Cancer Res.*, 46, 5339, 1986.
65. Kumar, C.S., Muthukumaran, G., Frost, L.J., Noe, M., Ahn, Y.H., Mariano, T.M., and Pestka, S., Molecular characterization of the murine interferon γ receptor cDNA, *J. Biol. Chem.*, 264, 17939, 1989.
66. Nakagawa, T., Nakagawa, N., Delsing, G.A., Volkman, D., and Kehrl, J.H., Demonstration and partial characterization of the interferon-γ receptor on human B lymphocytes, *J. Cell. Biochem.*, 40, 417, 1989.
67. Strickland, R.W., Wahl, L.M., and Finbloom, D.S., Corticosteroids enhance the binding of recombinant interferon-γ to cultured human monocytes, *J. Immunol.*, 137, 1577, 1986.
68. Aiyer, R.A., Serrano, L.E., and Jones, P.P., Interferon-γ binds to high and low affinity receptor components on murine macrophages, *J. Immunol.*, 136, 3229, 1986.
69. Gutch, M.J. and Reich, N.C., Repression of the interferon signal transduction pathway by the adenovirus *E1A* oncogene, *Proc. Natl. Acad. Sci. U.S.A.*, 88, 7913, 1991.
70. Yap, W.H., Teo, T.S., and Tan, Y.H., An early event in the interferon-induced transmembrane signaling process, *Science*, 234, 355, 1986.
71. Becton, D.L., Adams, D.O., and Hamilton, T.A., Characterization of protein kinase C activity in interferon γ treated murine peritoneal macrophages, *J. Cell. Physiol.*, 125, 485, 1985.
72. Ostrowski, J., Meier, K.E., Stanton, T.H., Smith, L.L., and Bomsztyk, K., Interferon-γ and interleukin-1α induce transient translocation of protein kinase C activity to membranes in a B-lymphoid cell line. Evidence for a protein kinase C-independent pathway in lymphokine-induced cytoplasmic alkalinization, *J. Biol. Chem.*, 263, 13786, 1988.

73. **Ito, M., Takami, Y., Tanabe, F., Shigeta, S., Tsukui, K., and Kawade, Y.,** Modulation of protein kinase C activity during inhibition of tumor cell growth by IFN-β and -γ, *Biochem. Biophys. Res. Commun.,* 150, 126, 1988.
74. **Mattila, P. and Renkonen, R.,** IFN-γ induces a phospholipase-D dependent triphasic activation of protein kinase C in endothelial cells, *Biochem. Biophys. Res. Commun.,* 189, 1732, 1992.
75. **Reich, N.C. and Pfeffer, L.M.,** Evidence for involvement of protein kinase-C in cellular response to interferon-α, *Proc. Natl. Acad. Sci. U.S.A.,* 87, 8761, 1990.
76. **Hannigan, G.E. and Williams, B.R.G.,** Signal transduction by interferon-α through arachidonic acid metabolism, *Science,* 251, 204, 1991.
77. **Offermanns, S. and Schultz, G.,** Tyrosine phosphorylation is an early and requisite signal induced by interferon-γ in HL-60 cells, *FEBS Lett.,* 310, 260, 1992.
78. **Velazquez, L., Fellous, M., Stark, G.R., and Pellegrini, S.,** A protein tyrosine kinase in the interferon α/β signaling pathway, *Cell,* 70, 313, 1992.
79. **Fu, X.F.,** A transcription factor with SH2 and SH3 domains is directly activated by an interferon-α-induced cytoplasmic protein tyrosine kinase(s), *Cell,* 70, 323, 1992.
80. **Chebath, J., Benech, A., Honavessian, A., Galabru, J., and Revel, M.,** Four different forms of interferon-induced 2'5'-oligo(A)synthetase identified by immunoblotting in human cells, *J. Biol. Chem.,* 262, 3852, 1987.
81. **David, S., Nissim, A., Chebath, J., and Salzberg, S.,** 2'-5'-Oligoadenylate synthetase gene expression in normal and murine sarcoma virus-transformed NIH 3T3 cells, *J. Virol.,* 63, 1116, 1989.
82. **Schwartz, E.L. and Nilson, L.A.,** Activation of 2',5'-oligoadenylate synthetase activity on induction of HL-60 leukemia cell differentiation, *Mol. Cell. Biol.,* 9, 3897, 1989.
83. **Beresini, M.H., Lempert, M.J., and Epstein, L.B.,** Overlapping polypeptide induction in human fibroblasts in response to treatment with interferon-α, interferon-β, interleukin 1α, interleukin 1β, and tumor necrosis factor, *J. Immunol.,* 140, 485, 1988.
84. **Czarniecki, C.W., Chiu, H.H., Wong, G.H.W., McCabe, S.M., and Palladino, M.A.,** Transforming growth factor-$β_1$ modulates the expression of class II histocompatibility antigens on human cells, *J. Immunol.,* 140, 4217, 1988.
85. **Rambaldi, A., Young, D.C., Herrmann, F., Cannistra, S.A., and Griffin, J.D.,** Interferon-γ induces expression of the interleukin 2 receptor gene in human monocytes, *Eur. J. Immunol.,* 17, 153, 1987.
86. **Collart, M.A., Belin, D., Vassalli, J.-D., de Kossodo, S., and Vasalli, P.,** γ Interferon enhances macrophage transcription of the tumor necrosis factor/cachectin, interleukin 1, and urokinase genes, which are controlled by short-lived repressors, *J. Exp. Med.,* 164, 2113, 1986.
87. **Farber, J.M.,** A macrophage mRNA selectively induced by γ-interferon encodes a member of the platelet factor 4 family of cytokines, *Proc. Natl. Acad. Sci. U.S.A.,* 87, 5238, 1990.
88. **Staeheli, P., Danielson, P., Haller, O., and Sutcliffe, J.G.,** Transcriptional activation of the mouse Mx gene by type I interferon, *Mol. Cell. Biol.,* 6, 4770, 1986.
89. **Kelly, J.M., Porter, A.C.G., Chernajowsky, Y., Gilbert, C.S., Stark, G.R., and Kerr, I.M.,** Characterization of a human gene inducible by α- and β-interferons and its expression in mouse cells, *EMBO J.,* 1601, 1986.
90. **Levy, D., Larner, A., Chaudhuri, A., Babiss, L.E., and Darnell, J.E., Jr.,** Interferon-stimulated transcription: isolation of an inducible gene and identification of its regulatory region, *Proc. Natl. Acad. Sci. U.S.A.,* 83, 8929, 1986.
91. **Samanta, H., Engel, D.A., Chao, H.M., Thakur, A., Garcia-Blanco, M.A., and Lengyel, P.,** Interferons as gene activators. Cloning of the 5' terminus and the control segment of an interferon activated gene, *J. Biol. Chem.,* 261, 1986.
92. **Blomstrom, D.C., Fahey, D., Kutny, R., Korant, B.D., and Knight, E., Jr.,** Molecular characterization of the interferon-induced 15-kDa protein: molecular cloning and nucleotide and amino acid sequence, *J. Biol. Chem.,* 261, 8811, 1986.
93. **Luster, A.D., Jhanwar, S.C., Chaganti, R.S.K., Kersey, J.H., and Ravetch, J.V.,** Interferon-inducible gene maps to a chromosomal band associated with a (4;11) translocation in acute leukemia cells, *Proc. Natl. Acad. Sci. U.S.A.,* 84, 2868, 1987.
94. **Hannigan, G. and Williams, B.R.G.,** Transcriptional regulation of interferon-responsive genes is closely linked to interferon receptor occupancy, *EMBO J.,* 5, 1607, 1986.
95. **Celada, A. and Schreiber, R.D.,** Role of protein kinase C and intracellular calcium mobilization in the induction of macrophage tumoricidal activity by interferon-γ, *J. Immunol.,* 137, 2373, 1986.

96. **Schindler, C., Shuai, K., Prezioso, V.R., and Darnell, J.E.,** Interferon-dependent tyrosine phosphorylation of a latent cytoplasmic transcription factor, *Science,* 257, 809, 1992.
97. **David, M. and Larner, A.C.,** Activation of transcription factor by interferon-α in a cell-free system, *Science,* 257, 813, 1992.
98. **Reis, L.F.L., Harada, H., Wolchok, J.D., Taniguchi, T., and Vilcek, J.,** Critical role of a common transcription factor, IRF-1, in the regulation of IFN-β and IFN-inducible genes, *EMBO J.,* 11, 185, 1992.
99. **Yu-Lee, L.-Y., Hrachovy, J.A., Stevens, A.M. and Schwarz, L.A.,** Interferon-regulatory factor 1 is an immediate-early gene under transcriptional regulation by prolactin in Nb2 T cells, *Mol. Cell. Biol.,* 10, 3087, 1990.
100. **Marshall, A.H., Alper, D., and Hiscott, J.,** Modulation of nuclear proto-oncogene expression and cellular growth in myeloid leukemic cells by human interferon α, *J. Cell. Physiol.,* 135, 324, 1988.
101. **Yaar, M., Peacocke, M., Cohen, M.S., and Gilchrest, B.A.,** Dissociation of proto-oncogene induction from growth response in normal human fibroblasts, *J. Cell. Physiol.,* 145, 39, 1990.
102. **Lehn, P., Sigaux, F., Grausz, D., Loiseau, P., Castaigne, S., Degos, L., Flandrin, G., and Dautry, F.,** The c-*myc* and c-*fos* expression during interferon-α therapy for hairy cell leukemia, *Blood,* 68, 967, 1986.
103. **Mohamed, A.N., Nakeff, A., Mohammad, R.M., KuKuruga, M., and Al-Katib, A.,** Modulation of c-*myc* oncogene expression by phorbol ester and interferon-γ: appraisal by flow cytometry, *Oncogene,* 3, 429, 1988.
104. **Jonak, G.J. and Knight, E., Jr.,** Selective reduction of c-*myc* mRNA in Daudi cells by human β interferon, *Proc. Natl. Acad. Sci. U.S.A.,* 81, 1747, 1984.
105. **Knight, E., Jr., Anton, E.A., Friedland, B., and Jonak, G.J.,** Regulation of c-myc proteins by interferon, in *Interferons as Cell Growth Inhibitors and Antitumor Factors,* Friedman, R.M., Merigan, T., and Sreevalsan, T., Eds., Alan R. Liss, New York, 1986, 403.
106. **Clemens, M.J., Tilleray, V.J., James, R., and Gewert, D.R.,** Relationship of cellular oncogene expression to inhibition of growth and induction of differentiation of Daudi cells by interferons or TPA, *J. Cell. Biochem.,* 38, 251, 1988.
107. **Einat, M., Resnitzky, D., and Kimchi, A.,** Close link between reduction of c-*myc* expression by interferon and G_0/G_1 arrest, *Nature,* 313, 597, 1985.
108. **Resnitzky, D. and Kimchi, A.,** Deregulated c-*myc* expression abrogates the interferon- and interleukin 6-mediated G_0/G_1 cell cycle arrest but not other inhibitory responses in M1 myeloblastic cells, *Cell Growth Differ.,* 2, 33, 1991.
109. **Osanto, S., Jansen, R., and Vloemans, M.,** Down-regulation of c-*myc* expression by interferon-γ and tumor necrosis factor-α precedes growth arrest in human melanoma cells, *Eur. J. Cancer,* 28A, 1622, 1992.
110. **Knight, E., Jr., Anton, E.D., Fahey, D., Friedland, B.K., and Jonak, G.J.,** Interferon regulates c-*myc* gene expression in Daudi cells at the post-transcriptional level, *Proc. Natl. Acad. Sci. U.S.A.,* 82, 1151, 1985.
111. **Dani, C., Mechti, N., Piechaczyk, M., Lebleu, B., Jeanteur, P., and Blanchard, J.M.,** Increased rate of degradation of c-myc mRNA in interferon-treated Daudi cells, *Proc. Natl. Acad. Sci. U.S.A.,* 82, 4896, 1985.
112. **Meadows, L.M., George, D.J., and Kaufman, R.E.,** Dissociation of thymidine incorporation and transferrin receptor expression from cell growth and c-myc accumulation in α-interferon-treated cells, *J. Biol. Response Modif.,* 9, 212, 1990.
113. **Jonak, G.J., Friedland, B.K., Anton, E.D., and Knight, E., Jr.,** Regulation of c-*myc* RNA and its proteins in Daudi cells by interferon-β, *J. Interferon Res.,* 7, 41, 1987.
114. **Sariban, E., Mitchell, T., Griffin, J., and Kufe, D.W.,** Effects of interferon-γ on proto-oncogene expression during induction of human monocytic differentiation, *J. Immunol.,* 138, 1954, 1987.
115. **Matsui, T., Takahashi, R., Mihara, K., Nakagawa, T., Koizumi, T., Nakao, Y., Sugiyama, T., and Fujita, T.,** Cooperative regulation of c-*myc* expression in differentiation of human promyelocytic leukemia induced by recombinant γ-interferon and 1,25-dihydroxyvitamin D_3, *Cancer Res.,* 45, 4366, 1985.
116. **Piacibello, W., Guerrasio, A., Salvetti, L., Aglietta, M., Saglio, G., and Gavosto, F.,** Human γ interferon modifies c-*myc* expression and growth patterns of U937 cell line but not of its subclone 1937, *Cell Biol. Int. Rep.,* 10, 467, 1986.

117. **Dron, M., Modjtahedi, N., Brison, O., and Tovey, M.G.,** Interferon modulation of c-*myc* expression in cloned Daudi cells: relationship to the phenotype of interferon resistance, *Mol. Cell. Biol.,* 6, 1374, 1986.
118. **Yarden, A. and Kimchi, A.,** Tumor necrosis factor reduces c-*myc* expression and cooperates with interferon-γ in HeLa cells, *Science,* 234, 1419, 1986.
119. **Pape, K.A. and Floyd-Smith, G.,** Effects of interferon-β on Daudi cells and on small cell lung carcinoma cells which over-express the c-*myc* oncogene, *Anticancer Res.,* 9, 1737, 1989.
120. **Bernards, R., Dessain, S.K., and Weinberg, R.A.,** N-*myc* amplification causes down-modulation of MHC class I antigen expression in neuroblastoma, *Cell,* 47, 667, 1986.
121. **Radzioch, D., Bottazzi, B., and Varesio, L.,** Augmentation of c-*fos* mRNA expression by activators of protein kinase C in fresh, terminally differentiated resting macrophages, *Mol. Cell. Biol.,* 7, 595, 1987.
122. **Radzioch, D. and Varesio, L.,** The c-*fos* messenger RNA expression in macrophages is downregulated by interferon-γ at the posttranscriptional level, *Mol. Cell. Biol.,* 11, 2718, 1991.
123. **Wan, Y.-J.Y., Levi, B.-Z., and Ozato, K.,** Induction of c-*fos* gene expression by interferon, *J. Interferon Res.,* 8, 105, 1988.
124. **Mehmet, H., Morris, C.M.G., Taylor-Papadimitriou, J., and Rozengurt, E.,** Interferon inhibition of DNA synthesis in Swiss 3T3 cells: dissociation from protein kinase C activation, *Biochem. Biophys. Res. Commun.,* 145, 1026, 1987.
125. **Hannigan, G.E. and Williams, B.R.G.,** Interferon-α activates binding of nuclear factors to a sequence element in the c-*fos* proto-oncogene 5′-flanking region, *J. Interferon Res.,* 12, 355, 1992.
126. **Dubois, M.-F., Vignal, M., Le Cunff, M., and Chany, C.,** Interferon inhibits transformation of mouse cells by exogenous cellular or viral oncogenes, *Nature,* 303, 433, 1983.
127. **Samid, D., Chang, E.H., and Fricdman, R.M.,** Development of transformed phenotype induced by a human *ras* oncogene is inhibited by interferon, *Biochem. Biophys. Res. Commun.,* 126, 509, 1985.
128. **Perucho, M. and Esteban, M.,** Inhibitory effect of interferon on the genetic and oncogenic transformation by viral and cellular genes, *J. Virol.,* 54, 229, 1985.
129. **Samid, D., Chang, E.H., and Friedman, R.M.,** Biochemical correlates of phenotypic reversion in interferon-treated mouse cells transformed by a human oncogene, *Biochem. Biophys. Res. Commun.,* 119, 21, 1984.
130. **Samid, D., Chang, E.H., Friedman, R.M., Schaff, Z., and Greene, J.J.,** Biological and morphological characteristics of phenotypic revertants appearing in interferon-treated mouse cells transformed by a human oncogene, *J. Exp. Pathol.,* 2, 211, 1985.
131. **Chang, E.H., Ridge, J., Black, R., Zou, Z.-Q., Masnyk, T., Noguchi, P., and Harford, J.B.,** Interferon-γ induces altered oncogene expression and terminal differentiation in A431 cells, *Proc. Soc. Exp. Biol. Med.,* 186, 319, 1987.
132. **Maran, A., Goldberg, I.D., and Steinberg, B.M.,** Induction of c-Ha-*ras* gene expression by double-stranded RNA and interferon requirement, *Mol. Cell. Biol.,* 10, 4424, 1990.
133. **Canivet, M., Mercier, G., Giron, M.-L., Emanoil-Ravier, R., and Périès, J.,** Differential regulation of v-Ki-ras, c-myc and IAP gene expression by interferon in a murine cell line transformed by Kirsten mouse sarcoma retrovirus, in *Interferons as Cell Growth Inhibitors and Antitumor Factors,* Friedman, R.M., Merigan, T., and Sreevalsan, T., Eds., Alan R. Liss, New York, 1986, 319.
134. **Lin, S.L., Garber, E.A., Wang, E., Caliguiri, L.A., Schellekens, H., Goldberg, A.R., and Tamm, I.,** Reduced synthesis of pp60^{src} and expression of the transformation-related phenotype in interferon-treated Rous sarcoma virus-transformed rat cells, *Mol. Cell. Biol.,* 3, 1656, 1983.
135. **Soslau, G., Bogucki, A.R., Gillespie, D., and Hubbell, H.R.,** Phosphoproteins altered by antiproliferative doses of human interferon-β in a human bladder carcinoma cell line, *Biochem. Biophys. Res. Commun.,* 119, 941, 1984.
136. **Rimoldi, D., Samid, D., Flessate, D.M., and Friedman, R.M.,** Transcriptional inhibition of Ha-*ras* in interferon-induced revertants of *ras* transformed mouse cells, *Cancer Res.,* 48, 5157, 1988.
137. **Samid, D., Flessate, D.M., and Friedman, R.M.,** Interferon-induced revertants of *ras*-transformed cells: resistance to transformation by specific oncogenes and retransformation by 5-azacytidine, *Mol. Cell. Biol.,* 7, 2196, 1987.
138. **Brouty-Boyé, D., Wybier-Franqui, J., Nardeux, P., Daya-Grosjean, L., Andeol, Y., and Suarez, H.G.,** Interferon-induced phenotypic changes in human tumor cells relative to the effects of interferon on c-*ras* oncogene expression, *J. Interferon Res.,* 6, 461, 1986.

139. **Chang, E.H., Black, R., Zou, Z.-Q., Masnyk, T., Ridge, J., Noguchi, P., and Harford, J.B.,** γ-Interferon modulates growth of A431 cells and expression of EGF receptors, in *Interferons as Cell Growth Inhibitors and Antitumor Factors,* Friedman, R.M., Merigan, T., and Sreevalsan, T., Eds., Alan R. Liss, New York, 1986, 335.
140. **Yi, T.-L. and Willman, C.L.,** Cloning of the murine c-*fgr* proto-oncogene cDNA and induction of c-*fgr* expression by proliferation and activation factors in normal bone marrow-derived monocytic cells, *Oncogene,* 4, 1081, 1989.
141. **Revel, M. and Chebath, J.,** Interferon-activated genes, *Trends Biochem. Sci.,* 11, 166, 1986.
142. **Saegusa, Y., Ziff, M., Welkovich, L., and Cavender, D.,** Effect of inflammatory cytokines on human endothelial cell proliferation, *J. Cell. Physiol.,* 142, 488, 1990.
143. **Besancon, F., Bourgeade, M.-F., and Testa, U.,** Inhibition of transferrin receptor expression by interferon-α in human lymphoblastoid cells and mitogen-induced lymphocytes, *J. Biol. Chem.,* 260, 13074, 1985.
144. **Bourgeade, M.-F., Silbermann, F., Thang, M.N., and Besancon, F.,** Reduction of transferrin receptor expression by interferon-α in a human cell line sensitive to its antiproliferative effect, *Biochem. Biophys. Res. Commun.,* 153, 897, 1988.
145. **Pietenpol, J.A., Howe, P.H., Cunningham, M.R., and Leof, E.B.,** Interferon α/β modulation of growth-factor-stimulated mitogenicity in AKR-2B fibroblasts, *J. Cell. Physiol.,* 141, 453, 1989.
146. **Zoon, K.C., Karasaki, Y., zur Nedden, D.L., Hu, R., and Arnheiter, H.,** Modulation of epidermal growth factor receptors by human α interferon, *Proc. Natl. Acad. Sci. U.S.A.,* 83, 8226, 1986.
147. **Forsberg, K., Paulsson, Y., and Westermark, B.,** Effect on platelet-derived growth factor-induced mitogenesis of double-stranded RNA: evidence for an autocrine growth inhibition mediated by interferon-β, *J. Cell. Physiol.,* 136, 266, 1988.
148. **Pelus, L.M., Ottmann, O.G., and Nocka, K.H.,** Synergistic inhibition of human marrow granulocyte-macrophage progenitor cells by prostaglandin E and recombinant interferon-α, -β, and -γ and an effect mediated by tumor necrosis factor, *J. Immunol.,* 140, 479, 1988.
149. **Williamson, B.D., Carswell, E.A., Rubin, B.Y., Prendergast, J.S., and Old, L.J.,** Human tumor necrosis factor produced by human B cell lines: synergistic cytotoxic interaction with human interferon, *Proc. Natl. Acad. Sci. U.S.A.,* 80, 5397, 1983.
150. **Tsujimoto, M., Feinman, R., and Vilcek, J.,** Differential effects of type I IFN and IFN-γ on the binding of tumor necrosis factor to receptors in two human cell lines, *J. Immunol.,* 137, 2272, 1986.
151. **Griffin, C.G. and Grant, B.W.,** Effects of recombinant interferons on human megakaryocyte growth, *Exp. Hematol.,* 18, 1013, 1990.
152. **Siegel, J.P.,** Effects of interferon-γ on the activation of human T lymphocytes, *Cell. Immunol.,* 111, 461, 1988.
153. **Brunda, M.J., Tarnowski, D., and Davatelis, V.,** Interaction of recombinant interferons with recombinant interleukin-2: differential effects on natural killer cell activity and interleukin-2-activated killer cells, *Int. J. Cancer,* 37, 787, 1986.
154. **Sayers, T.J., Mason, A.T., and Ortaldo, J.R.,** Regulation of human natural killer cell activity by interferon-γ: lack of a role in interleukin 2-mediated augmentation, *J. Immunol.,* 136, 2176, 1986.
155. **Defrance, T., Aubry, J.-P., Vanbervliet, B., and Banchereau, J.,** Human interferon-γ acts as a B cell growth factor in the anti-IgM antibody co-stimulatory assay but has no direct B cell differentiation activity, *J. Immunol.,* 137, 3681, 1986.
156. **Romagnani, S., Giudizi, M.G., Biagiotti, R., Almericogna, F., Mingari, C., Maggi, E., Liang, C.-M., and Moretta, L.,** Cell growth factor activity of interferon-γ: recombinant human interferon-γ promotes proliferation of anti-μ-activated human B lymphocytes, *J. Immunol.,* 136, 3513, 1986.
157. **Bichthuy, L.T. and Fauci, A.S.,** Recombinant interleukin-2 and γ-interferon act synergistically on distinct steps of in vitro terminal human B-cell maturation, *J. Clin. Invest.,* 77, 1173, 1986.
158. **Julius, M.H., Paige, C.J., Leanderson, T., and Cambier, J.C.,** Neither interleukin 2 nor γ interferon directly promote growth and differentiation of mouse B cells, *Scand. J. Immunol.,* 25, 195, 1987.
159. **Karray, S., Vazquez, A., Merle-Beral, H., Olive, D., Debre, P., and Galanaud, P.,** Synergistic effect of recombinant IL 2 and interferon-γ on the proliferation of human monoclonal lymphocytes, *J. Immunol.,* 138, 3824, 1987.
160. **Rambaldi, A., Young, D.C., Herrmann, F., Cannistra, S.A., and Griffin, J.D.,** Interferon-γ induces expression of the interleukin 2 receptor gene in human monocytes, *Eur. J. Immunol.,* 17, 153, 1987.

161. **Heyns, A., du P., Eldor, A., Vlodavsky, I., Kaiser, N., Fridman, R., and Panet, A.,** The antiproliferative effect of interferon and the mitogenic action of growth factors are independent cell cycle events: studies with vascular smooth muscle cells and endothelial cells, *Exp. Cell Res.*, 161, 297, 1985.
162. **Hosang, M.,** Recombinant interferon-γ inhibits the mitogenic effect of platelet-derived growth factor at a level distal to the growth factor receptor, *J. Cell. Physiol.*, 134, 396, 1988.
163. **Zagari, M., Hepler, J.R., Harris, C., and Herman, B.,** Inhibition of early platelet-derived growth factor responses in BALB/c-3T3 cells by interferon, *Biochem. Biophys. Res. Commun.*, 150, 1207, 1988.
164. **Garotta, G., Talmadge, K.W., Pink, J.R.L., Dewald, B., and Baggiolini, M.,** Functional antagonism between type I and type II interferons on human macrophages, *Biochem. Biophys. Res. Commun.*, 140, 948, 1986.
165. **Pitha, P.M.,** Interferons: a new class of tumor suppressor genes?, *Cancer Cells*, 2, 215, 1990.
166. **Michalevicz, R. and Revel, M.,** Interferons regulate the *in vitro* differentiation of multilineage lympho-myeloid stem cells in hairy cell leukemia, *Proc. Natl. Acad. Sci. U.S.A.*, 84, 2307, 1987.
167. **Glazer, R.I., Chapekar, M.S., Hartman, K.D., and Knode, M.C.,** Appearance of membrane-bound tyrosine kinase during differentiation of HL-60 leukemia cells by immune interferon and tumor necrosis factor, *Biochem. Biophys. Res. Commun.*, 140, 908, 1986.
168. **Sariban, E., Mitchell, T., and Kufe, D.,** Expression of the c-*fms* proto-oncogene during human monocytic differentiation, *Nature*, 316, 64, 1985.
169. **Onozaki, K., Urawa, H., Tamatani, T., Iwamura, Y., Hashimoto, T., Baba, T., Suzuki, H., Yamada, M., Yamamoto, S., Oppenheim, J.J., and Matsushima, K.,** Synergistic interactions of interleukin 1, interferon-β, and tumor necrosis factor in terminally differentiating a mouse myeloid leukemic cell line (M1), *J. Immunol.*, 140, 112, 1988.
170. **Hemmi, H. and Breitman, T.R.,** Combinations of recombinant human interferons and retinoic acid synergistically induce differentiation of the human promyelocytic leukemia cell line HL-60, *Blood*, 69, 501, 1987.
171. **Trinchieri, G., Rosen, M., and Perussia, B.,** Retinoic acid with tumor necrosis factor and immune interferon in inducing differentiation and growth inhibition of the human promyelocytic leukemic cell line HL-60, *Blood*, 69, 1218, 1987.
172. **Lin, J. and Sartorelli, A.C.,** Stimulation by interferon of the differentiation of human promyelocytic leukemia (HL-60) cells produced by retinoic acid and actinomycin D, *J. Interferon Res.*, 7, 379, 1987.
173. **Takuma, T., Takeda, K., and Konno, K.,** Synergism of tumor necrosis factor and interferon-γ in induction of differentiation of human myeloblastic leukemic ML-1 cells, *Biochem. Biophys. Res. Commun.*, 145, 514, 1987.
174. **McAchren, S.S., Jr., Salehi, Z., Weinberg, J.B., and Niedel, J.E.,** Transcription interruption may be a common mechanism of c-myc regulation during HL-60 differentiation, *Biochem. Biophys. Res. Commun.*, 151, 574, 1988.
175. **Symington, F.W.,** Lymphotoxin, tumor necrosis factor, and γ interferon are cytostatic for normal human keratinocytes, *J. Invest. Dermatol.*, 92, 798, 1989.
176. **Hori, K., Mihich, E., and Ehrke, M.J.,** Role of tumor necrosis factor and interleukin 1 in γ-interferon-promoted activation of mouse tumoricidal macrophages, *Cancer Res.*, 49, 2606, 1989.
177. **Tsai, S.-C.J. and Gaffney, E.V.,** Modulation of cell proliferation by human recombinant interleukin-1 and immune interferon, *J. Natl. Cancer Inst.*, 79, 77, 1987.
178. **Genot, E., Billard, C., Sigaux, F., Mathiot, C., Degos, L., Falcoff, E., and Kolb, J.-P.,** Proliferative response of hairy cells to B cell growth factor (BCGF): in vivo inhibition by interferon-α and in vitro effects of interferon-α, -β, and -γ, *Leukemia*, 1, 590, 1987.
179. **Skicki-Mullen, M.B., Markovic, S.N., and Murasko, D.M.,** Interferon-induced inhibition of Moloney sarcoma virus-transformed cells: requirement for T cells, *Cancer Res.*, 49, 522, 1989.
180. **Grabstein, K.H., Urdal, D.L., Tushinski, R.J., Mochizuki, D.Y., Price, V.L., Cantrell, M.A., Gillis, S., and Conlon, P.J.,** Induction of macrophage tumoricidal activity by granulocyte-macrophage colony-stimulating factor, *Science*, 232, 506, 1986.
181. **Hamilton, T.A., Jansen, M.M., Somers, S.D., and Adams, D.O.,** Effects of bacterial lipopolysaccharide on protein synthesis in murine peritoneal macrophages: relationship to activation for macrophage tumoricidal function, *J. Cell. Physiol.*, 128, 9, 1986.

182. **Saito, T., Berens, M.E., and Welander, C.E.,** Direct and indirect effects of human recombinant γ-interferon on tumor cells in a clonogenic assay, *Cancer Res.,* 46, 1142, 1986.
183. **Chen, E., Karr, R.W., Frost, J.P., Gonwa, T.A., and Ginder, G.D.,** Gamma interferon and 5-azacytidine cause transcriptional elevation of class I major histocompatibility complex gene expression in K562 leukemia cells in the absence of differentiation, *Mol. Cell. Biol.,* 6, 1698, 1986.
184. **Vogel, J., Kress, M., Khoury, G., and Jay, G.,** A transcriptional enhancer and an interferon-responsive sequence in major histocompatibility complex class I genes, *Mol. Cell. Biol.,* 6, 3550, 1986.
185. **Collins, T., Lapierre, L.A., Fiers, W., Strominger, J.L., and Pober, J.S.,** Recombinant human tumor necrosis factor increases mRNA levels and surface expression of HLA-A,B antigens in vascular endothelial cells and dermal fibroblasts *in vitro, Proc. Natl. Acad. Sci. U.S.A.,* 83, 446, 1986.
186. **Fransen, L., van der Heyden, J., Ruysschaert, R., and Fiers, W.,** Recombinant tumor necrosis factor: its effect and its synergism with interferon-γ on a variety of normal and transformed human cell lines, *Eur. J. Cancer Clin. Oncol.,* 22, 419, 1986.
187. **Feinman, R., Henriksen-DeStefano, D., Tsujimoto, M., and Vilcek, J.,** Tumor necrosis factor is an important mediator of tumor cell killing by human monocytes, *J. Immunol.,* 138, 635, 1987.
188. **Talmadge, J.E., Tribble, H.R., Pennington, R.W., Phillips, H., and Wiltrout, R.H.,** Immunomodulatory and immunotherapeutic properties of recombinant γ-interferon and recombinant tumor necrosis factor in mice, *Cancer Res.,* 47, 2563, 1987.
189. **Gerrard, T.L., Siegel, J.P., Dyer, D.R., and Zoon, K.C.,** Differential effects of interferon-α and interferon-γ on interleukin secretion by monocytes, *J. Immunol.,* 138, 2535, 1987.
190. **Brouty-Boyé, D., Wybier-Franqui, J., and Suarez, H.G.,** IFN-induced phenotypic changes in human tumor cells relative to the effect of IFN on oncogene expression, in *Interferons as Cell Growth Inhibitors and Antitumor Factors,* Friedman, R.M., Merigan, T., and Sreevalsan, T., Eds., Alan R. Liss, New York, 1986, 309.
191. **Tong, L.J., Yamaguchi, N., Kita, M., and Imanishi, J.,** Enhancement of the growth of human osteosarcoma cells by human interferon-γ, *Cell Struct. Funct.,* 17, 257, 1992.
192. **Sergiescu, D., Gerfaux, J., Joret, A.-M., and Chany, C.,** Persistent expression of v-*mos* oncogene in transformed cells that revert to nonmalignancy after prolonged treatment with interferon, *Proc. Natl. Acad. Sci. U.S.A.,* 83, 5764, 1986.
193. **Seliger, B., Kruppa, G., and Pfizenmaier, K.,** Murine γ interferon inhibits v-*mos*-induced fibroblast transformation via down regulation of retroviral gene expression, *J. Virol.,* 61, 2567, 1987.
194. **Öberg, F., Larsson, L.-G., Anton, R., and Nilsson, K.,** Interferon γ abrogates the differentiation block in v-*myc*-expressing U-937 monoblasts, *Proc. Natl. Acad. Sci. U.S.A.,* 88, 5567, 1991.
195. **Talcott, P.A., Koller, L.D., Woodard, L.F., and Whitbeck, G.A.,** Opposing effects of the interferon inducer, avridine: enhancement or suppression of tumor growth depending on treatment regimen, *Int. J. Immunopharmacol.,* 8, 553, 1986.
196. **Mistchenko, A.S., Diez, R.A., Romquin, N., Sanceau, J., and Witzerbin, J.,** Interferon-γ modulates retinoblastoma gene mRNA in monocytoid cells, *Int. J. Cancer,* 53, 87, 1993.
197. **Diaz, M.O., Rubin, C.M., Harden, A., Ziemin, S., Larson, R.A., Le Beau, M.M., and Rowley, J.D.,** Deletions of interferon genes in acute lymphoblastic leukemia, *N. Engl. J. Med.,* 322, 77, 1990.
198. **Einhorn, S., Grandér, D., Björk, O., Bröndum-Nielsen, K., and Söderhäll, S.,** Deletion of alpha-, beta-, and omega-interferon genes in malignant cells from children with acute lymphocytic leukemia, *Cancer Res.,* 50, 7781, 1990.
199. **James, C.D., He, J., Carlbom, E., Nordenskjold, M., Cavenee, W.K., and Collins, V.P.,** Chromosome 9 deletion mapping reveals interferon and interferon β-1 gene deletions in human glial tumors, *Cancer Res.,* 51, 1684, 1991.

Chapter 5

Tumor Necrosis Factors

I. INTRODUCTION

Proteins with selective cytotoxic properties for transformed cells are known under the generic name of cytotoxins.[1] Such proteins may be present in tumor necrosis serum and are capable of inhibiting metastasis of experimental tumors such as B16 mouse melanoma.[2] However, these proteins may have growth-stimulating properties in certain types of cells or under certain physiological conditions, and the generic name cytokines should be more conveniently applied to them. An important member of this family of proteins is lymphotoxin, also called tumor necrosis factor β (TNF-β), which is produced mainly by monocytes and macrophages.[3] Other members of the family are tumor necrosis factor α (TNF-α) and IFN-γ, as well as cytotoxins produced by lymphocytes, in particular by natural killer (NK) cells or their closely associated cells — the large granular lymphocytes (LGLs).[4] TNF-β, TNF-α, and IFN-γ can display inhibitory effects on the proliferation of nonhematic cells such as normal human basal keratinocytes without affecting cell viability.[5] TNF-α and TNF-β bind to the same cell surface receptor and have similar, but not identical, biological activities. Although they were initially considered as antitumor agents, TNF-α and TNF-β are "inflammatory cytokines" produced at the sites of inflammation by infiltrating mononuclear cells, and play a beneficial role in the resistance to different types of infectious and neoplastic processes. The physiologic effects of TNFs are exerted through the activation of multiple signal transduction pathways and may lead to changes in the expression of a large number of genes.

The cytotoxin family may include other agents in addition to TNF-α and TNF-β, but they remain poorly characterized. The cytotoxic effects of NK cells are mediated by a soluble factor, the NK cytotoxicity factor (NKCF), and the effects of LGLs by another factor, cytolysin.[6,7] NKCF is distinct from the TNFs and has been partially purified from human lymphocyte-conditioned medium.[8] A lymphotoxin, the cytotoxic T-lymphocyte toxin (CTL-toxin), is released by cloned cell lines of IL-2-dependent human cytotoxic T lymphocytes.[9] A lymphokine with inhibitory effects on tumor cells was named tumor migration inhibition factor (TMIF).[10] The structural and functional relationships between NKCF, cytolysin, the CTL-toxin, and TMIF remain to be established. An additional member of the cytotoxin/TNF family has been identified recently and shown to be a membrane protein with significant homology to TNF-α, TNF-β, and the ligand for the CD40 receptor.[11] The gene encoding this protein, called lymphotoxin β, is localized next to the TNF-α locus in the major histocompatibility complex (MHC). Cell surface complexes between the different types of lymphotoxins may be involved in immune regulation. In general, the processes associated with lymphokine-induced cytotoxicity involve complex interactions between different lymphokines and different cells, which include NK cells, macrophages, and particular subtypes of T cells.[12] The cells producing TNF-β and TNF-α may be different. Whereas TNF-α is produced mainly by monocytes and macrophages, TNF-β is produced by mitogen-activated T lymphocytes.[13,14] A cloned human lymphoblastoid cell line (K16ob) produces TNF-β constitutively.[15]

The biological effects of TNF-α and TNF-β are partially identical. The cytotoxins differ quantitatively, but not qualitatively, in their effects on polymorphonuclear neutrophil functions *in vitro,* and TNF-β may be less toxic than TNF-α *in vivo.*[16] Some of the important biological effects of TNF-β are due to its synergistic actions with TNF-α. The antiproliferative effects of TNF-α and TNF-β are synergistic in a clonogenic assay using RPMI-4788 cells, which were established from a human colon cancer.[17] Both TNF-α and TNF-β are able to induce fragmentation of tumor target cell DNA and act as mediators of cytolytic T-cell killing.[18] The synergy of IL-1 with IL-2 in the generation of lymphokine-activated NK cells is mediated by TNF-α and TNF-β.[19] TNF-α and TNF-β inhibit virus replication and induce resistance of different types of cells against RNA and DNA virus infection.[20] These effects are not mediated by IFN synthesis but may be synergized by IFNs.

Different tumor cells, even from the same type, may exhibit wide variability in their responses to cytotoxins or lymphokines, and no synergistic actions are observed in some cases. Human myelogenous leukemia cell lines, for example, show marked heterogeneity in their response to TNF-α and TNF-β, and one line (K-562) is highly resistant to these cytokines.[21] Moreover, no synergistic action may be seen when the same cells are simultaneously exposed to IFN-α or IFN-γ.

II. TUMOR NECROSIS FACTOR β

Tumor necrosis factor β (TNF-β), also called lymphotoxin, is a multifunctional cytokine produced by mitogen-stimulated lymphocytes.[22] EBV-infected human lymphoblastoid cell lines produce TNF-β constitutively and express high-affinity TNF-β receptors.[23] Thus, TNF-β functions as an autocrine growth factor for these cell lines. Constitutive production of TNF-β is observed in T-cell lines infected with HTLV-I or HTLV-II.[24] The TAT gene of the AIDS-associated agent, HIV-1, induces TNF-β production in human B-lymphoblastoid cells.[25]

A. STRUCTURE OF TNF-β AND THE TNF-β GENE

TNF-β was isolated from a human lymphoblastoid cell line (RPMI-1788) and was characterized as a 25-kDa glycoprotein composed of 171 amino acids.[26] TNF-β lacks cysteine residues and has one asparagine-linked glycosylation site at position 62. The structure of human TNF-β at a resolution of 1.9 Å has been determined.[27]

TNF-β is encoded by a gene located on human chromosome 6, at region 6p21.3, within the MHC locus and between the genes coding for C4 complement and HLA-B antigen.[28] A cDNA copy of this gene was expressed in *Escherichia coli,* and no homology was found between lymphotoxin and other proteins secreted by stimulated lymphocytes, such as IL-2, IL-3, and IFN-γ.[21] However, TNF-β is highly homologous to TNF-α, especially in the last exons which code for 80% of the secreted protein.[29] Moreover, the genes of both TNF-α and TNF-β are syntenic.[30]

The complete sequence of the mouse TNF-β gene, including 1200 bp of its 5' flanking region, has been reported.[31] RNA processing is a limiting step for IL-2-induced murine TNF-β expression.[32] The TNF-α/TNF-β gene cluster lies on mouse chromosome 17, closely linked to the H-2D end of the H-2 MHC locus. The 3' end of the murine TNF-β gene is separated by about 1.2 kb from the beginning of the TNF-α gene, and both genes are transcribed in similar orientations. Comparisons of the predicted amino acid sequences of murine and human TNF-β indicates that the proteins are about 72% homologous, with much greater sequence conservation in the carboxy-terminal portion.

B. FUNCTIONS OF TNF-β

TNF-β is a cytokine that exerts multiple effects on its target cells, including cell killing, growth stimulation, and induction of differentiation.[14] TNF-β can contribute to immunoregulation, defense against viral and parasitic infections, and rejection of tumors. TNF-β inhibits the locomotion and stimulates the oxygen-dependent respiratory burst and degranulation of neutrophils in response to specific exogenous stimuli.[33] The mechanisms by which TNF-β exerts such pleiotropic effects are little understood. In particular, it is not known if the cytotoxic and differentiation-inducing effects of TNF-β are exerted through a common mechanism.

The functions of TNF-β are similar or partially identical to those of TNF-α, and both cytokines appear to share a common cell surface receptor. Both TNF-β and TNF-α are involved as mediators in the mechanisms of inflammatory processes and both display antitumor actions. TNF-β and TNF-α stimulate fibroblasts to produce HGFs and exert a positive and negative influence on *in vitro* hematopoietic colony formation.[34] In general, TNF-β and TNF-α are qualitatively and quantitatively similar in their spectrum of biological actions.[35] Moreover, TNF-β and TNF-α share many physiological effects with IL-1, and specific effects of TNFs may be augmented by coincident generation of other cytokines, including IL-1 and IFN-γ. However, the genes encoding TNF-α and TNF-β may be differentially regulated in human T lymphocytes, suggesting some specific physiological properties of their respective products.[36]

C. ANTINEOPLASTIC EFFECTS OF TNF-β

Initially, TNF-α and TNF-β were described as having similar or identical cytotoxic activities, but more recent studies indicate that TNF-β is usually less active than TNF-α with respect to its antineoplastic effects. TNF-α and TNF-β have different antiproliferative properties on several human tumor cell lines, and higher concentrations of TGF-β are generally required for a half maximal antiproliferative effect.[37] Such differences are difficult to explain since both cytokines share a common receptor on the cell surface. However, the binding characteristics of TNF-α and TNF-β to their receptor may be partially different or there may be a modified receptor molecule capable of recognizing only one of the two cytokines.

III. TUMOR NECROSIS FACTOR α

Tumor necrosis factor α (TNF-α) is a potent cytokine that is produced mainly by macrophages and exhibits cytotoxicity for neoplastic cells.[38-45] It has an important role in the metabolic response to sepsis and was discovered through the consequences of bacterial infections on the evolution of tumors. Since the late 1800s it was known that certain tumors in patients with a concomitant bacterial infection may occasionally regress, which was attributed to tumor-necrosis activities elicited by bacterial toxins.[46] In 1962 it was shown that the serum of mice challenged with endotoxin contains a tumor necrotizing factor.[47] This factor is not produced by bacteria directly, but is produced and secreted by the host cells upon stimulation by bacterial toxins. A particular factor, which was later called tumor necrosis factor, was detected in sera from endotoxin-treated mice, rats, and rabbits that had been previously sensitized with the *Mycobacterium bovis* strain of bacillus Calmette-Guérin (BCG).[48] Sera from such animals causes hemorrhagic necrosis, and in some cases, complete regression of certain types of transplanted tumors such as methylcholanthrene (MCA)-induced tumors in mice.

An agent discovered through work related to the metabolic consequences of bacterial infections was termed cachectin. Human infection by Gram-negative pathogens may result in derangement of multiple functions including metabolic alterations, coagulopathy, fever, shock, and widespread tissue injury. For many years it was believed that bacterial pathogens or their products were directly responsible for these effects, which may lead to the demise of the host. Bacterial LPS have long been recognized as the agents that confer the cytotoxicity of Gram-negative pathogens. More recently, it became clear that the toxicity of LPS is dependent on the production of an endogenous factor by the host. Infection or endotoxemia in animals produces hypertriglyceridemia, which results from the accumulation of triglycerides in very low-density lipoproteins (VLDL) due to their delayed clearance from the circulation, and this effect is associated with suppression of both lipoprotein lipase and hepatic triglyceride lipase activities.[49] TNF-α and cachectin (the pyrogenic agent responsible for the hypertriglyceridemic state occurring in mammals during certain infections) are identical molecules.[50,51]

A. PRODUCTION OF TNF-α

The availability of human recombinant TNF-α has enabled the development of sensitive and specific radioimmunoassays for the detection and quantitation of the factor in tissues and body fluids. TNF-α is produced during the normal fetal and neonatal development of the rat,[52] and has also been detected in human amniotic fluid as well as in placental and decidual tissues.[53] Bioassay testing shows that most of the TNF-α present in human amniotic fluid is biologically inactive, whereas placental and decidual supernatants have biologic activity that correlates with TNF-α levels detected by radioimmunoassay. TNF-α is normally present in human peripheral blood, and injection of endotoxin to healthy men results in a marked increase in the levels of circulating TNF-α.[54] Elevation of plasma TNF-α concentrations occurs 60 to 90 min after i.v. injection of endotoxin, and flu-like symptoms of chills, headache, myalgias, and nausea are most severe when concentrations of circulating TNF-α are maximal. Other cytokines (IL-1β and IFN-γ) are not elevated in the blood after the injection of endotoxin.

Monocytes and macrophages are involved in the production of TNF-α. Human peripheral blood macrophages do not synthesize TNF-α constitutively, but can release the lymphokine very rapidly after the action of certain stimuli.[55] LPS-stimulated blood cells produce TNF-α, which can be detected thereafter in the plasma.[56] Circulating human peripheral blood granulocytes can synthesize and secrete TNF-α.[57] Human alveolar macrophages also have the capacity to produce TNF-α, and this capacity may be increased in macrophages isolated from patients with pulmonary sarcoidosis, a granulomatous inflammatory disease.[58]

IFN-γ activates human and murine macrophages to produce TNF-α in the presence of small amounts of LPS.[59] Human IFN-γ stimulates peripheral blood monocytes in culture to secrete TNF-α.[60] IFN-γ enhances transcriptional expression of the TNF-α gene in mouse peritoneal macrophages.[61] Expression of TNF-α and IFN-γ is induced in macrophages by *Nocardia rubra* cell wall skeleton, an immunotherapeutic agent developed for the treatment of malignant diseases.[62] Both TNF-α and IL-1 enhance cytotoxicity of normal human macrophages for tumor cells, but simultaneous treatment of the macrophages with the two cytokines results in a less than additive response, which is apparently due to downregulation of autocrine TNF-α induction by the action of IL-1.[63] It is thus clear that complex and highly coordinated mechanisms are involved in determining the physiologic effects of cytokines *in vivo*.

In addition to monocytes and macrophages, other hematic cells, including lymphoblastoid cells and lymphocytes, produce TNF-α.[38] Both TNF-α and TNF-β can be produced by murine B lymphocytes, but this production is restricted to certain differentiation stages of the B-cell lineage.[64] NK-sensitive, but not NK-resistant, tumor cell lines induce large granular lymphocytes (LGLs) to produce factors with cytotoxic and/or cytostatic activity, and one of these factors was identified as TNF-α.[65] The production of TNF-α by LGLs is enhanced by IFN-γ. TNF-α may also be produced by certain nonhematic cells, including TNF-α-resistant mouse fibroblasts.[66]

Physical, chemical, and biological agents of exogenous origin may have striking effects on the production of TNF-α. Exposure of human sarcoma cells to ionizing radiation *in vitro* may result in increased production of TNF-α mRNA and protein.[67] TNF-α enhances radiation lethality in both TNF-α-producing and -nonproducing tumor cells. These results suggest that, in addition to the direct cytotoxic effects caused by ionizing radiation on tumor cells, the radiation may cause lethal effects on these cells through production of TNF-α, which may act through autocrine or paracrine mechanisms.

Sendai virus induces human leukocytes to produce high levels of TNF-α, whose mRNA can represent as much as 0.6% of the total RNA in the stimulated cells.[68] The leukocytes exposed to Sendai virus also synthesize large amounts of IFN-α. Production of TNF-α gene transcripts by human peripheral blood mononuclear cells can be primed by BCG or other Gram-positive bacteria, and can be triggered or greatly stimulated thereafter by exposure of cells to LPS, phorbol ester, IL-2, IL-3, CSF-2, IFN-γ, and mitogens, which can act as primers or regulators of the production of both TNF-α and TNF-β.[69-71] Tumor-cell destruction associated with the action of IL-2, IL-3, CSF-2, and IFN-γ is mediated by TNF-α and TNF-β. Production of TNF-α by prostaglandins is also regulated by PGE_2.[72]

Both TNF-α and TNF-β are produced by some human tumor cell lines. About half of the tumor cell lines of various tissue origins were found to constitutively express TNF-α mRNA, and many of these cell lines concomitantly contained TNF-β mRNA.[73] Cell lines lacking TNF-α or TNF β gene expression can be induced by phorbol ester and/or cytokines to accumulate the respective mRNAs. The HL-60 human promyelocytic leukemia cell line produces and secretes TNF-α when triggered to differentiation by phorbol ester. TPA-induced production of TNF-α by HL-60 cells occurs at the transcriptional level and is regulated by metabolites of the archidonic acid pathway, including leukotriene B_4 and PGD_2.[74] Cytokines such as IFN-α, IFN-γ, TNF-β, and TNF-α itself induce transient TNF-α mRNA expression in HL-60 cells.[75] HL-60 cells are resistant to the cytotoxic, but not to the cytostatic, action of TNF-α.[76] TNF-α induces TNF-α transcripts and synthesis of a TNF-α-like protein in ZR-75-1 human breast carcinoma cells, which are themselves resistant to cytotoxicity elicited by exogenous TNF-α.[77] Thus, treatment of certain cells with TNF-α may result in both endogenous TNF-α expression and resistance to exogenous TNF-α cytotoxicity. The precise relationship between these two effects and the possible role of TNF-α and/or TNF-β production by tumor cells in the pathogenesis of neoplastic diseases is unknown.

B. TNF-α STRUCTURE AND THE TNF-α GENE

The genes coding for TNF-α and TNF-β are located on human chromosome 6, at region 6p21.1-p22, which corresponds to the locus of the MHC HLA complex.[78] The location of TNF-α and TNF-β genes is in fact within the segment between HLA-DR and HLA-A, or centromeric of HLA-DP. The biological significance of this synteny is not clear, but it is well known that some MHC haplotypes may predispose to susceptibility to a number of human diseases. In the mouse, the genes for TNF-α and TNF-β are closely linked on chromosome 17, being separated by approximately 1 kb of DNA, and are located on a region 70 kb upstream of the MHC H-2D gene.[79]

TNF-α is antigenically distinct from TNF-β and IFN-γ.[80,81] Human TNF-α was purified to homogeneity from serum-free tissue culture supernatants of HL-60 cells induced by phorbol ester.[82-84] Human TNF-α is secreted as a protein of 17,350 Da with 157 amino acid residues, and contains two cysteine residues at position 69 and 101 which are involved in disulfide linkage. Also, 36% of the amino acid sequences of TNF-α are identical to those of TNF-β, but the homology between the two molecules may be increased to 51% when conservative substitutions are considered.[84] The active form of TNF-α is trimeric, and the structure of the TNF-α trimer has been determined at 2.9 and 2.6 Å resolution by X-ray crystallography.[85,86] The TNF-α monomers associate about a threefold axis of symmetry to form a compact bell-shaped trimer. A shallow groove at the basis of the TNF-α trimer is probably the locus of interaction with the TNF-α receptor. The membrane-embedded TNF-α trimer has a central pore-like region and at least some of its physiological effects may be associated to its intrinsic ion channel-forming activity.[87] Site-directed mutational analysis has contributed to confirm that correct trimer formation is necessary for biological TNF-α activity and to define the receptor binding sites of the molecule.[88] Each TNF-α trimer has three receptor binding sites located at the intersubunit grooves, but the binding sites extend beyond the grooves to include other surface residues at the base of the TNF-α molecule.

In addition to the 17-kDa form of TNF-α, human monocytes contain a 26-kDa form of the protein that corresponds to a molecule encoded by the TNF-α gene, but in which the signal peptide is not removed from the protein.[89] The 26-kDa form of TNF-α is a transmembrane protein that is produced by activated monocytes and may function at the site of inflammation by either cell-to-cell contact or local release of a TNF-α secretory component. In contrast, septic shock and cachexia would result from either acute or chronic systemic activation of monocytes resulting in the widespread release of TNF-α into the circulation.

cDNAs encoding TNF-α have been cloned and expressed in both bacteria and eukaryotic cells.[90-95] The recombinant TNF-α protein can inhibit the proliferation of transformed cells *in vitro* and induces necrosis of murine tumors *in vivo*. The human protein was characterized as an essentially nonhelical and β-sheet-rich structure capable of forming oligomers.[94] Natural and recombinant TNF-α of human and murine origin exists predominantly in the form of biologically active trimers under physiological conditions.[96] The trimers bind to TNF-α receptors and elicit a cytotoxic response. Two cysteine residues form an intrapolypeptide bond in the human TNF-α molecule. Recombinant human TNF-α molecules with higher basicity on their amino-terminal region display broader cytotoxicity to tumor cells.[97]

The murine TNF-α gene has been cloned and expressed in mammalian cells as well as in *Escherichia coli*.[98,99] Nonrecombinant murine TNF-α purified from serum was characterized as a glycoprotein of 40 kDa composed of monomers of 16 to 18 kDa associated through noncovalent bonds.[100] Both molecular weight forms of murine TNF-α display cytotoxic and necrotizing activities. The 235-amino acid murine pre-TNF-α polypeptide is almost 80% homologous to the human pre-TNF-α protein. The murine pre-TNF-α polypeptide consists of a amino acid pre sequence followed by a mature TNF-α sequence of 156 amino acids. Human and mouse TNF-α are derived from a precursor polypeptide which contains 76 (human) or 79 (mouse) additional amino acids attached to the amino terminus of the mature factor protein. Whereas the human TNF-α protein is not glycosylated, the mature mouse TNF-α molecule is glycosylated. Both the human and murine recombinant TNF-α molecules have been shown to be compact trimers and glycosylation would not affect the degree of TNF-α polymerization.[101] The gene encoding rabbit TNF-α has also been cloned.[102]

Altered proteins produced by genetic engineering procedures that determine site-directed changes in specific points of the coding nucleotide sequences are designated "muteins". Such muteins may have one or more substitutions, additions, or deletions to the amino acid sequence of the parental protein. The construction of TNF-α muteins yield interesting results.[103] Deletion of the first four and seven amino acids from the amino terminus of the recombinant TNF-α molecule resulted in two- to threefold increase in its relative cytotoxicity on all TNF-α-sensitive cell lines tested. Deletion of the first eight amino acids led to a molecule with a specific activity at least as great as that of the parent, whereas deletion to the tenth amino acid residue led to a TNF-α molecule with slightly decreased relative cytotoxicity on the same cell lines. The results of these studies suggest that the amino-terminal region of the recombinant TNF-α molecule may contain the TNF-α binding site and/or may determine the magnitude of the interaction of the molecule with its cellular receptors.

C. THE TNF-α RECEPTOR

A high-affinity binding site determines cell susceptibility to the action of both TNF-α and TNF-β.[104,105] The two cytokines share a common receptor on the cell surface. TNF receptors are present on various types of cells, including human polymorphonuclear blood cells.[106] Although resting T lymphocytes lack specific binding sites for TNF-α, high-affinity receptors for the factor are induced *de novo* upon primary activation of T cells.[107] There is species specificity in the interaction of TNF-α with its receptor, as observed in a comparative study with murine and human cells.[108]

Truncated TNF-α lacking the ten amino-terminal residues display lower cytotoxicity on a variety of tumor cell lines and exhibit lower affinity for the TNF-α receptor on the ME-180 human cervical carcinoma-cell line.[109] Antibodies directed against the amino terminus of human TNF-α block the association of TNF-α with its receptors on the cell surface and inhibit the biological effects of TNF-α.[110] The results suggest that amino acid residues located on the amino-terminal region of the receptor are involved in the interaction of TNF-α with its receptor on the cell surface.

1. Structure and Function of the TNF-α Receptor

Purification and partial sequentiation of a TNF-α-binding protein from the serum of cancer patients led to the preparation of synthetic probes, which were used to isolate cDNA clones encoding a TNF-α receptor.[111] The receptor was characterized as a 415-amino acid protein with extracellular, transmembrane, and intracellular regions. The extracellular cysteine-rich domain of the TNF-α receptor shows homology to that of the NGF receptor and to the B-lymphocyte activation protein Bp50. A TNF-α receptor was isolated as a 68-kDa glycoprotein from human B-cell lines (UC/Hela 2-5 cells) that express 150,000 to 180,000 receptors per cell, and a cDNA for the human TNF-α receptor was cloned from these cells.[112] Lower molecular weight forms of the receptor may represent soluble forms of the intact receptor molecule which are shed from the cells. The physiological significance of soluble receptors for TNF-α and other cytokines is not known, but they may provide a protective mechanism against systemic activity of these potent agents. Increased serum levels of soluble TNF-α receptors are observed in some cancer patients.[113] The mechanisms of signal transduction by TNF-α after binding to its receptor on the cell surface are unknown. Cytoplasmic truncation of the TNF-α receptor abolishes signaling, but not induced shedding of the receptor.[114]

2. Molecular Heterogeneity of the TNF-α Receptor

Molecular heterogeneity of TNF-α binding sites has been observed in different types of human cells. Comparison of the structure of TNF-α receptors in different human cell types (peripheral blood granulocytes, foreskin fibroblasts, and a breast tumor) indicated that the factor binds to four cellular polypeptides of 138, 90, 75, and 54 kDa.[115] The 138-kDa protein was detected in the human breast carcinoma cell line MCF-7, which is highly responsive to the cytotoxic action of TNF-α. In the human histiocytic lymphoma cell line U-937, the TNF-α receptor has been identified as a glycoprotein of 65 to 80 kDa, and the number of binding sites per cell was calculated to be about 12,000.[116]

Distinct types of TNF-α receptors have been detected in different types of cells. The use of monoclonal antibodies against the TNF-α-binding proteins from HL-60 and U-937 cell lines suggested the existence of two distinct TNF-α receptor molecules that contribute to varying extents to the binding of TNF-α by different types of human cells.[117] Two major types of TNF-α receptors detected in human cells, termed A and B, have been characterized. The type A TNF-α receptor is represented by a 100-kDa protein and the type B receptor consists of a major cross-linked product of 70 to 75 kDa and a minor product of 95 kDa. The two types of receptors exhibit distinct distributions in different cell types. The type A TNF receptor is expressed in myeloid cells and the type B receptor is found in several epithelial cell lines. The two types of TNF-α receptors are regulated independently and both receptors are biologically active.[118] Both types of TNF-α receptors induce the activation of the transcription factor NF-κB.

Recent evidence shows the existence of two major types of TNF-α receptors in human cells: a 55-kDa molecule designated TNF-R1 or TNF-R55, and a 75-kDa molecule designated TNF-R2 or TNF-R75. Both types of receptors bind TNF-α and TNF-β with high affinity. The extracellular regions of TNF-R1 and TNF-R2 share about 30% amino acid identity and are characterized by the presence of four cysteine-rich repeat units that form the ligand-binding domain of the molecule. These receptors are phosphorylated in serine and threonine residues and are internalized after ligand binding.[119]

Both types of TNF receptors are expressed in a wide variety of cells, but TNF-R2 is expressed especially on cells of myeloid origin, and is strongly expressed on stimulated B and T cells.[120] TNF-R1 is expressed in most cell types, particularly in those susceptible to the cytotoxic action of TNF-α. There is evidence that the cytotoxic activity of TNF-α is mediated by TNF-R1.[121] The human larynx carcinoma cell line HEp-2 expresses only TNF-R1 receptors. Certain TNF-α mutants interact selectively with TNF-R1, and this interaction may be sufficient to trigger cytotoxic activity against transformed cells.[122] The TNF-R1 gene is located on human chromosome 12p13.[123] A third type of TNF receptor identified in human liver may be generated by posttranslational modification and recognizes TNF-α, but not TNF-β.[124] This type of receptor is not expressed in other organs and may explain, at least in part, the differences observed in the actions of the two lymphotoxins.

Two types of TNF-α receptor also exist in murine cells.[125] Like the human receptors, the two murine receptors, TNF-R1 and TNF-R2, are encoded by distinct genes which are located on the mouse chromosomes 4 and 6, respectively. The two murine TNF-α receptors share only modest sequence homology, which is restricted to the cysteine-rich, ligand-binding extracellular region of the molecule. No similarity exists in the leader, transmembrane, or cytoplasmic domains. The murine TNF-α receptors show strong homology to their human analogs and display similar ligand-binding characteristics. Genes encoding TNF receptors are presumably very ancient and the biological significance of TNF-α receptor heterogeneity is not understood.

3. Regulation of TNF-α Receptor Expression

The TNF-α-receptor complex at the cell surface, which has a molecular weight of about 100 kDa, is subjected to endocytosis and downregulatory phenomena. Transfer of the complex to lysosomes is followed by its degradation.[126] A diversity of factors and mechanisms participate in the regulation of TNF-α receptor expression. TNF-β strongly upregulates the expression of TNF-α receptors in human peripheral blood lymphocytes.[127] IL-2 may be a mediator in the regulation of TNF-α receptor expression in lymphocytes.[128]

Expression of TNF-α/β receptors is upregulated by IFN-γ in human peripheral blood lymphocytes.[129-131] Class I IFNs and IFN-γ may have opposite effects on the regulation of TNF receptor expression.[130] In HeLa cells IFN-α and IFN-β increase TNF-α binding, whereas in HT-29 cells these two IFNs either slightly decrease or have no effect on TNF-α binding. In contrast, IFN-γ increases TNF-α binding in the two cell lines, and this effect is antagonized by type I IFNs in HT-29 cells, but not in HeLa cells. In spite of the inhibitory effect of IFN-β on the IFN-γ-induced stimulation of TNF receptor expression, IFN-β does not inhibit the synergistic enhancement of TNF-α cytotoxicity by IFN-γ in HT-29 cells. These results suggest that modulation of TNF-α receptors may not be a major mechanism of synergism between IFN and TNF-α.

The presence of a TNF receptor is necessary, but insufficient to explain the sensitivity of target cells to the cytotoxic activity of TNF-α.[21,93,132] The lectin, concanavalin A, causes an increase in TNF receptors expressed in the human cervical carcinoma cell line ME-180 without changing receptor affinity, but in spite of the increased TNF-α binding, the cell killing induced by TNF-α is abolished by concanavalin A.[133] The mechanism of concanavalin A-induced inhibition of cell killing by TNF-α is unknown, but the lectin causes a decrease in the rate of internalization of the TNF receptor and inhibits the release or degradation of TNF-α by the cells. Cell lines completely resistant to the cytotoxic action of TNF-α may not differ from TNF-α-sensitive cell lines by the number or affinity of TNF-α binding sites or by the internalization and subsequent degradation of TNF-α receptors.[134] However, fibroblasts resistant to TNF-α may lack TNF-α receptors and produce a cytotoxic factor which would be identical to TNF-α.[66]

The molecular mechanisms of TNF receptor modulation are poorly understood, but there is evidence that protein kinase C may be involved in such modulation, probably via direct phosphorylation of the receptor protein.[135-140] A rapid loss of high-affinity TNF-α receptors occurs in activated T lymphocytes and other types of cells by the action of agents known to activate protein kinase C, including PMA and the calcium ionophore A23187, and this action is antagonized by an inhibitor of the enzyme.

4. TNF-α Inhibitors

A TNF-α inhibitory activity was detected in the urine of some febrile patients by using a cytotoxicity assay on the TNF-α-susceptible cell line L929.[141] Purification and characterization of this activity indicated that the TNF-α inhibitor is represented by a 33-kDa protein and that its biological activity on L929 cells is preserved in the presence of actinomycin D.[142] In contrast to TNF-α, TNF-β cytotoxicity is only slightly affected by the inhibitor. The mechanism of action of the inhibitor involves blocking of TNF-α binding to its receptor on the cell surface. Recent evidence indicates that this TNF-α inhibitor, termed TNFrI, is represented by a soluble form of the TNF-α receptor.[143] Serum ultrafiltrates from patients with different types of cancer may contain the TNF inhibitor/soluble TNF receptor molecule.[144]

A second TNF-α inhibitor, termed TNFrII, isolated from the human histiocytic lymphoma cell line U-937 is capable of inhibiting both TNF-α and TNF-β.[145] The cDNA sequence of TNFrII suggests that it also corresponds to a soluble fragment of a TNF receptor. Expression of the TNFrII cDNA sequence in COS-7 cells verified that it encodes a receptor for TNF that can give rise to a soluble inhibitor of TNF-α, presumably through proteolytic cleavage.

D. POSTRECEPTOR MECHANISMS OF ACTION OF TNF-α

The postreceptor mechanisms of action of TNF-α remain little characterized. Many different biochemical alterations have been observed in mammalian cells treated with TNF-α, but the precise role of each of these alterations is unknown. TNF-α-induced changes occur at the level of the membrane, the cytoplasm, and the nucleus as well as in cellular organelles. TNF-α can induce a depression of cytochrome P-450-dependent microsomal metabolism in mice.[146] Studies of the introduction of TNF-α directly into the cytoplasm of target cells by microinjection demonstrated that TNF-α is capable of killing the cells through some intracellular type of activity, suggesting that TNF-α may have important intracellular roles after its internalization into the cell.[147] Major steps in the TNF-α-mediated cytotoxicity cascade include G protein-coupled activation of phospholipases, generation of free radicals, and damage to nuclear DNA by endonucleases.[148] Ultimately, the cells may undergo apoptosis.

1. Production of cAMP and cGMP

The adenylyl cyclase system mediates at least some of the cellular actions of TNF-α. Exposure of human fibroblasts to TNF-α causes a rapid accumulation of intracellular cAMP and increases the activity of cAMP-dependent protein kinase.[149] The activated kinase phosphorylates histone HII-B *in vitro,* but the normal endogenous substrates of the TNF-α-activated enzyme have not been identified. In addition to its effect on cAMP, TNF-α can stimulate the production of cGMP in certain cellular systems, for example, in rat renal mesangial cells.[150]

2. Production of Prostaglandins

TNF-α stimulates the production of PGE_2 by vascular endothelial cells *in vitro*.[49] Mononuclear cells enhance the production of PGE_2 by polymorphonuclear leukocytes via TNF-α.[151] Synergistic interaction of TNF-α and IL-1 stimulate PGE_2 production and phospholipase A_2 release by human lung fibroblast cell lines and rat mesangial cells.[152,153] IL-1α and IL-1β are more potent than TNF-α in stimulating prostaglandin production in the latter system, but synergistic effects between TNF-α and IL-1α or IL-1β are observed when the factors are added together.

3. Production of Polyamines

The activity of ODC, a rate-limiting enzyme in polyamine biosynthesis, is suppressed by TNF-α in the A375 human melanoma cell line, whose growth is inhibited by TNF-α, and is increased in the U373 MG human melanoma cell line, whose growth is stimulated by TNF-α.[154] Putrescine, a product of the ODC reaction and a precursor of polyamines, can partially overcome the growth-inhibitory effect of TNF-α, which suggests that ODC activity is an important component of the antiproliferative action of TNF-α.

4. Membrane GTP Binding and GTPase Activity

In the human leukemia cell line HL-60 and the mouse fibroblast cell line L929, TNF-α stimulates membrane GTP binding and GTPase activity in a dose- and time-dependent manner.[155] The GTPase activity stimulated by TNF-α is sensitive to pertussis toxin and the cytosolic effects of TNF-α are inhibited by this toxin. These results suggest that TNF-α transduces signals at the cell membrane level through the activity of a G protein.

5. Intracellular Calcium

The role of intracellular Ca^{2+} in the cytotoxic effects of TNF-α is poorly understood. Studies on TNF-α-mediated lysis of tumor cells using the calcium chelator, EGTA, and a compound capable of blocking intracellular Ca^{2+} mobilization suggest the existence of a Ca^{2+}-independent lytic pathway, in which secreted or membrane-bound TNF-α may interact with the target cells and ultimately results in DNA degradation and target cell lysis.[156] Thus, TNF-α-mediated tumor cell lysis can take place in Ca^{2+}-free medium and in the absence of intracellular Ca^{2+} mobilization.

6. Phospholipid and Sphingolipid Metabolism

Little is known of the possible role of phospholipid metabolism in the cellular mechanism of action of TNF-α. TNF-α induces activation and translocation of protein kinase C in some, but not all, target cells.[157] Moreover, different profiles of protein kinase C translocation are observed in different cell lines treated with TNF-α. The mechanism of TNF-α-induced protein kinase C activation, as well as the possible physiological role of this activation, are unclear. Although TNF-α causes translocation of protein kinase C to the membrane of cultured human amniotic cells (WISH cells), activation of protein kinase C is not required for TNF-α to induce a decrease in EGF binding to the cells.[158]

In human synovial cells, TNF-α stimulates arachidonic acid release and phospholipid metabolism.[159] Treatment of rat chondrocytes with TNF-α or IL-1 results in a dose-dependent stimulation of membrane-associated phospholipase activity in both the secreted and membrane-associated form.[160] The mechanism by which TNF-α and IL-1 activate phospholipase remains to be determined. In the murine osteoblast cell line MC3T3-E1, TNF-α activates phospholipase C and increases the metabolism of 1,2-diacylglycerol to liberate arachidonate for prostaglandin synthesis.[161] The cytotoxic effects of TNF-α may be associated with activation of phospholipase D.[162]

Sphingolipids may have a role in the mechanism of TNF-α action. In a cell-free system, TNF-α induced a reduction in the membrane content of sphingomyelin and an increase in ceramide concentrations with increased ceramide-activated protein kinase activity.[163] Such results suggest that the TNF-α signaling pathway may involve sphingomyelin hydrolysis to ceramide by a sphingomyelinase and stimulation of a ceramide-activated protein kinase.

7. Protein Phosphorylation

TNF-α, as well as the calcium ionophore A23187, induces the phosphorylation of a 27-kDa cellular protein in a time- and concentration-dependent manner in several types of cells (HeLa, ME 180, and bovine aortic endothelial cells).[164] However, this phosphorylation is not observed in L929 cells, for which TNF-α is highly cytotoxic, suggesting that it may play a role in actions other than the induction of cell death by TNF-α. Three 28-kDa proteins phosphorylated by TNF-α in bovine aortic endothelial cells were identified as stress proteins whose phosphorylation is also enhanced by arsenite.[165] As stress proteins often play a protective role, phosphorylation of these proteins in endothelial cells may be responsible for their resistance to TNF-α. A 28-kDa protein which is rapidly phosphorylated by TNF-α in the ME-180 human cervical carcinoma cell line was identified as a cap-binding protein.[166,167] Cap-binding proteins play an essential role in the translational machinery of the cell, mediating the interaction of mRNAs with polyribosomes. The protein phosphorylated by TNF-α is the eukaryotic initiation factor 4E, a 24- to 28-kDa ATP-Mg^{2+}-independent cap-binding protein. Overexpression of this factor may result in the expression of malignant transformation, suggesting that E4 may be the product of a putative proto-oncogene.[168] The EGF receptor, which is the product of the c-*erb*-B1 proto-oncogene, is phosphorylated on tyrosine residues by the TNF-α receptor in human tumor cells.[169,170] Since the TNF-α receptor does not possess tyrosine kinase activity, this phosphorylation must depend on the secondary activation of cellular tyrosine kinases.

8. Transcriptional Effects

Some actions of TNF-α may be exerted at the transcriptional level by modifying the expression of distinct genes.[171] Both TNF-α and IL-1 are importantly involved as mediators of the hepatic acute-phase response to inflammation and tissue injury.[172] This response is associated with the activation or inactivation of individually regulated specific genes in the liver, which takes place at the transcriptional level. TNF-α induces in cultured human foreskin fibroblasts the synthesis of two proteins of 36 kDa (p36) and 42 kDa (p42), and this synthesis is prevented by actinomycin D.[173] Whereas p42 appears to be stable, p36 turns over within a few hours. The physiological roles of these proteins is unknown.

The TNF-α gene is closely linked to the MHC locus on human chromosome 6 and it is interesting to note that TNF-α may have important effects on the expression of class I MHC antigens on the cell surface. TNF-α increases both the mRNA levels and the cell surface expression of HLA-A and HLA-B antigens in human vascular endothelial cells and dermal fibroblasts *in vitro*.[174] The increase in specific mRNA level is blocked by cycloheximide. These results suggest that *in vivo* TNF-α may enhance the participation of the immune system, especially of cytolytic T lymphocytes, in the destruction of virally altered or neoplastic cells. Induction of MHC antigens by TNF-α may be mediated by the increased production of other cytokines.

Differential screening with molecular probes has facilitated the isolation of cDNA sequences that are stimulated by TNF-α in human fibroblasts (FS-4 cell line).[175] Eight distinct TNF-α-stimulated gene sequences were partially sequenced and compared with known sequences. One of these sequences was identical with IL-8 and another corresponded to the gene encoding the monocyte chemotactic and activating factor. Two sequences were identical to the genes coding for collagenase and stromelysin, respectively. The other sequences showed no homologies with known genes.

9. Effect of TNF-α on Proto-Oncogene Expression

The levels of expression of particular proto-oncogenes may be altered by TNF-α acting either alone or in combination with other growth factors. Exposure of quiescent human FS-4 fibroblasts to TNF-α and/or IL-1 results in a marked and rapid increase the levels of c-*fos* and c-*myc* mRNA, and this effect is increased by treatment with cycloheximide.[176] TNF-α stimulates transcription of the collagenese gene, and this effect is mediated by a prolonged stimulation of c-*jun* proto-oncogene expression.[177] The Jun protein is a major component of the transcription factor AP-1, and downregulation of human elastin gene expression by TNF-α may involve suppression of promoter activity by AP-1.[178] In mouse 3T3-L1 fibroblasts TNF-α stimulates transcription of the c-*fos*, c-*jun*, and *jun*-B proto-oncogenes, as well as that of the gene for β-actin.[179] This effect is reminiscent of that of the serum-derived growth factors, and is associated with increased glucose transport and induction of glucose transporter in the plasma membrane.

In fresh human renal cancer cells and renal cancer cell lines, TNF-α stimulates c-*jun* and *jun*-B gene expression.[180] The mitogenic response to TNF-α requires c-Jun/AP-1.[181]

HeLa cells respond to TNF-α with growth arrest at the G_0-G_1 transition of the cycle, and this effect is accompanied by reduced expression of c-*myc* mRNA.[182] The inhibitory effect of TNF-α on c-*myc* expression in HeLa cells does not depend on protein synthesis and is enhanced in the presence of IFN-γ. TNF-α inhibits the expression of both c-*myc* and c-*myb* mRNA in various human leukemia cell lines, including HL-60 promyelocytic leukemia cells, where it induces a process of differentiation.[183] The effect of TNF-α on c-*myc* expression in HL-60 cells occurs primarily at the level of transcription and is independent of protein synthesis. Expression of the c-*fms*/CSF-1 receptor in HL-60 cells is stimulated by TNF-α by both transcriptional and posttranscriptional mechanisms.[184] PGE_2 and cAMP may be involved in regulating the transcriptional activation of the c-*fms*/CSF-1 receptor gene by TNF-α.

Treatment of v-*mos*- and c-*myc*-transformed NIH/3T3 cells with recombinant murine TNF-α in noncytotoxic concentrations causes a strong inhibition of both proliferative capacity in monolayer culture and colony formation in soft agar, and these effects are preceded by a selective reduction in the steady-state mRNA levels of the respective oncogenes used for transformation.[185] The transcriptional activity of the LTR-controlled v-*mos* and c-*myc* genes was not altered, but a decreased half-life of the respective mRNAs suggests that TNF-α in this system primarily affects the stability of v-*mos* and c-*myc* gene transcripts. In contrast, v-H-*ras*-transformed cells exhibit little sensitivity to TNF-α treatment and no downregulation of v-H-*ras* mRNA is observed in these cells during treatment with TNF-α.

10. Cytotoxic Effects of TNF-α

TNF-α has been recognized as a monocyte-derived protein with direct cytotoxic effects on a diversity of cell types. The mechanism of TNF-α cytotoxicity is little understood, but there is evidence that it requires protein synthesis and is abolished in the presence of protein synthesis inhibitors. The cytostatic effects of TNF-α on the human breast cancer cell line, T47D, are exerted at the G_1 to S phase of the cycle via an intracellular mechanism which is largely independent of protein kinase C, protein kinase A, calmodulin, and the phosphatases PP1 or PP2B.[186] In the murine TA1 adipogenic cell line, as well as in HeLa cells and NIH/3T3 fibroblasts, TNF-α cytotoxicity appears to be mediated by lipoxygenase metabolites of arachidonic acid, which may directly or indirectly operate via the generation of superoxide anions.[187] Glucocorticoids can exert a protective effect, inhibiting the cytotoxic action of TNF-α on cells such as the murine fibroblastic cell line L929, and this protection is also dependent on *de novo* synthesis of proteins.[188] Interaction *in vivo* between glucocorticoids and TNF-α may play a modulating role in certain inflammatory processes.

11. TNF-α-Induced Proteins

Treatment of sensitive cells with TNF-α results in the synthesis of a set of proteins with molecular weight of 80, 67, and 56 kDa, the induction of which is also observed when the cells are treated with IFN.[189] Whereas the induction of the 80- and 56-kDa proteins after TNF-α treatment is dependent on the synthesis of an intermediary protein, that of the 67-kDa protein may occur by a direct action of TNF-α. The intermediary protein responsible for the induction of the 80-kDa protein by TNF-α is IFN-$β_1$ or an antigenically related molecule, and the 80-kDa protein could play a role in mediating the antiviral effects of TNF-α.

12. Effects of TNF-α on DNA Synthesis

Although TNF-α is directly cytotoxic to a variety of tumor cells and cell lines, in certain biological systems TNF-α can stimulate DNA synthesis and cell proliferation. TNF-α stimulates, for example, the growth of diploid human FS-4 fibroblasts maintained in a chemically defined, serum-free medium.[190,191] Simultaneous addition of TNF-α and EGF to cells grown in serum-free medium may result in synergistic stimulation of DNA synthesis and cell growth. Administration of small doses of TNF-α to intact rats *in vivo* results in a significant increase in DNA synthesis in the liver, which may be related to an increase in DNA polymerase-α activity.[192]

E. PHYSIOLOGIC EFFECTS OF TNF-α

TNF-α is a hormone-like cytokine that has important effects on a variety of organs and tissues. It is involved in hematopoietic, immune, and inflammatory processes and has important effects on blood vessels and blood coagulation. In addition, TNF-α exerts physiologic effects in liver, bone, cartilage, muscle, and other tissues.

1. Hematopoietic, Immune, and Inflammatory Processes

The physiological effects of TNF-α are multiple and include different types of cells and tissues. TNF-α participates, in concert with other cytokines and CSFs, in the regulation of hematopoiesis.[193] It may display either stimulating or inhibiting effects on hematopoietic processes, depending on the particular type of cell and the predominant physiologic conditions.[194] The proliferation of human bone marrow granulocyte-macrophage CFUs is synergistically inhibited by PGE, IFN, and TNF-α.[195] In addition to its effect on hematopoietic processes, TNF-α may alter the peripheral distribution of blood cells. Injection of TNF-α to the rat results in induction of lymphopenia and neutropenia, which may be due to transient intravascular margination of the circulating cells.[196] However, TNF-α has no direct chemoattractant effect *in vitro* on neutrophils or monocytes.[197]

TNF-α shares with IFN many of the systemic and local effects of IL-1, including fever and acute phase changes.[198,199] It has an important role in the cellular processes associated with immune and inflammatory responses, including the acute phase response.[200,201] A single injection of TNF-α into human adult subjects can reproduce the symptoms observed in endotoxic shock or the cachexia of chronic infection, including fever, tachycardia, and hypotension.[202] These alterations may be associated with TNF-α-induced production of endogenous agents such as IL-1 and PGE_2.[203-206] However, the effects of TNF-α on IL-1 production vary according to the doses: at higher doses of TNF-α macrophages produce no IL-1, but at intermediate doses TNF-α induces an increase in IL-1 production.[207] At lower doses, TNF-α induces the production of a factor that synergizes with IL-1.

TNF-α and IL-1 share many biological activities in spite of their different structural features and their action through binding to different cellular receptors.[208] Some of the biological effects of TNF-α in diverse cell types could be mediated by the generation of IL-1. The synthesis of serum amyloid A in the liver and other tissues is stimulated by TNF-α although to a lesser extent that the stimulation induced by IL-1.[209] It is not known whether TNF-α acts directly upon serum amyloid A-synthesizing cells or indirectly via IL-1 production. Serum amyloid A is a sensitive and quantitative indicator of inflammation.

Administration of TNF-α to intact animals may result in the production of marked effects on blood cell populations. Injection of human TNF-α to mice causes striking changes in peripheral blood leukocyte populations.[210] The changes consist of early mild lymphocytosis followed by lymphopenia and a parallel neutropenia followed by neutrophilia. The changes are both relative and absolute and are similar to those produced by injection of LPS, suggesting that LPS may act through release of TNF-α.

TNF-α has an immunoregulatory role and is similar to IL-1 in facilitating the proliferation of human mature T cells.[211] Multiple stimulatory activities are exerted by TNF-α on activated human T cells, including the expression of HLA-DR antigens and high-affinity IL-2 receptors.[107] TNF-α may directly induce IL-2 receptor expression and does not appear to act via an indirect mechanism in this induction.[212] As a consequence, T cells exposed to TNF-α exhibit an enhanced proliferative response to IL-2. TNF-α and TNF-β synergize with suboptimal levels of IL-2 in the generation of LAK cell activity, and this action is inhibited by TGF-β.[213,214] TNF-α is effective as a costimulator of IL-2-dependent IFN-γ production.[107] The antiviral effects of TNF-α and IL-1 are mediated by the production of IFN-$β_1$ and are neutralized by anti-IFN-β serum.[215,216]

Complex interactions between different types of cytokines may be important for the physiological effects of TNF-α. TNF-α may be considered as an important immunomodulator and mediator of monocyte cytotoxicity induced by itself, IFN-γ, and IL-2.[217] TNF-α and IFN-γ may act synergistically in upregulating the expression of class I MHC mRNA and protein in vascular endothelium as well as in pancreatic β cells, and may have a role in amplifying the targeting and destruction of β cells by cytotoxic T cells in the insulitis lesion associated with type I diabetes.[218,219] An effector molecule involved in monocyte-mediated cytotoxicity, the monocyte-derived cytotoxic factor (MDCF), may be similar or identical to TNF-α.[220] TNF-α selectively inhibits the stimulation of human B cells by EBV, abrogating both the proliferation of B cells and the secretion of immunoglobulins.[221] The cytostatic effect of TNF-α on EBV-activated human B cells is dependent on the presence of macrophages.

TNF-α is an autocrine growth regulator during macrophage differentiation.[222] Both TNF-α and TNF-β may act as helper factors that facilitate macrophage activation and may enhance the tumor toxicity of preactivated macrophages.[223] However, the TNFs are not capable of inducing a direct activation of macrophages. TNF-α induces down-modulation of CSF-1 receptors on murine macrophages, and an interaction between TNF-α and CSF-1 may be important for macrophage activation.[224]

Granulocytes have specific high-affinity receptors for TNF-α, and TNF-α release by mononuclear phagocytes may contribute to granulocyte activation and aggregation during inflammation.[225] Both TNF-α and IL-1 stimulate the passage of neutrophils from the vascular bed to the interstitial tissue, even in the absence of an externally applied chemotactic gradient.[226] TNF-α augments the production of ornithine by peritoneal macrophages.[227] Ornithine and its decarboxylation product, putrescine, potentiate immune responses *in vivo*. Treatment of peritoneal exudate cells with TNF-α augments the capacity of these cells to immunize mice *in vivo*. TNF-α also possesses intrinsic collagenolytic activity, inducing a rapid collagen turnover in granulation tissue.[228]

TNF-α has antiviral effects and induces resistance against a diversity of RNA and DNA viruses, including vesicular stomatitis virus (VSV), encephalomyocarditis virus (EMCV), and herpes simplex virus (HSV).[229-231] Human TNF-α enhances nonspecific resistance of animals to various bacterial and fungal infections, which may be explained by its action on nonspecific immunity processes involving macrophages and polymorphonuclear cells.[232] Pretreatment of rats with both TNF-α and IL-1 favorably alters lung glutathione redox status, decreasing lung injury and enhancing survival of animals exposed to hyperoxia.[233]

TNF-α and TNF-β have important effects on polymorphonuclear neutrophil functions, stimulating their migration and superoxide anion production.[234] Human neutrophils possess elevated numbers of high-affinity TNF-α receptors which are internalized after ligand binding.[235] This binding inhibits the migration of neutrophils and activates them to produce superoxide anion, which acts as a toxic oxygen radical. TNF-α-activated neutrophils are capable of inflicting a marked disruption of human endothelial cell monolayers and inhibit the proliferative activity of these cells. Low concentrations of TNF-α cause aggregation and activation of granulocytes.[225] The results suggest that interactions between TNF-α, neutrophils, and endothelial cells may play a major role in the development of inflammatory reactions. In addition, TNF-α stimulates myelopoiesis (granulopoiesis) and can protect mice against lethal irradiation.[236] However, TNF-α may have inhibitory effects on the growth of neutrophil cells. Recombinant human TNF-α suppresses the growth of neutrophil colonies at concentrations that do not affect monocyte-macrophage or eosinophil colonies.[237]

Chronic inflammatory diseases are frequently associated with decreased red blood cell mass. TNF-α and IL-1, produced by monocytes/macrophages, have been implicated in the anemia of chronic disease. Chronic administration of *Salmonella* endotoxin or sublethal quantities of TNF-α to rats results in a significant decrease in the red blood cell mass.[238] The TNF-α-induced anemia is related to a decreased red blood cell synthesis and a reduced life span of circulating red blood cells.

The role of TNF-α in parasitic diseases is unknown, but there is evidence that TNF-α may be involved in the mechanisms of host immune response to some parasites. TNF-α inhibits the growth of malaria parasites *in vivo* but not *in vitro*.[239]

2. Blood Vessels and Blood Coagulation

Many of the physiological actions of TNF-α *in vivo* may be related to its action on the blood vessels. In addition to the well-known action of TNF-α on endothelial cells, vascular smooth-muscle cells, which are the most abundant cell type in blood vessels, also respond to TNF-α as well as to TNF-β.[240] Both factors induce transient accumulation of IL-1 mRNA by adult human vascular smooth-muscle cells maintained in *in vitro* culture. Treatment of the cells with TNF-α also results in increased secretion of IL-1, release of prostaglandin (PGE_2), and induction of the gene coding for (2′-5′)-oligoadenylate synthetase, an enzyme that may mediate the antiproliferative and antiviral actions of IFN.

TNF-α produced and secreted by macrophages is an angiogenic factor.[241] It can induce capillary blood-vessel formation in the rat cornea and the developing chick chorioallantoic membrane at very low doses. *In vitro,* TNF-α stimulates chemotaxis of bovine adrenal capillary endothelial cells and induces cultures of these cells grown on type 1 collagen gels to form capillary-tube-like structures. These findings suggest that TNF-α may have a role in inflammation and wound repair by stimulating new blood vessel growth. However, TNF-α may cause morphologic changes in, growth inhibition of, and cytotoxicity against vascular endothelial cells.[242] Under certain conditions, TNF-α inhibits capillary growth by a direct cytostatic and cytotoxic action on microvascular endothelial cells.[243] An inhibiting effect of TNF-α on angiogenesis may be responsible, at least in part, for suppression of tumor growth.

In certain tumor tissues TNF-α could have a dual role: stimulating tumor development by promoting vessel growth and inducing tumor regression by mechanisms associated with cytotoxicity. TNF-α is able to suppress the *in vitro* tumor-induced endothelial cell motility, but not the spontaneous one.[244,245] Histological evaluation of the hemorrhagic necrosis induced by human TNF-α suggests that the primary lesion induced by the factor in experimental tumors (Meth A mouse sarcomas) is due to its action on the tumor vasculature and/or the vasculature surrounding the tumor, and not to its direct effects on tumor cells.[246] However, although these changes may mediate, at least in part, the TNF-α-induced hemorrhagic necrosis of transplanted tumors, there is evidence that TNF-α has direct activity against transformed cells.

Human TNF-α, either alone or in combination with IL-1, can influence hemostatic/thrombotic activities at the blood-vascular interface.[247] The endothelial-directed actions of TNF-α may be relevant to intravascular coagulation and hemorrhagic tumor necrosis.[248] Coagulation disorders are frequently observed after exposure of animals to endotoxin or TNF-α, suggesting that TNF-α may affect the hemostatic balance. The fibrinolytic system may be altered by the action of TNF-α. The major fibrinolytic enzyme is plasmin, which is generated from its zymogen, plasminogen, by one or two distinct plasminogen activators, termed the urokinase-type and the tissue-type plasminogen activators.[249] In turn, the levels of activity of plasminogen activators are modulated by the action of two specific and fast-acting plasminogen activator inhibitors (PAIs), PAI-1 and PAI-2. PAI-1 is found in plasma and platelets, as well as in the conditioned media of endothelial cells and other types of cells maintained in culture *in vitro*.[250] PAI-2 is found in both monocytes and granulocytes and is an intracellular nonglycosylated protein.[251]

TNF-α suppresses secreted fibrinolytic activity of cells such as the HT-1080 human fibrosarcoma cell line.[252] These cells constitutively express the urokinase-type and the tissue-type plasminogen activator as well as PAI-1 and PAI-2. The effect of TNF-α on HT-1080 cells is mediated by the transcriptional induction of both PAIs in concert with suppression of tissue-type plasminogen activator gene expression. TNF-α induces PAI-1 and the urokinase-type plasminogen activator mRNA and protein in the human carcinoma cell line T-CAR1, whereas the tissue-type plasminogen activator is not affected or is slightly decreased.[253] Both TNF-α and IL-1 induce PAI-1 mRNA and suppress secreted tissue-type plasminogen activator in bovine aortic endothelial cells.[254] PAI-2 is a major protein induced in human fibroblasts and SK-MEL-109 melanoma cells by TNF-α.[255] The TNF-α-mediated reprogramming of gene transcription may induce an antifibrinolytic state, which may cooperate with the induction of procoagulant activity to stabilize the fibrin deposits commonly found in inflamed tissues.[252] These changes may also be important in the evolution of malignant diseases.

3. Bone, Cartilage, and Muscle

TNF-α may exert important effects on bone tissue, where it acts as a mitogenic agent stimulating DNA synthesis and bone cell growth.[256] TNF-α and TNF-β, as well as IL-1α, have an important role in bone reabsorption and remodelation.[257] Both TNF-α and IL-1α stimulate mouse osteoblastoma-like cells to produce prostaglandin (PGE_2) and a macrophage colony-stimulating activity that may be involved in osteoclastic bone resorption.[258] At the same time, TNF-α and IL-1 inhibit alkaline phosphatase activity, which may lead to decreased bone formation. The stimulatory effect of TNF-α, observed on osteoblastic collagen synthesis, is secondary to its mitogenic effect, and chronic exposure to TNF-α may inhibit osteoblastic function and stimulates collagen degradation. TNF-α stimulates the resorption and inhibits the synthesis of proteoglycan in cartilage.[259] The factor may mediate changes of skeletal muscle plasma membrane potential.[260]

4. Endocrine and Reproductive Systems

TNF-α may have important effects on the endocrine system, including the hypophysis and the gonads. In rat pituitary cells incubated *in vitro*, TNF-α stimulates the release of ACTH, TSH, and growth hormone, but not prolactin.[261,262] These effects are accompanied by a decrease in the intracellular concentrations of cAMP and are partially blocked by the prostaglandin synthesis inhibitor, indomethacin, which suggests that the mechanism of action of TNF-α on the pituitary cells may be via stimulation of prostaglandin release. TNF-α may affect pituitary growth hormone secretion *in vivo* and *in vitro* by direct interaction with specific receptors present in the gland.[263] On the other hand, the stimulation of rat anterior pituitary cells by hypothalamic factors, including ACTH, LH, growth hormone, and prolactin, is inhibited by TNF-α.[264] The CRF-stimulated secretion of ACTH is inhibited by TNF-α in a dose-dependent manner. This inhibitory effect may contribute to the increased mortality observed in cases of severe septic shock with high levels of circulating TNF-α.

The possible role of TNF-α in the regulation of gonadal functions is suggested by the results from several studies. TNF-α enhances the inhibitory effect of IL-1β on Leydig cell steroidogenesis.[265] TNF-α has been localized immunohistochemically in the ovary of the rat and cow, and granulosa cells appear to be a source of TNF-α. Incubation of preovulatory follicles from cyclic proestrus rats with various doses of TNF-α demonstrated that TNF-α stimulates the production of progesterone.[266] Follicular androstenedione production was inhibited by low doses of TNF-α *in vitro*, whereas estradiol production was unaffected. The action of FSH on rat ovarian granulosa cells is attenuated *in vitro* by TGF-α at sites proximal, but not distal, to cAMP generation.[267] Locally produced TNF-α could have a role in ovarian steroidogenesis and follicular development *in vivo* through a paracrine type of mechanism, attenuating the action of gonadotropins.

TNF-α may be involved in regulating the production of specific growth factors by different types of cells. TNF-α markedly stimulates the synthesis and secretion of NGF in quiescent cultures of mouse fibroblasts, which is a result of an increase in the NGF mRNA level.[268] Basic FGF and EGF, but not PDGF, exert a similar effect in this system.

F. TNF-α AS A GROWTH FACTOR

TNF-α has cytostatic or cytolytic effects on only some tumor cell lines; other cell lines may not respond to the growth-inhibitory action of TNF-α, and the growth of some normal cells, including human fibroblasts, is enhanced when TNF-α is added to the medium.[93] TNF-α is a direct mitogen for the fibroblasts and is largely responsible for the monocyte-derived stimulation of these cells observed *in vitro*.[269,270] TNF-α is also a direct mitogen for rat hepatocytes.[271] The growth factor-like effects of TNF-α are associated with metabolic changes. Stimulation of glucose utilization occurs in a number of rat tissues (spleen, liver, kidney, skin, lung, and intestine) after the infusion of nonlethal doses of TNF-α.[272]

The effects of TNF-α on cell proliferation can be either enhanced or suppressed by other growth factors. TNF-α-induced stimulation of cellular growth in confluent cultures of human diploid fibroblasts maintained in serum-free medium is enhanced by insulin.[190] Stimulation of DNA synthesis of mouse hepatocytes in primary culture by TNF-α can be suppressed by TGF-β and IL-6.[273] The mitogenic action of TNF-α on cultured human fibroblasts is associated with a TNF-α-induced increase in the expression of EGF receptors on the cell surface, which is due to increased EGF receptor synthesis without changes in the affinity of the receptor molecule.[274] In addition, TNF-α induces the expression of transferrin receptors on the surface of human fibroblasts, which may be required for its mitogenic effects on these cells.[275] TNF-α and EGF may generate similar or identical intracellular signals for the stimulation of cellular growth and the regulation of transferrin receptor expression. Thus TNF-α may be considered primarily as a growth factor, since stimulation of cell growth is probably a normal function of TNF-α. The growth-promoting action of TNF-α on diploid human fibroblasts (WI-38 cells) is suppressed in a dose-dependent manner by TGF-β through mechanisms requiring *de novo* protein synthesis.[276]

TNF-α may act synergistically with IFN-γ in the regulation of morphology, function, and growth of particular tissues or cellular systems, including various normal and transformed human and murine cell lines.[277-279] IFN-γ, and to a lesser extent IFN-α and IFN-β, potentiate the cytotoxic effects of TNF-α.[131] The antiviral effects of TNF-α on human fibroblasts are mediated by IFN-β.[280] Both TNF-α and TNF-β have the ability to induce differentiation of human myeloid leukemia cell lines in synergy with IFN-γ.[281] HL-60 human leukemia cells possess receptors for TNF-α, and TNF-α can act in synergy with IFN-β and calcitriol to induce the monocytic differentiation of these cells.[282] Differentiation of HL-60 cells into the monocytic pathway induced by TNF-α and IFN-γ is accompanied by the appearance of a membrane-bound tyrosine kinase activity.[283] TNF-α and IFN-γ may act singly as well as in combination to alter the morphology and behavior of human endothelial cells, inducing cell elongation and overlapping, rearrangement of actin filaments, and loss of the fibronectin matrix.[284] Human IFN-γ stimulates the production of TNF-α by human peripheral blood monocytes in culture.[60] Combined treatment with TNF-α and suboptimal doses of IFN-γ may be useful for the control of metastatic cancer *in vivo*.[285] However, no synergistic action between TNFs and IFNs is seen in certain types of cells, for example, in human leukemia cell lines.[21]

TNF-α induces expression of mRNAs for different types of CSFs in cultures of human umbilical vein endothelial cells.[286] Human TNF-α stimulates the expression of CSF-2 transcripts and the production and secretion of CSF-2 in hematopoietic tissue, normal human lung fibroblasts, and vascular endothelial cells as well as in cells of several malignant tissues.[286-288] TNF-α acts as an inducer of IFN-β$_2$/IL-6, which may represent a homeostatic negative feedback mechanism in the control of cell proliferation.[289]

G. GROWTH-INHIBITING AND CELL-KILLING EFFECTS OF TNF-α

TNF-α displays inhibitory effects on the proliferation of various types of cells. For example, TNF-α is a rapid, irreversible, and extremely potent inhibitor of erythroid progenitors (CFU-E and BFU-E) and hematopoietic cell lines expressing features of the erythroid lineage (K562 and HE2) or the granulocyte-macrophage lineage (HL-60).[290] The inhibitory action of TNF-α on these cells does not require accessory cells such as lymphocytes or macrophages. The presence of TNF-α receptors on hematopoietic cells is required, but is not sufficient by itself to confer sensitivity to TNF-α. The majority (80 to 95%) of HEL cells express TNF-α receptors while only 40 to 60% are inhibited by TNF-α. The mechanisms involved in the growth-inhibitory effects of TNF-α are unknown. The antiproliferative activity of TNF-α and

TNF-β on the human cervical carcinoma cell line, ME-180, is suppressed by either EGF and TGF-α by mechanisms not involving downregulation of TNF receptors.[291] These results suggest that production of growth factors by certain tumor cells may account for their TNF-α-resistant phenotype.

TNF-α can induce cell death (apoptosis) in sensitive cells. In the C3HA murine cell line, TNF-α induces cytolysis without a change in nuclear integrity, and this effect is associated with an early loss of stress fibers in perinuclear areas of the cytoplasm, including disruption of microfilaments.[292] The dissolution of microfilaments is followed by cytoplasmic alteration, decrease in cell volume, and lysis of the cytoplasmic membrane.

H. CACHECTIN-RELATED ACTIVITIES OF TNF-α

Cachexia is a syndrome characterized by marked anorexia and weight loss accompanied by alterations in lipid and protein metabolism. It is frequently associated with severe chronic inflammation and malignant diseases. Despite food intake, cachexia is potentially lethal. A factor named cachectin, detected in the blood of cachectic animals, is identical to TNF-α. Injection of sublethal doses of cachectin/TNF-α to animals may result in cachexia through stimulation of the breakdown of energy stores in the body.

TNF-α secreted by activated macrophages and monocytes can inhibit lipoprotein lipase (LPL) activity.[50,293,294] LPL catalyzes the hydrolysis of lipoprotein-derived triacylglycerol, providing fatty acids for storage or catabolism in various tissues, including adipose tissue, heart, and liver. LPL is synthesized within the adipocytes and is secreted by these cells. The enzyme is activated by apoprotein C-II, a protein present in very low-density lipoproteins (VLDL) and low-density lipoproteins (LDL). LPL activity in adipose tissue allows the accumulation of fatty acids, which are reesterified in adipocytes, to form stored triacylglycerol. Exposure of 3T3-L1 adipocytes to TNF-α stimulates lipolysis and suppresses LPL activity.[295] The amount of LPL mRNA is reduced in TNF-α-treated 3T3-L1 adipocytes, indicating that the molecular basis for the loss of LPL activity is a significant decrease in LPL transcripts available for translation.[296]

Administration of TNF-α to intact rats may result in stimulation of hepatic lipid synthesis and hyperlipidemia, with increased levels of triglycerides and cholesterol in the plasma.[297,298] Factors other than TNF-α are involved in the origin of cachexia. Alterations in lipid metabolism, with lipid mobilization, are not a distinctive property of TNF-α but may be produced by a diversity of cytokines, including IFNs.[299] The lipogenic effect of TNF-α in the liver may be mediated by IL-6.[300] The inhibitory effect of cachectin on LPL activity is limited to adipose tissue; in other tissues, specially in the liver, cachectin may induce increased LPL activity.[301]

Anorexia occurs frequently in animals treated with TNF-α and it may have an important role in the cachectin-related activities of this cytokine. However, little is known about the mechanisms involved in the anorectic effect of TNF-α. This effect of TNF-α could be exerted at the level of the central nervous system, the peripheral level, or both. Studies performed on intact rats with central or peripheral injection of TNF-α suggest that it may produce its anorectic effect at peripheral sites, possibly through mediators which remain to be identified.[302]

1. Role of TNF-α in Infectious Diseases

TNF-α may have an important role in infectious diseases of either bacterial or viral origin. TNF-α is a potent pyrogen and is responsible, at least in part, for the hypertriglyceridemia and other metabolic changes observed in mammals during some infections. However, injection of TNF-α into mice may result in hypothermic activity, similar to the hypothermia induced by endotoxin.[303] The hypothermic activity of TNF-α is not mediated via the induction of IL-1 production by mononuclear phagocytes. Systemic release of TNF-α, which may occur in endotoxemic states, can initiate shock and tissue injury.[304] Glucocorticoid hormones, which strongly antagonize the effects of endotoxin if they are administered before infections or endotoxemic insult, completely abolish TNF-α biosynthesis at both the transcriptional and translational levels.

Antiviral activity of TNF-α may serve to limit some viral infections. Resistance of cells to TNF-α during viral infections may depend on specific viral functions. A 14.7-kDa (14.7K) protein from the adenovirus E3 transcription unit may inhibit cytolysis by TNF-α.[305] Cells infected with group C human adenovirus mutants that do not synthesize the 14.7K protein are lysed by TNF-α, whereas uninfected cells and cells infected by adenoviruses that synthesize 14.7K are not lysed. On the other hand, adenovirus infection may enhance the susceptibility of some cells to lysis by TNF-α. Expression of the adenovirus E1A oncogene in NIH/3T3 increases their susceptibility to TNF-α-induced killing.[306]

2. Role of TNF-α in Cancer-Associated Cachexia

TNF-α may have an important role in the development of cachectic states that are frequently associated with cancer. Injection of a constructed tumor cell line that continuously secretes recombinant human TNF-α into nude mice results in marked anorexia associated with severe weight loss and cachexia.[307] However, in spite of continued exposure to recombinant human TNF-α, the mice develop a resistance to the factor and resume their pretreatment food intake and weight.[308] Chronic administration of sublethal doses of TNF-α to rats induces a syndrome similar to disease-associated cachexia, with symptoms including anorexia, weight loss, depletion of whole-body protein and lipid stores, reduction of red blood cell mass, leukocytosis, and tissue inflammation.[309] The rats can become tolerant to these effects, increasing their food intake and gaining weight despite the continuous administration of TNF-α. However, the mechanism of this tolerance is unknown and experimental observations suggest that TNF-α is a mediator of anorexia in tumor-bearing rats.[310]

If TNF-α is shown to be an important mediator of cancer-associated cachexia, antagonists to this factor may prove to be useful adjuvants in the treatment of cancer patients. However, the precise role of TNF-α in cancer-associated cachexia is not clear. Whereas TNF-α-like cytotoxicity is present in the serum of patients with septicemia, it is usually absent in the serum of untreated cancer patients.[311] No TNF-α was detected in the serum from 19 cancer patients who had lost up to 40% of premorbid body weight.[312] Administration of recombinant human TNF-α to noncachectic patients with a variety of malignant neoplasms (as part of a phase I trial of TNF-α as an antineoplastic agent) indicated that the cytokine stimulates certain of the metabolic disturbances seen in cancer patients, especially alterations in amino acid metabolism.[201] However, it is not clear whether the observed alterations are responsible for the development of the cachexia associated with human cancer.

I. EFFECTS OF TNF-α ON TUMOR CELL GROWTH

TNF-α displays cytotoxic (cytostatic and/or cytolytic) effects against a diversity of neoplastic cells of human and nonhuman origin. The antitumor activity of TNF-α results from a combination of its direct cytostatic effect on tumor cells and indirect effects involving host immune mechanisms.[313,314] Tumors are frequently infiltrated by macrophages, which may represent a defense reaction of the organism against the tumor. Unfortunately, only a small proportion of macrophages infiltrating tumors such as human colorectal carcinomas produce TNF-α even when the tumor is heavily infiltrated by the macrophages, suggesting that the natural population of these cells is suboptimally activated.[315] Thus, the potential antitumor properties of TNF-α may be exploited for its use in human cancer therapy.

1. Tumor Regression by TNF-α Treatment

The potential benefits of TNF-α for cancer treatment have been explored in a number of experimental and clinical studies. Inhibition of neoplastic cell growth induced by treatment with purified human TNF-α has been observed in human cell lines as well as in human solid tumors passaged in nude mice.[316,317]

Murine TNF-α displays clear necrotizing effects on Meth A sarcomas transplanted into BALB/c female mice.[100] Complete regression of MCA-induced fibrosarcomas was observed in mice treated with recombinant TNF-α and some of the treated mice remained free of tumors for over 400 d, whereas the median survival of control mice was 28 to 39 d.[318] Partial tumor regression was observed in mice receiving transplanted human ovarian carcinoma cells (NIH:OVCAR-3), but no cures were obtained in this model.

TNF-α exhibits antineoplastic effect against various types of primarily cultured human cancer cells as well as on a variety of human and murine transformed cell lines.[278,319] The sensitivity of tumor cell lines to TNF-α, however, shows wide variation and some cell lines are rather resistant to the factor.[126] Cells expressing high levels of proto-oncogene products, for example, NIH/3T3 cells with amplified expression of the c-*neu*/*erb*-B2 gene, show resistance to TNF-α.[320] Moreover, the antiproliferative effect of TNF-α is not specific for neoplastic cells since normal cells also may be inhibited, although to a lesser extent than the tumor cells. Although TNF-α suppresses the *in vitro* growth of human leukemia progenitor cells, it also has some inhibitory effect on the growth of granulocyte-macrophage and erythroid progenitor cells.[321] Cooperation between TNF-α and IL-1 may be required for the induction of differentiation in neoplastic cells such as the M1 mouse myeloid leukemia cell line.[322] Human and mouse TNFs behave similarly regarding the *in vitro* cytostatic/cytolytic activity and show only weak species specificity.

Organotypic culture may be used for assessing the antitumor effects of TNF-α.[323] This system differs from the usual tissue culture by the fact that the cells are not adherent to an "artificial" substrate, so that they are located in a more physiological environment. It involves, for example, fragments of normal heart tissue to which the melanoma cells adhere, then proliferate and invade. Treatment of B16B16 mouse melanoma cells maintained in heart organotypic culture with a combination of TNF-α and IFN-γ during 4 to 7 d resulted in selective killing of the tumor cells without damage to the normal heart cells. Eventually, the treatment may result in complete elimination of the melanoma cells with no apparent toxicity of the normal heart tissue.

Intralesional application of recombinant human TNF-α may induce tumor regression in patients with advanced malignant disease.[324] The local tumor regressions observed in some patients suggest a higher efficacy of local vs. systemic TNF-α treatment, where such dramatic tumor responses are not seen even at higher total doses. However, the duration of the response is usually short, implying a development of resistance to the effects of TNF-α.

2. Mechanisms of the Antineoplastic Effects of TNF-α

The mechanisms involved in the antineoplastic effects of TNF-α are only partially understood. TNF-α may act directly on the tumor cells or indirectly through activation of the immune system or other mechanisms. Most probably, the antitumor effects exerted by TNF-α *in vivo* represent the result of both types of mechanisms. An analysis of the relationship between TNF-α receptor occupancy and the kinetics of cell death conducted in the TNF-α-sensitive L929.10 murine fibrosarcoma cell line indicated that TNF-α-induced tumor cell death is a sequential, multiphasic process which includes events that are either dependent or independent of receptor occupancy.[325] Three sequential phases were defined by rates of cell death following the addition of TNF-α: the induction phase, the burst phase, and the slow lytic phase. The induction phase, which extends for several hours, is the initial event during which no cell death can be detected after the addition of TNF-α to the cell culture. The burst phase is characterized by a rapid increase in the loss of cell viability, but not all of the cells of the population die during the burst phase. The remaining cells undergo cytolysis at a much slower rate, during the final lytic phase. These three phases were also observed in other sensitive target tumor cells such as the ME-180 human cervical carcinoma cell line.

TNF-α-mediated autocrine inhibition of cell proliferation may contribute to the maintenance of the stable phase of chronic myelogenous leukemia (CML). Unlike the progenitor cells from normal donors, myeloid progenitor cells from CML patients with chronic leukemia constitutively express TNF-α mRNA and secrete functional TNF-α protein. This endogenous TNF-α may impede the growth of CML cells, as suggested by the effect of a monoclonal antibody to TNF-α, which neutralizes bioactive TNF-α and increases DNA synthesis in the CML cells.[326]

The mechanisms of the direct antitumor effects of TNF-α are little understood but may include damage of liposome membranes in the tumor cells. TNF-α induces membrane damage as assessed by the rapid release of dye encapsulated in the liposomes.[327] IFN-γ induces very slow leakage of dye from the liposomes, suggesting that it cause less membrane damage than TNF-α, but TNF-α and IFN-γ may display synergistic effects in the induction of this damage.

The nucleus may be a major target for the cytotoxic action of TNF-α. Treatment of sensitive cells with TNF-α at relatively high doses may result in degradation of their cellular DNA into fragments that are multiples of 200 bp.[328] DNA fragmentation occurring in tumor cells exposed to TNF-α is due to activation of endogenous endonucleases and may be responsible, at least in part, for the antitumor effects of TNF-α. The rate at which DNA fragmentation occurs correlates with the rate at which cells respond to the cytotoxic effect of the lymphokine. Studies with epipodophyllotoxins, which inhibit the rejoining activity of DNA topoisomerase II, suggest that this enzyme may also play a key role, in addition to endonucleases, in nuclear changes related to the cell death induced by both TNF-α and TNF-β.[329] However, the role of DNA fragmentation in the antitumor effects of TNFs is not clear. Differentiation of HL-60 human leukemia cells induced by TNF-α is accompanied by the release of DNA fragments.[330] The process of differentiation of HL-60 cells is blocked by inhibiting energy metabolism and is associated with only slight effects on proliferation and little or no cytotoxicity.

The antitumor effects of TNF-α are related, in part, to mechanisms other than direct cytotoxicity against the tumor cells, as indicated by the fact that no clear correlation exists between the TNF-α receptor number in the tumor and sensitivity to TNF-α.[331] Immune mechanisms may be important in the antitumor effects of TNF-α. TNF-α enhances the expression of genes associated with the expression of HLA antigens in human tumor cells.[332] Immunogenic MCA-induced sarcomas may undergo a complete regression in mice treated with human TNF-α, whereas nonimmunogenic tumors do not suffer complete regression, although both immunogenic and nonimmunogenic tumors undergo hemorrhagic necrosis after TNF-α administration.[333] TNF-α may act as an autocrine signal during the activation of tumoricidal macrophages.[334]

Natural cytotoxic cell activity, but not natural killer cell activity, is partially mediated in the mouse by TNF-α.[335] Anti-TNF-α antibody can block natural cytotoxic lysis of target cells and there is strong evidence that natural cytotoxic cells and TNF-α activate the same lytic mechanism within target cells and that TNF-α mediates the lytic activity of natural cytotoxic effector cells.[336] Tumor cells selected either *in vivo* or *in vitro* for natural cytotoxic resistance are also selected for TNF-α resistance. Thus, natural cytotoxic and TNF-α lysis of target cells may have similar, if not identical, lytic mechanisms.

TNF-α is a potent effector molecule for tumor cell killing mediated by activated macrophages.[337,338] Tumor cell variants with genetically acquired resistance to the destroying action of activated macrophages have a selective resistance to TNF-α produced by these cells. At least in certain systems, all of the classical tumorigenic effects of macrophages can be accounted for by the production and release of TNF-α. Acquisition of cytotoxicity against tumor cells such as the WEHI 164 murine fibrosarcoma cell line by circulating monocytes is associated with the production of TNF-α.[339] Monocytes present in human peripheral blood are not spontaneously cytotoxic for the tumor cells, but acquire cytotoxicity upon exposure to endotoxin or endotoxin-like agonists. Activation of macrophage tumoricidal properties by TNF-α requires the cooperation of other cytokines.[340] IFN-γ increases the cytotoxicity of monocytes against tumor cells by sensitizing the target cells to the lytic action of TNF-α.[337]

The streptococcal preparation, OK-432, has been used as an immunomodulating agent and may have antitumor activity in cancer patients. The mechanisms of OK-432-induced tumor regression are not understood, but it has been shown that OK-432 induces a cytostatic activity in the sera of some cancer patients and that this activity is partially represented by TNF-α.[341]

3. Sensitivity of Tumor Cells to TNF-α

Tumor cells are highly variable in their sensitivity to TNF-α. Whereas cell lines established from solid tumors of either human or murine origin are frequently sensitive to TNF-α, many different human and murine leukemia and lymphoma cell lines are resistant to TNF-α as defined by cell viability, cell proliferation, or uptake of thymidine and uridine.[342] In general, human leukemia cell lines exhibit great heterogeneity in their response to TNFs, and their sensitivity to TNFs may not be correlated to variation in TNF binding or morphological characteristics.[21] The resistance of human epithelial tumor cell lines to TNF-α may be associated with a constitutive production of TNF-α mRNA and protein by these cells.[343] There is evidence that constitutive production of small amounts of TNF-α by neoplastic cell lines may correlate with reduced tumorigeneticity and reduced invasiveness *in vivo*.[344]

The sensitivity of different types of transformed cells to the cytostatic and cytolytic effects of TNF-α shows great variation. For example, clone A from established AS-653 spindle-cell sarcoma sublines derived from MCA-induced rat fibrosarcoma exhibits high metastatic potential to lymph nodes and its growth is completely inhibited by continuous exposure to low concentrations of TNF-α, whereas clone G from the same cells exhibits low metastatic potential and its growth is not inhibited by high concentrations of TNF-α.[345] The cytotoxicity of TNF-α on clone A of AS-653 cells is time- and concentration-dependent, but the mechanism of antitumor effect of TNF-α on these cells is not due to inhibition of DNA and RNA synthesis. Different types of mechanisms may be responsible for the resistance of tumor cells to TNF-α. Using selection procedures, two distinct types of TNF-α-resistant variants were derived from the TNF-α-sensitive murine fibrosarcoma cell line L929s.[346] Whereas a first type of cells constitutively produced TNF-α and lacked TNF-α receptors, a second type of cell did not produce detectable amounts of TNF-α and did not exhibit consistent differences in the number or binding activity of surface TNF-α receptors. The second type of cells became sensitive to TNF-α-mediated cell lysis in the presence of actinomycin D, cycloheximide, or IFN-γ, suggesting that some protein synthesis-dependent protection mechanism was active in these cells. However, the nature of this salvage pathway could not be elucidated.

4. Undesirable and Dangerous Effects of TNF-α

The clinical use of TNF-α is limited by the occurrence of various undesirable side effects produced by the physiological activity of TNF-α.[347] Not only tumor cells, but also normal cells may be damaged by the cytotoxic effects of TNF-α.[348] Tumor-cell populations may develop resistance to TNF-α. Even clonal tumor-cell populations, i.e., tumor cells derived from a single cell, for example, from a single human renal cell carcinoma, exhibit a heterogeneous response to the cytotoxic effects of human TNF-α.[349]

TNF-α may not inhibit, but may have stimulating effects on the growth of certain neoplastic cells. TNF-α can induce proliferation of tumor cells such as neoplastic B cells from human CLL.[350] It also stimulates, through an autocrine mechanism, the proliferation of several human neuroblastoma cell lines.[351] In murine systems, a brief exposure to human TNF-α can increase the replication of leukemogenic retroviruses.[352] Thus, TNF-α is potentially dangerous and great caution should be exerted with the clinical use of TNF-α for therapeutic purposes.

5. Combination of TNF-α with Other Agents

The biological parameters responsible for sensitivity or resistance to TNF-α in defined systems *in vitro* or in intact animals are poorly understood. Combination of TNF-α with other cytokines may result in a synergistic enhancement of the antitumor effects. Small concentrations of murine TNF-α and IFN-γ can act synergistically, but not separately, to induce antitumor cytotoxic activation of peritoneal macrophages against the TNF-α-insensitive tumor cell line L5178Y.[353] A combination of small concentrations of IFN-γ and IL-1 is ineffective in this system. The mechanisms by which different cytokines, acting in particular combinations at small concentrations but that are by themselves ineffective, are able to activate the antitumor effects of macrophages are not known, but these findings may have clinical and therapeutic implications.

Certain human tumor cell lines that are not sensitive or are slightly sensitive to TNF-α alone may become sensitive when IFN-γ is present as well.[277] A combination of TNF-α/IFN-γ treatment has a synergistic cytotoxic effect on some human colon carcinoma cell lines.[354] IFN-γ may enhance the effectiveness of TNF-α in some of these cell lines, but not conversely. In contrast, nontransformed human cell lines may be insensitive to TNF-α even in the presence of IFN-γ. Human TNF-α may have additive therapeutic activity for metastatic tumors *in vivo* when administered in conjunction with suboptimal doses of IFN-γ.[355] The combined treatment of murine tumors with TNF-α and IL-2 may give better results than the treatment with either cytokine alone.[356] The mechanisms of the synergistic effects between TNF-α and IFN-γ or IL-2 may involve some immunomodulatory changes.

Combined treatment with TNF-α and IFN-γ may be effective for antitumor therapy *in vivo*. Established B16BL6 mouse melanoma tumors *in vivo* can be induced to necrotize and regress by a combined systemic treatment with human TNF-α and murine IFN-γ.[357] A similar combined treatment could be useful in AIDS patients or in individuals infected with the HIV virus. Infection of lymphoid cells by HIV may result in the deficient production of cytokines that would otherwise eliminate the virus. Treatment of cells with a combination of TNF-α and IFN-γ reduces their susceptibility to infection with HIV, and suppresses the production of HIV mRNA and core protein p24 as well as the production of infectious HIV.[358]

Chemotherapeutic agents could be combined with TNF-α for the treatment of neoplastic diseases. In the intradermally transplanted Meth A sarcoma system in mice, adriamycin, cyclophosphamide, and 5-fluorouracil enhance the number of complete tumor regressions when combined with low doses of TNF-α.[359] A potentiation of the TNF-α-induced tumor necrosis by the chemotherapeutic agents, especially by cyclophosphamide, was revealed by histological analyses. Human TNF-α may enhance the cytotoxicity against cultured malignant cells (the murine fibrosarcoma cell line L929) of DNA topoisomerase II-target drugs such as actinomycin D, adriamycin, teniposide, and etoposide.[360] These results suggest that TNF-α may be a useful adjuvant to this class of drugs, which are known to possess antitumor activity.

An important problem with the use of either TNF-α or TNF-α inducers for cancer treatment is the occurrence of side effects. This could be circumvented in some cases by the simultaneous administration of certain drugs. Nonsteroidal antiinflammatory drugs (acetylsalicylate, indomethacin, and phenylbutazone) can protect mice injected with viable *Listeria monocytogenes* or powdered *Corynebacterium parvum* and challenged with LPS against the lethal effect of endotoxin without affecting the animals to produce TNF-α.[361]

6. Tumor-Promoting Effects of TNF-α

TNF-α may have a biphasic effect on the growth of certain tumor cells and under certain conditions, partially depending on the dose, it may enhance tumor-cell growth.[362] In BALB/3T3 fibroblasts, TNF-α acts as a tumor promoter.[363] TNF-α may promote the survival and proliferation of tumor cells in two types of human B-cell malignancy: hairy-cell leukemia and B-cell chronic lymphocytic leukemia.[364] Coexpression of TNF-α and its receptor is observed frequently in human ovarian cancer, suggesting that TNF-α may promote the growth in these tumors by an autocrine or paracrine mechanism.[365] Thus, TNF-α may act in certain cases as a tumor growth factor and great caution must be observed in clinical trials involving the therapeutic application of TNF-α.

7. Differentiation-Inducing Effects of TNFs on Tumor Cells

TNF-α and TNF-β can induce the differentiation of certain types of transformed cells. TNF-α is identical with a differentiation-inducing factor that was identified as a lymphokine produced by mitogen-stimulated T cells and that induces differentiation of human myeloid leukemia cells into the monocyte/macrophage pathway.[366] The capability of TNF-α to induce tumor-cell differentiation may depend on its concentration. High-affinity binding concentrations of TNF-α induce the differentiation of M1 human myeloblastic leukemia and HL-60 human promyelocytic leukemia cells, whereas low-affinity binding concentrations abolish this effect in a concentration-dependent manner.[367] In certain types of cells, TNF-α acts not as an inducer but as an inhibitor of differentiation. It strongly inhibits the differentiation of mouse 3T3-L1 preadipocytes into mature adipocytes.[368] TNF-β induces the terminal differentiation of the human leukemia cell lines HL-60 and THP-1.[369]

The differentiation-inducing effects of TNF-α on tumor cells may be associated with altered proto-oncogene expression, but the biological significance of these changes is unknown. Induction of HL-60 cell monocytic differentiation by TNF-α is associated with increased expression of c-*fos* mRNA and protein product.[370]

However, other studies suggested that c-*fos* gene expression may not be functionally linked to HL-60 cell differentiation. Phorbol ester-resistant KG-1a cells can be induced to monocytic differentiation by TNF-α.[371] Simultaneous treatment with TNF-α and calcitriol results in synergistic effects on the induction of HL-60 cell differentiation and the reduction of c-*myc* mRNA levels.[372] TNF-α and retinoic acid may have synergistic effects in the induction of HL-60 cell differentiation.[373] Low concentrations of TNF-α and retinoic acid, inactive in inducing differentiation when used separately, are able to induce complete differentiation of HL-60 cells into both the monocyte-macrophage or the granulocyte phenotype. IFN-γ may also contribute to this induction, but it acts through a mechanism different from that of TNF-α. While the differentiation of HL-60 cells induced by TNF-α is associated with decreased expression of the c-*myc* gene, the differentiation induced by IFN-γ is independent of c-*myc* expression.[374] The decreased expression of c-*myc* induced by TNF-α in HL-60 cells is associated with interruption of the c-*myc* gene transcription. IFN-γ and TNF-α potentiate, in a synergistic manner, the differentiation-inducing effects of calcitriol on the myeloid leukemia-derived human cells lines HL-60, ML3, and U-937.[373] The differentiation-inducing effect of TNF-α on murine myeloid leukemia M1 cells may be mediated by an increased expression of IFN-$β_1$.[375]

IV. TUMOR MIGRATION INHIBITING FACTOR

A lymphokine with inhibitory effects on tumor cells has been named tumor migration inhibiting factor (TMIF).[376] This inhibitory lymphokine is distinct from another migration inhibition factor which acts on nonneoplastic cells, mainly on macrophages. TMIF can reversibly inhibit the migration of tumor cells both *in vivo* and *in vitro*. In addition, TMIF is capable of inhibiting the binding of tumor cells to endothelial monolayers. TMIF is apparently a low molecular weight protein and has been detected in the serum and urine from some patients with multiple myeloma, but not in patients with adenocarcinoma of the breast. It was suggested that TMIF is a member of a novel class of lymphokine mediators, termed neomodulins, which have the common task of influencing functional properties of tumor cells.

V. TUMOR-KILLING FACTOR

The tumor-killing factor (TKF) is a tumor-specific cytotoxic protein that was purified to homogeneity from the culture medium of the J774.1 murine macrophage-like cell line.[377] This cell line does not produce TKF under the usual culture conditions, but starts to produce it when a lectin purified from the hemolymph of *Sarcophaga peregrina* (flesh fly) larvae is added to the medium. *Sarcophaga* lectin itself has an antitumor effect on transplanted syngeneic and allogeneic murine tumors.[378] However, the antitumor effect of this lectin is mediated mainly by the induction of TKF secretion by specific cells. *Sarcophaga* lectin-binding proteins of 170 and 110 kDa are present on the surface of mouse macrophages.[379] Antibody against TKF inhibits the cytotoxic activities produced *in vitro* by mouse peritoneal macrophages and *in vivo* in the serum of tumor-bearing mice in response to *Sarcophaga* lectin.[380]

The TKF is a protein of 45-kDa, similar to TNF-α.[377] TKF has a trimeric structure. Dissociation of this structure into 15-kDa monomeric units, produced either spontaneously or by the action of macrophages, results in inactivation of the biological effects of the protein.[381] There are specific receptors for TKF on the surface of various types of cells, but not all cells possessing TKF receptors are sensitive to TKF.[382] After binding, TKF-receptor complexes are internalized and fusion of the resulting endosomes with lysosomes are required for the expression of the cytotoxic activity of TKF. The normal function of TKF is unknown.

REFERENCES

1. **Billingham, M.E.J.,** Cytokines as inflammatory mediators, *Br. Med. Bull.,* 43, 350, 1987.
2. **Watanabe, N., Niitsu, Y., Sone, H., Neda, H., Yamaguchi, N., and Urushikazi, I.,** Inhibitory effect of tumor necrosis serum on the metastasis of B-16 mouse melanoma, *Jpn. J. Cancer Res.,* 76, 989, 1985.
3. **Fair, D.S., Jeffes, E.W.B., III, and Granger, G.A.,** Release of LT molecules with restricted physical heterogeneity by a continuous human lymphoid cell line in vitro, *Cell. Immunol.,* 16, 185, 1979.
4. **Wright, S.C. and Bonavida, B.,** Studies on the mechanism of natural killer (NK) cell-mediated cytotoxicity. I. Release of cytotoxic factors specific for NK-sensitive target cells (NKCF) during co-culture of NK effector cells with NK target cells, *J. Immunol.,* 129, 433, 1982.
5. **Symington, F.W.,** Lymphotoxin, tumor necrosis factor, and γ interferon are cytostatic for normal human keratinocytes, *J. Invest. Dermatol.,* 92, 798, 1989.
6. **Herberman, R.B., Reynolds, C.W., and Ortaldo, J.R.,** Mechanism of cytotoxicity by natural killer (NK) cells, *Annu. Rev. Immunol.,* 4, 651, 1986.
7. **Grossman, Z. and Herberman, R.B.,** Natural killer cells and their relationship to T cells: hypothesis on the role of T-cell receptor gene rearrangement on the course of adaptive differentiation, *Cancer Res.,* 46, 2651, 1986.
8. **Bialas, T., Kolitz, J., Levi, E., Polivka, A., Oez, S., Miller, G., and Welte, K.,** Distinction of partially purified human natural killer cytotoxic factor from recombinant human tumor necrosis factor and recombinant human lymphotoxin, *Cancer Res.,* 48, 891, 1988.
9. **Green, L.M., Reade, J.L., Ware, C.F., Devlin, P.E., Liang, C.-M., and Devlin, J.J.,** Cytotoxic lymphokines produced by cloned human cytotoxic T lymphocytes. II. A novel CTL-produced cytotoxin that is antigenically distinct from tumor necrosis factor and α-lymphotoxin, *J. Immunol.,* 137, 3488, 1986.
10. **Cohen, M.C. and Cohen, S.,** The role of lymphokines in neoplastic disease, *Hum. Pathol.,* 17, 264, 1986.
11. **Browning, J.L., Ngam-ek, A., Lawton, P., DeMarinis, J., Tizard, R., Chow, E.P., Hession, C., O'Brine-Greco, B., Foley, S.F., and Ware, C.F.,** Lymphotoxin β, a novel member of the TNF family that forms a heteromeric complex with lymphotoxin on the cell surface, *Cell,* 72, 847, 1993.
12. **Ting, C.-C., Yang, S.S., and Hargrove, M.E.,** Lymphokine-induced cytotoxicity: characterization of effectors, precursors, and regulatory ancillary cells, *Cancer Res.,* 46, 513, 1986.
13. **Evans, C.H.,** Lymphotoxin — an immunologic hormone with anticarcinogenic and antitumor activity, *Cancer Immunol. Immunother.,* 12, 181, 1982.
14. **Paul, N.L. and Ruddle, N.H.,** Lymphotoxin, *Annu. Rev. Immunol.,* 6, 407, 1988.
15. **Yamanaka, H.I. and Karpas, A.,** Identity of human B-cell line cytotoxic lymphokine with tumor necrosis factor type β, *Proc. Natl. Acad. Sci. U.S.A.,* 86, 1343, 1989.
16. **Figari, I.S., Mori, N.A., and Palladino, M.A., Jr.,** Regulation of neutrophil migration and superoxide production by recombinant tumor necrosis factors α and β: comparison to recombinant interferon-γ and interleukin-1α, *Blood,* 70, 979, 1987.
17. **Miyake, M., Fuchimoto, S., and Orita, K.,** Synergistic effect of natural human tumor necrosis factors α and β in the clonogenic assay, *Exp. Cell Biol.,* 56, 297, 1988.
18. **Schmid, D.S., Hornung, R., McGrath, K.M., Paul, N., and Ruddle, N.H.,** Target cell DNA fragmentation is mediated by lymphotoxin and tumor necrosis factor, *Lymphokine Res.,* 6, 195, 1987.
19. **Lazemby, A.W., Roth, J.A., Owen-Schaub, L.G., and Grimm, E.A.,** IL-1 synergy with IL-2 in the generation of lymphokine activated killer cells is mediated by TNF-α and TNF-β (lymphotoxin), *Cytokine,* 4, 479, 1992.
20. **Wong, G.H.W. and Goeddel, D.V.,** Tumour necrosis factors α and β inhibit virus replication and synergize with interferons, *Nature,* 323, 819, 1986.
21. **Beran, M., Andersson, B.S., Kelleher, P., Whalen, K., McCredie, K., and Gutterman, J.,** Diversity of the effect of recombinant tumor necrosis factors α and β on human myelogenous leukemia cell lines, *Blood,* 69, 721, 1987.

22. **Aggarwal, B.B.,** Human lymphotoxin, *Methods Enzymol.,* 116, 441, 1985.
23. **Estrov, Z., Kurzrock, R., Pocsik, E., Pathak, S., Kantarjian, H.M., Zipf, T.F., Harris, D., Talpaz, M., and Aggarwal, B.B.,** Lymphotoxin is an autocrine growth factor for Epstein-Barr virus-infected B cell lines, *J. Exp. Med.,* 177, 763, 1993.
24. **Nakajima, T., Kitamura, K., Yamashita, N., Mizushima, Y., Delespesse, G., and Lai, R.B.,** Constitutive expression and production of tumor necrosis factor-β in T-cell lines infected with HTLV-I and HTLV-II, *Biochem. Biophys. Res. Commun.,* 191, 371, 1993.
25. **Sastry, K.J., Reddy, R.H.R., Pandita, R., Totpal, K., and Aggarwal, B.B.,** HIV-1 TAT gene induces tumor necrosis factor-β (lymphotoxin) in a human B-lymphoblastoid cell line, *J. Biol. Chem.,* 265, 20091, 1990.
26. **Gray, P.W., Aggarwal, B.B., Benton, C.V., Bringman, T.S., Henzel, W.J., Jarrett, J.A., Leung, D.W., Moffat, B., Ng, P., Svedersky, L.P., Palladino, M.A., and Nedwin, G.E.,** Cloning and expression of cDNA for human lymphotoxin, a lymphokine with tumour necrosis activity, *Nature,* 312, 721, 1984.
27. **Eck, M.J., Ultsch, M., Rinderknecht, E., Devos, A.M., and Sprang, S.R.,** The structure of human lymphotoxin (tumor necrosis factor-β) at 1.9 Å resolution, *J. Biol. Chem.,* 267, 2119, 1992.
28. **Evans, A.M., Petersen, J.W., Sekhon, G.S., and DeMars, R.,** Mapping of prolactin and tumor necrosis factor-β genes on human chromosome 6p using lymphoblastoid cell deletion mutants, *Somat. Cell Mol. Genet.,* 15, 203, 1989.
29. **Nedwin, G.E., Naylor, S.L., Sakaguchi, A.Y., Smith, D., Jarrett-Nedwin, J., Pennica, D., Goeddel, D.V., and Gray, P.W.,** Human lymphotoxin and tumour necrosis factor genes: structure, homology and chromosomal localization, *Nucleic Acids Res.,* 13, 6361, 1985.
30. **Nedwin, G.E., Jarrett-Nedwin, J., Smith, D.H., Naylor, S.L., Sakaguchi, A.Y., Goeddel, D.V., and Gray, P.W.,** Structure and chromosomal localization of the human lymphotoxin gene, *J. Cell. Biochem.,* 29, 171, 1985.
31. **Gardner, S.M., Mock, B.A., Hilgers, J., Huppi, K.E., and Roeder, W.D.,** Mouse lymphotoxin and tumor necrosis factor: structural analysis of the cloned genes, physical linkage, and chromosomal position, *J. Immunol.,* 139, 476, 1987.
32. **Weil, D., Brosset, S., and Dautry, F.,** RNA processing is a limiting step for murine tumor necrosis factor β expression in response to interleukin-2, *Mol. Cell. Biol.,* 10, 5865, 1990.
33. **Ferrante, A., Nandoskar, M., Bates, E.J., Goh, D.H.B., and Beard, L.J.,** Tumour necrosis factor β (lymphotoxin) inhibits locomotion and stimulates the respiratory burst and degranulation of neutrophils, *Immunology,* 63, 507, 1988.
34. **Zucali, J.R., Broxmeyer, H.E., Gross, M.A., and Dinarello, C.A.,** Recombinant human tumor necrosis factors α and β stimulate fibroblasts to produce hemopoietic growth factors in vitro, *J. Immunol.,* 140, 840, 1988.
35. **Pober, J.S., Lapierre, L.A., Stolpen, A.H., Brock, T.A., Springer, T.A., Fiers, W., Bevilacqua, M.P., Mendrick, D.L., and Gimbrone, M.A., Jr.,** Activation of cultured human endothelial cells by recombinant lymphotoxin: comparison with tumor necrosis factor and interleukin 1 species, *J. Immunol.,* 138, 3319, 1987.
36. **English, B.K., Weaver, W.M., and Wilson, C.B.,** Different regulation of lymphotoxin and tumor necrosis factor genes in human lymphocytes-T, *J. Biol. Chem.,* 266, 7108, 1991.
37. **Browning, J. and Ribolini, A.,** Studies on the differing effects of tumor necrosis factor and lymphotoxin on the growth of several tumor lines, *J. Immunol.,* 143, 1859, 1989.
38. **Old, L.J.,** Tumor necrosis factor, *Science,* 230, 630, 1985.
39. **Beutler, B. and Cerami, A.,** Cachectin (tumor necrosis factor): a macrophage hormone governing cellular metabolism and inflammatory response, *Endocr. Rev.,* 9, 57, 1988.
40. **Kunkel, S.L., Remick, D.G., Strieter, R.M., and Larrick, J.W.,** Mechanisms that regulate the production and effects of tumor necrosis factor-α, *Crit. Rev. Immunol.,* 9, 93, 1989.
41. **Beutler, B.,** The complex regulation and biology of TNF (cachectin), *Crit. Rev. Oncogenesis,* 2, 9, 1990.
42. **Vilcek, J. and Lee, T.H.,** Tumor necrosis factor — new insights into the molecular mechanisms of its multiple actions, *J. Biol. Chem.,* 266, 7313, 1991.
43. **Fiers, W.,** Tumor necrosis factor — characterization at the molecular, cellular and in vivo level, *FEBS Lett.,* 285, 199, 1991.
44. **Camussi, G., Albano, E., Tetta, C., and Bussolino, F.,** The molecular action of tumor necrosis factor-α, *Eur. J. Biochem.,* 202, 3, 1991.

45. **Van der Poll, T. and Sauerwein, H.P.,** Tumor necrosis factor: its role in the metabolic response to sepsis, *Clin. Sci.,* 84, 247, 1993.
46. **Nauts, H.C., Fowler, G.A.A., and Bogatko, F.H.,** A review of the influence of bacterial infection and of bacterial products (Coley's toxins) on malignant tumors in man, *Acta Med. Scand.,* Suppl. 276, 5, 1953.
47. **O'Malley, W.E., Achinstein, B., and Shear, M.J.,** Action of bacterial polysaccharide on tumors. II. Damage of sarcoma 37 by serum of mice treated with *Serratia marcescens* polysaccharide, and induced tolerance, *J. Natl. Cancer Inst.,* 29, 1169, 1962.
48. **Carswell, E.A., Old, L.J., Kassel, R.L., Green, S., Fiore, N., and Williamson, B.,** An endotoxin-induced serum factor that causes necrosis of tumors, *Proc. Natl. Acad. Sci. U.S.A.,* 72, 3666, 1975.
49. **Kawakami, M., Murase, T., Itakura, H., Yamada, N., Ohsawa, N., and Takaku, F.,** Lipid metabolism in endotoxic rats: decrease in hepatic triglyceride lipase activity, *Microbiol. Immunol.,* 30, 849, 1986.
50. **Beutler, B., Greenwald, D., Hulmes, J.D., Chang, M., Pan, Y.-C.E., Mathison, J., Ulevitch, R., and Cerami, A.,** Identity of tumour necrosis factor and the macrophage-secreted factor cachectin, *Nature,* 316, 552, 1985.
51. **Beutler, B., Krochin, N., Milsark, I.W., Leudke, C., and Cerami, A.,** Control of cachectin (tumor necrosis factor) synthesis: mechanisms of endotoxin resistance, *Science,* 232, 977, 1986.
52. **Yamasu, K., Onoe, H., Soma, G.-I., Oshima, H., and Mizuno, D.-I.,** Secretion of tumor necrosis factor during fetal and neonatal development of the mouse: ontogenic inflammation, *J. Biol. Response Modif.,* 8, 644, 1989.
53. **Jäättelä, M., Kuusela, P., and Saksela, E.,** Demonstration of tumor necrosis factor in human amniotic fluids and supernatants of placental and decidual tissues, *Lab. Invest.,* 58, 48, 1988.
54. **Michie, H.R., Monogue, K.R., Spriggs, D.R., Revhaug, A., O'Dwyer, S., Dinarello, C.A., Cerami, A., Wolff, S.M., and Wilmore, D.W.,** Detection of circulating tumor necrosis factor after endotoxin administration, *N. Engl. J. Med.,* 318, 1481, 1988.
55. **Hofsli, E., Lamvik, J., and Nissen-Meyer, J.,** Evidence that tumor necrosis factor (TNF) is not constitutively present in vivo. The association of TNF with freshly isolated monocytes reflects a rapid in vitro production, *Scand. J. Immunol.,* 28, 435, 1988.
56. **Strieter, R.M., Remick, D.G., Ham, J.M., Colletti, L.M., Lynch, J.P. III, and Kunkel, S.L.,** Tumor necrosis factor-α gene expression in human whole blood, *J. Leukocyte Biol.,* 47, 366, 1990.
57. **Dubravec, D.B., Spriggs, D.R., Mannick, J.A., and Rodirck, M.L.,** Circulating human peripheral blood granulocytes synthesize and secrete tumor necrosis factor α, *Proc. Natl. Acad. Sci. U.S.A.,* 87, 6758, 1990.
58. **Bachwich, P.R., Lynch, J.P., III, Larrick, J., Spengler, M., and Kunkel, S.L.,** Tumor necrosis factor production by human sarcoid alveolar macrophages, *Am. J. Pathol.,* 125, 421, 1986.
59. **Gilford, G.E. and Lohmann-Matthes, M.-L.,** Gamma interferon priming of mouse and human macrophages for induction of tumor necrosis factor production by bacterial lipopolysaccharide, *J. Natl. Cancer Inst.,* 78, 121, 1987.
60. **Scuderi, P., Sterling, K.E., Raitano, A.B., Grogan, T.M., and Rippe, R.A.,** Recombinant interferon-γ stimulates the production of human tumor necrosis factor *in vitro, J. Interferon Res.,* 7, 155, 1987.
61. **Collart, M.A., Belin, D., Vassalli, J.-D., de Kossodo, S., and Vasalli, P.,** γ Interferon enhances macrophage transcription of the tumor necrosis factor/cachectin, interleukin 1, and urokinase genes, which are controlled by short-lived repressors, *J. Exp. Med.,* 164, 2113, 1986.
62. **Izumi, S., Hirai, O., Hayashi, K., Konishi, Y., Okuhara, M., Kohsaka, M., Aoki, H., and Yamamura, Y.,** Induction of a tumor necrosis factor-like activity by *Nocardia rubra* cell wall skeleton, *Cancer Res.,* 47, 1785, 1987.
63. **Smith, D.M., Lackides, G.A., and Epstein, L.B.,** Coordinated induction of autocrine tumor necrosis factor and interleukin 1 in normal human monocytes and the implications for monocyte-mediated cytotoxicity, *Cancer Res.,* 50, 3146, 1990.
64. **Laskov, R., Lancz, G., Ruddle, N.H., McGrath, K.M., Specter, S., Klein, T., Djeu, J.Y., and Friedman, H.,** Production of tumor necrosis factor (TNF-α) and lymphotoxin (TNF-β) by murine pre-B and B cell lymphomas, *J. Immunol.,* 144, 3424, 1990.
65. **Peters, P.M., Ortaldo, J.R., Shalaby, M.R., Svedersky, L.P., Nedwin, G.E., Bringman, T.S., Hass, P.E., Aggarwal, B.B., Herberman, R.B., Goeddel, D.V., and Palladino, M.A.,** Natural killer-sensitive targets stimulate production of TNF-α but not TNF-β (lymphotoxin) by highly purified human peripheral blood large granular lymphocytes, *J. Immunol.,* 137, 1592, 1986.

66. **Rubin, B.Y., Anderson, S.L., Sullivan, S.A., Williamson, B.D., Carswell, E.A., and Old, L.J.,** Nonhematopoietic cells selected for resistance to tumor necrosis factor produce tumor necrosis factor, *J. Exp. Med.,* 164, 1350, 1986.
67. **Hallahan, D.E., Spriggs, D.R., Beckett, M.A., Kufe, D.W., and Weichselbaum, R.R.,** Increased tumor necrosis factor α mRNA after cellular exposure to ionizing radiation, *Proc. Natl. Acad. Sci. U.S.A.,* 86, 10104, 1989.
68. **Berent, S.L., Torczynski, R.M., and Bollon, A.P.,** Sendai virus induces high levels of tumor necrosis factor mRNA in human peripheral leukocytes, *Nucleic Acids Res.,* 14, 8997, 1986.
69. **Cannistra, S.A., Vellenga, E., Groshek, P., Rambaldi, A., and Griffin, J.D.,** Human granulocyte-monocyte colony-stimulating factor and interleukin 3 stimulate monocyte cytotoxicity through a tumor necrosis factor-dependent mechanism, *Blood,* 71, 672, 1988.
70. **Nedwin, G.E., Svedersy, L.P., Bringman, T.S., Palladino, M.A., Jr., and Goeddel, D.V.,** Effect of interleukin 2, interferon-γ, and mitogens on the production of tumor necrosis factors α and β, *J. Immunol.,* 135, 2492, 1985.
71. **Satoh, M., Shimada, Y., Inagawa, H., Minagawa, H., Kajigawa, T., Oshima, H., Abe, S., Yamazaki, M., and Mizuno, D.,** Priming effect of interferons and interleukin 2 on endogenous production of tumor necrosis factor in mice, *Jpn. J. Cancer Res.,* 77, 342, 1986.
72. **Kunkel, S.L., Wiggins, R.C., Chensue, S.W., and Larrick, J.,** Regulation of macrophage tumor necrosis factor production by prostaglandin E_2, *Biochem. Biophys. Res. Commun.,* 137, 404, 1986.
73. **Krönke, M., Hensel, G., Schlüter, C., Scheurich, P., Schütze, S., and Pfizenmaier, K.,** Tumor necrosis factor and lymphotoxin gene expression in human tumor cell lines, *Cancer Res.,* 48, 5417, 1988.
74. **Horiguchi, J., Spriggs, D., Imamaura, K., Stone, R., Luebbers, R., and Kufe, D.,** Role of arachidonic acid metabolism in transcriptional induction of tumor necrosis factor gene expression by phorbol ester, *Mol. Cell. Biol.,* 9, 252, 1989.
75. **Hensel, G., Männel, D.N., Pfizenmaier, K., and Krönke, M.,** Autocrine stimulation of TNF-α mRNA expression in HL-60 cells, *Lymphokine Res.,* 6, 119, 1987.
76. **Darzynkiewicz, Z., Carter, S.P., and Old, L.J.,** Effect of recombinant tumor necrosis factor on HL-60 cells: cell-cycle specificity and synergism with actinomycin D, *J. Cell. Physiol.,* 130, 328, 1987.
77. **Spriggs, D., Ikamura, K., Rodriguez, C., Horiguchi, J., and Kufe, D.W.,** Induction of tumor necrosis factor expression and resistance in a human breast tumor cell line, *Proc. Natl. Acad. Sci. U.S.A.,* 84, 6563, 1987.
78. **Spies, T., Morton, C.C., Nedospasov, S.A., Fiers, W., Pious, D., and Strominger, J.L.,** Genes for the tumor necrosis factors α and β are linked to the human major histocompatibility complex, *Proc. Natl. Acad. Sci. U.S.A.,* 83, 8699, 1986.
79. **Müller, U., Jongeneel, C.V., Nedospasov, S.A., Lindahl, K.F., and Steinmetz, M.,** Tumour necrosis factor and lymphotoxin genes close to *H-2D* in the mouse major histocompatibility complex, *Nature,* 325, 265, 1987.
80. **Stone-Wolff, D.S., Yip, Y.K., Chroboczek Kelker, H., Le, J., Henriksen-DeStefano, D., Rubin, B.Y., Rinderknecht, E., Aggarwal, B.B., and Vilcek, J.,** Interrelationships of human interferon-γ with lymphotoxin and monocyte cytotoxin, *J. Exp. Med.,* 159, 828, 1984.
81. **Chroboczek Kelker, H., Oppenheim, J.D., Stone-Wolff, D., Henriksen-deStefano, D., Aggarwal, B.B., Stevenson, H.C., and Vilcek, J.,** Characterization of human tumor necrosis factor produced by peripheral blood monocytes and its separation from lymphotoxin, *Int. J. Cancer,* 36, 69, 1985.
82. **Pennica, D., Nedwin, G.E., Hayflick, J.S., Seeburg, P.H., Derynck, R., Palladino, M.A., Kohr, W.J., Aggarwal, B.B., and Goeddel, D.V.,** Human tumour necrosis factor: precursor structure, expression and homology to lymphotoxin, *Nature,* 312, 724, 1984.
83. **Aggarwal, B.B., Kohr, W.J., Hass, P.E., Moffat, B., Spencer, S.A., Henzel, W.J., Bringman, T.S., Nedwin, G.E., Goeddel, D.V., and Harkins, R.N.,** Human tumor necrosis factor: production, purification, and characterization, *J. Biol. Chem.,* 260, 2345, 1985.
84. **Aggarwal, B.B. and Kohr, W.J.,** Human tumor necrosis factor, *Methods Enzymol.,* 116, 448, 1985.
85. **Jones, E.Y., Stuart, D.I., and Walker, N.P.C.,** Structure of tumour necrosis factor, *Nature,* 338, 225, 1989.
86. **Eck, M.J. and Sprang, S.R.,** The structure of tumor necrosis factor-α at 2.6 Å resolution. Implications for receptor binding, *J. Biol. Chem.,* 264, 17595, 1989.
87. **Kagan, B.L., Baldwin, R.L., Munoz, D., and Wisnieski, B.J.,** Formation of ion-permeable channels by tumor necrosis factor-α, *Science,* 255, 1427, 1992.

88. Zhang, X.-M., Weber, I., and Chen, M.-J., Site-directed mutational analysis of human tumor necrosis factor-α receptor binding site and structure-functional relationship, *J. Biol. Chem.*, 267, 24069, 1992.
89. Kriegler, M., Perez, C., DeFay, K., Albert, I., and Lu, S.D., A novel form of TNF/cachectin is a cell surface cytotoxic transmembrane protein: ramifications for the complex physiology of TNF, *Cell*, 53, 45, 1988.
90. Shirai, T., Yamaguchi, H., Ito, H., Todd, C.W., and Wallace, R.B., Cloning and expression in *Escherichia coli* of the gene for human tumour necrosis factor, *Nature*, 313, 803, 1985.
91. Wang, A.M., Creasey, A.A., Ladner, M.B., Lin, L.S., Strickler, J., Van Arsdell, J.N., Yamamoto, R., and Mark, D.F., Molecular cloning of the complementary DNA for human tumor necrosis factor, *Science*, 228, 149, 1985.
92. Marmenout, A., Fransen, L., Tavernier, J., Van der Heyden, J., Tizard, R., Kawashima, E., Shaw, A., Johnson, M.-J., Semon, D., Müller, R., Ruysschaert, M.-R., Van Vliet, A., and Fiers, W., Molecular cloning and expression of human tumor necrosis factor and comparison with mouse tumor necrosis factor, *Eur. J. Biochem.*, 152, 515, 1985.
93. Sugarman, B.J., Aggarwal, B.B., Hass, P.E., Figari, I.S., Palladino, M.A., Jr., and Shepard, H.M., Recombinant human tumor necrosis factor-α: effects on proliferation of normal and transformed cells in vitro, *Science*, 230, 943, 1985.
94. Davis, J.M., Narachi, M.A., Alton, N.K., and Arakawa, T., Structure of human tumor necrosis factor α derived from recombinant DNA, *Biochemistry*, 26, 1322, 1987.
95. Korn, J.H., Mory, Y., Ziberstein, A., Holtmann, H., Revel, M., and Wallach, D., Cloning of genomic DNA for tumor necrosis factor and efficient expression in CHO cells, *Lymphokine Res.*, 7, 349, 1988.
96. Smith, R.A. and Baglioni, C., The active form of tumor necrosis factor is a trimer, *J. Biol. Chem.*, 262, 6951, 1987.
97. Soma, G.-I., Kitahara, N., Tsuji, Y., Kato, M., Oshima, H., Gatanaga, T., Inagawa, H., Noguchi, K., Tanabe, Y., and Mizuno, D., Improvement of cytotoxicity of tumor necrosis factor (TNF) by increase in basicity of its N-terminal region, *Biochem. Biophys. Res. Commun.*, 148, 629, 1987.
98. Fransen, L., Müller, R., Marmenout, A., Tavernier, J., Van der Heyden, J., Kawashima, E., Chollet, A., Tizard, R., Van Heuverswyn, H., Van Vliet, A., Ruysschaert, M.-R., and Fiers, W., Molecular cloning of mouse tumour necrosis factor cDNA and its eukaryotic expression, *Nucleic Acids Res.*, 13, 4417, 1985.
99. Pennica, D., Hayflick, J.S., Bringman, T.S., Palladino, M.A., and Goeddel, D.V., Cloning and expression in *Escherichia coli* of the cDNA for murine tumor necrosis factor, *Proc. Natl. Acad. Sci. U.S.A.*, 82, 6060, 1985.
100. Haranaka, K., Carswell, E.A., Williamson, B.D., Prendergast, J.S., Satomi, N., and Old, L.J., Purification, characterization, and antitumor activity of nonrecombinant mouse tumor necrosis factor, *Proc. Natl. Acad. Sci. U.S.A.*, 83, 3949, 1986.
101. Wingfield, P., Pain, R.H., and Craig, S., Tumour necrosis factor is a compact trimer, *FEBS Lett.*, 211, 179, 1987.
102. Ito, H., Shirai, T., Yamamoto, S., Akir, M., Kawahara, S., Todd, C.W., and Wallace, R.B., Molecular cloning of the gene encoding rabbit tumor necrosis factor, *DNA*, 5, 157, 1986.
103. Creasey, A.A., Doyle, L.V., Reynolds, M.T., Jung, T., Lin, L.S., and Vitt, C.R., Biological effects of recombinant human tumor necrosis factor and its novel muteins on tumor and normal cell lines, *Cancer Res.*, 47, 145, 1987.
104. Kull, F.C., Jr., Jacobs, S., and Cuatrecasas, P., Cellular receptor for ^{125}I-labeled tumor necrosis factor: specific binding, affinity labeling, and relationship to sensitivity, *Proc. Natl. Acad. Sci. U.S.A.*, 82, 5756, 1985.
105. Baglioni, C., McCandless, S., Tavernier, J., and Fiers, W., Binding of human tumor necrosis growth factor to high affinity receptors on HeLa and lymphoblastoid cells sensitive to growth inhibition, *J. Biol. Chem.*, 260, 13395, 1985.
106. Pichyangkul, S., Schick, D., Jian, F., Berent, S., Bollon, A., and Kahn, A., Binding of tumor necrosis factor α (TNF-α) to high-affinity receptors on polymorphonuclear cells, *Exp. Hematol.*, 15, 1055, 1987.
107. Scheurich, P., Thoma, B., Ücer, U., and Pfizenmaier, K., Immunoregulatory activity of recombinant human tumor necrosis factor (TNF)-α: induction of TNF receptors on human T cells and TNF-α mediated enhancement of T cell responses, *J. Immunol.*, 138, 1786, 1987.

108. **Smith, R.A., Kirstein, M., Fiers, W., and Baglioni, C.,** Species specificity of human and murine tumor necrosis factor, *J. Biol. Chem.,* 261, 14871, 1986.
109. **Carlino, J.A., Lin, L.S., and Creasey, A.A.,** Use of a sensitive receptor binding assay to discriminate between full-length and truncated human recombinant tumor necrosis factor proteins, *J. Biol. Chem.,* 262, 958, 1987.
110. **Socher, S.H., Riemen, M.W., Martinez, D., Friedman, A., Tai, J., Quintero, J.C., Garsky, V., and Oliff, A.,** Antibodies against amino acids 1–15 of tumor necrosis factor block its binding to cell surface receptor, *Proc. Natl. Acad. Sci. U.S.A.,* 84, 8829, 1987.
111. **Schall, T.J., Lewis, M., Koller, K.J., Lee, A., Rice, G.C., Wong, G.H.W., Gatanaga, T., Granger, G.A., Lentz, R., Raab, H., Kohr, W.J., and Goeddel, D.V.,** Molecular cloning and expression of a receptor for human tumor necrosis factor, *Cell,* 61, 361, 1990.
112. **Heller, R.A., Song, K., Onasch, M.A., Fischer, W.H., Chang, D., and Ringold, G.M.,** Complementary DNA cloning of a receptor for tumor necrosis factor and demonstration of a shed form of the receptor, *Proc. Natl. Acad. Sci. U.S.A.,* 87, 6151, 1990.
113. **Aderka, D., Engelmann, H., Hornik, V., Skornick, Y., Levo, Y., Wallach, D., and Kushtai, G.,** Increased serum levels of soluble receptors for tumor necrosis factor in cancer patients, *Cancer Res.,* 51, 5602, 1991.
114. **Brake-Busch, C., Nophar, Y., Kemper, O., Engelmann, H., and Wallach, D.,** Cytoplasmic truncation of the p55 tumour necrosis factor (TNF) receptor abolishes signaling, but not induced shedding of the receptor, *EMBO J.,* 11, 943, 1992.
115. **Creasey, A.A., Yamamoto, R., and Vitt, C.R.,** A high molecular weight component of the human tumor necrosis factor receptor is associated with cytotoxicity, *Proc. Natl. Acad. Sci. U.S.A.,* 84, 3293, 1987.
116. **Tsujimoto, M., Feinman, R., Kohase, M., and Vilcek, J.,** Characterization and affinity crosslinking of receptors for tumor necrosis factor on human cells, *Arch. Biochem. Biophys.,* 249, 563, 1986.
117. **Brockhaus, M., Schoenfeld, H.-J., Schlaeger, E.-J., Hunziker, W., Lesslauer, W., and Loetscher, H.,** Identification of two types of tumor necrosis factor receptors on human cell lines by monoclonal antibodies, *Proc. Natl. Acad. Sci. U.S.A.,* 87, 3127, 1990.
118. **Hohmann, H.-P., Brockhaus, M., Baeuerle, P.A., Remy, R., Kolbeck, R., and van Loon, A.P.G.M.,** Expression of the types A and B tumor necrosis factor (TNF) receptors is independently regulated, and both receptors mediate activation of the transcription factor NF-kappa B. TNF-α is not needed for induction of a biological effect via TNF receptors, *J. Biol. Chem.,* 265, 22409, 1990.
119. **Pennica, D., Lam, V.T., Mize, N.K., Weber, R.F., Lewis, M., Fendly, B.M., Lipari, M.T., and Goeddel, D.V.,** Biochemical properties of the 75-kDa tumor necrosis factor receptor. Characterization of ligand binding, internalization, and receptor phosphorylation, *J. Biol. Chem.,* 267, 21172, 1992.
120. **Heller, R.A., Song, K., Fan, N., and Chang, D.J.,** The p70 tumor necrosis factor receptor mediates cytotoxicity, *Cell,* 70, 47, 1992.
121. **Tartaglia, L.A., Rothe, M., Hu, Y.F., and Goeddel, D.V.,** Tumor necrosis factor's cytotoxic activity is signaled by the p55 TNF receptor, *Cell,* 73, 213, 1993.
122. **Van Ostade, X., Vandenabeele, P., Everaerdt, B., Loetscher, H., Gentz, R., Brockhaus, M., Lesslauer, W., Tavernier, J., Brouckaert, P., and Fiers, W.,** Human TNF mutants with selective activity on the p55 receptor, *Nature,* 361, 266, 1993.
123. **Fuchs, P., Strehl, S., Dworzak, M., Himmler, A., and Ambros, P.F.,** Structure of the human TNF receptor 1 (p60) gene (TNFR1) and localization to chromosome 12p13, *Genomics,* 13, 219, 1992.
124. **Schwalb, D.M., Han, H.-M., Marino, M., Warren, R., Porter, A., Goh, C., Fair, W.R., and Donner, D.B.,** Identification of a new receptor subtype for tumor necrosis factor-α, *J. Biol. Chem.,* 268, 9949, 1993.
125. **Goodwin, R.G., Anderson, D., Jerzy, R., Davis, T., Brannan, C.I., Copeland, N.G., Jenkins, N.A., and Smith, C.A.,** Molecular cloning and expression of the type 1 and type 2 murine receptors for tumor necrosis factor, *Mol. Cell. Biol.,* 11, 3020, 1991.
126. **Peetre, C., Gullberg, U., Nilsson, E., and Olsson, I.,** Effects of recombinant tumor necrosis factor on proliferation and differentiation of leukemic and normal hemopoietic cells in vitro, *J. Clin. Invest.,* 78, 1694, 1986.
127. **Owen-Schaub, L.B., de Mars, M., Murphy, E.C., Jr., and Grimm, E.A.,** TNF-β (lymphotoxin) strongly upregulates TNF-α gene expression in human peripheral blood lymphocytes, *Lymphokine Res.,* 9, 491, 1990.

128. **Owen-Schaub, L.B., Crump, W.L., III, Morin, G.I., and Grimm, E.A.,** Regulation of lymphocyte tumor necrosis factor receptors by IL-2, *J. Immunol.,* 143, 2236, 1989.
129. **Aggarwal, B.B., Eessalu, T.E., and Hass, P.E.,** Characterization of receptors for human tumour necrosis factor and their regulation by γ-interferon, *Nature,* 318, 665, 1985.
130. **Tsujimoto, M. and Vilcek, J.,** Tumor necrosis factor receptors in HeLa cells and their regulation by interferon-γ, *J. Biol. Chem.,* 261, 5384, 1986.
131. **Aggarwal, B.B. and Eesalu, T.E.,** Induction of receptors for tumor necrosis factor-α by interferons is not a major mechanism for their synergistic cytotoxic response, *J. Biol. Chem.,* 262, 10000, 1987.
132. **Lehmann, V. and Dröge, W.,** Demonstration of membrane receptors for human natural and recombinant ^{125}I-labeled tumor necrosis factor on HeLa cell clones and their role in tumor cell sensitivity, *Eur. J. Biochem.,* 158, 1, 1986.
133. **Aggarwal, B.B., Traquina, P.R., and Eesalu, T.E.,** Modulation of receptors and cytotoxic response of tumor necrosis factor-α by various lectins, *J. Biol. Chem.,* 261, 13652, 1986.
134. **Tsujimoto, M., Yip, Y.K., and Vilcek, J.,** Tumor necrosis factor: specific binding and internalization in sensitive and resistant cells, *Proc. Natl. Acad. Sci. U.S.A.,* 82, 7626, 1985.
135. **Scheurich, P., Unglaub, R., Maxeiner, B., Thoma, B., Zugmaier, G., and Pfizenmaier, K.,** Rapid modulation of tumor necrosis factor membrane receptors by activators of protein kinase C, *Biochem. Biophys. Res. Commun.,* 141, 855, 1986.
136. **Aggarwal, B.B. and Eesalu, T.E.,** Effect of phorbol esters on down-regulation and redistribution of cell surface receptors for tumor necrosis factor-α, *J. Biol. Chem.,* 262, 16450, 1987.
137. **Johnson, S.E. and Baglioni, C.,** Tumor necrosis factor receptors and cytocidal activity are down-regulated by activators of protein kinase C, *J. Biol. Chem.,* 263, 5686, 1988.
138. **Unglaub, R., Maxeiner, B., Thoma, B., Pfizenmaier, K., and Scheurich, P.,** Downregulation of tumor necrosis factor (TNF) sensitivity via modulation of TNF binding capacity by protein kinase C activators, *J. Exp. Med.,* 166, 1788, 1987.
139. **Gessani, S., McCandless, S., and Baglioni, C.,** Downregulation of tumor necrosis factor receptors of macrophages by interferons and interleukin-1. Role of protein kinase C activation, *J. Biol. Regul. Homeost. Agents,* 2, 166, 1988.
140. **Galeotti, T., Boscoboinik, D., and Azzi, A.,** Regulation of the TNF-α receptor in human osteosarcoma cells. Role of microtubules and of protein kinase C, *Arch. Biochem. Biophys.,* 300, 287, 1993.
141. **Seckinger, P., Isaaz, S., and Dayer, J.-M.,** A human inhibitor of tumor necrosis factor α, *J. Exp. Med.,* 167, 1511, 1988.
142. **Seckinger, P., Isaaz, S., and Dayer, J.-M.,** Purification and biologic characterization of a specific tumor necrosis factor α inhibitor, *J. Biol. Chem.,* 264, 11966, 1989.
143. **Seckinger, P., Zhang, J.-H., Hauptmann, B., and Dayer, J.-M.,** Characterization of a tumor necrosis factor α (TNF-α) inhibitor: evidence of immunological cross-reactivity with the TNF receptor, *Proc. Natl. Acad. Sci. U.S.A.,* 87, 5188, 1990.
144. **Gatanaga, T., Hwang, C., Kohr, W., Cappuccini, F., Lucci, J.A., III, Jeffes, E.W.B., Lentz, R., Tomich, J., Yamamoto, R.S., and Granger, G.A.,** Purification and characterization of an inhibitor (soluble tumor necrosis factor receptor) for tumor necrosis factor and lymphotoxin obtained from the serum ultrafiltrates of human cancer patients, *Proc. Natl. Acad. Sci. U.S.A.,* 87, 8781, 1990.
145. **Kohno, T., Brewer, M.T., Baker, S.L., Schwartz, P.E., King, M.W., Hale, K.K., Squires, C.H., Thompson, R.C., and Vannice, J.L.,** A second tumor necrosis factor receptor gene product can shed a naturally occurring tumor necrosis factor inhibitor, *Proc. Natl. Acad. Sci. U.S.A.,* 87, 8331, 1990.
146. **Ghezzi, P., Saccardo, B., and Bianchi, M.,** Recombinant tumor necrosis factor depresses cytochrome P-450-dependent microsomal metabolism in mice, *Biochem. Biophys. Res. Commun.,* 136, 316, 1986.
147. **Smith, M.R., Munger, W.E., Kung, H.-F., Takacs, L., and Durum, S.K.,** Direct evidence for an intracellular role for tumor necrosis factor-α. Microinjection of tumor necrosis factor kills target cells, *J. Immunol.,* 144, 162, 1990.
148. **Larrick, J.W. and Wright, S.C.,** Cytotoxic mechanism of tumor necrosis factor-α, *FASEB J.,* 4, 3215, 1990.
149. **Zhang, Y., Lin, J.-X., and Vilcek, J.,** Enhancement of cAMP levels and protein kinase activity by tumor necrosis factor and interleukin 1 in human fibroblasts: role in the induction of interleukin 6, *Proc. Natl. Acad. Sci. U.S.A.,* 85, 6802, 1988.
150. **Pfeilschifter, J. and Schwarzenbach, H.,** Interleukin-1 and tumor necrosis factor stimulate cGMP formation in rat renal mesangial cells, *FEBS Lett.,* 273, 185, 1990.

151. **Akama, H., Ichikawa, Y., Matsushita, Y., Shinozawa, T., and Homma, M.,** Mononuclear cells enhance prostaglandin E_2 production of polymorphonuclear leukocytes via tumor necrosis factor α, *Biochem. Biophys. Res. Commun.,* 168, 857, 1990.
152. **Pfeilschifter, J., Pignat, W., Vosbeck, K., and Märki, F.,** Interleukin 1 and tumor necrosis factor synergistically stimulate prostaglandin synthesis and phospholipase A2 release from rat mesangial cells, *Biochem. Biophys. Res. Commun.,* 159, 385, 1989.
153. **Elias, J.A., Gustilo, K., Baeder, W., and Freundlich, B.,** Synergistic stimulation of fibroblast prostaglandin production by recombinant interleukin 1 and tumor necrosis factor, *J. Immunol.,* 138, 3812, 1987.
154. **Endo, Y., Matsushima, K., Onozaki, K., and Oppenheim, J.J.,** Role of ornithine decarboxylase in the regulation of cell growth by IL-1 and tumor necrosis factor, *J. Immunol.,* 141, 2342, 1989.
155. **Imamura, K., Sherman, M.L., Spriggs, D., and Kufe, D.,** Effect of tumor necrosis factor on GTP binding and GTPase activity in HL-60 and L929 cells, *J. Biol. Chem.,* 263, 10247, 1988.
156. **Hasegawa, Y. and Bonavida, B.,** Calcium-independent pathway of tumor necrosis factor-mediated lysis of target cells, *J. Immunol.,* 142, 2670, 1989.
157. **Schütze, S., Nottrott, S., Pfizenmaier, K., and Krönke, M.,** Tumor necrosis factor signal transduction. Cell-type-specific activation and translocation of protein kinase C, *J. Immunol.,* 144, 2604, 1990.
158. **Katoh, T., Karasaki, Y., Hirano, H., Gotoh, S., and Higashi, K.,** Translocation of protein kinase C to membranes induced by TNF does not cause the inhibition of EGF binding to human WISH cells, *Biochem. Biophys. Res. Commun.,* 168, 690, 1990.
159. **Godfrey, R.W., Johnson, W.J., and Hoffstein, S.T.,** Recombinant tumor necrosis factor and interleukin-1 both stimulate human synovial cell arachidonic acid release and phospholipid metabolism, *Biochem. Biophys. Res. Commun.,* 142, 235, 1987.
160. **Suffys, P., Van Roy, F., and Fiers, W.,** Tumor necrosis factor and interleukin 1 activate phospholipase in rat chondrocytes, *FEBS Lett.,* 232, 24, 1988.
161. **Rapuano, B.E. and Bockman, R.S.,** Tumor necrosis factor-α stimulates phosphatidylinositol breakdown by phospholipase C to coordinately increase the levels of diacylglycerol, free arachidonic acid and prostaglandins in an osteoblast (MC3T3-E1) cell line, *Biochim. Biophys. Acta,* 1091, 374, 1991.
162. **De Valck, D., Beyaert, R., Van Roy, F., and Fiers, W.,** Tumor necrosis factor cytotoxicity is associated with phospholipase D activation, *Eur. J. Biochem.,* 212, 491, 1993.
163. **Dressler, K.A., Mathias, S., and Kolesnik, R.N.,** Tumor necrosis factor-α activates the sphingomyelin signal transduction pathway in a cell-free system, *Science,* 255, 1715, 1992.
164. **Hepburn, A., Demolle, D., Boeynaems, J.-M., Fiers, W., and Dumont, J.E.,** Rapid phosphorylation of a 27-kDa protein induced by tumor necrosis factor, *FEBS Lett.,* 227, 175, 1988.
165. **Robaye, B., Hepburn, A., Lecocq, R., Fiers, W., Boeynaems, J.-M., and Dumont, J.E.,** Tumor necrosis factor-α induces the phosphorylation of 28-kDa stress proteins in endothelial cells: possible role in protection against cytotoxicity?, *Biochem. Biophys. Res. Commun.,* 163, 301, 1989.
166. **Marino, M.W., Pfeffer, L.M., Guidon, P.T., Jr., and Donner, D.B.,** Tumor necrosis factor induces phosphorylation of a 28-kDa mRNA cap-binding protein in human cervical carcinoma cells, *Proc. Natl. Acad. Sci. U.S.A.,* 86, 8417, 1989.
167. **Marino, M.W., Feld, L.J., Jaffe, E.A., Pfeffer, L.M., Han, H.-M., and Donner, D.B.,** Phosphorylation of the proto-oncogene product eukaryotic initiation factor 4E is a common cellular response to tumor necrosis factor, *J. Biol. Chem.,* 266, 2685, 1991.
168. **Lazaris-Karatzas, A., Montine, K.S., and Sonenberg, N.,** Malignant transformation by a eukaryotic initiation factor subunit that binds to mRNA 5' cap, *Nature,* 345, 542, 1990.
169. **Donato, N.J., Gallick, G.E., Steck, P.A., and Rosenblum, M.G.,** Tumor necrosis factor modulates epidermal growth factor receptor phosphorylation and kinase activity in human tumor cells, *J. Biol. Chem.,* 264, 20474, 1989.
170. **Donato, N.J., Rosenblum, M.G., and Steck, P.A.,** Tumor necrosis factor regulates tyrosine phosphorylation on epidermal growth factor receptors in A431 carcinoma cells: evidence for a distinct mechanism, *Cell Growth Differ.,* 3, 259, 1992.
171. **Schütze, S., Scheurich, P., Schlüter, C., Ücer, U., Pfizenmaier, K., and Krönke, M.,** Tumor necrosis factor-induced changes of gene expression in U037 cells. Differentiation-dependent plasticity of the responsive state, *J. Immunol.,* 140, 3000, 1988.
172. **Perlmutter, D.H., Dinarello, C.A., Punsal, P.I., and Colten, H.R.,** Cachectin/tumor necrosis factor regulates hepatic acute-phase gene expression, *J. Clin. Invest.,* 78, 1349, 1986.

173. Kirstein, M. and Baglioni, C., Tumor necrosis factor induces synthesis of two proteins in human fibroblasts, *J. Biol. Chem.*, 261, 9565, 1986.
174. Collins, T., Lapierre, L.A., Fiers, W., Strominger, J.L., and Pober, J.S., Recombinant human tumor necrosis factor increases mRNA levels and surface expression of HLA-A,B antigens in vascular endothelial cells and dermal fibroblasts *in vitro, Proc. Natl. Acad. Sci. U.S.A.*, 83, 446, 1986.
175. Lee, T.H., Lee, G.W., Ziff, E.B., and Vilcek, J., Isolation and characterization of eight tumor necrosis factor-induced gene sequences from human fibroblasts, *Mol. Cell. Biol.*, 10, 1982, 1990.
176. Lin, J.-X. and Vilcek, J., Tumor necrosis factor and interleukin-1 cause a rapid and transient stimulation of c-*fos* and c-*myc* mRNA levels in human fibroblasts, *J. Biol. Chem.*, 262, 11908, 1987.
177. Brenner, D.A., O'Hara, M., Angel, P., Chojkier, M., and Karin, M., Prolonged activation of *jun* and collagenase genes by tumour necrosis factor-α, *Nature*, 337, 661, 1989.
178. Kahari, V.M., Chen, Y.Q., Bashir, M.M., Rosenbloom, J., and Uitto, J., Tumor necrosis factor-α down-regulates human elastin gene expression. Evidence for the role of AP-1 in the suppression of promoter activity, *J. Biol. Chem.*, 267, 26134, 1992.
179. Cornelius, P., Marlowe, M., Lee, M.D., and Pekala, P.H., The growth factor-like effects of tumor necrosis factor-α. Stimulation of glucose transport activity and induction of glucose transporter and immediate early gene expression in 3T3-L1 preadipocytes, *J. Biol. Chem.*, 265, 20506, 1990.
180. Koo, A.S., Chiu, R., Soong, J., Dekernion, J.B., and Belldegrun, A., The expression of c-jun and junB mRNA in renal cell cancer and in vitro regulation by transforming growth factor β1 and tumor necrosis factor α1, *J. Urol.*, 148, 1314, 1992.
181. Brach, M.A., Gruss, H.J., Sott, C., and Herrmann, F., The mitogenic response to tumor necrosis factor alpha requires c-Jun/AP-2, *Mol. Cell. Biol.*, 13, 4284, 1993.
182. Yarden, A. and Kimchi, A., Tumor necrosis factor reduces c-*myc* expression and cooperates with interferon-γ in HeLa cells, *Science*, 234, 1419, 1986.
183. Schachner, J., Blick, M., Freireich, E., Gutterman, J., and Beran, M., Suppression of c-*myc* and c-*myb* expression in myeloid cells lines treated with recombinant tumor necrosis factor-α, *Leukemia*, 2, 749, 1988.
184. Sherman, M.L., Weber, B.L., Datta, R., and Kufe, D.W., Transcriptional and posttranscriptional regulation of macrophage-specific colony stimulating factor gene expression by tumor necrosis factor. Involvement of arachidonic acid metabolites, *J. Clin. Invest.*, 85, 442, 1990.
185. Seliger, B., Stark, G., and Pfizenmaier, K., Tumor necrosis factor-α affects LTR-controlled oncogene expression in transformed mouse fibroblasts at the post-transcriptional level, *J. Immunol.*, 141, 2138, 1988.
186. Pusztai, L., Lewis, C.E., and McGee, J.O.D., Growth arrest of the breast cancer cell line, T47D, by TNF-α; cell cycle specificity and signal transduction, *Br. J. Cancer*, 67, 290, 1993.
187. Chang, D.J., Ringold, G.M., and Heller, R.A., Cell killing and induction of manganous superoxide dismutase by tumor necrosis factor-α is mediated by lipoxygenase metabolites of arachidonic acid, *Biochem. Biophys. Res. Commun.*, 188, 538, 1992.
188. Tsujimoto, M., Okamura, N., and Adachi, H., Dexamethasone inhibits the cytotoxic activity of tumor necrosis factor, *Biochem. Biophys. Res. Commun.*, 153, 109, 1988.
189. Rubin, B.Y., Anderson, S.L., Lunn, R.M., Richardson, N.K., Hellermann, G.R., Smith, L.J., and Old, L.J., Tumor necrosis factor and IFN induce a common set of proteins, *J. Immunol.*, 141, 1180, 1988.
190. Vilcek, J., Palombella, V.J., Henriksen-DeStefano, D., Swenson, C., Feinman, R., Hirai, M., and Tsujimoto, M., Fibroblast growth enhancing activity of tumor necrosis factor and its relationship to other polypeptide growth factors, *J. Exp. Med.*, 163, 632, 1986.
191. Palombella, V.J., Mendelsohn, J., and Vilcek, J., Mitogenic action of tumor necrosis factor in human fibroblasts: interaction with epidermal growth factor and platelet-derived growth factor, *J. Cell. Physiol.*, 135, 23, 1988.
192. Feingold, K.R., Soued, M., Grunfeld, C., Moser, A.H., Verdier, J.A., and DoVale, H.G., Tumor necrosis factor stimulates DNA synthesis in the liver of intact cells, *Biochem. Biophys. Res. Commun.*, 153, 576, 1988.
193. Akahane, K., Hosoi, T., Urabe, A., Kawakami, M., and Takaku, F., Effects of recombinant human tumor necrosis factor (rhTNF) on normal human and mouse hemopoietic progenitor cells, *Int. J. Cell Cloning*, 5, 16, 1987.
194. Chen, B.D.-M. and Mueller, M., Recombinant tumor necrosis factor enhances the proliferative responsiveness of murine peripheral macrophages to macrophage colony-stimulating factor but inhibits their proliferative responsiveness to granulocyte-macrophage colony-stimulating factor, *Blood*, 75, 1627, 1990.

195. **Pelus, L.M., Ottmann, O.G., and Nocka, K.H.,** Synergistic inhibition of human marrow granulocyte-macrophage progenitor cells by prostaglandin E and recombinant interferon-α, -β, and -γ and an effect mediated by tumor necrosis factor, *J. Immunol.*, 140, 479, 1988.
196. **Ulich, T.R., del Castillo, J., Ni, R.-X., Bikhazi, N., and Calvin, L.,** Mechanisms of tumor necrosis factor α-induced lymphopenia, neutropenia, and biphasic neutrophilia: a study of lymphocyte recirculation and hematologic interactions of TNF α with endogenous mediators of leukocyte traffiking, *J. Leukocyte Biol.*, 45, 155, 1989.
197. **Schell-Frederick, E., Tepass, T., Lorscheidt, G., Pfreundschuh, M., Schaadt, M., and Diehl, V.,** Effects of recombinant tumor necrosis factor (rHuTNFα) on human neutrophils and monocytes: in vitro, ex vivo and in vivo, *Eur. J. Haematol.*, 43, 286, 1989.
198. **Dinarello, C.A.,** Interleukins, tumor necrosis factors (cachetin), and interferons as endogenous pyrogens and mediators of fever, *Lymphokines*, 14, 1 1987.
199. **Okusawa, S., Gelfand, J.A., Ikejima, T., Connolly, R.J., and Dinarello, C.A.,** Interleukin 1 induces shock-like state in rabbits. Synergism with tumor necrosis factor and the effect of cyclooxygenase inhibition, *J. Clin. Invest.*, 81, 1162, 1988.
200. **Warren, R.S., Donner, D.B., Starnes, H.F., Jr., and Brennan, M.F.,** Modulation of endogenous hormone action by recombinant human necrosis factor, *Proc. Natl. Acad. Sci. U.S.A.*, 84, 8619, 1987.
201. **Warren, R.S., Starnes, H.F., Jr., Gabrilove, J.L., Oettgen, H.F., and Brennan, M.F.,** The acute metabolic effects of tumor necrosis factor administration in humans, *Arch. Surg.*, 122, 1396, 1987.
202. **Starnes, H.F., Jr., Warren, R.S., Jeevanandam, M., Gabrilove, J.L., Larchian, W., Oettgen, H.R., and Brennan, M.F.,** Tumor necrosis factor and the acute metabolic response to tissue injury in man, *J. Clin. Invest.*, 82, 1321, 1988.
203. **Le, J., Weinstein, D., Gubler, U., and Vilcek, J.,** Induction of membrane-associated interleukin 1 by tumor necrosis factor in human fibroblasts, *J. Immunol.*, 138, 2137, 1987.
204. **Bachwich, P.R., Chensue, S.W., Larrick, J.W., and Kunkel, S.L.,** Tumor necrosis factor stimulates interleukin-1 and prostaglandin E_2 production in resting macrophages, *Biochem. Biophys. Res. Commun.*, 136, 94, 1986.
205. **Nawroth, P.P., Bank, I., Handley, D., Cassimeris, J., Chess, L., and Stern, D.,** Tumor necrosis factor/cachectin interacts with endothelial cell receptors to induce release of interleukin 1, *J. Exp. Med.*, 163, 1363, 1986.
206. **Dinarello, C.A., Cannon, J.G., Wolff, S.M., Bernheim, H.A., Beutler, B., Cerami, A., Figari, I.S., Palladino, M.A., Jr., and O'Connor, J.V.,** Tumor necrosis factor (cachectin) is an endogenous pyrogen and induces production of interleukin 1, *J. Exp. Med.*, 163, 1433, 1986.
207. **Hoffman, M.K.,** The effects of tumor necrosis factor on the production of interleukin-1 by macrophages, *Lymphokine Res.*, 5, 255, 1986.
208. **Le, J. and Vilcek, J.,** Tumor necrosis factor and interleukin 1: cytokines with multiple overlapping biological activities, *Lab. Invest.*, 56, 234, 1987.
209. **Sipe, J.D., Vogel, S.N., Douches, S., and Neta, R.,** Tumor necrosis factor/cachectin is a less potent inducer of serum amyloid A synthesis than interleukin 1, *Lymphokine Res.*, 6, 93, 1987.
210. **Remick, D.G., Larrick, J., and Kunkel, S.L.,** Tumor necrosis factor-induced alterations in circulating leukocyte populations, *Biochem. Biophys. Res. Commun.*, 141, 818, 1986.
211. **Yokota, S., Geppert, T.D., and Lipsky, P.E.,** Enhancement of antigen- and mitogen-induced human T lymphocyte proliferation by tumor necrosis factor-α, *J. Immunol.*, 140, 531, 1988.
212. **Lee, J.C., Truneh, A., Smith, M.F., Jr., and Tsang, K.Y.,** Induction of interleukin 2 receptor (TAC) by tumor necrosis factor in YT cells, *J. Immunol.*, 139, 1935, 1987.
213. **Espevik, T., Figari, I.S., Ranges, G.E., and Palladino, M.A., Jr.,** Transforming growth factor-β_1 (TGF-β_1) and recombinant human tumor necrosis factor-α reciprocally regulate the generation of lymphokine-activated killer cell activity. Comparison between natural porcine platelet-derived TGF-β_1 and TGF-β_2, and recombinant human TGF-β_1, *J. Immunol.*, 140, 2312, 1988.
214. **Owen-Schaub, L.B., Gutterman, J.U., and Grimm, E.A.,** Synergy of tumor necrosis factor and interleukin 2 in the activation of human cytotoxic lymphocytes: effect of tumor necrosis factor α and interleukin 2 in the generation of human lymphokine-activated killer cells cytotoxicity, *Cancer Res.*, 48, 788, 1988.
215. **Van Damme, J., De Ley, M., Van Snick, J., Dinarello, C.A., and Billiau, A.,** The role of interferon-β_1 and the 26-kDa protein (interferon-β_2) as mediators of the antiviral effect of interleukin 1 and tumor necrosis factor, *J. Immunol.*, 139, 1867, 1987.

216. Ito, M. and O'Malley, J.A., Antiviral effects of recombinant human tumor necrosis factor, *Lymphokine Res.*, 6, 309, 1987.
217. Philip, R. and Epstein, L.B., Tumour necrosis factor as immunomodulator and mediator of monocyte cytotoxicity induced by itself, γ-interferon and interleukin-1, *Nature*, 323, 86, 1986.
218. Campbell, I.L., Oxbrow, L., West, J., and Harrison, L.C., Regulation of MHC protein expression in pancreatic β-cells by interferon-γ and tumor necrosis factor-α, *Mol. Endocrinol.*, 2, 101, 1988.
219. Johnson, D.R. and Pober, J.S., Tumor necrosis factor and immune interferon synergistically increase transcription of HLA class I heavy- and light-chain genes in vascular endothelium, *Proc. Natl. Acad. Sci. U.S.A.*, 87, 5183, 1990.
220. Nissen-Meyer, J., Austgulen, R., and Espevik, T., Comparison of recombinant tumor necrosis factor and the monocyte-derived cytotoxic factor involved in monocyte-mediated cytotoxicity, *Cancer Res.*, 47, 2251, 1987.
221. Janssen, O. and Kabelitz, D., Tumor necrosis factor selectively inhibits activation of human B cells by Epstein-Barr virus, *J. Immunol.*, 140, 125, 1988.
222. Witsell, A.L. and Schook, L.B., Tumor necrosis factor-α is an autocrine growth regulator during macrophage differentiation, *Proc. Natl. Acad. Sci. U.S.A.*, 89, 4754, 1992.
223. Heidenreich, S., Weyers, M., Gong, J.-H., Sprenger, H., Nain, M., and Gemsa, D., Potentiation of lymphokine-induced macrophage activation by tumor necrosis factor-α, *J. Immunol.*, 140, 1511, 1988.
224. Shieh, J.-H., Peterson, R.H.F., Warren, D.J., and Moore, M.A.S., Modulation of colony-stimulating factor-1 receptors on macrophages by tumor necrosis factor, *J. Immunol.*, 143, 2534, 1989.
225. Larrick, J.W., Graham, D., Toy, K., Lin, L.S., Senyk, G., and Fendly, B.M., Recombinant tumor necrosis factor causes activation of human granulocytes, *Blood*, 69, 640, 1987.
226. Maizel, A.L. and Mehta, S.R., Effect of interleukin 1 on human thymocytes and purified human T cells, *J. Exp. Med.*, 153, 470, 1980.
227. Dröge, W., Benninghoff, B., and Lehmann, V., Tumor necrosis factor augments the immunogenicity and the production of L-ornithine by peritoneal macrophages, *Lymphokine Res.*, 6, 111, 1987.
228. Nakagawa, H., Kitagawa, H., and Aikawa, Y., Tumor necrosis factor stimulates gelatinase and collagenase production by granulation tissue in culture, *Biochem. Biophys. Res. Commun.*, 142, 791, 1987.
229. Wong, G.H.W. and Goeddel, D.V., Tumour necrosis factors α and β inhibit virus replication and synergize with interferons, *Nature*, 323, 819, 1986.
230. Mestan, J., Digel, W., Mittnacht, S., Hillen, H., Blohm, D., Möller, A., Jacobsen, H., and Kirchner, H., Antiviral effects of recombinant tumour necrosis factor *in vitro*, *Nature*, 323, 816, 1986.
231. Arakawa, T., Hsu, Y.-R., Toth, E., and Stebbing, N., The antiviral activity of recombinant human tumor necrosis factor-α, *J. Interferon Res.*, 7, 103, 1987.
232. Parant, M., Parant, F., Vinit, M.-A., and Chelid, L., Action protectrice du "tumor necrosis factor" (TNF) obtenu par recombinaison génétique contre l'infection expérimentale bactérienne ou fongique, *C. R. Acad. Sci. Paris*, 304, 1, 1987.
233. White, C.W., Ghezzi, P., Dinarello, C.A., Caldwell, S.A., McMurthy, I.F., and Repine, J.E., Recombinant tumor necrosis factor/cachectin and interleukin 1 pretreatment decreases lung oxidized glutathione accumulation, lung injury, and mortality in rats exposed to hyperoxia, *J. Clin. Invest.*, 79, 1868, 1987.
234. Figari, I.S., Mori, N.A., and Palladino, M.A., Jr., Regulation of neutrophil migration and superoxide production by recombinant tumor necrosis factors-α and -β: comparison to recombinant interferon-γ and interleukin-1α, *Blood*, 70, 979, 1987.
235. Shalaby, M.R., Palladino, M.A., Jr., Hirabayashi, S.E., Eesalu, T.E., Lewis, G.D., Shepard, H.M., and Aggarwal, B.B., Receptor binding and activation of polymorphonuclear neutrophils by tumor necrosis factor-α, *J. Leukocyte Biol.*, 41, 196, 1987.
236. Urbaschek, R., Männel, D.N., and Urbaschek, B., Tumor necrosis factor induced stimulation of granulopoiesis and radioprotection, *Lymphokine Res.*, 6, 179, 1987.
237. Murase, T., Hotta, T., Ohno, R., and Saito, H., Predominant suppression of neutrophil colony growth by recombinant human tumor necrosis factor, *Proc. Soc. Exp. Biol. Med.*, 186, 188, 1987.
238. Moldawer, L.L., Marano, M.A., Wei, H., Fong, Y., Silen, M.L., Kuo, G., Manogue, K.R., Vlassara, H., Cohen, H., Cerami, A., and Lowry, S.F., Cachectin/tumor necrosis factor-α alters red blood cell kinetics and induces anemia in vivo, *FASEB J.*, 3, 1637, 1989.
239. Taverne, J., Tavernier, J., Fiers, W., and Playfair, J.H.L., Recombinant tumor necrosis factor inhibits malaria parasites *in vivo* but not *in vitro*, *Clin. Exp. Immunol.*, 67, 1, 1987.

240. **Warner, S.J.C. and Libby, P.,** Human vascular smooth muscle cells: target for and source of tumor necrosis factor, *J. Immunol.,* 142, 100, 1989.
241. **Leibovich, S.J., Polverini, P.J., Shepard, H.M., Wiseman, D.M., Shively, V., and Nuseir, N.,** Macrophage-induced angiogenesis is mediated by tumour necrosis factor-α, *Nature,* 329, 630, 1987.
242. **Sato, N., Goto, T., Haranaka, K., Satomi, N., Nariuchi, H., Mano-Hirano, Y., and Sawasaki, Y.,** Actions of tumor necrosis factor on cultured vascular endothelial cells: morphologic modulation, growth inhibition, and cytotoxicity, *J. Natl. Cancer Inst.,* 76, 1113, 1986.
243. **Sato, N., Fukuda, K., Nariuchi, H., and Sagara, N.,** Tumor necrosis factor inhibiting angiogenesis in vitro, *J. Natl. Cancer Inst.,* 79, 1383, 1987.
244. **Mano-Hirano, Y., Sato, N., Sawasaki, Y., and Goto, T.,** Inhibition of tumor-induced migration of bovine capillary endothelial cells by recombinant human tumor necrosis factor, *Proc. Jpn. Acad.,* B62, 235, 1986.
245. **Mano-Hirano, Y., Sato, N., Sawasaki, Y., Haranaka, K., Satomi, N., Nariuchi, H., and Goto, T.,** Inhibition of tumor-induced migration of bovine capillary endothelial cells by mouse and rabbit tumor necrosis factor, *J. Natl. Cancer Inst.,* 78, 115, 1987.
246. **Palladino, M.A., Jr., Shalaby, M.R., Kramer, S.M., Ferraiolo, B.L., Baughman, R.A., Deleo, A.B., Crase, D., Marafino, B., Aggarwal, B.B., Figari, I.S., Liggitt, D., and Patton, J.S.,** Characterization of the antitumor activities of human tumor necrosis factor-α and the comparison with other cytokines: induction of tumor-specific immunity, *J. Immunol.,* 138, 4023, 1987.
247. **Bevilacqua, M.P., Pober, J.S., Majeau, G.R., Fiers, W., Cotran, R.S., and Gimbrone, M.A., Jr.,** Recombinant tumor necrosis factor induces procoagulant activity in culture human vascular endothelium: characterization and comparison with the actions of interleukin 1, *Proc. Natl. Acad. Sci. U.S.A.,* 83, 4533, 1986.
248. **Shimomura, K., Manda, T., Mukumoto, S., Kobayashi, K., Nakano, K., and Mori, J.,** Recombinant human tumor necrosis factor-α: thrombus formation is a cause of anti-tumor activity, *Int. J. Cancer,* 41, 243, 1988.
249. **Dano, K., Andreasen, P.A., Grondahl-Hansen, J., Kristensen, P., Nielsen, L.S., and Skriver, L.,** Plasminogen activators, tissue degradation and cancer, *Adv. Cancer Res.,* 44, 139, 1985.
250. **Erickson, L.A., Hekman, C.M., and Loskutoff, D.J.,** The primary plasminogen activator inhibitors in endothelial cells, platelets, serum and plasma are immunologically related, *Proc. Natl. Acad. Sci. U.S.A.,* 82, 8710, 1985.
251. **Wohlwend, A., Belin, D., and Vassalli, J.-D.,** Plasminogen activator-specific inhibitors produced by human monocyte/macrophages, *J. Exp. Med.,* 165, 320, 1987.
252. **Medcalf, R.L., Kruithof, E.K.O., and Schleuning, W.-D.,** Plasminogen activator inhibitor 1 and 2 are tumor necrosis factor/cachectin-responsive genes, *J. Exp. Med.,* 168, 751, 1988.
253. **Georg, B., Helseth, E., Lund, L.R., Skandsen, T., Riccio, A., Dano, K., Unsgaard, G., and Andreasen, P.A.,** Tumor necrosis factor-α regulates mRNA for urokinase-type plasminogen activator and type-1 plasminogen activator inhibitor in human neoplastic cell lines, *Mol. Cell. Endocrinol.,* 61, 87, 1989.
254. **Schleef, R., Bevilacqua, R., Sawdey, M.P., Gimbrone, M.A., and Loskutoff, D.J.,** Cytokine activation of vascular endothelium: effects on tissue-type plasminogen activator and type 1 plasminogen activator inhibitor, *J. Biol. Chem.,* 263, 5797, 1988.
255. **Pytel, B.A., Peppel, K., and Baglioni, C.,** Plasminogen activator inhibitor type-2 is a major protein induced in human fibroblasts and SK-MEL-109 melanoma cells by tumor necrosis factor, *J. Cell. Physiol.,* 144, 416, 1990.
256. **Canalis, E.,** Effects of tumor necrosis factor on bone formation *in vitro, Endocrinology,* 121, 1596, 1987.
257. **Thomson, B.A., Mundy, G.R., and Chambers, T.J.,** Tumor necrosis factors α and β induce osteoblastic cells to stimulate osteoclastic bone resorption, *J. Immunol.,* 138, 775, 1987.
258. **Sato, K., Fujii, Y., Ono, M., Nomura, H., and Shizume, K.,** Production of interleukin 1α-like factor and colony-stimulating factor by a squamous cell carcinoma of the thyroid (T3M-5) derived from a patient with hypercalcemia and leukocytes, *Cancer Res.,* 47, 6474, 1987.
259. **Saklatvala, J.,** Tumour necrosis factor α stimulates resorption and inhibits synthesis of proteoglycan in cartilage, *Nature,* 322, 547, 1986.
260. **Tracey, K.J., Lowry, S.F., Beutler, B., Cerami, A., Albert, J.D., and Shires, G.T.,** Cachectin/tumor necrosis factor mediates changes of skeletal muscle plasma membrane potential, *J. Exp. Med.,* 164, 1368, 1986.

261. **Milenkovic, L., Rettori, V., Snyder, G.D., Beutler, B., and McCann, S.M.,** Cachectin alters anterior pituitary hormone release by a direct action *in vitro*, *Proc. Natl. Acad. Sci. U.S.A.,* 86, 2418, 1989.
262. **Walton, P.E. and Cronin, M.J.,** Tumor necrosis factor-α inhibits growth hormone secretion from cultured anterior pituitary cells, *Endocrinology,* 125, 925, 1989.
263. **Elsasser, T.H., Caperna, T.J., and Fayer, R.,** Tumor necrosis factor-α affects growth hormone secretion by a direct pituitary interaction, *Proc. Soc. Exp. Biol. Med.,* 198, 547, 1991.
264. **Gaillard, R.C., Turnill, D., Sappino, P., and Muller, A.F.,** Tumor necrosis factor α inhibits the hormonal response of the pituitary gland to hypothalamic releasing factors, *Endocrinology,* 127, 101, 1990.
265. **Calkins, J.H., Guo, H., Sigel, M.M., and Lin, T.,** Tumor necrosis factor-α enhances inhibitory effects of interleukin-1β on Leydig cell steroidogenesis, *Biochem. Biophys. Res. Commun.,* 166, 1313, 1990.
266. **Roby, K.F. and Terranova, P.F.,** Tumor necrosis factor α alters follicular steroidogenesis *in vitro*, *Endocrinology,* 123, 2952, 1988.
267. **Adashi, E.Y., Resnick, C.E., Croft, C.S., and Payne, D.W.,** Tumor necrosis factor α inhibits gonadotropin hormonal action in nontransformed ovarian granulosa cells. A modulatory noncytotoxic property, *J. Biol. Chem.,* 264, 11591, 1989.
268. **Hattori, A., Tanaka, E., Murase, K., Ishida, N., Chatani, Y., Tsujimoto, M., Hayashi, K., and Kohno, M.,** Tumor necrosis factor stimulates the synthesis and secretion of biologically active nerve growth factor in non-neuronal cells, *J. Biol. Chem.,* 268, 2577, 1993.
269. **Austgulen, R., Espevik, T., Nissen-Meyer, J.,** Fibroblast growth-stimulatory activity released from human monocytes: the contribution of tumour necrosis factor, *Scand. J. Immunol.,* 26, 621, 1987.
270. **Paulsson, Y., Austgulen, R., Hofsli, E., Heldin, C.-H., Westermark, B., and Nissen-Meyer, J.,** Tumor necrosis factor-induced expression of platelet-derived growth factor A-chain messenger RNA in fibroblasts, *Exp. Cell Res.,* 180, 490, 1989.
271. **Beyer, H.S. and Theologides, A.,** Tumor necrosis factor-α is a direct hepatocyte mitogen in the rat, *Biochem. Mol. Biol. Int.,* 29, 1, 1993.
272. **Mészéros, K., Lang, C.H., Bagby, G.J., and Spitzer, J.J.,** Tumor necrosis factor increases in vivo glucose utilization of macrophage-rich tissues, *Biochem. Biophys. Res. Commun.,* 149, 1, 1987.
273. **Satoh, M. and Yamazaki, M.,** Tumor necrosis factor stimulates DNA synthesis of mouse hepatocytes in primary culture and is suppressed by transforming growth factor β and interleukin-6, *J. Cell Physiol.,* 150, 134, 1992.
274. **Palombella, V.J., Yamashiro, D.J., Maxfield, F.R., Decker, S.J., and Vilcek, J.,** Tumor necrosis factor increases the number of epidermal growth factor receptors on human fibroblasts, *J. Biol. Chem.,* 262, 1950, 1987.
275. **Hori, T., Kashiyama, S., Oku, N., Hayakawa, M., Shibamoto, S., Tsujimoto, M., Nishihara, T., and Ito, F.,** Effects of tumor necrosis factor on cell growth and expression of transferrin receptors in human fibroblasts, *Cell Struct. Funct.,* 13, 425, 1988.
276. **Kamijo, R., Takeda, K., Naguno, M., and Konno, K.,** Suppression of TNF-stimulated proliferation of diploid fibroblasts and TNF-induced cytotoxicity against transformed fibroblasts by TGF-β, *Biochem. Biophys. Res. Commun.,* 158, 155, 1989.
277. **Fransen, L., van der Heyden, J., Ruysschaert, R., and Fiers, W.,** Recombinant tumor necrosis factor: its effect and its synergism with interferon-γ on a variety of normal and transformed human cell lines, *Eur. J. Cancer Clin. Oncol.,* 22, 419, 1986.
278. **Fransen, L., Ruysschaert, M.-R., van der Heyden, J., and Fiers, W.,** Recombinant tumor necrosis factor: species specificity for a variety of human and murine transformed cell lines, *Cell. Immunol.,* 100, 260, 1986.
279. **Broxmeyer, H.E., Williams, D.E., Lu, L., Cooper, S., Anderson, S.L., Beyer, G.S., Hoffman, R., and Rubin, B.Y.,** The suppressive influences of human tumor necrosis factors on bone marrow hematopoietic progenitor cells from normal donors and patients with leukemia: synergism of tumor necrosis factor and interferon-γ, *J. Immunol.,* 136, 4487, 1986.
280. **Reis, L.F.L., Le, J., Hirano, T., Kishimoto, T., and Vilcek, J.,** Antiviral action of tumor necrosis factor in human fibroblasts is not mediated by B cell stimulatory factor 2/IFN-β_2, and is inhibited by specific antibodies to IFN-β, *J. Immunol.,* 140, 1566, 1988.
281. **Trinchieri, G., Kobayashi, M., Rosen, M., Louden, R., Murphy, M., and Perusia, B.,** Tumor necrosis factor and lymphotoxin induce differentiation of human myeloid cell lines in synergy with immune interferon, *J. Exp. Med.,* 164, 1206, 1986.

282. **Weinberg, J.B. and Larrick, J.W.,** Receptor-mediated monocytoid differentiation of human promyelocytic cells by tumor necrosis factor: synergistic actions with interferon-γ and 1,25-dihydroxyvitamin D_3, *Blood,* 70, 994, 1987.
283. **Glazer, R.I., Chapekar, M.S., Hartman, K.D., and Knode, M.C.,** Appearance of membrane-bound tyrosine kinase during differentiation of HL-60 leukemia cells by immune interferon and tumor necrosis factor, *Biochem. Biophys. Res. Commun.,* 140, 908, 1986.
284. **Stolpen, A.H., Guinan, E.C., Fiers, W., and Pober, J.S.,** Recombinant tumor necrosis factor and immune interferon act singly and in combination to recognize human vascular endothelial cell monolayers, *Am. J. Pathol.,* 123, 16, 1986.
285. **Talmadge, J.E., Phillips, H., Schindler, J., Tribble, H., and Pennington, R.,** Systematic preclinical study on the therapeutic properties of recombinant human interleukin 2 for the treatment of metastatic disease, *Cancer Res.,* 47, 5725, 1987.
286. **Seelentag, W.K., Mermod, J.-J., Montesano, R., and Vassalli, P.,** Additive effects of interleukin 1 and tumour necrosis factor-α on the accumulation of the three granulocyte and macrophage colony-stimulating factor mRNAs in human endothelial cells, *EMBO J.,* 6, 2261, 1987.
287. **Broudy, V.C., Kaushansky, K., Segal, G.M., Harlan, J.M., and Adamson, J.W.,** Tumor necrosis factor type α stimulates human endothelial cells to produce granulocyte/macrophage colony-stimulating factor, *Proc. Natl. Acad. Sci. U.S.A.,* 83, 7467, 1986.
288. **Munker, R., Gasson, J., Ogawa, M., and Koeffler, H.P.,** Recombinant human TNF induces production of granulocyte-macrophate colony-stimulating factor, *Nature,* 323, 79, 1986.
289. **Kohase, M., Henrik-DeStefano, D., May, L.T., Vilcek, J., and Sehgal, P.B.,** Induction of $β_2$-interferon by tumor necrosis factor: a homeostatic mechanism in the control of cell proliferation, *Cell,* 45, 659, 1986.
290. **Roodman, G.D., Bird, A., Hutzler, D., and Montgomery, W.,** Tumor necrosis factor-α and hematopoietic progenitors: effects of tumor necrosis factor on the growth of erythroid progenitors CFU-E and BFU-E and the hematopoietic cell lines K562, HL60, and HEL cells, *Exp. Hematol.,* 15, 928, 1987.
291. **Sugarman, B.J., Lewis, G.D., Eessalu, T.E., Aggarwal, B.B., and Shepard, H.M.,** Effects of growth factors on the antiproliferative activity of tumor necrosis factors, *Cancer Res.,* 47, 780, 1987.
292. **Scanlon, M., Laster, S.M., Wood, J.G., and Gooding, L.R.,** Cytolysis by tumor necrosis factor is preceded by a rapid and specific dissolution of microfilaments, *Proc. Natl. Acad. Sci. U.S.A.,* 86, 182, 1989.
293. **Price, S.R., Olivecrona, T., and Pekala, P.H.,** Regulation of lipoprotein lipase synthesis in 3T3-L1 adipocytes by cachectin. Further proof for identity with tumour necrosis factor, *Biochem. J.,* 240, 601, 1986.
294. **Porat, O.,** The effect of tumor necrosis factor α on the activity of lipoprotein lipase in adipose tissue, *Lymphokine Res.,* 8, 459, 1989.
295. **Kawakami, M., Murase, T., Ogawa, H., Ishibashi, S., Mori, N., Takaku, F., and Shibata, S.,** Human recombinant TNF suppresses lipoprotein lipase activity and stimulates lipolysis in 3T3-L1 cells, *J. Biochem.,* 101, 331, 1987.
296. **Cornelius, P., Enerback, S., Bjursell, G., Olivecrona, T., and Pekala, P.H.,** Regulation of lipoprotein lipase mRNA content in 3T3-L1 cells by tumour necrosis factor, *Biochem. J.,* 249, 765, 1988.
297. **Feingold, K.R. and Grunfeld, C.,** Tumor necrosis factor-α stimulates hepatic lipogenesis in the rat in vivo, *J. Clin. Invest.,* 80, 184, 1987.
298. **Feingold, K.R., Serio, M.K., Adi, S., Moser, A.H., and Grunfeld, C.,** Tumor necrosis factor stimulates hepatic lipid synthesis and secretion, *Endocrinology,* 124, 2336, 1989.
299. **Patton, J.S., Shepard, H.M., Wilking, H., Lewis, G., Aggarwal, B.B., Eessalu, T.E., Gavin, L.A., and Grunfeld, C.,** Interferons and tumor necrosis factors have similar catabolic effects on 3T3 L1 cells, *Proc. Natl. Acad. Sci. U.S.A.,* 83, 8313, 1986.
300. **Grunfeld, C., Adi, S., Soued, M., Moser, A., Fiers, W., and Feingold, K.R.,** Search for mediators of the lipogenic effects of tumor necrosis factor: potential role for interleukin 6, *Cancer Res.,* 50, 4233, 1990.
301. **Semb, H., Peterson, J., Tavernier, J., and Olivecrona, T.,** Multiple effects of tumor necrosis factor on lipoprotein lipase *in vivo, J. Biol. Chem.,* 262, 8390, 1987.
302. **Bodnar, R.J., Pasternak, G.W., Mann, P.E., Paul, D., Warren, R., and Donner, D.B.,** Mediation of anorexia by human recombinant tumor necrosis factor through a peripheral action in the rat, *Cancer Res.,* 49, 6280, 1989.
303. **Männel, D.N., Falk, W., and Northoff, H.,** Endotoxic activities of tumor necrosis factor independent of IL1 secretion by macrophages/monocytes, *Lymphokine Res.,* 6, 151, 1987.

304. Tracey, K.J., Beutler, B., Lowry, S.F., Merryweather, J., Wolpe, S., Milsark, I.W., Hariri, R.J., Fahey, T.J., III, Zentella, A., Albert, J.D., Shires, G.T., and Cerami, A., Shock and tissue injury induced by recombinant human cachectin, *Science,* 234, 470, 1986.
305. Gooding, L.R., Elmore, L.W., Tollefson, A.E., Brady, H.A., and Wold, W.S.M., A 14,700 MW protein from the E3 region of adenovirus inhibits cytolysis by tumor necrosis factor, *Cell,* 53, 341, 1988.
306. Chen, M.-J., Holskin, B., Strickler, J., Gorniak, J., Clark, M.A., Johnson, P.J., Mitcho, M., and Shalloway, D., Induction by *E1A* oncogene expression of cellular susceptibility to lysis by TNF, *Nature,* 330, 581, 1987.
307. Oliff, A., Defeo-Jones, D., Boyer, M., Martinez, D., Kiefer, D., Vuocolo, G., Wolfe, A., and Socher, S.H., Tumors secreting human TNF/cachectin induce cachexia in mice, *Cell,* 50, 555, 1987.
308. Socher, S.H., Friedman, A., and Martinez, D., Recombinant human tumor necrosis factor induces acute reductions in food intake and body weight in mice, *J. Exp. Med.,* 167, 1957, 1988.
309. Tracey, K.J., Wei, H., Manogue, K.R., Fong, Y., Hesse, D.G., Nguyen, H.T., Kuo, G.C., Beutler, B., Cotran, R.S., Cerami, A., and Lowry, S.F., Cachectin/tumor necrosis factor induces cachexia, anemia, and inflammation, *J. Exp. Med.,* 167, 1211, 1988.
310. Stovroff, M.C., Fraker, D.L., Swedenborg, J.A., and Norton, J.A., Cachectin/tumor necrosis factor: a possible mediator of cancer anorexia in the rat, *Cancer Res.,* 48, 4567, 1988.
311. Waage, A., Espevik, T., and Lamvik, J., Detection of tumour necrosis factor-like cytotoxicity in serum from patients with septicemia but not from untreated cancer patients, *Scand. J. Immunol.,* 24, 739, 1986.
312. Socher, S.H., Martinez, D., Craig, J.B., Kuhn, J.G., and Oliff, A., Tumor necrosis factor not detectable in patients with clinical cancer cachexia, *J. Natl. Cancer Inst.,* 80, 595, 1988.
313. Tomazic, V.J., Farha, M., Loftus, A., and Elias, G.E., Antitumor activity of recombinant tumor necrosis factor on mouse fibrosarcoma in vivo and in vitro, *J. Immunol.,* 140, 4056, 1988.
314. Schreiber, H., Gressler, V.H., Teng, M.N., Rothstein, J.L., and Rowley, D.A., Cytokines as effectors in tumor immunity, *Immunol. Allergy Clin. N. Am.,* 10, 747, 1990.
315. Beissert, S., Bergholz, M., Waase, I., Lepsien, G., Schauer, A., Pfizenmaier, K., and Krönke, M., Regulation of tumor necrosis factor gene expression in colorectal adenocarcinoma: *in vivo* analysis by *in situ* hybridization, *Proc. Natl. Acad. Sci. U.S.A.,* 89, 5064, 1989.
316. Nobuhara, M., Kanamori, T., Ashida, Y., Ogino, H., Horisawa, Y., Nakayama, K., Asami, T., Iketani, M., Noda, K., Andoh, S., and Kurimoto, M., The inhibition of neoplastic cell proliferation with human natural tumor necrosis factor, *Jpn. J. Cancer Res.,* 78, 193, 1987.
317. Munker, R. and Koeffler, P., In vitro action of tumor necrosis factor on myeloid leukemia cells, *Blood,* 69, 1102, 1987.
318. Creasey, A.A., Reynolds, M.T., and Laird, W., Cures and partial regression of murine and human tumors by recombinant human tumor necrosis factor, *Cancer Res.,* 46, 5687, 1986.
319. Watanabe, N., Niitsu, Y., Neda, H., Sone, H., Yamaucyi, N., Umetsu, T., and Urushizaki, I., Antitumor effect of tumor necrosis factor against various primarily cultured human cancer cells, *Jpn. J. Cancer Res.,* 76, 1115, 1985.
320. Hudziak, R.M., Lewis, G.D., Shalaby, R.F., Eessalu, T.E., Aggarwal, B.B., Ullrich, A., and Shepard, H.M., Amplified expression of the HER2/ERBB2 oncogene induces resistance to tumor necrosis factor α in NIH 3T3 cells, *Proc. Natl. Acad. Sci. U.S.A.,* 85, 5102, 1988.
321. Murase, T., Hotta, T., Saito, H., and Ohno, R., Effect of recombinant human tumor necrosis factor on the colony growth of human leukemia progenitor cells and normal hematopoietic progenitor cells, *Blood,* 69, 467, 1987.
322. Tamatani, T., Urawa, H., Hashimoto, T., and Onozaki, K., Tumor necrosis factor as an interleukin 1-dependent differentiation inducing factor (D-factor) for mouse myeloid leukemic cells, *Biochem. Biophys. Res. Commun.,* 143, 390, 1987.
323. Mareel, M., Dragonetti, C., Tavernier, J., and Fiers, W., Tumor-selective cytotoxic effects of murine tumor necrosis factor (TNF) and interferon γ (IFN-γ) in organ culture of B16 melanoma cells and heart tissue, *Int. J. Cancer,* 42, 470, 1988.
324. Bartsch, H.H., Pfizenmaier, K., Schroeder, M., and Nagel, G.A., Intralesional application of recombinant human tumor necrosis factor α induces local tumor regression in patients with advanced malignancies, *Eur. J. Cancer Clin. Oncol.,* 25, 287, 1989.
325. Coffman, F.D., Green, L.M., and Ware, C.F., The relationship of receptor occupancy to the kinetics of cell death mediated by tumor necrosis factor, *Lymphokine Res.,* 7, 371, 1988.

326. **Duncombe, A.S., Heslop, H.E., Turner, M., Meager, A., Priest, R., Exley, T., and Brenner, M.K.,** Tumor necrosis factor mediates autocrine growth inhibition in a chronic leukemia, *J. Immunol.,* 143, 3828, 1989.
327. **Yoshimura, T. and Sone, S.,** Different and synergistic actions of human tumor necrosis factor and interferon-γ in damage of liposome membranes, *J. Biol. Chem.,* 262, 4597, 1987.
328. **Rubin, B.Y., Smith, L.J., Hellerman, G.R., Lunn, R.M., Richardson, N.K., and Anderson, S.L.,** Correlation between the anticellular and DNA fragmenting activities of tumor necrosis factor, *Cancer Res.,* 48, 6006, 1988.
329. **Coffman, F.D., Green, L.M., Godwin, A., and Ware, C.F.,** Cytotoxicity mediated by tumor necrosis factor in variant subclones of the ME-180 cervical carcinoma line: modulation by specific inhibitors of DNA topoisomerase II, *J. Cell. Biochem.,* 39, 95, 1989.
330. **Elias, L., Moore, P.B., and Rose, S.M.,** Tumor necrosis factor induced DNA fragmentation of HL-60 cells, *Biochem. Biophys. Res. Commun.,* 157, 963, 1988.
331. **Manda, T., Shinomura, K., Mukumoto, S., Kobayashi, K., Mizota, T., Hirai, O., Matsumoto, S., Oku, T., Nishigaki, F., Mori, J., and Kikuchi, H.,** Recombinant human tumor necrosis factor-α: evidence of an indirect mode of antitumor activity, *Cancer Res.,* 47, 3707, 1987.
332. **Pfizenmaier, K., Scheurich, P., Schlüter, C., and Krönke, M.,** Tumor necrosis factor enhances HLA-A, B, C and HLA-DR gene expression in human tumor cells, *J. Immunol.,* 138, 975, 1987.
333. **Asher, A., Mulé, J.J., Reichert, C.M., Shiloni, E., and Rosenberg, S.A.,** Studies on the anti-tumor efficacy of systemically administered recombinant tumor necrosis factor against several murine tumors in vivo, *J. Immunol.,* 138, 963, 1987.
334. **Mace, K.F., Ehrke, M.J., Hori, K., Maccubbin, D.L., and Mihich, E.,** Role of tumor necrosis factor in macrophage activation and tumoricidal activity, *Cancer Res.,* 48, 5427, 1988.
335. **Ortaldo, J.R., Mason, L.L., Mathieson, B.J., Liang, S.-M., Flick, D.A., and Herberman, R.B.,** Mediation of mouse natural cytotoxic activity by tumour necrosis factor, *Nature,* 321, 700, 1986.
336. **Patek, P.Q., Lin, Y., and Collins, J.L.,** Natural cytotoxic cells and tumor necrosis factor activate similar lytic mechanisms, *J. Immunol.,* 138, 1641, 1987.
337. **Feinman, R., Henriksen-DeStefano, D., Tsujimoto, M., and Vilcek, J.,** Tumor necrosis factor is an important mediator of tumor cell killing by human monocytes, *J. Immunol.,* 138, 635, 1987.
338. **Urban, J.L., Shepard, H.M., Rothstein, J.L., Sugarman, B.J., and Schreiber, H.,** Tumor necrosis factor: a potent effector molecule for tumor cell killing by activated macrophages, *Proc. Natl. Acad. Sci. U.S.A.,* 83, 5233, 1986.
339. **Kornbluth, R.S. and Eddington, T.S.,** Tumor necrosis factor production by human monocytes is a regulated event: induction of TNF-α-mediated cellular cytotoxicity by endotoxin, *J. Immunol.,* 137, 2585, 1986.
340. **Hori, K., Ehrke, M.J., Mace, K., Maccubbin, D., Doyle, M.J., Otsuka, Y., and Mihich, E.,** Effect of recombinant human tumor necrosis factor on the induction of murine macrophage tumoricidal activity, *Cancer Res.,* 47, 2793, 1987.
341. **Kokunai, I., Shimano, T., Sekimoto, K., Takeda, T., Kobayashi, T., Yayoi, E., Yamamoto, A., and Mori, T.,** Induction of tumor necrosis factor by administration of OK-432 in cancer patients, *J. Clin. Lab. Immunol.,* 21, 169, 1986.
342. **Hahn, C.J., Ovak, G.M., Donovan, R.M., and Pauly, J.L.,** Effect of human recombinant tumor necrosis factor on the growth of different human and mouse long-term hematopoietic cell lines, *J. Leukocyte Biol.,* 40, 21, 1986.
343. **Spriggs, D.R., Imamura, K., Rodriguez, C., Sariban, E., and Kufe, D.W.,** Tumor necrosis factor expression in human epithelial tumor cell lines, *J. Clin. Invest.,* 81, 455, 1988.
344. **Vanhaesebroeck, B., Mareel, M., Van Roy, F., Grooten, J., and Fiers, W.,** Expression of the tumor necrosis factor gene in tumor cells correlates with reduced tumorigenicity and reduced invasiveness in vivo, *Cancer Res.,* 51, 2229, 1991.
345. **Ishihara, J., Saijo, N., Sasaki, Y., Nakano, H., Ozaki, A., Tatakashi, H., Sakurai, M., Nakagawa, K., Iigo, M., Kanzawa, F., Hoshi, A., Hong, W.S., Jett, J.R., and Takahashi, T.,** The different effects of recombinant human tumor necrosis factor on rat fibrosarcoma sublines, *Cancer Immunol. Immunother.,* 24, 185, 1987.
346. **Vanhaesebroeck, B., Van Bladel, S., Lenaerts, A., Suffys, P., Beyaert, R., Lucas, R., Van Roy, F., and Fiers, W.,** Two discrete types of tumor necrosis factor-resistant cells derived from the same cell line, *Cancer Res.,* 51, 2469, 1991.

347. **Bollon, A.P., Berent, S.L., Torczynski, R.M., Hill, N.O., Lemeshev, Y., Hill, J.M., Jia, F.L., Joher, A., Pichyangkul, S., and Khan, A.,** Human cytokines, tumor necrosis factor, and interferons: gene cloning, animal studies, and clinical trials, *J. Cell. Biochem.,* 36, 353, 1988.
348. **Abboud, S.L., Gerson, S.L., and Berger, N.A.,** The effect of tumor necrosis factor on normal human hematopoietic progenitors, *Cancer,* 60, 2965, 1987.
349. **Heicappell, R., Naito, S., Ichinose, Y., Creasey, A.A., Lin, L.S., and Fidler, I.J.,** Cytostatic and cytolytic effects of human recombinant tumor necrosis factor on human renal cell carcinoma cell lines derived from a single surgical specimen, *J. Immunol.,* 138, 1634, 1987.
350. **Digel, W., Stefanic, M., Schöniger, W., Buck, C., Raghavachar, A., Frickhofen, N., Heimpel, H., and Porzsolt, F.,** Tumor necrosis factor induces proliferation of neoplastic B cells from chronic lymphocytic leukemia, *Blood,* 73, 1242, 1989.
351. **Goillot, E., Combaret, V., Ladenstein, R., Baubet, D., Blay, J.-Y., Philip, T., and Favrot, M.C.,** Tumor necrosis factor as an autocrine growth factor for neuroblastoma, *Cancer Res.,* 52, 3194, 1992.
352. **Yagi, M.J., Holland, J.F., and Bekesi, J.G.,** Tumor necrosis factor enhances murine SL3-3 retrovirus replication, *J. Clin. Lab. Immunol.,* 24, 129, 1987.
353. **Chen, L., Suzuki, Y., and Wheelock, E.F.,** Interferon-γ synergizes with tumor necrosis factor and with interleukin 1 and requires the presence of both monokines to induce antitumor cytotoxic activity in macrophages, *J. Immunol.,* 139, 4096, 1987.
354. **Schiller, J.H., Bittner, G., Storer, B., and Willson, J.K.V.,** Synergistic antitumor effects of tumor necrosis factor and γ-interferon on human colon carcinoma cell lines, *Cancer Res.,* 47, 2809, 1987.
355. **Talmadge, J.E., Phillips, H., Schindler, J., Tribble, H., and Pennington, R.,** Systematic preclinical study on the therapeutic properties of recombinant human interleukin 2 for the treatment of metastatic disease, *Cancer Res.,* 47, 5725, 1987.
356. **Winkelhake, J.L., Stampfl, S., and Zimmerman, R.J.,** Synergistic effects of combination therapy with human recombinant interleukin-2 tumor necrosis factor in murine tumor models, *Cancer Res.,* 47, 3948, 1987.
357. **Brouckaert, P.G.G., Leroux-Roels, G.G., Guisez, Y., Tavernier, J., and Fiers, W.,** *In vivo* anti-tumor activity of recombinant human and murine TNF, alone and in combination with murine IFN-γ, on a syngeneic murine melanoma, *Int. J. Cancer,* 38, 763, 1986.
358. **Wong, G.H.W., Krowka, J.F., Stites, D.P., and Goeddel, D.V.,** In vitro anti-human immunodeficiency virus activities of tumor necrosis factor-α and interferon-γ, *J. Immunol.,* 140, 120, 1988.
359. **Regenass, U., Müller, M., Curschellas, E., and Matter, A.,** Anti-tumor effects of tumor necrosis factor in combination with chemotherapeutic agents, *Int. J. Cancer,* 39, 266, 1987.
360. **Alexander, R.B., Nelson, W.G., and Coffey, D.S.,** Synergistic enhancement by tumor necrosis factor of *in vitro* cytotoxicity from chemotherapeutic drugs targeted at DNA topoisomerase II, *Cancer Res.,* 47, 2403, 1987.
361. **Ha, D.K.K., Cheng, C.P., Fung, K.P., Choy, Y.M., and Lee, C.Y.,** Effect of anti-inflammatory drugs on the production of tumour necrosis factor and lipopolysaccharide-induced mortality in mice, *Cancer Lett.,* 34, 291, 1987.
362. **Lewis, G.D., Aggarwal, B.B., Eesalu, T.E., Sugarman, B.J., and Shepard, H.M.,** Modulation of the growth of transformed cells by human tumor necrosis factor-α and interferon-γ, *Cancer Res.,* 47, 5382, 1987.
363. **Komori, A., Yatsunami, J., Sugamuna, M., Okabe, S., Abe, S., Sakai, A., Sasaki, K., and Fujiki, H.,** Tumor necrosis factor acts as a tumor promoter in BALB/3T3 cell transformation, *Cancer Res.,* 53, 1982, 1993.
364. **Cordingley, F.T., Bianchi, A., Hoffbrand, A.V., Reittie, J.E., Heslop, H.E., Vyakarnam, A., Turner, M., Meager, A., and Brenner, M.K.,** Tumour necrosis factor as an autocrine tumour growth factor for chronic B-cell malignancies, *Lancet,* 1, 969, 1988.
365. **Naylor, M.S., Stamp, G.W.H., Foulkes, W.D., Eccles, D., and Balkwill, F.R.,** Tumor necrosis factor and its receptors in human ovarian cancer. Potential role in disease progression, *J. Clin. Invest.,* 91, 2194, 1993.
366. **Takeda, K., Iwamoto, S., Sugimoto, H., Takuma, T., Kawatani, N., Noda, M., Masaki, A., Morise, H., Arimura, H., and Konno, K.,** Identity of differentiation inducing factor and tumour necrosis factor, *Nature,* 323, 338, 1986.
367. **Ishikura, H., Hori, K., and Bloch, A.,** Differential biologic effects resulting from bimodal binding of recombinant human tumor necrosis factor to myeloid leukemia cells, *Blood,* 73, 419, 1989.

368. **Kawakami, M., Watanabe, N., Ogawa, H., Kato, A., Sando, H., Yamada, N., Murase, T., Takaku, F., Shibata, S., and Oda, T.,** Cachectin/TNF kills or inhibits the differentiation of 3T3-L1 cells according to developmental stage, *J. Cell. Physiol.,* 138, 1, 1989.
369. **Hemmi, H., Nakamura, T., Tamura, K., Shimizu, Y., Kato, S., Miki, T., Takahashi, N., Muramatsu, M., Numao, N., and Sugamura, K.,** Lymphotoxin: induction of terminal differentiation of the human myeloid leukemia cell lines HL-60 and THP-1, *J. Immunol.,* 138, 664, 1987.
370. **Squinto, S.P., Doucet, J.P., Block, A.L., Morrow, S.L., and Davenport, W.D., Jr.,** Induction of macrophage-like differentiation of HL-60 leukemia cells by tumor necrosis factor-α: potential role of *fos* expression, *Mol. Endocrinol.,* 3, 409, 1989.
371. **Kharbanda, S., Nakamura, T., Datta, R., Sherman, M.L., and Kufe, D.,** Induction of monocytic differentiation by tumor necrosis factor in phorbol ester-resistant KG-1a cells, *Cancer Commun.,* 2, 327, 1990.
372. **Katakami, Y., Nakao, Y., Katakami, N., Koizumi, T., Ogawa, R., Yamada, H., Takai, Y., and Fujita, T.,** Cooperative effects of tumor necrosis factor-α and 1,25-dihydroxyvitamin D_3 on growth inhibition, differentiation, and c-*myc* reduction in human promyelocytic leukemia cell line HL-60, *Biochem. Biophys. Res. Commun.,* 152, 1151, 1988.
373. **Trinchieri, G., Rosen, M., and Perussia, B.,** Induction of differentiation of human myeloid cell lines by tumor necrosis factor in cooperation with 1α,25-dihydroxyvitamin D_3, *Cancer Res.,* 47, 2236, 1987.
374. **McAchren, S.S., Jr., Salehi, Z., Weinberg, J.B., and Niedel, J.E.,** Transcription interruption may be a common mechanism of c-myc regulation during HL-60 differentiation, *Biochem. Biophys. Res. Commun.,* 151, 574, 1988.
375. **Onozaki, K., Urawa, H., Tamatani, T., Iwamura, Y., Hashimoto, T., Baba, T., Suzuki, H., Yamada, M., Yamamoto, S., Oppenheim, J.J., and Matsushima, K.,** Synergistic interactions of interleukin 1, interferon-β, and tumor necrosis factor in terminally differentiating a mouse myeloid leukemic cell line (M1), *J. Immunol.,* 140, 112, 1988.
376. **Cohen, M.C. and Cohen, S.,** The role of lymphokines in neoplastic disease, *Hum. Pathol.,* 17, 264, 1986.
377. **Itoh, A., Ohsawa, F., and Natori, S.,** Purification of a cytotoxic protein produced by the murine macrophage-like cell line J774.1 in response to *Sarcophaga* lectin, *J. Biochem.,* 99, 9, 1986.
378. **Itoh, A., Iizuka, K., and Natori, S.,** Antitumor effect of *Sarcophaga* lectin on murine transplanted tumors, *Jpn. J. Cancer Res.,* 76, 1027, 1985.
379. **Okhuma, Y., Komano, H., and Natori, S.,** Participation of common surface receptor(s) in the activation of murine macrophages by *Sarcophaga* lectin and wheat germ agglutinin, *Cancer Res.,* 46, 3648, 1986.
380. **Itoh, A., Ohsawa, F., Ohkuma, Y., and Natori, S.,** Participation of tumor killing factor in the antitumor effect of *Sarcophaga* lectin, *FEBS Lett.,* 201, 37, 1986.
381. **Nakai, M. and Natori, S.,** Rapid inactivation of tumor killing factor *in vitro*, *J. Biochem.,* 101, 303, 1987.
382. **Ohsawa, F. and Natori, S.,** Analysis of murine cellular receptors for tumor-killing factor, *Cancer Res.,* 47, 42, 1987.

Chapter 6

Erythropoietic Growth Factors

I. INTRODUCTION

The process of formation of red blood cells (erythropoiesis) occurs through a series of sequential stages which involve the proliferation and progressive differentiation of different types of erythroid cells (Figure 1). In the mammalian organism, this complex process takes place in the fetal liver and the adult bone marrow, and its final result is the production of an enormous number of mature erythrocytes whose main function is the transport of oxygen from the lung to peripheral tissues. A normal person of 70 kg has approximately 2.3×10^{13} red blood cells that are synthesized at a rate of about 2.3×10^6/s. Hypoxic stress induces a marked increase in the rate of erythrocyte production. Erythrocytes have a finite life span and aged cells from the erythrocyte population are eliminated and continuously replaced by freshly produced mature erythrocytes. An insufficient production of erythrocytes, or an increased destruction or loss of these cells, may result in anemia. Peripheral tissue hypoxia, due to blood loss or decreased atmospheric oxygen at high altitudes, induces an increase in erythrocyte production.

Erythropoiesis is subjected to multiple control mechanisms which involve hormones, growth factors, iron supply, oxygen tension, and other endogenous and exogenous agents. Erythropoietin is the most important and specific regulator of erythropoiesis. Its action takes place mainly from the stages of colony-forming units erythroid (CFU-E) to basophilic erythroblast. CFU-Es are highly responsive to erythropoietin and can generate human erythroblast colonies in approximately 7 days. In addition to erythropoietin, other endogenous factors are involved in the stimulation of erythroid progenitor cell proliferation and differentiation. Testosterone is one such substance because it cooperates with erythropoietin in the regulation of RNA synthesis in marrow cells.[1,2] CSF-2, CSF-3, and IL-3 are all able to initiate proliferation of the earlier erythroid precursors, and other HGFs may have a role in controlling the proliferation of erythroid precursors through the subsequent stages of differentiation.[3] IL-3 is capable of stimulating the full development of many erythroid burst-forming units (BFU-E) *in vitro,* even in the absence of serum and erythropoietin.[4] However, IL-3 alone is unable to support the terminal differentiation of cells from the erythroid lineage, which requires the action of erythropoietin.[5]

IGF-I and/or insulin is required for the production of CFU-E *in vitro.*[6] A heparin-binding erythroid cell-stimulating factor (ECSF) from fetal bovine serum is identical with IGF-II.[7] IGF-II is captured in the extracellular matrix and is able to act in a manner similar to that of FGF, IL-3, or CSF-2. The TGF-α receptor may cooperate with the estrogen receptor in the regulation of chicken erythroid progenitor self-renewal.[8]

It is thus clear that many hormones and growth factors are capable of regulating the proliferation and differentiation of erythroid cells *in vitro.* However, the respective roles of testosterone, estrogen, IL-3, IGF-I, IGF-II, insulin, TGF-α, erythropoietin, and other hormones and growth factors in erythropoiesis occurring in the intact animal are unknown. IL-3 and other factors may be the stimulus for early erythroid progenitor proliferation, and erythropoietin may act later in the maturation progression. The cellular mechanisms involved in the regulation of erythropoiesis by hormones and growth factors also are unknown, but there is evidence that changes at the level of gene expression may have an important role in such complex processes.

Both common and specific transcription factors may be involved in the regulation of gene expression in cells committed to the erythroid lineage. One of these factors, the erythroid transcription factor NF-E2, is a hematopoietic-specific basic leucine zipper protein.[9] The expression of certain proto-oncogenes may be altered during erythropoiesis. Expression of the c-*myc* gene decreases during erythroid differentiation and this change shows a good correlation with an increased expression of transferrin receptors in the maturing cells.[10] However, the precise role of the products of c-*myc* and other proto-oncogenes in erythropoiesis is unknown.

II. ERYTHROID-POTENTIATING ACTIVITY

Erythroid-potentiating activity (EPA) is a growth factor with burst-promoting activity (BPA), i.e., it stimulates the growth of early erythroid progenitors referred to as BFU-E, which gives rise to colonies

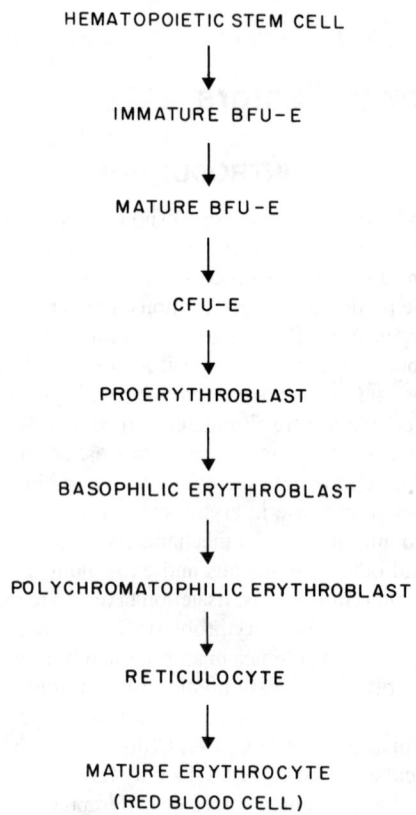

Figure 6.1 Stages of normal erythroid differentiation.

of hemoglobinized cells. Human EPA specifically stimulates the growth of peripheral blood- and bone marrow-derived erythroid precursors from mouse and man. However, the physiological activities of EPA *in vivo* are unknown. The EPA molecule has strong protease inhibitory properties and is also referred to as the tissue inhibitor of metalloproteinases (TIMP).[11] The TIMP is a major inhibitor of matrix metalloproteinases and is secreted in high amounts by differentiating cells. The precise relationship between the mitogenic and enzyme-inhibitory activities of EPA is not understood.

EPA is a 28-kDa glycoprotein which specifically stimulates cells of the erythroid lineage. Results of studies performed with an EPA cDNA clone indicate that human EPA is encoded by a single gene of 3 kb, interrupted by at least two introns.[12] The gene encoding EPA has been assigned to human chromosome X and is localized in the region Xp11.1-p11.4.[13] A major retroviral core protein has been identified as structurally related to EPA.[14]

EPA may be involved in autocrine regulation of the growth of the K562 human erythroleukemia cell line.[15] EPA mRNA and protein is produced by K562 cells, and these cells possess EPA receptors of 32 kDa. Treatment of K562 cells with phorbol ester results in megakaryoblastic differentiation and markedly increased EPA/TIMP secretion, which is preceded by enhanced c-*fos* and c-*jun* proto-oncogene transcription and formation of the AP-1 transcription factor.[16]

III. ERYTHROID BURST-PROMOTING ACTIVITY

An erythropoiesis-stimulating factor, the erythroid burst-promoting activity (EBPA), was purified from the membranes of normal, unstimulated human peripheral blood lymphocytes.[17,18] Release of EBPA by lymphocytes may contribute to the regulation of erythropoietic activity from precursor cells located in the vicinity. EBPA is a 28-kDa glycoprotein which stimulates erythroid burst formation in serum-free human bone marrow culture and exhibits no apparent synergistic interactions with other growth factors. It is distinct from EPA and is devoid of GM-CSF activity, and has negligible effect on the formation of human megakaryocytes and mixed hematopoietic clones. EBPA is exfoliated from lymphocyte surface membrane components and acts on the earliest committed erythroid progenitor cells. However, the exact physiological role of EBPA is not understood. Studies related to the effects of recombinant human erythropoietin on serum-free cultures of hematopoietic cells have demonstrated that erythropoietin itself, in the absence of EBPA, has the ability to induce burst formation of primitive erythroid progenitors.[19]

Clinical hypothyroidism is often complicated by anemia and this defect can be corrected by administration of thyroid hormone alone. BFU-E is particularly sensitive to the effect of thyroid hormone, and these effects are mediated by the release of soluble EBPA-like molecules from accessory cells in culture.[20] One of these molecules may be represented by EBPA itself.

IV. ERYTHROPOIETIN

Erythropoietin is centrally involved in the regulation of red blood cell formation.[21-29] It one of the few characterized substances that has been shown to be involved with a specific effect on a single pathway of cell differentiation. With only rare exceptions, erythropoiesis in mammals is absolutely dependent on erythropoietin. Under normal conditions the rate of red cell production is adjusted to the oxygen demand and supply in the peripheral tissues. This adjustment is accomplished by a feedback circuit linking oxygen sensors in the tissues to the erythroid cells in the bone marrow, and mediated by the red cells in one direction and the hormone, erythropoietin, in the opposite direction. Consequently, the level of erythropoietin in blood must be inversely related to the number of circulating red cells.[30]

A. ORIGIN AND SYNTHESIS OF ERYTHROPOIETIN

Synthesis of erythropoietin in the whole animal is increased in response to lowered tissue oxygen tension (hypoxia) and decreased under conditions of hyperoxia. The major sites of oxygen sensing and erythropoietin production are the liver during fetal life and the kidney in the adult. Kidney mass loss associated with chronic renal failure and other renal diseases may result in anemia due to decreased production of erythropoietin. Transcripts of the human erythropoietin gene have been detected in the kidney as well as in the fetal and adult liver.[31] Tissue hypoxia due to anemia or bleeding, as well as by the injection of cobalt chloride, can induce the accumulation of erythropoietin mRNA in the rat kidney and liver.[32-34] In adult rats and mice, the accumulation of erythropoietin mRNA upon stimulation by cobalt injection occurs almost exclusively in the kidney. Erythropoietin mRNA appears in the kidney between 3 and 6 h after injection of cobalt. The production of erythropoietin in the kidney is regulated, at least in part, at the transcriptional level, but the mechanisms by which changes in kidney oxygen tension modulate expression of the erythropoietin gene is unknown. The human erythropoietin gene contains promoter and enhancer elements that are appropriately responsive to hypoxia and cobalt.[35] Both transcriptional and posttranscriptional mechanisms may be involved in regulating erythropoietin mRNA levels. The stability of erythropoietin mRNA is modulated by the transcription and translation of rapidly cycling gene product(s).[36]

The human cell line RC-1 is characterized by the continuous production of erythropoietin.[37] Two established human hepatoma cell lines (Hep3B and HepG2) synthesize large amounts of erythropoietin mRNA and protein in response to hypoxia or $CoCl_2$.[38] Erythropoietin has been purified to homogeneity from the urine of patients with severe aplastic anemia.[39]

B. BIOLOGICAL EFFECTS OF ERYTHROPOIETIN

Erythropoietin is the primary factor regulating red blood cell formation in mammals and some other animals.[21-29] It is both a mitogen and a survival factor for erythropoietic cells.[40] The concentration of erythropoietin in the blood is of approximately 0.01 nM under normal conditions and is increased under conditions of hypoxia. Erythropoietin exerts its physiological activities through binding to specific receptors on erythroid progenitor cells, which results in the induction of progenitor cell differentiation into mature erythrocytes. Erythroid progenitors (CFU-E) are abundant in the fetal liver and IGF-I is involved in the regulation of erythropoietin-stimulated proliferation and differentiation of these progenitors.[41] Incorporation of thymidine in cell cultures of erythroid cells from fetal calf and rat livers reaches the highest values when both erythropoietin and IGF-I are added simultaneously to the medium.[42] In addition to its effect on DNA synthesis and cell proliferation, in erythropoietin-sensitive erythroid precursors the hormone is involved in the maintenance of cell viability and maturation through stimulation of RNA and protein synthesis.[43] The effect of erythropoietin on the differentiation of erythroid cells may be independent from those related to the stimulation of DNA synthesis. Cell division is not required for the commitment of CFU-E cells to differentiation by erythropoietin.[44]

Erythropoietin is not only involved in the production of erythrocytes but also in preventing the programmed death (apoptosis) of erythroid progenitors by retarding DNA breakdown, thus promoting the survival of erythroid cells.[45,46]

In addition to its effects on erythropoiesis, erythropoietin can stimulate megakaryocyte colony formation in semisolid culture medium. High-affinity binding sites for erythropoietin are present on rodent megakaryocytes.[47] However, studies with a recombinant human erythropoietin preparation on murine megakaryocyte colony formation, using serum-free and serum-containing culture systems, have demonstrated that erythropoietin alone is insufficient for megakaryocyte colony growth and that it requires a factor present in serum to stimulate megakaryocyte colony formation.[48] IL-3 may be required by erythropoietin to stimulate megakaryocyte colony formation.

Human erythropoietin has a mitogenic and positive chemotactic effect on endothelial cells.[49] The hormone exerts in a dose-dependent fashion a proliferative effect on human umbilical-vein endothelial cells and bovine adrenal capillary endothelial cells, and binding studies revealed the existence of a large number of receptors with high affinity for erythropoietin.

C. STRUCTURE OF ERYTHROPOIETIN AND THE ERYTHROPOIETIN GENE

Erythropoietin is a glycoprotein which has been purified from the plasma of animals made artificially anemic and from the urine of severely anemic patients. The gene coding for erythropoietin is located on human chromosome region 7q21.[50] The human gene has been cloned and its expression in a mammalian system (CHO cells) yielded a secreted product with full biological activity.[31,51,52]

The circulating human hormone is composed of 165 amino acids and has two disulfide bonds which are essential for biological activity.[53] The hormone has one site with *O*-linked and three sites with *N*-linked oligosaccharides, which are also required for full biological activity *in vivo*. The calculated molecular weight of the polypeptide moiety of the human erythropoietin molecule is 18,398 Da.[54] Recombinant human erythropoietin is equivalent to the natural hormone in its physiological action,[55] and is free of major side effects when applied therapeutically. The recombinant hormone is a potent stimulus for erythroid and multilineage colony formation *in vitro*.[56]

The erythropoietin gene from the *Cynomolgus* monkey *(Macaca fascicularis)* was cloned from a kidney cDNA library.[57] It encodes a 168-amino acid mature protein. Upon transfection into CHO cells, the monkey erythropoietin gene directed the synthesis of a biologically active glycosylated protein of 34-kDa. The monkey gene exhibits 92% homology to the human gene, and the homology at the amino acid level is 94%. Cloning and sequencing of the mouse erythropoietin gene also indicates a high degree of amino acid sequence conservation between the mouse and human hormone.[58,59] Erythropoietin exhibits no significant homology with any known protein. However, the amino-terminal portion of an erythropoietin-like polypeptide (ELP) isolated from bovine fetal serum shows sequence homology with the low density lipoprotein (LDL) receptor as well as with two proteins of the Epstein-Barr virus.[60]

D. THE ERYTHROPOIETIN RECEPTOR

The physiologic action of erythropoietin is initiated by its binding to a high-affinity receptor on the cell surface.[61-64] Specific binding sites for erythropoietin were first detected in erythroid progenitor cells obtained from the spleen of mice treated with the so-called anemic strain of F-MuLV.[65-67] The number of erythropoietin binding sites varies according to the differentiation state of the erythroid cells. Primitive human BFU-E have a much lower number of erythropoietin receptors than cells from CFU-E.[68] The BFU-E develop an increased concentration of the receptors in association with their maturation to CFU-E and the loss of proliferative capacity. Erythropoietin receptors expressed in erythroid cells and the placentas of human, mouse, and rat are similar.[69]

The erythropoietin receptor is a member of the cytokine receptor superfamily, which includes the receptors for IL-2, IL-3, IL-4, IL-5, IL-6, IL-7, CSF-2, and CSF-3. In spite of their structural similarities, the downstream signaling mechanisms of these receptors, at least in part, are different.[70] The murine erythropoietin receptor, as deduced from the cloned cDNA, is a polypeptide composed of 507 amino acids which comprises an extracellular ligand-binding domain of 223 amino acids, a single transmembrane domain of 24 amino acids, and a cytoplasmic domain of 236 amino acids. The extracellular domain of the receptor protein contains five cysteine residues. Residues between Pro-353 and His-362 and between Gln-278 and Leu-308, which are conserved among the hematopoietin/cytokine receptor superfamily, would be the functionally essential cytoplasmic domains of the receptor molecule.[71] Mutational substitution of amino acids from a conserved cytoplasmic region of the receptor, proximal to the transmembrane domain, completely abolishes all the functions of the receptor including the induction of mitogenesis, the phosphorylation of cellular proteins, and the expression of immediate-early genes such as c-*myc*, c-*fos*, and *egr*-1.[72]

cDNAs for the human erythropoietin receptor have been isolated and characterized.[73,74] The human gene is located on chromosome 19p and contains 8 exons spread over 6 kb of DNA. It encodes a polypeptide of 508 amino acids that exhibits a high degree of homology (over 80%) to the murine protein. Recombinant human erythropoietin binds to normal human bone marrow mononuclear cells that may contain two classes of binding sites, one of high affinity and the other of low affinity.[75] Extremely low numbers of erythropoietin receptors (four to six sites per cell) are present in human erythroleukemic cell lines, for example, in human K562 cells. The cloning, expression, and biologic characterization of the human erythropoietin receptor has been reported.[76,77] The derived 508-amino acid sequence is highly homologous to the murine receptor, particularly in the extracellular domain. Erythropoietin can induce tyrosine phosphorylation of the carboxy-terminal portion its own receptor in human erythropoietin-responsive cells.[78] Although the precise role of this modification is not understood, it may be responsible, at least in part, for the transductional mechanisms of erythropoietin action.

A model for the subunit structure and activation of the receptor for erythropoietin has been proposed.[79] The human and murine receptor may contain other components in addition to the 66-kDa polypeptide of 507/508 amino acids.[80] In particular, two polypeptides of approximately 85 and 100 kDa, which are unrelated to the 66-kDa polypeptide, could be subunits of the receptor molecule. In the hematopoietic cell line TF-1, established from the marrow cells of a patient with erythroleukemia, the receptor appears to be represented by two types of molecules of 105 kDa and 90 kDa.[81] The results from some studies suggest that the murine erythropoietin receptor consists of two subunits bridged by disulfide bonds.[82,83] However, the precise structure and function of the 85- and 100-kDa polypeptides are not clear as yet. Proteolytic digestion of the receptor present in the mouse spleen yields identical fragments from the 100- and 85-kDa proteins, suggesting that the sequences of these two proteins is similar or identical. The 85-kDa polypeptide is derived by proteolytic cleavage of the 100-kDa receptor.[84]

Expression of the mouse erythropoietin receptor gene depends on specific sequences contained in its 5'-flanking promoter region.[85] No TATA or CAAT boxes characteristic of many tissue-specific genes are present in the vicinity of the transcription initiation sites of the erythropoietin receptor gene, but the gene has potential binding sites for the ubiquitous Sp-1 and the erythroid-specific GATA-1 transcription factors.[64]

Occupancy of a relatively small number of high-affinity receptors for erythropoietin may be sufficient for eliciting a response in sensitive cells. The mouse erythroleukemia cell line SKT6 can be induced to differentiate by treatment with erythropoietin despite the fact that it expresses a small number of erythropoietin receptors.[86] Only 15 molecules of erythropoietin bound to the receptor on the surface of SKT6 cells may be sufficient to generate a specific cellular response. The receptor-binding site of erythropoietin is located at the carboxyl-terminal domain of the hormone molecule.[87] After binding to its receptor on the surface of erythroid cells, the hormone is internalized and degraded, probably in the lysosomal compartment of the cell.[88]

Erythropoietin receptors may be expressed by hematopoietic cells not pertaining to the erythroid lineage. High-affinity receptors for erythropoietin have been detected in bone marrow cells from patients with various hematological disorders.[89] Megakaryocytes and some mononuclear cells, probably representing early erythroid precursors, as well as immature cells of the myeloid lineage can bind erythropoietin, but no binding is detected in mature erythrocytes. In general, erythropoietin binding is confined to 4 to 5% of human marrow cells. The biological significance of erythropoietin binding to mature cells from nonerythroid lineages is not understood. The only nonerythroid cells in human bone marrow that bind significant amounts of erythropoietin may be the megakaryocytes, and the binding increases with the maturation of these cells.[90] IL-3-dependent cell lines from the myeloid and mast-cell lineages express functional erythropoietin receptors, and this expression is modulated by IL-3.[91,92] Erythropoietin exerts a mitogenic and positive chemotactic effect on human and bovine endothelial cells, which appear to express high-affinity erythropoietin receptors represented by a 45-kDa protein.[49]

The possible role of the erythropoietin receptor in hematologic human diseases such as polycytemia vera, familial erythrocytosis, and congenital red blood cell aplasia is unknown. A truncated erythropoietin receptor may be the cause of dominantly inherited benign human erythrocytosis.[93]

E. POSTRECEPTOR MECHANISMS OF ACTION OF ERYTHROPOIETIN

Little is known about the postreceptor events of erythropoietin action. Changes in adenylyl cyclase activity and/or $[Ca^{2+}]_i$ could have a role in the mechanisms of erythropoietin action, but these changes may be insufficient per se to elicit the proliferation of erythropoietin-responsive erythroblasts.[94] The erythropoietin-stimulated increase in $[Ca^{2+}]_i$ occurs in late, but not in early, human erythroid precursors and may have a role in erythroblast differentiation rather than proliferation.[95] Erythropoietin action on responsive erythroid cells does not seem to depend on acute changes in $[Ca^{2+}]_i$.[96] Studies with an erythropoietin- and IL-3-dependent subclone of the murine cell line DA-1 have shown that cAMP is not a second messenger for the action of erythropoietin or IL-3 on these cells.[97] Phosphorylation of an erythroid membrane protein of 43 kDa (pp43) is rapidly altered by erythropoietin.[98] Rapid activation of protein kinase C by erythropoietin may occur in the nucleus of erythroid progenitor cells.[99] Phosphorylation of cellular proteins on tyrosine may have an important role in the mechanism of action of erythropoietin. There is a correlation between the mitogenic effect of erythropoietin in DA-3 cells (an IL-3-dependent cell line derived from M-MuLV-induced leukemia) and the phosphorylation of a 72-kDa protein.[100] Erythropoietin induces tyrosine phosphorylation and kinase activity of the c-Fps/Fes proto-oncogene product in human erythropoietin-responsive cells.[101] Since the receptor of erythropoietin lacks the sequences that characterize tyrosine kinases, the receptor may be coupled to cellular tyrosine kinases. Tyrosine phosphorylation of the carboxy-terminal portion of the erythropoietin receptor may determine the association of the receptor with cellular proteins containing SH2 domains, such as the phosphatidylinositol 3-kinase (PI 3-kinase).[102]

Ras proteins may be involved in the mechanism of action of erythropoietin. Stimulation of a human erythroleukemic cell line (HEL cells) with erythropoietin resulted in a rapid increase in the amount of GTP bound to endogenous p21 Ras protein.[103] The Ras activation by erythropoietin may be associated with stimulation of tyrosine-protein kinases, tyrosine phosphorylation of GTPase activating protein (GAP), and inhibition of GAP activity.

Erythropoietin-induced maturation of MEL cells is associated with an increase in the number of transferrin receptors, but the rate of iron uptake from transferrin remains constant and the amount of transferrin internalized during the steady-state binding of transferrin does not change.[104] IL-1 antagonizes some of the late postreceptor events of erythropoietin action.[105] Porphobilinogen deaminase is the key enzyme induced by erythropoietin during normal erythroid differentiation, and the control of heme synthesis appears to be at the level of tetrapyrrole synthesis.[106] The effect of erythropoietin on the increase of porphobilinogen deaminase appears to be at the level of transcription.

The physiologic effects of erythropoietin are related, at least in part, to selective alterations in gene expression and induction of DNA synthesis in target cells such as erythroblasts.[107-109] The hormone stimulates the activity of RNA polymerases and induces the synthesis of globin mRNA in immature erythroblasts. Testosterone may synergize the effects of erythropoietin for hemoglobin synthesis.[110] The molecular mechanism by which erythropoietin induces DNA synthesis and mitosis in target cells is unknown, but the hormone is required only in the G_1 phase for the cells to progress through the cell cycle.[111]

The possible role of proto-oncogenes in the mechanisms of action of erythropoietin is unknown. Expression of c-*myc* by a protein kinase C-dependent pathway is an early response to erythropoietin in both normal and leukemic murine erythroid cells.[112,113] Among eight proto-oncogenes examined during *in vitro* differentiation of human BFU-E, c-*myc*, and c-*fos* proto-oncogene expression decreased during differentiation.[113] Addition of erythropoietin together with EBPA induced c-*myc* and c-*fos* gene expression in serum-free cultured progenies of BFU-E. In two murine cell lines which expressed c-*myc* and c-*myb* transcripts before stimulation, and which responded to erythropoietin in different ways, erythropoietin induced c-*fos* and c-*myb* RNA, whereas c-*myc* RNA remained unchanged.[114] The results suggested that the c-*fos* gene is involved in the early signaling system of erythropoietin, and that the c-*myb* gene is involved in erythroid differentiation but not in proliferation.

F. ERYTHROPOIETIN AND NEOPLASTIC TRANSFORMATION

Human erythroblastic leukemia cells differ from normal erythropoietic cells by both an autonomous growth in relation to specific growth factors and a relative blockage in their terminal differentiation.[116] Leukemic erythroid clonogenic cells arise from expansion of erythroid progenitors at different stages of differentiation, i.e., from early or late BFU-E, or from more mature progenitors which are represented by CFU-E. The autonomous growth of human erythroleukemia cells may be associated in some cases to an autocrine secretion of erythropoietin.[117]

Erythropoietin-like activity is produced in tumor cells such as human renal cell and hepatocellular carcinomas.[118] Studies with *in situ* hybridization have indicated that tumor cells of epithelial origin are the site of erythropoietin production in patients with renal adenocarcinoma and polycythemia.[119] Erythropoiesis in chronic myelogenous leukemia is generally erythropoietin-dependent.[120] The retroviruses H-MuSV and K-MuSV, which contain the v-H-*ras* and v-K-*ras* oncogenes, respectively, can alter the growth of erythroid cells *in vitro,* inducing erythropoietin-dependent proliferation.[121] In this system, self-renewal appears to be restricted despite the presence of the retrovirus, and the cells eventually undergo extensive hemoglobinization, indicating that they can reach a state of terminal differentiation. A variant from the Rauscher erythroleukemia cell line (Red 5-1.5), which contains erythropoietin receptors, exhibits differentiation markers upon treatment with erythropoietin, including increased RNA and DNA synthesis, stimulated incorporation of iron into protein, and formation of hemoglobin-containing colonies.[122]

Erythroid cells transformed by several oncogene-transducing avian retroviruses may have lost their dependence on erythropoietin, both for self-renewal and differentiation. Different oncogenes are active in inducing this phenomenon, including v-*erb*-A, v-*erb*-B, v-*src*, v-*fps*, v-*ets*, and v-*myb*.[123] The mechanisms responsible for the oncogene-induced acquisition of growth factor independency are unknown, but one possibility is that the oncogene protein products might function by mimicking the interaction between the growth factor and its receptor. Avian retroviruses integrated near the c-*erb*-B proto-oncogene of erythroblastosis cells can activate the expression of this gene (which is the same as the EGF receptor) and can produce erythropoietin-independent growth of these cells.[124,125]

Infection of mice with the polycythemia-inducing strain of Friend murine leukemia virus, F-MuLV, causes the emergence of new erythroid precursors which proliferate *in vitro* to form colonies and even become differentiated, but that do not require the addition of erythropoietin to proliferate and synthesize hemoglobin *in vitro*.[126] F-MuLV forms a complex with a replication-defective virus, the spleen focus-forming virus (SFFV), and the complex formed by the two viruses can acutely induce an erythroleukemia in mice. There are two forms of SFFV, one of them a polycythemia-inducing variant ($SFFV_P$) and the other an anemia-inducing variant ($SFFV_A$). Both variants of SFFV are capable of inducing alterations in cell proliferation and differentiation through the product of their *env* gene, which encodes a 55-kDa glycoprotein (gp55). $SFFV_P$ induces lethal erythroleukemia *in vivo* and erythropoietin-independent burst formation *in vitro*.[127,128] Erythropoietin-dependent cells infected with $SFFV_P$ do not secrete erythropoietin and possess normal erythropoietin receptors.[129]

Cells infected with the $SFFV_P$ virus, but not cells infected with other retroviruses, acquire the ability to grow in the absence of erythropoietin. This action is not associated with an autocrine mechanism involving the synthesis and secretion of erythropoietin, but is due to a direct interaction between the gp55 protein and the erythropoietin receptor.[130,131] This interaction is capable of generating a growth signal from within the cell, which may be regulated by a protein encoded by the murine gene *Fv*-2.[132] SFFV-induced activation of the erythropoietin receptor in murine cell lines results in constitutive phosphorylation on tyrosine of a 97-kDa protein.[133] The 97-kDa protein also is rapidly phosphorylated in response to IL-2, IL-3, and several growth factors.

The erythroleukemia cell line IW32, which was originated by F-MuLV-induced transformation, constitutively synthesizes high amounts of erythropoietin and contains a rearranged and amplified erythropoietin locus.[134] The abnormal gene contained in IW32 cells is more sensitive to DNase I than the normal gene, which suggests that the transcriptionally active gene is the rearranged one. However, the activation of the erythropoietin gene in IW32 cells is apparently not associated with F-MuLV provirus insertion near the gene.

The activated erythropoietin receptor may display oncogene-like properties. A point mutation at codon 129 of the murine erythropoietin receptor results in constitutive activation of the receptor, and proerythroblast cells expressing the altered receptor have rearranged and inactivated p53 gene expression and are capable of inducing erythroleukemia upon injection into mice.[135]

V. ERYTHROID DIFFERENTIATION FACTOR

Murine erythroleukemia (MEL) cells can be induced to erythroid differentiation in a dose-dependent manner by a polypeptide factor extracted from the conditioned medium of phorbol ester-treated human monocyte-like cell line THP-1.[136] This factor, termed erythroid differentiation factor (EDF), is a member of the TGF-β protein family.

EDF is a 25-kDa protein with a primary structure which corresponds to a homodimer of two $β_A$ chains of inhibin,[137] a physiologic inhibitor of FSH secretion.[138] In fact, the primary structure of EDF is identical to that of activin A, a gonadal protein with FSH-releasing activity. EDF mRNA is expressed in the bone marrow. Biologically active EDF has been obtained from CHO cells expressing a plasmid that contains a cDNA copy of the EDF gene.[139]

EDF can induce hemoglobin synthesis and inhibit the growth of murine erythroleukemia cells (Friend cells) and the human erythroleukemia cell line K-562. It can also enhance colony formation of normal human erythroid progenitors *in vitro* in the presence of erythropoietin. The maximum effect of EDF is obtained at concentrations within the nanomolar range. EDF display differentiation-inducing activity for murine Friend erythroleukemia cells and K-562 human erythroleukemia cells. Native and recombinant EDF proteins possess FSH-releasing activity when assayed in an *in vitro* system of cultured anterior pituitary cells. Administration of EDF increases the frequency of erythropoietic precursors (CFU-E and BFU-E) in normal and anemic (bled) mice.[140] EDF/activin A and follistatin (an endogenous inhibitor of FSH secretion) may have opposing actions in the regulation of erythropoiesis.[141] Expression of EDF/activin A is induced during human monocyte activation,[142] but the precise physiological significance of this expression is unknown.

EDF receptors characterized in murine erythroleukemia cells are represented by proteins of 115, 51, and 42 kDa.[143] The exact relationship between these three proteins with EDF receptor activity is unknown. The postreceptor mechanism of EDF action may involve the activation of phosphoinositide breakdown with generation of inositol trisphosphate, which would result in the intracellular mobilization of Ca^{2+} from a nonmitochondrial trigger pool.[144]

Treatment of K-562 cells with EDF induces an increase in the levels of c-*fos* mRNA which begin within 3 h and reach levels 8 to 18 times higher than those existing in basal conditions within 72 h.[145] The levels of c-*myc* and c-*fms* mRNA decrease in a transient manner, being restored within 48 h. In contrast, the levels of c-*myb* and c-*abl* mRNA decrease within 1 h during EDF treatment, before growth inhibition of the cells become apparent. The exact relationship between changes in proto-oncogene expression and growth inhibition and differentiation of K-562 remains to be clarified.

EDF induces hemoglobin synthesis in neoplastic hematopoietic cell lines such as K-562 human erythroleukemia cells with concomitant reduction of their proliferation, indicating that it induces erythroid terminal differentiation of these cells. This effect is preceded by changes in the levels of expression of several proto-oncogenes, as well as by a reduction in the expression of transferrin receptors. The mechanism of EDF-induced erythroid differentiation is unknown, but it may be related to a reduction of transferrin and erythropoietin receptors.

REFERENCES

1. **Perretta, M., Waissbluth, L., Ludwig, U., and Garrido, F.,** Hormonal control of RNA polymerases in rat bone marrow nuclei. The action of erythropoietin and testosterone, *Arch. Biol. Med. Exp.,* 13, 247, 1980.
2. **Perretta, M., Waissbluth, L., Ludwig, U., Garrido, F., Garrido, A., and Ronco, A.M.,** Different RNA species stimulated by testosterone and erythropoietin in isolated bone marrow nuclei obtained from polycythemic and anemic rats, *J. Steroid Biochem.,* 14, 537, 1981.
3. **Metcalf, D. and Nicola, N.A.,** The regulatory factors controlling murine erythropoiesis in vitro, in *Aplastic Anemia: Stem Cell Biology and Advances in Treatment,* Alan R. Liss, New York, 1984, 93.
4. **Goodman, J.W., Hall, E.A., Miller, K.L., and Shinpock, S.G.,** Interleukin 3 promotes erythroid burst formation in "serum-free" cultures without detectable erythropoietin, *Proc. Natl. Acad. Sci. U.S.A.,* 82, 3291, 1985.
5. **Suda, J., Suda, T., Kubota, K., Ihle, J.N., Saito, M., and Miura, Y.,** Purified interleukin-3 and erythropoietin support the terminal differentiation of hemopoietic progenitors in serum-free culture, *Blood,* 67, 1002, 1986.
6. **Sawada, K., Krantz, S.B., Dessypris, E.N., Koury, S.T., and Sawyer, S.T.,** Human colony-forming units-erythroid do not require accessory cells, but do require direct interaction with insulin-like growth factor I and/or insulin for erythroid development, *J. Clin. Invest.,* 83, 1701, 1989.
7. **Li, Q., Blacher, R., Esch, F., and Congote, L.F.,** A heparin-binding erythroid cell stimulating factor from fetal bovine serum has the N-terminal sequence of insulin-like growth factor II, *Biochem. Biophys. Res. Commun.,* 166, 557, 1990.
8. **Schroeder, C., Gibson, L., Nordström, C., and Beug, H.,** The estrogen receptor cooperates with the TGF-α receptor (c-erbB) in regulation of chicken erythroid progenitor self-renewal, *EMBO J.,* 12, 951, 1993.
9. **Andrews, N.C., Erdjument-Bromage, H., Davidson, M.B., Tempst, P., and Orkin, S.H.,** Erythroid transcription factor NF-E2 is a haematopoietic-specific basic leucine zipper protein, *Nature,* 362, 722, 1993.

10. **Umemura, T., Umene, K., Nishimura, J., Fukumaki, Y., Sasaki, Y., and Ibayashi, H.,** Expression of c-*myc* oncogene during differentiation of human burst-forming unit, erythroid (BFU-E), *Biochem. Biophys. Res. Commun.,* 135, 521, 1986.
11. **Docherty, A.J.P., Lyons, A., Smith, B.J., Wright, E.M., Stephens, P.E., and Harris, T.J.R.,** Sequence of human tissue inhibitor of metalloproteinases and its identity to erythroid-potentiating activity, *Nature,* 318, 66, 1985.
12. **Gasson, J.C., Golde, D.W., Kaufman, S.E., Westbrook, S.E., Westbrook, C.A., Hewick, R.M., Kaufman, R.J., Wong, G.G., Temple, P.A., Leary, A.C., Brown, E.L., Orr, E.C., and Clark, S.C.,** Molecular characterization and expression of the gene encoding human erythroid-potentiating activity, *Nature,* 315, 768, 1985.
13. **Huebner, K., Isobe, M., Gasson, J.C., Golde, D.W., and Croce, C.M.,** Localization of the gene encoding human erythroid-potentiating activity to chromosome region X11.1-Xp11.4, *Am. J. Hum. Genet.,* 38, 819, 1986.
14. **Patarca, R. and Haseltine, W.A.,** A major retroviral core protein related to EPA and TIMP, *Nature,* 318, 390, 1985.
15. **Avalos, B.R., Kaufman, S.E., Tomonaga, M., Williams, R.E., Golde, D.W., and Gasson, J.C.,** K562 cells produce and respond to human erythroid-potentiating activity, *Blood,* 71, 1720, 1988.
16. **Alitalo, R., Partanen, J., Pertovaara, L., Hölttä, E., Sistonen, L., Andersson, L., and Alitalo, K.,** Increased erythroid potentiating activity/tissue inhibitor of metalloproteinases and *jun/fos* transcription factor complex characterize tumor promoter-induced megakaryoblastic differentiation of K562 leukemia cells, *Blood,* 75, 1974, 1990.
17. **Feldman, L., Cohen, C.M., Riordan, M.A., and Dainiak, N.,** Purification of a membrane-derived human erythroid growth factor, *Proc. Natl. Acad. Sci. U.S.A.,* 84, 6775, 1987.
18. **Dainiak, N., Najman, A., Kreczko, S., Baillou, C., Mier, J., Feldman, L., Gorin, N.C., and Duhamel, G.,** B-lymphocytes as a source of cell surface growth-promoting factors for hematopoietic progenitors, *Exp. Hematol.,* 15, 1086, 1987.
19. **Misago, M., Chiba, S., Tsukada, J., Kikuchi, M., and Eto, S.,** Effect of recombinant erythropoietin on human BFU-E in serum-free cultures, *Acta Haematol. Jpn.,* 51, 967, 1988.
20. **Dainiak, N., Sutter, D., and Kreczko, S.,** L-Triiodothyronine augments erythropoietic growth factor release from peripheral blood and bone marrow leukocytes, *Blood,* 68, 1289, 1986.
21. **Goldwasser, E.,** Erythropoietin and the differentiation of red blood cells, *Fed. Proc.,* 34, 2285, 1975.
22. **Finch, C.A.,** Erythropoiesis, erythropoietin, and iron, *Blood,* 60, 1241, 1982.
23. **Goldwasser, E.,** Erythropoietin and its mode of action, *Blood Cells,* 10, 147, 1984.
24. **Eckhardt, K.-U. and Bauer, C.,** Erythropoietin in health and disease, *Eur. J. Clin. Invest.,* 19, 117, 1989.
25. **Erslev, A.J.,** Erythropoietin, *Leukemia Res.,* 14, 683, 1990.
26. **Krantz, S.B.,** Erythropoietin, *Blood,* 77, 419, 1991.
27. **Jelkmann, W.,** Erythropoietin: structure, control of production, and function, *Physiol. Rev.,* 72, 449, 1992.
28. **Koury, M.J. and Bondurant, M.C.,** The molecular mechanism of erythropoietin action, *Eur. J. Biochem.,* 210, 649, 1992.
29. **Tabbara, I.A.,** Erythropoietin — biology and clinical applications, *Arch. Int. Med.,* 153, 298, 1993.
30. **Erslev, A.J., Caro, J., Birgegard, G., Silver, R., and Miller, O.,** The biogenesis of erythropoietin, *Exp. Hematol.,* 8 (Suppl. 8), 1, 1980.
31. **Jacobs, K., Shoemaker, C., Rudersdorf, R., Neill, S.D., Kaufman, R.J., Mufson, A., Seehra, J., Jones, S.S., Hewick, R., Fritsch, E.F., Kawakita, M., Shimizu, T., and Miyake, T.,** Isolation and characterization of genomic and cDNA clones of human erythropoietin, *Nature,* 313, 806, 1985.
32. **Beru, N., McDonald, J., Lacombe, C., and Goldwasser, E.,** Expression of the erythropoietin gene, *Mol. Cell. Biol.,* 6, 2571, 1986.
33. **Bondurant, M.C. and Koury, M.J.,** Anemia induces accumulation of erythropoietin mRNA in the kidney and liver, *Mol. Cell. Biol.,* 6, 2731, 1986.
34. **Schuster, S.J., Badiavas, E.V., Costa-Giomi, P., Weinman, R., Erslev, A.J., and Caro, J.,** Stimulation of erythropoietin gene transcription during hypoxia and cobalt exposure, *Blood,* 73, 13, 1989.
35. **Imagawa, S., Goldberg, M.A., Doweiko, J., and Bunn, H.F.,** Regulatory elements of the erythropoietin gene, *Blood,* 77, 278, 1991.

36. **Goldberg, M.A., Gaut, C.C., and Bunn, H.F.,** Erythropoietin mRNA levels are governed by both the rate of gene transcription and posttranscriptional events, *Blood,* 77, 271, 1991.
37. **Sherwood, J.B. and Shouval, D.,** Continuous production of erythropoietin by an established human renal carcinoma cell line: development of the cell line, *Proc. Natl. Acad. Sci. U.S.A.,* 83, 165, 1986.
38. **Goldberg, M.A., Glass, G.A., Cunningham, J.M., and Bunn, H.F.,** The regulated expression of erythropoietin by two human hepatoma cell lines, *Proc. Natl. Acad. Sci. U.S.A.,* 84, 7972, 1987.
39. **Matsushita, J., Kawakita, M., Shibuya, K., Koishihara, Y., Sakaguchi, M., and Takatsuki, A.,** Human urinary erythropoietin: preparation with high potency, *Acta Haematol.,* 84, 169, 1990.
40. **Spivak, J.L., Pham, T., Isaacs, M., and Hankins, W.D.,** Erythropoietin is both a mitogen and a survival factor, *Blood,* 77, 1228, 1991.
41. **Akahane, K., Tojo, A., Tobe, K., Kasuga, M., Urabe, A., and Takaku, F.,** Binding properties and proliferative potency of insulin-like growth factor I in fetal mouse liver cells, *Exp. Hematol.,* 15, 1068, 1987.
42. **Congote, L.F.,** Effects of insulin-like growth factor I, platelet-derived growth factor, fibroblast growth factor, and transforming growth factor-β on thymidine incorporation into fetal liver cells, *Exp. Hematol.,* 15, 936, 1987.
43. **Koury, M.J. and Bondurant, M.C.,** Maintenance by erythropoietin of viability and maturation of murine erythroid precursor cells, *J. Cell. Physiol.,* 137, 65, 1988.
44. **Noguchi, T., Fukumoto, H., Mishina, Y., and Obinata, M.,** Differentiation of erythroid progenitor (CFU-E) cells from mouse fetal liver cells and murine erythroleukemia (TSA8) cells without proliferation, *Mol. Cell. Biol.,* 8, 2604, 1988.
45. **Koury, M.J. and Bondurant, M.C.,** Erythropoietin retards DNA breakdown and prevents programmed death in erythroid progenitor cells, *Science,* 248, 378, 1990.
46. **Kelley, L.L., Koury, M.J., and Bondurant, M.C.,** Regulation of programmed death in erythroid progenitor cells by erythropoietin: effects of calcium and or protein and RNA syntheses, *J. Cell. Physiol.,* 151, 487, 1992.
47. **Fraser, J.K., Tan, A.S., Lin, F.-K., and Berridge, M.V.,** Expression of specific high-affinity binding sites for erythropoietin on rat and mouse megakaryocytes, *Exp. Hematol.,* 17, 10, 1989.
48. **Tsukada, J., Misago, M., Sato, T., Kikuchi, M., Oda, S., Chiba, S., and Eto, S.,** The effect of recombinant erythropoietin on murine megakaryocyte colony formation, *Int. J. Cell Cloning,* 5, 401, 1987.
49. **Anagnostou, A., Lee, E.S., Kessimian, N., Levinson, R., and Steiner, M.,** Erythropoietin has a mitogenic and positive chemotactic effect on endothelial cells, *Proc. Natl. Acad. Sci. U.S.A.,* 87, 5978, 1990.
50. **Law, M.L., Cai, G.-Y., Lin, F.-K., Wei, Q., Huang, S.-Z., Hartz, J.H., Morse, H., Lin, C.-H., Jones, C., and Kao, F.-T.,** Chromosomal assignment of the human erythropoietin gene and its DNA polymorphism, *Proc. Natl. Acad. Sci. U.S.A.,* 83, 6920, 1986.
51. **Lin, F.-K., Suggs, S., Lin, C.-H., Browne, J.K., Smalling, R., Egrie, J.C., Chen, K.K., Fox, G.M., Martin, F., Stabinsky, Z., Badrawi, S.M., Lai, P.-H., and Goldwasser, E.,** Cloning and expression of the human erythropoietin gene, *Proc. Natl. Acad. Sci. U.S.A.,* 82, 7580, 1985.
52. **Powell, J.S., Berkner, K.L., Lebo, R.V., and Adamson, J.W.,** Human erythropoietin gene high level of expression in stably transfected mammalian cells and chromosome localization, *Proc. Natl. Acad. Sci. U.S.A.,* 83, 6465, 1986.
53. **Shimizu, T., Miyake, T., Pilch, A.M., Mantel, C., and Murphy, M.J., Jr.,** Biochemical properties of human urinary megakaryocyte colony-stimulating factor and erythropoietin: the role of sulfhydryl groups and disulfide bonds, *Exp. Cell Biol.,* 54, 286, 1986.
54. **Lai, P.-H., Everett, R., Wang, F.-F., Arakawa, T., and Goldwasser, E.,** Structural characterization of human erythropoietin, *J. Biol. Chem.,* 261, 3116, 1986.
55. **Egrie, J.C., Strickland, T.W., Lane, J., Aoki, K., Cohen, A.M., Smalling, R., Trail, G., Lin, F.K., Browne, J.K., and Hines, D.K.,** Characterization and biological effects of recombinant human erythropoietin, *Immunobiology,* 172, 213, 1986.
56. **Ganser, A., Völkers, B., Scigalla, P., and Hoelzer, D.,** Effect of human recombinant erythropoietin on human hemopoietic progenitor cells in vitro, *Klin. Wochenschr.,* 66, 236, 1988.
57. **Lin, F.-K., Lin, C.-H., Lai, P.-H., Browne, J.K., Egrie, J.C., Smalling, R., Fox, G.M., Chen, K.K., Castro, M., and Suggs, S.,** Monkey erythropoietin gene: cloning, expression and comparison with the human erythropoietin gene, *Gene,* 44, 201, 1986.

58. **McDonald, J.D., Lin, F.-K., and Goldwasser, E.,** Cloning, sequencing, and evolutionary analysis of the mouse erythropoietin gene, *Mol. Cell. Biol.,* 6, 842, 1986.
59. **Shoemaker, C.B. and Mitsock, L.D.,** Murine erythropoietin gene: cloning, expression, and human gene homology, *Mol. Cell. Biol.,* 6, 849, 1986.
60. **Congote, L.F.,** The N-terminal portion of an erythropoietin-like peptide from fetal bovine serum has sequence homology with the LDL receptor and two proteins of the Epstein-Barr virus, *Biochem. Biophys. Res. Commun.,* 133, 404, 1985.
61. **D'Andrea, A.D. and Zon, L.I.,** Erythropoietin receptor. Subunit structure and activation, *J. Clin. Invest.,* 86, 681, 1990.
62. **Winkelmann, J.C.,** The human erythropoietin receptor, *Int. J. Cell Cloning,* 10, 254, 1992.
63. **Barber, D.L. and D'Andrea, A.D.,** The erythropoietin receptor and the molecular basis of signal transduction, *Semin. Hematol.,* 29, 293, 1992.
64. **Youssoufian, H., Longmore, G., Neumann, D., Yoshimura, A., and Lodish, H.F.,** Structure, function, and activation of the erythropoietin receptor, *Blood,* 81, 2223, 1993.
65. **Krantz, S.B. and Goldwasser, E.,** Specific binding of erythropoietin to spleen cells infected with the anemia strain of Friend virus, *Proc. Natl. Acad. Sci. U.S.A.,* 81, 7574, 1984.
66. **Sawyer, S.T., Krantz, S.B., and Luna, J.,** Identification of the receptor for erythropoietin by cross-linking to Friend virus-infected erythroid cells, *Proc. Natl. Acad. Sci. U.S.A.,* 84, 3690, 1987.
67. **Mayeux, P., Billat, C., and Jacquot, R.,** Murine erythroleukaemia cells (Friend cells) possess high-affinity binding sites for erythropoietin, *FEBS Lett.,* 211, 229, 1987.
68. **Sawada, K., Krantz, S.B., Dai, C.-H., Koury, S.T., Horn, S.T., Glick, A.D., and Civin, C.I.,** Purification of human blood burst-forming units-erythroid and demonstration of the evolution of erythropoietin receptors, *J. Cell. Physiol.,* 142, 219, 1990.
69. **Sawyer, S.T., Krantz, S.B., and Sawada, K.,** Receptors for erythropoietin in mouse and human erythroid cells and placenta, *Blood,* 74, 103, 1989.
70. **Yamamura, Y., Kageyama, Y., Matuzaki, T., Noda, M., and Ikawa, Y.,** Distinct downstream signaling mechanism between erythropoietin receptor and interleukin-2 receptor, *EMBO J.,* 11, 4909, 1992.
71. **Chiba, T., Kishi, A., Sugiyama, M., Amanuma, H., Machide, M., Nagata, Y., and Todokoro, K.,** Functionally essential cytoplasmic domain of the erythropoietin receptor, *Biochem. Biophys. Res. Commun.,* 186, 1236, 1992.
72. **Miura, O., Cleveland, J.L., and Ihle, J.N.,** Inactivation of erythropoietin receptor function by point mutations in a region having homology with other cytokine receptors, *Mol. Cell. Biol.,* 13, 1788, 1993.
73. **Noguchi, C.T., Bae, K.S., Chin, K., Wada, Y., Schechter, A.N., and Hankins, W.D.,** Cloning of the human erythropoietin receptor gene, *Blood,* 78, 2548, 1991.
74. **Maouche, L., Tournamille, C., Hattab, C., Boffa, G., Cartron, J.-P., and Chrétien, S.,** Cloning of the gene encoding the human erythropoietin receptor, *Blood,* 78, 2557, 1991.
75. **Hoshino, S., Teramura, M., Takahashi, M., Motoji, T., Oshimi, K., Ueda, M., and Mizoguchi, H.,** Expression and characterization of erythropoietin receptors on normal human bone marrow cells, *Int. J. Cell Cloning,* 7, 156, 1989.
76. **Winkelmann, J.C., Penny, L.A., Deaven, L.L., Forget, B.G., and Jenkins, R.B.,** The gene for the human erythropoietin receptor: analysis of the coding sequence and assignment to chromosome 19p, *Blood,* 76, 24, 1990.
77. **Jones, S.S., D'Andrea, A.D., Haines, L.L., and Wong, G.G.,** Human erythropoietin receptor: cloning, expression, and biologic characterization, *Blood,* 76, 31, 1990.
78. **Dusant-Erfourt, I., Casadevall, N., Lacombe, C., Müller, O., Billat, C., Fischer, S., and Mayeux, P.,** Erythropoietin induces the tyrosine phosphorylation of its own receptor in human erythropoietin-responsive cells, *J. Biol. Chem.,* 267, 10670, 1992.
79. **D'Andrea, A.D. and Zon, L.I.,** Erythropoietin receptor — structure and activation, *J. Clin. Invest.,* 86, 681, 1990.
80. **Tojo, A., Fukamachi, H., Saito, T., Kasuga, M., Urabe, A., and Takaku, F.,** Induction of the receptor for erythropoietin in murine erythroleukemia cells after dimethyl sulfoxide treatment, *Cancer Res.,* 48, 1818, 1988.
81. **Kitamura, T., Tojo, A., Kuwaki, T., Chiba, S., Miyazono, K., Urabe, A., and Takaku, F.,** Identification and analysis of human erythropoietin receptors on a factor-dependent cell line, TF-1, *Blood,* 73, 375, 1989.

82. Sasaki, R., Yanagawa, S., Hitomi, K., and Chiba, H., Characterization of erythropoietin receptor of murine erythroid cells, *Eur. J. Biochem.*, 168, 43, 1987.
83. McCaffery, P.J., Fraser, J.K., Lin, F.-K., and Berridge, M.V., Subunit structure of the erythropoietin receptor, *J. Biol. Chem.*, 264, 10507, 1989.
84. Sawyer, S.T., The two proteins of the erythropoietin receptor are structurally similar, *J. Biol. Chem.*, 264, 13343, 1989.
85. Youssoufian, H., Zon, L.I., Orkin, S.H., D'Andrea, A.D., and Lodish, H.F., Structure and transcription of the mouse erythropoietin receptor gene, *Mol. Cell. Biol.*, 10, 3675, 1990.
86. Todokoro, K., Kanazawa, S., Amanuma, H., and Ikawa, Y., Specific binding of erythropoietin to its receptor on responsive mouse erythroleukemia cells, *Proc. Natl. Acad. Sci. U.S.A.*, 84, 4126, 1987.
87. Fibi, M.R., Stuber, W., Hintzobertreis, P., Luben, G., Krumwieh, D., Siebold, B., Zettlmeiss, G., and Kupper, H.A., Evidence for the location of the receptor binding site of human erythropoietin at the carboxyl-terminal domain, *Blood*, 77, 1203, 1991.
88. Sawyer, S.T., Krantz, S.B., and Goldwasser, E., Binding and receptor-mediated endocytosis of erythropoietin in Friend virus-infected erythroid cells, *J. Biol. Chem.*, 262, 5554, 1987.
89. Rosenlöf, K., Fyhrquist, F., and Pekonen, F., Receptors for recombinant erythropoietin in human bone marrow cells, *Scand. J. Clin. Lab. Invest.*, 47, 823, 1987.
90. Fraser, J.K., Lin, F.-K., and Berridge, M.V., Expression of high affinity receptors for erythropoietin on human bone marrow cells and on the human erythroleukemic cell line, HEL., *Exp. Hematol.*, 16, 836, 1988.
91. Sakaguchi, M., Koishihara, Y., Tsuda, H., Fujimoto, K., Shibuya, K., Kawakita, M., and Takatsuki, K., The expression of functional erythropoietin receptors on an interleukin-3 dependent cell line, *Biochem. Biophys. Res. Commun.*, 146, 7, 1987.
92. Tsao, C.-J., Tojo, A., Fukamachi, H., Kitamura, T., Saito, T., Urabe, A., and Takaku, F., Expression of the functional erythropoietin receptors on interleukin 3-dependent murine cell lines, *J. Immunol.*, 140, 89, 1988.
93. de la Chapelle, A., Traskelin, A.L., and Juvonen, E., Truncated erythropoietin receptor causes dominantly inherited benign human erythrocytosis, *Proc. Natl. Acad. Sci. U.S.A.*, 90, 4495, 1993.
94. Bonatou-Tzedaki, S.A., Sohi, M.K., and Arnstein, K.R.V., The role of cAMP and calcium in the stimulation of proliferation of immature erythroblasts by erythropoietin, *Exp. Cell Res.*, 170, 276, 1987.
95. Miller, B.A., Cheung, J.Y., Tillotson, D.L., Hope, S.M., and Scaduto, R.C., Jr., Erythropoietin stimulates a rise in intracellular-free calcium concentration in single BFU-E derived erythroblasts at specific stages of differentiation, *Blood*, 73, 1188, 1989.
96. Imagawa, S., Smith, B.R., Palmer-Crocker, R., and Bunn, H.F., The effect of recombinant erythropoietin on intracellular free calcium in erythropoietin-responsive cells, *Blood*, 73, 1452, 1989.
97. Tsuda, H., Sawada, T., Sakaguchi, M., Kawakita, M., and Takatsuki, K., Mode of action of erythropoietin (Epo) in an Epo-dependent murine cell line. I. Involvement of adenosine 3′,5′-cyclic monophosphate not as a second messenger but as a regulator of cell growth, *Exp. Hematol.*, 17, 211, 1989.
98. Choi, H.-S., Wojchowski, D.M., and Sytkowski, A.J., Erythropoietin rapidly alters phosphorylation of pp43, an erythroid membrane protein, *J. Biol. Chem.*, 262, 2933, 1987.
99. Mason-Garcia, M., Weill, C.L., and Beckman, B.S., Rapid activation by erythropoietin of protein kinase C in nuclei of erythroid progenitor cells, *Biochem. Biophys. Res. Commun.*, 168, 490, 1990.
100. Miura, O., D'Andrea, A., Kabat, D., and Ihle, J.N., Induction of tyrosine phosphorylation by the erythropoietin receptor correlates with mitogenesis, *Mol. Cell. Biol.*, 11, 4895, 1991.
101. Hanazono, Y., Chiba, S., Sasaki, K., Mano, H., Yazaki, Y., and Hirai, H., Erythropoietin induces tyrosine phosphorylation and kinase activity of the c-*fps/fes* proto-oncogene product in human erythropoietin-responsive cells, *Blood*, 81, 3193, 1993.
102. Damen, J.E., Mui, A.L.F., Puil, L., Pawson, T., and Krystal, G., Phosphatidylinositol 3-kinase associates, via its SRC homology-2 domains, with the activated erythropoietin receptor, *Blood*, 81, 3204, 1993.
103. Torti, M., Marti, K.B., Altschuler, D., Yamamoto, K., and Lapetina, E.G., Erythropoietin induces p21^{ras} activation and p120GAP tyrosine phosphorylation in human erythroleukemia cells, *J. Biol. Chem.*, 267, 8293, 1992.
104. Sawyer, S.T. and Krantz, S.B., Transferrin receptor number, synthesis, and endocytosis during erythropoietin-induced maturation of Friend virus-infected erythroid cells, *J. Biol. Chem.*, 261, 9187, 1986.

105. Schooley, J.C., Kullgren, B., and Allison, A.C., Inhibition by interleukin-1 of the action of erythropoietin on erythroid precursors and its possible role in the pathogenesis of hypoplastic anaemias, *Br. J. Haematol.*, 67, 11, 1987.
106. Beru, N. and Goldwasser, E., The regulation of heme biosynthesis during erythropoietin-induced erythroid differentiation, *J. Biol. Chem.*, 260, 9251, 1985.
107. Powsner, E.R. and Berman, L., Effect of erythropoietin on DNA synthesis by erythroblasts in vitro, *Blood*, 30, 189, 1967.
108. Conkie, D., Kleiman, L., Harrison, P.R., and Paul, J., Increase in the accumulation of globin mRNA in immature erythroblasts in response to erythropoietin in vivo or in vitro, *Exp. Cell Res.*, 93, 315, 1975.
109. Piantadosi, C.A., Dickerman, H.W., and Spivak, J.L., Sequential activation of splenic nuclear RNA polymerases by erythropoietin, *J. Clin. Invest.*, 57, 20, 1976.
110. Perretta, M., Valladares, L., Garrido, F., Valenzuela, D., and Ludwig, U., Hormonal control of gene expression: differential activation of rat bone marrow RNA polymerases by erythropoietin and testosterone, *Arch. Biol. Med. Exp.*, 12, 309, 1979.
111. Tsuda, H., Sawada, T., Kawakita, M., and Takatsuki, K., Mode of action of erythropoietin (Epo) in an Epo-dependent murine cell line. II. Cell cycle-dependency of Epo action, *Exp. Hematol.*, 17, 218, 1989.
112. Spangler, R., Bailey, S.C., and Sytkowski, A.J., Erythropoietin increases c-*myc* messenger RNA by a protein kinase C-dependent pathway, *J. Biol. Chem.*, 266, 681, 1991.
113. Spangler, R. and Sytkowski, A.J., The c-*myc* is an erythropoietin early response gene in normal erythroid cells: evidence for a protein kinase C-mediated signal, *Blood*, 79, 52, 1992.
114. Umemura, T., Umene, K., Takahira, H., Takeichi, N., Katsuno, M., Fukumaki, Y., Nishimura, J., Sakaki, Y., and Ibayashi, H., Hematopoietic growth factors (BPA and Epo) induce the expressions of c-*myc* and c-*fos* proto-oncogenes in normal human erythroid progenitors, *Leukemia Res.*, 12, 187, 1988.
115. Tsuda, H., Aso, N., Sawada, T., Hata, H., Kawakita, M., Mori, K.J., and Takatsuki, K., Alteration of nuclear proto-oncogene expression by erythropoietin (Epo) in Epo-responsive murine cell lines, *Int. J. Cell Cloning*, 9, 123, 1991.
116. Mitjavila, M.T., Villeval, J.L., Cramer, P., Henri, A., Gasson, J., Krystal, G., Tulliez, M., Berger, R., Breton-Gorius, J., and Vainchenker, W., Effects of granulocyte-macrophage colony-stimulating factor and erythropoietin on leukemic erythroid colony formation in human early erythroblastic leukemias, *Blood*, 70, 965, 1987.
117. Mitjavila, M.-T., Le Couedic, J.-P., Casadevall, N., Navarro, S., Villeval, J.-L., Dubart, A., and Vanchenker, W., Autocrine stimulation by erythropoietin and autonomous growth of human erythroid leukemic cells in vitro, *J. Clin. Invest.*, 88, 789, 1991.
118. Okabe, T., Urabe, A., Kato, T., Chiba, S., and Takaku, F., Production of erythropoietin-like activity by human renal and hepatic carcinomas in cell culture, *Cancer*, 55, 1918, 1985.
119. Da Silva, J.-L., Lacombe, C., Bruneval, P., Casadevall, N., Leporrier, M., Camilleri, J.-P., Bariety, J., Tambourin, P., and Varet, B., Tumor cells are the site of erythropoietin synthesis in human renal cancers associated with polycythemia, *Blood*, 75, 577, 1990.
120. Greenberg, B.R., Hirasuna, J.D., and Woo, L., In vitro response to erythropoietin in erythroblastic transformation of chronic myelogenous leukemia, *Exp. Hematol.*, 8, 52, 1980.
121. Hankins, W.D. and Scolnick, E.M., Harvey and Kirsten sarcoma viruses promote the growth and differentiation of erythroid precursor cells *in vitro*, *Cell*, 26, 91, 1981.
122. Weiss, T.L., Barker, M.E., Selleck, S.E., and Wintroub, B.U., Erythropoietin binding and induced differentiation of Rauscher erythroleukemia cell line Red 5-1.5, *J. Biol. Chem.*, 264, 1804, 1989.
123. Beug, H., Kahn, P., Vennström, B., Hayman, M.J., and Graf, T., How do retroviral oncogenes induce transformation in avian erythroid cells?, *Proc. R. Soc. London*, B226, 121, 1985.
124. Raines, M.A., Lewis, W.G., Crittenden, L.B., and Kung, H.-J., The c-*erbB* activation in avian leukosis virus-induced erythroblastosis: clustered integration sites and the arrangement of provirus in the c-*erbB* alleles, *Proc. Natl. Acad. Sci. U.S.A.*, 82, 2287, 1985.
125. Beug, H., Hayman, M.J., Raines, M.B., Kung, H.J., and Vennström, B., Rous-associated virus 1-induced erythroleukemic cells exhibit a weakly transformed phenotype in vitro and release c-*erbB*-containing retroviruses unable to transform fibroblasts, *J. Virol.*, 57, 1127, 1986.
126. Horoszewicz, J.S., Leong, S.S., and Carter, W.A., Friend leukemia: rapid development of erythropoietin-independent hematopoietic precursors, *J. Natl. Cancer Inst.*, 54, 265, 1975.
127. Ruscetti, S. and Wolff, L., Spleen focus-forming virus: relationship of an altered envelope gene to the development of a rapid erythroleukemia, *Curr. Top. Microbiol. Immunol.*, 112, 21, 1984.

128. **Aaronson, S.A. and Pierce, J.M.**, Molecular mimicry of growth factors by products of tumor viruses, *Cancer Cells,* 2, 212, 1990.
129. **Ruscetti, S.K. and Ruscetti, F.W.**, Apparent epo-independence of erythroid cells infected with the polycythemia-inducing strain of Friend spleen focus-forming virus is not due to epo production or change in number or affinity of epo receptors, *Leukemia,* 3, 703, 1989.
130. **Ruscetti, S.K., Janesch, N.J., Chakraborti, A., Sawyer, S.T., and Hankins, W.D.**, Friend spleen focus-forming virus induces factor independence in an erythropoietin-dependent erythroleukemia cell line, *J. Virol.,* 64, 1057, 1990.
131. **Yoshimura, A., D'Andrea, A.D., and Lodish, H.F.**, Friend spleen focus-forming virus glycoprotein gp55 interacts with the erythropoietin receptor in the endoplasmic reticulum and affects receptor metabolism, *Proc. Natl. Acad. Sci. U.S.A.,* 87, 4139, 1990.
132. **Hoatlin, M.E., Kozak, S.L., Lilly, F., Chakraborti, A., Kozak, C.A., and Kabat, D.**, Activation of erythropoietin receptors by Friend viral gp55 and by erythropoietin and down-modulation by the murine $Fv\text{-}2^r$ resistance gene, *Proc. Natl. Acad. Sci. U.S.A.,* 87, 9985, 1990.
133. **Showers, M.O., Moreau, J.-F., Linnekin, D., Druker, B., and D'Andrea, A.D.**, Activation of the erythropoietin receptor by the Friend spleen focus-forming virus gp55 glycoprotein induces constitutive protein tyrosine phosphorylation, *Blood,* 80, 3070, 1992.
134. **McDonald, J., Beru, N., and Goldwasser, E.**, Rearrangement and expression of erythropoietin genes in transformed mouse cells, *Mol. Cell. Biol.,* 7, 365, 1987.
135. **Longmore, G.D. and Lodish, H.F.**, An activating mutation in the murine erythropoietin receptor induces erythroleukemia in mice: a cytokine receptor superfamily oncogene, *Cell,* 67, 1089, 1991.
136. **Eto, Y., Tsuji, T., Takezawa, M., Takano, S., Yokogawa, Y., and Shibai, H.**, Purification and characterization of erythroid differentiation factor (EDF) isolated from human leukemia cell line THP-1, *Biochem. Biophys. Res. Commun.,* 142, 1095, 1987.
137. **Murata, M., Eto, Y., Shibai, H., Sakai, M., and Muramatsu, M.**, Erythroid differentiation factor is encoded by the same mRNA as that of the inhibit β_A chain, *Proc. Natl. Acad. Sci. U.S.A.,* 85, 2434, 1988.
138. **Ying, S.-Y.**, Inhibins and activins: chemical properties and biological activity, *Proc. Soc. Exp. Biol. Med.,* 186, 253, 1987.
139. **Murata, M., Onomichi, K., Eto, Y., Shibai, H., and Muramatsu, M.**, Expression of erythroid differentiation factor (EDF) in Chinese hamster ovary cells, *Biochem. Biophys. Res. Commun.,* 151, 230, 1988.
140. **Shizaki, M., Sakai, R., Tabuchi, M., Eto, Y., Kosaka, M., and Shibai, H.**, In vivo treatment with erythroid differentiation factor (EDF/activin A) increases erythroid precursors (CFU-E and BFU-E) in mice, *Biochem. Biophys. Res. Commun.,* 165, 1155, 1989.
141. **Shizaki, M., Sakai, R., Tabuchi, M., Nakamura, T., Sugino, K., Sugino, H., and Eto, Y.**, Evidence for the participation of endogenous activin A/erythroid differentiation factor in the regulation of erythropoiesis, *Proc. Natl. Acad. Sci. U.S.A.,* 89, 1553, 1992.
142. **Eramaa, M., Hurme, M., Stenman, U.H., and Ritvos, O.**, Activin-A/erythroid differentiation factor is induced during human monocyte activation, *J. Exp. Med.,* 176, 1449, 1992.
143. **Hino, M., Tojo, A., Miyazono, K., Miura, Y., Chiba, S., Eto, Y., Shibai, H., and Takaku, F.**, Characterization of cellular receptors for erythroid differentiation factor on murine erythroleukemia cells, *J. Biol. Chem.,* 264, 10309, 1989.
144. **Shibata, H., Ogata, E., Etoh, Y., Shibai, H., and Kojima, I.**, Erythroid differentiation factor stimulates hydrolysis of polyphosphoinositide in Friend erythroleukemia cells, *Biochem. Biophys. Res. Commun.,* 146, 187, 1987.
145. **Miyamoto, Y., Kosaka, M., Eto, Y., Shiba, H., and Saito, S.**, Effect of erythroid differentiation factor on erythroid differentiation and proliferation of K-562 cells, *Biochem. Biophys. Res. Commun.,* 168, 1149, 1990.

Chapter 7

Platelet-Derived Growth Factor

I. INTRODUCTION

Platelets circulating in the peripheral blood derive from bone marrow megakaryocytes. The functions of platelets are manifold. They contain and release several factors which include platelet-derived growth factor (PDGF), IFN-γ, platelet factor-4 (PF-4), platelet-derived endothelial cell growth factor (PD-ECGF), β-thromboglobulin, platelet basic proteins, and a platelet-derived vascular permeability factor which may influence both normal and tumor cells.[1,2] PDGF is a potent mitogenic factor released by platelets.[3-17]

II. STRUCTURE OF PDGF AND THE PDGF GENES

Human PDGF is a heterodimeric glycoprotein of approximately 30 kDa. It is composed of two peptide chains, termed PDGF-A chain or PDGF-1 and PDGF-B chain or PDGF-2, respectively.[18-20] The two chains of PDGF are linked by disulfide bonds and are of similar size. Sequence homology of approximately 60% exists between the two chains of PDGF, suggesting that their gene sequences have a common ancestral origin.[21,22] The dimer structure is important for the biological activity of the PDGF molecule since reduction irreversibly inactivates PDGF. The factor is secreted in different cells as a heterodimer or as a mixture of homodimers. A CHO cell line that stably expresses transfected human PDGF precursor genes produces three dimeric combinations of PDGF chains: the PDGF-AB heterodimer and PDGF-AA and PDGF-BB homodimers.[23] The major part of PDGF purified from human platelets has a heterodimeric structure (PDGF-AB).[24] Two amino acid residues of the PDGF-B chain, arginine 27 and isoleucine 30, are crucially involved in recognition and activation.[25] These two residues are included in the region of the PDGF-B sequence (residues 24 to 63) which is responsible for the transforming ability of the polypeptide.

A. THE PDGF GENES

The gene encoding PDGF-A resides on human chromosome 7.[26] The PDGF-A gene was localized to human chromosome region 7, at region 7p21-p22.[27] In an independent study, the gene was localized to human chromosome band 7q11.23,[28] but the assignation of the *PDGFA* gene to chromosome band 7p22 was confirmed recently.[29,30] The nucleotide sequence of a cloned PDGF-A gene predicts a precursor polypeptide of 23 kDa and 211 amino acids.[26,27] The promoter region of the human PDGF-A gene has been characterized.[31] Expression of the PDGF-A gene is transcriptionally repressed by the WT1 tumor suppressor protein.[32] The gene encoding PDGF-B is located on human chromosome 22, at region 22q13.1, and is identical with the c-*sis* proto-oncogene.[33,34] The human c-*sis*/PDGF-B gene, which is 14 kb in length and contains 6 exons, has been cloned and sequenced.[35]

The different chromosome localizations of the genes encoding the two chains of PDGF suggest that their transcriptional expression may be regulated in different ways. Comparison of the PDGF-A and PDGF-B gene expression in human leukemia cells and normal human monocytes indicates that, in fact, these two genes are differentially regulated, although they share common control mechanisms at the posttranscriptional level.[36] The 3'-noncoding sequences of genes may play an important role in controlling gene expression, and it is thus interesting to observe that the untranslated 3' regions of the mRNAs coding for the two chains of PDGF contain only distantly related sequences.[37] An intriguing feature of the cDNA coding for the PDGF-A chain is the existence of two extremely long T-rich stretches in the untranslated 3' region. The intron-exon structures of the PDGF-A- and -B-chain genes are very similar. Two functionally different A-chain precursors, which differ by the presence or absence of a basic carboxyl terminus, are generated as a result of alternative mRNA splicing events, which include or exclude exon 6.[27]

B. MOLECULAR FORMS OF PDGF

PDGF activity consists of several isoforms of different molecular weights. Two active fractions, PDGF-I and PDGF-II, were obtained by gel filtration,[38] but additional forms of PDGF may exist.[39,40] PDGF-I is a 31-kDa protein which contains 7% carbohydrate, and PDGF-II is also a glycoprotein but is about 28 kDa and contains 4% carbohydrate.[38] The two isoforms of PDGF have equal mitogenic activity, amino acid composition, and immunological reactivity. PDGF-I may be identical to a 31-kDa PDGF-A chain homodimer mitogen (PDGF-AA) which is secreted by human endothelial cells.[41] A similar or identical homodimer is produced by myogenic cells.[42] Although normal human fibroblasts express PDGF-A chain mRNA only transiently upon mitogenic stimulation, constitutive expression of PDGF-A mRNA and PDGF-AA homodimers was found in a cell strain derived from patients with progeria (Hutchinson-Gilford syndrome), which is characterized by premature aging.[43] In addition, these cells expressed reduced levels of c-*fos* mRNA when stimulated with PDGF.

The PDGF-A chain synthesized by normal human endothelial cells differs from that synthesized by a transformed human glial cell line by an amino acid sequence at the carboxy terminus corresponding to a 69-bp deletion of the transcript.[44] This difference is probably generated by alternative RNA splicing in the transformed glial cell line, but its possible biological significance is unknown since both polypeptides are mitogenically active. Dissociation of the chemotactic and mitogenic activities of PDGF may be produced by human neutrophil elastase.[45] Porcine and human PDGF have very similar physicochemical characteristics.[46,47]

The B chain of human PDGF (PDGF-B or PDGF-2) corresponds to the primary translational product of the c-*sis* proto-oncogene, which is a 26-kDa polypeptide, $p26^{c\text{-}sis}$.[48] This product is processed to yield a disulfide-linked homodimer, $p56^{c\text{-}sis}$, which is further processed to a 35-kDa dimer, $p35^{c\text{-}sis}$. Like the v-Sis product, the c-Sis/PDGF-B product undergoes N-linked glycosylation, implying processing through the endoplasmic reticulum. The c-Sis/PDGF-B product possesses the functional properties of PDGF.

Homodimers of either chain of PDGF, i.e., PDGF-AA and PDGF-BB, bind to a single type of PDGF receptor and act as true mitogens by stimulating the kinase activity of the receptor.[49] Thus, PDGF homodimers can be considered as authentic growth factors. A factor called glioma-derived growth factor I (GDGF-I) is similar or identical to a PDGF-A homodimer and binds to the PDGF receptor on human fibroblasts; however, it has only limited mitogenic activity and has low ability to stimulate receptor autophosphorylation.[50] PDGF-AA and PDGF-BB are equivalent mitogens for vascular smooth-muscle cells, but they exhibit major differences in the binding and phosphorylation patterns towards these cells.[51] A novel growth factor, termed vascular permeability factor (VPF), is a 189-amino acid polypeptide, similar in structure to PDGF-B.[52] VPF is active in increasing blood vessel permeability, endothelial cell growth, and angiogenesis. Thus, different PDGF-like growth factors may have different functional activities, which could be mediated via different receptors and postreceptor mechanisms.

III. PRODUCTION OF PDGF AND PDGF-LIKE POLYPEPTIDES

PDGF is synthesized in the megakaryocyte, transported in blood by the α-granules of platelets, and is released during blood clotting. Interestingly, a megakaryocytic tumor cell line (CHRF-288), which was derived from an infant with megakaryoblastic leukemia and was propagated in nude mice, displayed little activity similar to PDGF when assayed either biochemically or by poly A+ RNA analysis.[53] CHRF-288 cells synthesize large amounts of a basic FGF-like and a TGF-β-like factor. It is not known whether CHRF-288 cells were arrested at a developmental stage prior to the normal expression of PDGF or whether transformation suppressed the synthesis of PDGF. In addition to megakaryocytes, PDGF is synthesized by other types of cells of hematopoietic origin, including monocytes and macrophages, as well as by arterial smooth-muscle cells, endothelial cells, and embryonic cells. Adherence of circulating monocytes to the endothelium, which is a prerequisite for their migration into injured tissues and their conversion into tissue macrophages, depends on an increase in PDGF-B mRNA and is associated with increases in c-*fos*, c-*jun*, and *egr*-2 mRNA.[54] In healing vascular grafts of baboons, PDGF mRNA and protein are expressed by intimal cells, and the synthesized PDGF-like proteins may contribute to regulate the proliferation of vascular smooth-muscle cells within the graft intima.[55]

Expression of PDGF mRNA involves both positive and negative regulation at the level of transcription, and the genes coding for the PDGF-A and PDGF-B/c-Sis chains are subjected to differential regulation. Stimulation of human umbilical vein endothelial cells with acidic FGF/HBGF-1 results in the production of PDGF-A chain mRNA but not PDGF-B mRNA.[56] Transcript levels of PDGF-A and PDGF-B/c-*sis* genes are independently regulated in cultured rat aortic smooth-muscle cells.[57] Increased PDGF-A chain expression occurs in human uterine smooth-muscle cells during the physiologic hypertrophy of pregnancy.[58] Distinct combinations of the PDGF-A and PDGF-B chains may be produced in response to different signals and may play different roles in the formation and maintenance of various types of cells. Cultured cells subjected to nonoptimal conditions selectively express PDGF-B mRNA and polypeptide, which may allow their survival and growth.[59]

Endothelial cells are a rich source of PDGF. A cDNA clone homologous to the v-*sis* oncogene was isolated and partially sequenced from human endothelial cells.[35] These cells express c-*sis*/PDGF-related transcripts, whose levels are increased in conditions favoring cellular proliferation and decreased in conditions favoring cellular differentiation.[60] Expression of A and B chains of PDGF is differentially regulated by endogenous and exogenous agents in cultured microvascular endothelial cells.[61] Human microvascular endothelial cells of renal (glomerular) origin, express increased levels of mRNAs for the A and B chains of PDGF when stimulated by phorbol ester, thrombin, or TGF-β, whereas stimulation with agents that elevate cAMP results in decreased levels of these mRNAs.[62-64] IFN-γ and basic FGF suppress the accumulation of PDGF-B/c-*sis* mRNA, and to a lesser extent PDGF-A mRNA, in endothelial cells derived from the human umbilical cord.[65,66] Expression of transcripts for the PDGF-A and PDGF-B/c-Sis chains in human glomerular mesangial cells is induced by PDGF itself as well as by EGF, TGF-α, basic FGF, and TNF-α, which exert mitogenic effects in the mesangial cells.[67] EGF, basic FGF, and TNF-α also stimulate these cells to secrete a PDGF-like factor. Furthermore, anti-PDGF antibody partially abrogates the mitogenic effect of EGF, suggesting that PDGF synthesis in mesangial cells is at least partly responsible for cell growth induced by other growth factors.

The results of these studies suggest that PDGF may be an effector molecule in the mitogenic response to different types of growth stimuli. However, PDGF does not appear to be a universal mediator of the mitogenic actions elicited by other growth factors. TGF-β, while inducing both PDGF-A and PDGF-B mRNAs, is not mitogenic in the mesangial cells, indicating that its effect on PDGF-related mRNA levels can be dissociated from DNA synthesis. TNF-α induces expression of PDGF-A mRNA and PDGF-like protein in FS-4 human fibroblasts, but the mitogenic effects of TNF-α on these cells appear to be direct and may not be mediated by PDGF-like molecules.[68]

Small amounts of PDGF (average of 17.5 ng/ml) are present in human serum[69] where it is bound to α_2-macroglobulin in the form of a complex.[70,71] The physiological role of this complex has not been established, but it may contribute to regulate the action of PDGF upon binding of PDGF to its receptor and to prevent the entrance of large amounts of free PDGF into the systemic circulation from sites of injury. The levels of PDGF in plasma are undetectable. PDGF is cleared very rapidly from the plasma compartment after release from the platelet. The half-life of radioiodinated human PDGF injected i.v. into baboons is less than 2 min.[69]

A 35-kDa polypeptide, called colostrum basic growth factor (CBGF), was identified in the colostrum of goats, cows, and sheep.[72] Although the functions of CBGF are unknown, its chemical and biological properties are very similar to those of PDGF. A mitogen secreted by cultured bovine pituitary follicule stellate cells, termed vascular endothelial cell growth factor (VEGF), is a 46-kDa homodimeric glycoprotein which exhibits structural homology to the PDGF A and B chains and the v-Sis oncoprotein.[73,74]

A diversity of PDGF-like molecules is produced in cells from different types of tumors, but similar or identical proteins are produced by cells that are not transformed such as endothelial cells, rat smooth-muscle cells, rat glomerular mesangial cells, and human lung fibroblasts.[40,75,76] Cultures of nontransformed monkey kidney epithelial cells of the BSC-1 line constitutively express the c-*sis* gene and secrete a protein that is a PDGF-B homodimer.[77] Cultured human microvascular endothelial cells produce and secrete a PDGF-like mitogen that is a 31-kDa homodimer of PDGF-A chains (PDGF-1 homodimer).[78] The normal PDGF-A chain precursor from human umbilical vein endothelial cells lacks the 15 carboxy-terminal highly basic amino acids encoded by a larger cDNA derived from a human clonal glioma cell line.[79] These two different species of PDGF A chains are generated by alternative RNA splicing and may possess different biological activities. Modified low-density lipoprotein (acetyl-LDL) induces a profound and specific suppression in the production of a PDGF-like product by cultured endothelial cells.[80]

A PDGF-like protein produced by cultured rat aortic smooth-muscle cells is developmentally regulated, being secreted by cells isolated from 13- to 18-day-old rats (pups), but not from 3-month-old animals (adults).[81] A similar protein is synthesized by adult rat arterial smooth-muscle cells in primary culture when modulated from contractile to synthetic phenotype, which gives the cells the ability to synthesize DNA and divide upon stimulation with serum or growth factors.[82] The arterial smooth-muscle cells express PDGF-A chain mRNA, secrete a PDGF-like mitogen, and bind exogenous PDGF in a phenotype- and growth state-dependent fashion.[83] These cells are thus able to promote their own growth in an autocrine or paracrine manner. However, in a study with cultured primate (baboon) aortic smooth-muscle cells it was found that both the PDGF-A and PDGF-B genes are transcribed, but the cells do not secrete mitogenic activity characteristic of native PDGF.[84] These results suggest that the expression of PDGF mitogenic activity is regulated, at least in part, by translational and/or posttranslational mechanisms.

Smooth-muscle cells derived from the intima of injured rat arteries are distinct from quiescent medial smooth-muscle cells derived from unmanipulated vessels. Intimal smooth-muscle cells secrete fivefold greater amounts of PDGF-like activity into conditioned medium in culture, have fewer receptors for PDGF, and are not mitogenically stimulated by exogenous purified PDGF.[85] These results suggest that proliferation of arterial smooth-muscle cells *in vivo,* either in young animals or following injury in adults, may be controlled, at least in part, by the local production of PDGF-like molecules in a manner similar to that observed in transformed cells.

Transcripts of the PDGF-B/c-*sis* proto-oncogene are elevated in human atherosclerotic lesions compared to the normal artery.[86] PDGF-like proteins, including PDGF-A homodimers, are produced by smooth-muscle cells from human atherosclerotic plaques.[87,88] The possible role of PDGF and PDGF-like proteins in atherosclerotic processes is unknown.

A myogenic cell line (L6J1), primary skeletal myoblasts, and primary adult arterial smooth-muscle cells express the PDGF-A gene, but not the PDGF-B/c-*sis* gene.[42] All these cells, in a manner similar to that of endothelial cells, produce a PDGF-A homodimer which has structural and immunologic properties similar to those of PDGF. The PDGF-A homodimer may stimulate proliferation of skeletal myoblasts and arterial smooth-muscle cells in an autocrine or paracrine manner.

PDGF and/or PDGF-like peptides may be importantly involved in physiological processes associated with wound healing, acting as potent microattractants and mitogens for cells of the local connective tissue. Two peptides related to PDGF have been identified in human wound fluid.[89] These PDGF-related peptides have a molecular weight of 16 to 17 and 34 to 36 kDa, respectively, and are not represented by PDGF-A or PDGF-B chains. They display chemotactic and mitogenic activities for NIH/3T3 cells *in vitro*. No authentic PDGF chains were detected in the human wound fluid samples collected from female patients who had undergone radical mastectomy for tumor removal.

A significant proportion of the mitogenic activity secreted by human alveolar or peritoneal macrophages is represented by PDGF-like products derived from the normal expression of the c-*sis* proto-oncogene.[90,91] Activated human blood monocytes, but not resting monocytes, release a mediator that attracts smooth-muscle cells and cooperates with other mediators to stimulate fibroblast proliferation. This mediator is PDGF or a very similar substance, and may be a product of c-*sis* gene transcription.[92] The results suggest that expression of the c-*sis* gene plays an important role in the normal processes of host defense and in the pathogenesis of nonmalignant inflammatory disorders.[91]

PDGF-like peptides are present in the nervous system. The PDGF-A chain gene is expressed by mammalian neurons during development and in maturity, and the PDGF-B chain gene is expressed in neurons of the central nervous system and the posterior pituitary gland.[93,94] It may be concluded that PDGF and PDGF-like molecules are widely expressed in a diversity of normal and transformed cells and tissues, but the precise role of PDGF and the PDGF-like peptides in these cells and tissues is little understood.

IV. FUNCTIONS OF PDGF

PDGF is indispensable for the growth *in vitro,* and probably also *in vivo,* of cells derived from connective tissue. PDGF is the most potent mitogenic agent for cells of mesenchymal origin, including fibroblasts, vascular smooth-muscle cells, and glial cells. Other types of cells may also exhibit mitogenic responses to PDGF. Coexpression of PDGF-B chain and the PDGF-β receptor in isolated pancreatic islet cells stimulates DNA synthesis.[95] The *in vivo* effects of PDGF are understood incompletely, but PDGF stimulates different metabolic and functional cellular activities, including commitment to DNA synthesis and induction of proliferation in different types of cells under certain physiological conditions. Expression of PDGF and PDGF-like molecules is subject to developmental regulation, suggesting an important role for these molecules in normal developmental processes.

PDGF may have an important role in wound healing and in the complex processes associated with tissue repair following injury. Studies with reconstituted fibrillar collagen gels *in vitro* showed that the structure of the extracellular matrix may influence the proliferative response of cells such as human skin fibroblasts to serum and purified PDGF.[96] This modulation may involve the expression of PDGF receptors and may operate *in vivo,* for example, during wound healing. PDGF alone appears to be of limited value in accelerating wound repair *in vivo,* but in combination with other growth factors, including EGF and IGF-I, it is able to modulate the normal healing process.[97] An interaction between PDGF and TGF-β may be important in wound healing processes, but PDGF and TGF-β enhance tissue repair activities by distinct mechanisms.[98] Whereas TGF-β transiently attracts fibroblasts into the wound and may stimulate collagen synthesis directly, PDGF is a more potent chemoattractant for wound macrophages and fibroblasts and stimulates these cells to express endogenous growth factors, including TGF-β, which, in turn, stimulates new collagen synthesis and sustained enhancement of wound healing over a more prolonged period of time. PDGF-AA homodimers are potent chemoattractants for fibroblasts and neutrophils, and for monocytes activated by lymphocytes or cytokines.[99] PDGF-AA homodimer is the predominant isoform in human platelets and acute human wound fluid.[100]

The effects of PDGF have been extensively evaluated *in vitro* in systems involving different types of cells. PDGF alone cannot initiate proliferation of quiescent BALB/c 3T3 mouse cells, but transient treatment of them with PDGF followed by plasma results in DNA synthesis and cell growth.[101] In this system PDGF act as a competence factor, stimulating the initial events in the replicative response by priming cells to the mitogenic action of progression factors contained in platelet-poor plasma.[102] The amount of PDGF per cell, rather than PDGF concentration, regulates the mitogenic response.[103] Heparin potentiates the growth-stimulatory effects of PDGF on cultured human skin fibroblasts, but the mechanism of this potentiation remains unexplained.[104]

Fibroblasts derived from patients with Werner's syndrome (an autosomal recessive disorder which is characterized by an apparent acceleration of the processes associated with aging) show a markedly attenuated response to the mitogenic effects of PDGF and FGF.[105] This blunted response is not due to a decreased number of receptors, but appears to be localized in pathways beyond binding of the growth factors to the cell surface. Moreover, Werner's syndrome fibroblasts exhibit a normal mitogenic response to fetal bovine serum, but not to adult serum, suggesting that the fetal serum contains a growth-promoting activity that is not present in serum from adult rats.

PDGF stimulates *in vitro* chemotaxis of human neutrophils and monocytes, and may act as a negative modulator of receptor-mediated activation of neutrophil oxidative burst and as an activator of phagocytosis.[106,107] PDGF may have an important role in processes such as tissue regeneration, wound healing, and inflammatory response at sites of injury or thrombosis. PDGF may be involved in the tissue remodeling that occurs in conjunction with chronic rejection of heart transplants.[108] Endogenous PDGF appears to be involved in occlusions of the coronary arteries that may occur after angioplasty of bypass surgery.[109] These occlusions are associated with accumulation of neointimal smooth-muscle cells, which is also a prominent feature of atherosclerosis in general.

V. THE PDGF RECEPTOR

The effects of PDGF at the cellular level are initiated by its interaction with specific high-affinity receptors.[110] PDGF receptors are phosphotyrosine-containing glycoproteins of 160 to 180 kDa, located on the cell surface.[111,112] Interaction of PDGF with its receptor is associated with activation of a protein-tyrosine kinase intrinsic to the PDGF-receptor complex.[113-116] Dimerization of the PDGF receptor upon ligand binding is intimately associated with activation of the PDGF receptor kinase.[117] Studies with PDGF chain-specific antibodies and ligand mutagenesis proved that PDGF is bivalent, but high-affinity PDGF binding can occur through a single ligand subunit.[118]

Cell surface expression of the PDGF receptor is an essential prerequisite for the initiation of the cellular actions of PDGF. The receptors are present in mesenchymal cells and in cells of glial origin, including smooth-muscle cells and connective tissue cells such as human and murine fibroblasts.[119] In the human and primate kidney, PDGF receptors localize to mesangial, parietal epithelial, and interstitial cells.[120] Human microvascular endothelial cells express PDGF receptors.[121] The receptors have also been detected in certain tumor cells, for example, in human osteosarcoma cells.[122] In bone marrow, stromal cells are a structural and functional support for hematopoiesis, and PDGF receptors, as well as EGF receptors, are normally expressed in these cells.[123] PDGF receptors are usually not found in blood cells or epithelial cells, but aberrant expression of PDGF receptors was detected in an anaplastic thyroid carcinoma cell line (C 643), whose thyroid epithelial origin was confirmed by the expression of thyroglobulin mRNA.[124] Interestingly, PDGF can act as a chemoattractant for the ciliated protozoan *Tetrahymena*, where it induces a rapid increase in RNA and DNA synthesis.[125] PDGF binding sites contained on the *Tetrahymena* cell surface may represent part of an evolutionary ancient regulatory mechanism.

A. THE PDGF RECEPTOR GENE

The murine PDGF receptor gene was cloned and its complete nucleotide sequence was determined.[126] The human PDGF receptor gene was also cloned and sequenced.[127] The 5.45-kb human cDNA clone predicts a 1106-amino-acid polypeptide, including the cleavable signal sequence. The overall amino acid sequence similarity of the murine and human PDGF receptor protein is 85%. The PDGF receptor gene was mapped to human chromosome 5, at region 5q31-q32, which is not far from the loci of the CSF-2 gene and the c-*fms*/CSF-1 receptor proto-oncogene.[126] In fact, the c-*fms*/CSF-1 receptor gene and the PDGF receptor genes are physically linked in a head-to-tail array and are separated by less than 500 bp on human chromosome 5q.[128] In addition to these two genes, human chromosome 5q contains the structural genes for IL-3, CSF-2, IL-5, and CSF-1. The gene for the β_2-adrenergic receptor is also located on the same chromosome region.[129]

Cross-competition binding studies have revealed the existence of more than one form of the PDGF receptor related to combinations of two types of PDGF receptor subunits, termed α and β subunits.[130] Both subunits have been cloned and sequenced,[131] and it has been recognized that they are encoded by separate genes. The gene encoding the PDGF receptor α subunit maps to human chromosome region 4q11-q12, in close proximity to the c-*kit* proto-oncogene.[132] The c-*kit* gene encodes a cell surface receptor protein with tyrosine kinase activity.[133] The PDGF receptor gene previously mapped to human chromosome region 5q31-q32, corresponds to the locus for the β subunit of the receptor.

B. BIOSYNTHESIS AND STRUCTURE OF THE PDGF RECEPTOR

A number of PDGF-related proteins have been identified in cultured human skin fibroblasts.[134-138] The human PDGF receptor is synthesized in the form of a 145-kDa precursor which is converted to a 165-kDa glycosylated form, and this form is further processed to molecules in the range of 170 to 180 kDa, which would represent the mature forms of the receptor. Smaller proteins detected with the PDGF receptor-specific antibody PR7212, including a 130-kDa protein, may represent degradation forms of the PDGF receptor originated by limited proteolysis.

The PDGF receptor gene located on mouse chromosome 5 is expressed as a single 5.2-kb mRNA species in different mouse cells such as fibroblasts, placenta, lung, and fetal kidney.[139] The receptor is synthesized in BALB/c 3T3 cells as a 160-kDa precursor that is converted to a mature form of 180 kDa within 30 to 45 min after synthesis.[140-142] The mature PDGF receptor molecule is a membrane glycoprotein which contains phosphotyrosine. Alterations in the oligosaccharide component of the PDGF receptor molecule may be responsible for the heterogeneity observed in the receptor present in BALB/c 3T3 cells.[143] The mature 180-kDa form of the PDGF receptor has a half-life of 3 h in the absence of the ligand, and its degradation is enhanced by the binding of PDGF. The PDGF receptor was also purified to homogeneity on a large scale from porcine uterus.[144]

Binding of PDGF to its receptor on the surface of normal or transformed cells can be blocked by competitive inhibition with protamine sulfate.[145] PDGF and protamine sulfate share several properties in common, both being extremely basic proteins with a predominance of basic amino acids. The polyanionic compound, suramin, can inhibit the interaction between PDGF and its receptor.[146,147] Suramin also alters the interaction of other growth factors (TGF-β, FGF, and EGF) with their receptors on the cell surface.[148] It is not known whether suramin binds free ligands and/or disrupts ligand/receptor interactions. Certain plasma PDGF-binding proteins are capable of inhibiting binding of PDGF to its cell surface receptors.[71]

C. MOLECULAR FORMS OF THE PDGF RECEPTOR

Although in earlier studies the existence of a single class of cell-surface PDGF receptor was assumed, recent evidence indicates the existence of different PDGF receptor isoforms: A-type or PDGF α-receptor, B-type or PDGF β-receptor, and A/B-type or PDGF α/β-receptor.[149-151] The PDGF receptor isoforms can be distinguished by their ligand binding specificity. The B-type receptor binds only PDGF-BB homodimers, whereas the A-type or A/B-type binds both PDGF-AA and PDGF-BB homodimers as well as PDGF-AB heterodimers (Figure 1). Expression of different PDGF receptor isoforms exhibits tissue specificity and developmental regulation. The mouse type-A PDGF receptor has been sequenced and its tissue expression has been determined, as well as its correlation with a metastatic phenotype.[152] During late neurogenesis in the nervous system of the rat, type-A PDGF receptors expression is restricted to glial cells of the oligodendrocyte lineage.[153] Human dermal fibroblasts in culture express high amounts of the B-type receptor, in comparison to the A-type receptor. The B-type receptor may be responsible for most PDGF receptor phosphorylation. A-type and B-type PDGF receptors activate unique and common signal transduction pathways.[154] Some of the known PDGF-induced cellular effects are transduced only by the B-type receptor.

PDGF receptor heterogeneity is related to the existence of two different subunit components of the receptor molecule. The receptor consists of combinations of α and β subunits which are encoded by distinct genes and dimerize to form three distinct receptor molecules that differ in their ability to bind the

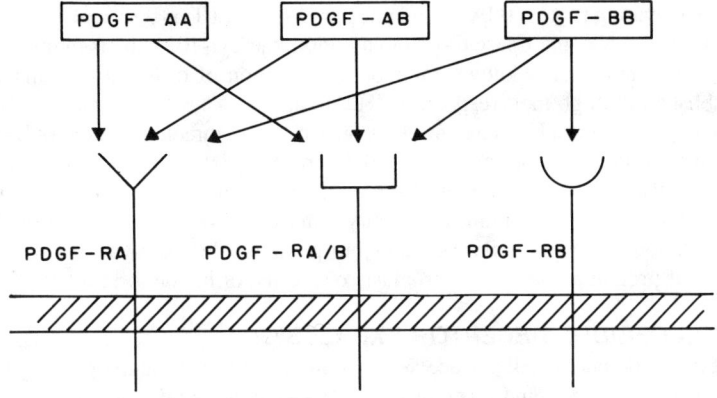

Figure 7.1 Binding of PDGF isoforms to different types of PDGF receptors.

three PDGF isoforms (PDGF-AA, PDGF-BB, and PDGF-AB).[137] The receptor α subunit binds either the A or B chain of PDGF, whereas the β subunit binds only the B-chain of PDGF. Thus αα receptors bind all three PDGF isoforms, αβ receptors bind PDGF-AB and PDGF-BB, and ββ receptors bind only PDGF-BB. The clonal human glioma cell line U-343 MGA 3IL expresses only the A-type PDGF receptor, and both PDGF-AA and PDGF-BB mediate, through their binding to this receptor, protein tyrosine phosphorylation, EGF receptor transmodulation, and a mitogenic response.[130] cDNAs for the α and β subunits of the human PDGF receptor have been cloned and sequenced.[131] Analysis of a cDNA clone encoding the α-subunit/A-chain of the human PDGF receptor predicts a 1089-residue receptor molecule which exhibits 44% overall amino acid similarity with the β-subunit/B-chain of the receptor.[138] Two PDGF-A chains, termed short and long A chains, generated by alternative RNA splicing of exon 6 of the A-chain gene, are expressed in a variety of normal tissues.[155] The different PDGF receptors have a similar domain organization, with five Ig-like extracellular domains and an intracellular split tyrosine kinase domain.

The PDGF receptor α subunit gene is closely linked to the *W/c-kit* locus on mouse chromosome 5 and the mouse patch *(Ph)* mutation is associated with a deletion in the gene.[156] Patch heterozygotes have a spotting phenotype that is similar to those of some of the *W* mutant alleles, although there is no evidence of a hematological defect. Presumptive homozygotes, produced in crosses between heterozygotes, display gross anatomical abnormalities and die midway through gestation.

D. PHOSPHORYLATION OF THE PDGF RECEPTOR

The PDGF receptor has a ligand-binding domain on the outside of the membrane and an effector domain inside. The cytoplasmic part of the receptor complex has an associated tyrosine kinase activity. The PDGF-stimulated kinase activity is not dependent on Ca^{2+} or cyclic nucleotides, but requires Mn^{2+}.[114] The mature PDGF receptor molecule is phosphorylated on both tyrosine and serine after PDGF stimulation.[157] Autophosphorylation of the receptor on tyrosine after PDGF binding has been ascertained by using monoclonal antibody to phosphotyrosine.[158] Studies with monoclonal antibodies which recognize the external domains of porcine and human PDGF receptors suggest that direct interaction with the PDGF binding site is not necessary for activation of the PDGF receptor kinase, since these antibodies do not inhibit binding of [^{125}I]-PDGF to its receptor, indicating that they do not recognize the receptor binding site for PDGF, but stimulate the receptor-associated tyrosine kinase activity in a dose-dependent manner.[159]

Association of the PDGF receptor with specific cellular proteins is most important for signal transduction. The Tyr-825 residue of the PDGF receptor is importantly involved in autophosphorylation, and this modification, as well as specific changes in receptor conformation, is required for the transduction of a PDGF-elicited signal.[160] The PDGF receptor displays PDGF-stimulatable tyrosine kinase activity and is able to phosphorylate various substrates, including angiotensin II and a Src-related peptide.[161] Members of the Src family of tyrosine kinases associate with activated PDGF receptors — and the Tyr-857 residue, but not the Tyr-751 residue, of the receptor molecule is required for efficient association.[162] The different tyrosyl residues of the PDGF receptor may exhibit distinct associations with specific cellular proteins. For the human PDGF receptor β subunit: phosphorylation at Tyr-740 and Tyr-751 is necessary for stable association with phosphatidylinositol 3-kinase (PI 3-kinase), phosphorylation of Tyr-771 permits binding of the Ras GTPase activating protein (GAP), and phosphorylation at Tyr-1009 and Tyr-1021 is important for stable association with phospholipase C-γ.[163] In addition, the Tyr-1021 site is required for the binding of a 64-kDa protein complex of unknown function. Association of different proteins with the PDGF receptor are established through their respective SH2 domains.

Protein kinase C, which phosphorylates proteins on serine and threonine, may not be involved in the regulation of the ligand-binding properties of the PDGF receptor.[164] This conclusion was deduced from the fact that TPA, which is a direct activator of protein kinase C, has little or no effect on the properties of the PDGF receptor, including its number, affinity, internalization, and degradation. PDGF-induced tyrosine phosphorylation of the PDGF receptor and phosphoinositide hydrolysis are unaffected by PMA-induced activation of protein kinase C in fibroblasts of murine or human origin.[165]

E. REGULATION OF PDGF RECEPTOR EXPRESSION

PDGF receptor expression on the cell surface depends on binding of the autologous ligand, which leads to a rapid internalization of the ligand-receptor complex — a process referred to as down-regulation. In addition, the level of PDGF receptor expression is modulated by heterologous ligands (transmodulation). Although several growth factors are capable of inducing transmodulation of PDGF receptor expression, TGF-β is the most potent one with this effect.[166] Moreover, TGF-β may differentially regulate the expression of PDGF-binding sites and the mitogenic responsiveness toward the three molecular isoforms of PDGF (PDGF-AA, PDGF-BB, and PDGF-AB). Treatment of Swiss 3T3 cells with TGF-β leads to an almost complete loss of PDGF-AA binding and results in a reduced mitogenic response to PDGF-AA. In contrast, binding of PDGF-BB is only reduced by about 50% in the cells treated with TGF-β. In addition to growth factors, other substances may influence the cellular responses to PDGF. Stimulation of fibroblastic cell proliferation by PDGF is enhanced synergistically by receptor-recognized $α_2$-macroglobulin.[167]

Little is known about the biochemical mechanisms involved in the induction of PDGF receptor expression. Cultured rat Schwann cells proliferate in response to PDGF only if simultaneously cultured in the presence of agents, such as forskolin, that elevate the intracellular concentrations of cAMP.[168] This response is associated with cAMP-mediated induction of PDGF receptor mRNA and protein. In addition, cAMP-mediated induction of the PDGF receptor in Schwann cells results in enhanced ligand-dependent receptor autophosphorylation and in enhanced PDGF-induced activation of c-*fos* proto-oncogene expression. A mechanism dependent on Ca^{2+} influx and protein kinase C activation may operate in the differential response of PDGF receptor isoforms to PDGF-AA in BALB/c 3T3 cells.[169]

F. INTERNALIZATION AND PROCESSING OF THE PDGF RECEPTOR

After binding to its receptor, PDGF is internalized and degraded in the lysosomes, but the fate of the PDGF receptor after internalization is unknown.[170] PDGF receptors are subjected to downregulation after incubation of cells with PDGF, which may serve to impede excessive cell proliferation by an eventually prolonged exposure to the growth factor. However, PDGF receptors can turn over quite rapidly from the cell surface pool in the absence of the ligand.[143] Incompletely processed PDGF receptors may show functional integrity, being capable of mediating the mitogenic activity of PDGF.[134]

VI. TRANSDUCTIONAL MECHANISMS OF PDGF ACTION

The transductional mechanisms involved in the cellular effects of PDGF may include activation of Ras proteins as well as alterations in protein phosphorylation, phosphoinositide metabolism, intracellular Ca^{2+} distribution, monovalent ion fluxes, guanine nucleotide binding proteins, and prostacyclin synthesis.

A. RAS PROTEINS

The transductional mechanisms of action of PDGF involve as an essential component the activation of Ras proteins. In the G54 cell line, a derivative of Swiss 3T3 cells that overexpresses normal c-H-Ras protein, PDGF-induced DNA synthesis is accompanied by an increase in the formation of Ras-GTP complexes, suggesting that these complexes are involved in the transmission of the mitogenic signal elicited by PDGF.[171] A specific protein, Grb2, links the ligand-activated PDGF receptor tyrosine kinase (and other tyrosine kinase receptors) to Ras through its SH2 domain.[172,173] Grb2 is a small, widely expressed protein, whose entire sequence is composed of a single SH2 domain flanked by two SH3 domains. Grb2 binds directly to a Ras exchange factor, Sos1, through its two SH3 domains, and Sos1 activates the Ras signaling pathway.[174]

Mutational analysis of the PDGF receptor indicates that the PDGF receptor-stimulated signaling pathways for the activation of Ras may be different in different types of cells.[175] In the CHO cell line, mutation of the tyrosine residues that are recognized by the PI 3-kinase renders the PDGF receptor incapable of activating Ras protein. On the other hand, in a pro-B-cell line, BaF3, either the PI 3-kinase, GAP, or phospholipase C-γ binding site of the PDGF receptor is dispensable for the activation of Ras protein. Therefore, several different PDGF receptor-mediated signaling pathways may function upstream of Ras, and the extent of the contribution of each pathway for the regulation of Ras protein activation may differ among different types of cells.[175]

B. PROTEIN PHOSPHORYLATION

Phosphorylation of specific cellular proteins on tyrosine is an essential component of the transductional mechanisms of PDGF action.[114,176] However, little is known about the cellular substrates whose phosphorylation is physiologically significant in relation to the action of PDGF on its target cells. A 85-kDa protein is rapidly phosphorylated in mouse fibroblasts treated with PDGF.[177] PDGF induces rapid and sustained tyrosine phosphorylation of phospholipase C-γ (PLC-γ/PLC-II) in quiescent BALB/c 3T3 cells.[178] This enzyme is involved in phosphoinositide hydrolysis and generation of intracellular second messengers. PDGF forms transient complexes with PLC-γ as well as with the products of some proto-oncogenes, including the Raf-1 protein and three members of the Src family, c-Src, c-Yes, and Fyn.[179] The tyrosine-specific kinase activity of these proteins is increased after PDGF stimulation of quiescent fibroblasts, coincident with their association with the PDGF receptor. Phosphorylation on specific tyrosine residues of the plasma membrane- and cytoskeleton-associated protein, calpactin I (annexin II), is induced by PDGF.[180] Calpactin I is also phosphorylated by oncoproteins of the *src* gene family. The use of synthetic peptides derived from the sequence surrounding Tyr-857 in the human PDGF β-receptor molecule showed that oligopeptides of only five amino acids, lacking acidic residues, can function as substrates for the receptor kinase.[181]

In addition to tyrosine phosphorylation, PDGF may stimulate the phosphorylation of specific cellular proteins on serine and threonine residues, which occurs through indirect mechanisms, by the action of secondarily activated protein kinases with specificity for serine/threonine residues. A nuclear protein of 64 kDa, termed pp64, is phosphorylated on serine and threonine residues by the action of PDGF on NRK cells.[182] The pp64 nuclear protein is additionally phosphorylated on tyrosine in SSV-transformed NRK cells. TPA, but not EGF or insulin, induce the phosphorylation of nuclear pp64.

The role of phosphotyrosine formation in the transductional mechanisms of action of PDGF is not totally clear. The mouse and human PDGF receptor contain an insert, the kinase insert, which is recognized by sequence similarity to other known tyrosine kinases. Expression in CHO cells, that normally lack PDGF receptors, of a transfected PDGF receptor containing an artificial deletion of the receptor tyrosine kinase insert is unable to elicit a mitogenic response, in spite of the fact that the transfectants exhibit PDGF binding, receptor downregulation, and tyrosine phosphorylation, as well as other transductional mechanisms related to PDGF action such as phosphatidylinositol hydrolysis, pH alteration, and an increase in $[Ca^{2+}]_i$.[183] The extent of PDGF-dependent tyrosine phosphorylation of the PDGF receptor from sparse vs. confluent human foreskin fibroblasts is quite similar in spite of the fact that sparse fibroblasts show a greater mitogenic response to PDGF than do confluent fibroblasts.[184] Sparse and confluent fibroblasts have the same number of PDGF receptors per cell and the apparent affinities of the two populations of receptors are similar. It is thus apparent that tyrosine phosphorylation of the PDGF receptor may not be tightly correlated to the PDGF mitogenic signal and that other biochemical changes may have an important role in the transduction of the PDGF-elicited signal.

C. PHOSPHOINOSITIDE METABOLISM AND TRANSLOCATION OF CA^{2+}

Transductional mechanisms of PDGF action include changes in phosphoinositide metabolism and intracellular mobilization of calcium. Stimulation of the proliferation of BALB/c 3T3 cells by PDGF is associated with activation of phospholipase C, which results in the hydrolysis of phosphatidylinositol 4,5-bisphosphate, increased production of 1,2-diacylglycerol, and subsequent activation of protein kinase C.[185,186] Stable physical association occurs in mouse BALB/c 363 cells between the PDGF receptor and the enzyme PLC-II/PLC-γ, which results in tyrosine phosphorylation and activation of the enzyme.[177,187] PDGF may promote translocation of PLC-II/PLC-γ from the cytosol to the plasma membrane.[188] In Rat-2 cells, PDGF increases the tyrosine phosphorylation and the activity of two PLC-γ subtypes, PLC-$γ_1$ and PLC-$γ_2$.[189] PLC-$γ_1$ mediates PDGF-induced phosphoinositide hydrolysis, and phosphorylation of this enzyme on the Tyr-783 residue is essential for its activation.[190] PLC-$γ_2$ is involved in signal transduction of PDGF in VSM cells.[191] An alternative pathway for 1,2-diacylglycerol production in PDGF-stimulated murine cells is by its synthesis from monoacylglycerol.[192]

The results of studies with a monoclonal antibody specific for phosphatidylinositol 4,5-bisphosphate strongly suggest that phosphatidylinositol breakdown is crucially involved in the elicitation and sustaining of cell proliferation induced by PDGF and bombesin, but is not essential for the mitogenic effects of FGF, EGF, insulin, and serum.[193,194] In the human osteosarcoma cell line MG-63-LS, PDGF, but not EGF or FGF, activate the inositol trisphophate/diacylglycerol second-messenger system in a dose-dependent manner, and this effect is inhibited by preincubation of the cells with TGF-β.[195] The inhibitory effect of TGF-β on the growth of MG-63-LS cells may be indirect, and may be exerted through interference with the generation of inositol trisphosphate.

PDGF rapidly stimulates phosphatidylinositol kinase activity and breakdown of polyphosphoinositides in human and mouse fibroblasts, with a severalfold increase in intracellular levels of inositol 1,4,5-trisphosphate and mobilization of Ca^{2+}.[196-199] These changes involve activation of protein kinase C, but their possible role in the mitogenic effects of PDGF is not clear, however. Although PDGF stimulates phospholipase C activity both *in vitro* and in living cells, studies using a molecular vector that overexpressed the PLC-II/PLC-γ suggested that other enzymes may be crucially involved in PDGF-induced signaling and DNA synthesis.[200] A correlation between PDGF-stimulated generation of inositol 1,4,5-trisphosphate, a rise in $[Ca^{2+}]_i$, and mitogenesis was not observed in this system. Studies with the tyrosine kinase inhibitor, genistein, indicate that accumulation of inositol phosphates, an increase in $[Ca^{2+}]_i$, and activation of protein kinase C may not be required for PDGF-induced DNA synthesis in mouse fibroblasts.[201]

Other phosphoinositide metabolic pathways may be regulated by PDGF action in different types of cells. PDGF stimulates synthesis of phosphatidylinositol 3,4,5-trisphosphate by activating the PI 3-kinase and mediating the translocation of the enzyme from the cytosol.[202,203] PDGF stimulates in NIH/3T3 cells the hydrolysis of phosphatidylcholine by activation of phospholipase D, resulting in the formation of phosphatidic acid, which is converted to diacylglycerol by the action of the enzyme, phosphatidic acid phosphohydrolase.[204] Phosphatidic acid may be an important intracellular mediator in the signaling transductional mechanisms of PDGF. In PDGF-stimulated mouse fibroblasts, phosphatidic acid accumulation, rather than a 1,2-diacylglycerol increase, correlates with mitogenesis.[205] Phosphatidic acid has an inhibitory effect on two regulatory proteins, inhibiting Ras GAP activity and increasing GTPase-inhibiting protein, which may result in an increase in Ras activity by keeping Ras in the form of a GTP complex. Ras activation occurs in PDGF-stimulated cells, and this activation may result in increased cell proliferation.

Calcium may be involved in mediating the cellular actions of PDGF. Release of Ca^{2+} from intracellular sequestration sites may be a mechanism by which PDGF stimulates cell growth.[206] Addition of PDGF to cultures of quiescent mouse fibroblasts induces a rapid increase in the $[Ca^{2+}]_i$, and the calcium ionophores A23187 and ionomycin can mimic the actions of PDGF on these cells, including an increase in c-*myc* gene expression.[207] An early, transient increase in $[Ca^{2+}]_i$ is required for the mitogenic effects of PDGF.[208] This increase is associated with a decline in cell pH_i by a later cell alkalinization.[209] Studies using digital image analysis of intracellular Fura-2 fluorescence to measure the $[Ca^{2+}]_i$ in individual BALB/c 3T3 cells indicate that an increase in the $[Ca^{2+}]_i$ is necessary for PDGF-stimulated mitogenesis.[210] In contrast, this increase is not necessary for the mitogenic action of FGF in the same cells. NIH/3T3 cells transformed by the EJ c-H-*ras* oncogene exhibit a reduced capacity to generate inositol 1,4,5-trisphosphate in response to PDGF, and the PDGF-induced Ca^{2+} mobilization is also altered in these cells.[211,212] Such alterations suggest that the p21 product of the mutant c-H-*ras* gene may uncouple the PDGF receptor from phospholipase C, which may lead to a decrease of phospholipase A_2, with diminished arachidonate release and prostaglandin biosynthesis.

Phospholipase C-mediated hydrolysis of phosphatidylcholine may be an important step in PDGF-stimulated DNA synthesis.[213] PDGF, as well as serum and phorbol esters, stimulate within seconds the hydrolysis of phosphatidylcholine, which results in generation of diacylglycerol and phosphocholine.[214] Production of diacylglycerol from phosphatidylcholine may provide additional mechanisms for the regulation of protein kinase C. PDGF stimulation of phospholipid hydrolysis results in increased release of PGE_2 and arachidonate. Cells expressing high levels of a mutant Ras protein exhibit a deficient activity of phospholipases C and A_2 and a reduction in PDGF-stimulated release of PGE_2 and arachidonate.[215,216] Further studies are required to elucidate the role of phospholipid metabolism in the transductional mechanisms of PDGF action.

D. NA+/H+ ANTIPORT AND CYTOPLASMIC ALKALINIZATION

PDGF-induced generation of 1,2-diacylglycerol can activate the Na$^+$/H$^+$ antiport, which may result in alkalinization of the cytoplasm.[196] This alkalinization is independent of changes in cytoplasmic Ca^{2+}.[209] Phorbol ester (PMA) blocks the activation of Na$^+$/H$^+$ exchange by PDGF or serum.[217] Activation of Na$^+$/H$^+$ exchange by PDGF may not require the intermediate activation of protein kinase C. The continued ability of PDGF to stimulate DNA synthesis in BALB/c 3T3 fibroblasts in the face of sustained cytoplasm acidification and the absence of protein kinase C activity suggests that cytosolic alkalinization and protein kinase C activation are not essential for PDGF-induced competence to proliferation.[218] In addition to the Na$^+$/H$^+$ antiporter and the Na$^+$,K$^+$-ATPase, PDGF stimulates the transport of ions into the cell through activation of a nonselective cation channel.[219]

E. ARACHIDONIC ACID AND PROSTACYCLIN

PDGF stimulates a biphasic mobilization of arachidonic acid in Swiss 3T3 cells, and this effect may depend on the action of phospholipase A$_2$.[220] Prostacyclin (PGI$_2$), a major archidonic acid metabolite produced by endothelial cells, is a potent vasodilator and inhibitor of platelet aggregation and release.[221] However, PDGF does not cause increased synthesis of PGI$_2$ in cultured endothelial cells of human or bovine origin.[222]

F. MODULATION OF CELLULAR RESPONSES TO PDGF

Different determinants of the PDGF molecule may be related to different cellular responses after interaction with the specific cell-surface receptors. For example, reduction of the native 32,000-Da PDGF to its constituent polypeptide chains (14,000- and 17,000-Da components) causes a loss of the ability to stimulate cell proliferation, but all the activity as a chemotactic agent for human neutrophils and monocytes is wholly retained.[223] Neutrophil elastase abolishes the chemotactic activity of PDGF for fibroblasts but has no effect on its chemotactic activity for monocytes, or on its mitogenic activity for 3T3 cells, or its capacity to bind to 3T3 cells.[45] The results obtained in these experiments suggest that the biological effects of PDGF can be modulated selectively by factors that might be released at the same sites as PDGF.

VII. EFFECTS OF PDGF ON EGF ACTION

A fundamental effect of PDGF in certain cellular systems is to increase the sensitivity of cells to EGF.[224] The mechanisms responsible for this phenomenon are not clear, however. The synergistic action of PDGF and EGF could provide a growth control *in vivo* through a PDGF-induced alteration of the sensitivity of cells to EGF, but at least some effects of PDGF are independent from EGF.[225]

PDGF mimics phorbol ester action on the phosphorylation of the EGF receptor at Thr-654 in WI-38 human fetal lung fibroblasts.[226] Since Thr-654 is the major site of phosphorylation of the EGF receptor catalyzed by protein kinase C, these results are consistent with the hypothesis that PDGF stimulates protein kinase C activity and that some of the effects of PDGF may be mediated by an increase in the intracellular levels of 1,2-diacylglycerol and free Ca^{2+} resulting from the hydrolysis of phosphatidylinositol 4,5-bisphosphate. The effect of PDGF on the phosphorylation of the EGF receptor is similar to that observed when cells are treated with phorbol ester or exogenous diacylglycerol. However, PDGF, phorbol esters, and diacylglycerol increase the phosphorylation of the EGF receptor at sites in addition to Thr-654, which suggests that these agents may affect the activity of cellular protein kinases other than kinase C but are also capable of phosphorylating the EGF receptor. The physiological role of the phosphorylation of the EGF receptor at different sites is not understood. The effects of PDGF and TPA on EGF receptor phosphorylation may exhibit specificity for different types of cells such as human skin fibroblasts and human lung fibroblasts.[227] Consequently, the exact biological significance of the heterologous regulation of EGF receptor expression is not understood. In any case, the effect of PDGF on EGF receptor phosphorylation is an example of the complex interactions existing between growth factors and proto-oncogene protein products.[226] The B chain of PDGF is the product of the c-*sis* proto-oncogene and the EGF receptor is the product of the c-*erb*-B proto-oncogene.

Addition of PDGF or phorbol ester to cultured human fetal lung fibroblasts causes an inhibition of the EGF-dependent phosphorylation of the EGF receptor on tyrosine.[226] This result represents an apparent paradox to data indicating that tyrosine phosphorylation of the EGF receptor is essential for its activation and that both PDGF and phorbol ester enhance the mitogenic effects of EGF.

In mouse BALB/c 3T3 cells and human foreskin fibroblasts, PDGF action correlates with a substantial loss of EGF receptor expression on the cell surface.[228,229] This effect is unidirectional since EGF does not decrease PDGF receptors. Although both PDGF and phorbol ester (PMA) cause a rapid, transient, protein synthesis-independent reduction in EGF binding capacity, the mechanism by which PDGF modulates EGF binding in mouse fibroblasts is apparently different from that of PMA.[230] Whereas PMA allows EGF binding activity to recover, PDGF induces a secondary and protein synthesis-dependent decline in EGF binding capacity.

VIII. POSTTRANSDUCTIONAL MECHANISMS OF ACTION OF PDGF

After binding to its receptor, PDGF initiates a cascade of events that may lead to cells competent to DNA synthesis and proliferation under the stimulus of specific hormones and growth factors. A diversity of biochemical, functional, and morphological changes may be observed in cellular systems *in vitro* after stimulation with PDGF.[4,7] Biochemical alterations induced by PDGF in cultured mouse fibroblasts include changes in ion and amino acid transport, glycolysis, and protein and prostaglandin synthesis. At least in some systems, the B chain of PDGF alone may be sufficient for mitogenesis.[231] In contrast to the manifold effects produced by PDGF *in vitro*, administration of PDGF to male Wistar rats results in only moderate metabolic and enzymatic changes affecting the hepatic pyruvate content, the cytosolic phosphorylation potential, and inducing increased glucose-6-phosphate dehydrogenase activity in the liver.[232] The reasons for the different effects of PDGF observed *in vivo* and *in vitro* are unknown.

A. PROTEIN PHOSPHORYLATION

The cellular actions of PDGF are mediated by the tyrosine kinase activity of the PDGF-receptor complex.[113-116] A number of cellular proteins are phosphorylated on tyrosine in response to PDGF,[233,234] including proteins of approximately 300, 200, 115, 72, 54, 45, and 35 kDa.[157] The respective functions of these proteins are unknown. Phosphorylation of the ribosomal protein S6 on serine residues is also stimulated by PDGF.[235] Some of the cellular proteins phosphorylated by the action of PDGF may be involved in the intracellular transmission of the PDGF-induced mitogenic signal, and may also be substrates for the protein products of oncogenes and proto-oncogenes with a similar type of kinase activity.[42] Stimulation of quiescent NRK cells with PDGF or TPA, but not EGF, results in the rapid phosphorylation of a nuclear protein of 64 kDa (pp64), and this process is apparently mediated by a PDGF-activated serine/threonine kinase.[236] The precise structure and function of pp64 remain to be elucidated, but it is not associated with the chromatin and can not be extracted from the nucleus with DNase or RNase.

B. CYTOSKELETAL CHANGES

PDGF induces structural changes in the cytoskeleton. Rearrangement of preformed microfilaments induced by PDGF in BALB/c 3T3 cells is accompanied by phosphorylation of the myosin light chain, which depends on the intrinsic kinase activity of the PDGF receptor.[237] Microfilament and microtubule rearrangements may be important for transduction of the mitogenic response to PDGF and other growth factors.

Rapid and reversible time- and dose-dependent alterations in the distribution of vinculin and actin occur in fibroblasts and porcine vascular smooth-muscle cells stimulated by PDGF.[238,239] Within 2.5 min of exposure to PDGF, vinculin disappears from adhesion plaques while actin, in the form of stress fibers, becomes disrupted a few minutes thereafter. These changes are preceded by a PDGF-stimulated rapid increase in the $[Ca^{2+}]_i$. Adhesion plaques (focal contacts) are regions where actin microfilaments terminate in cells such as cultured fibroblasts and where the plasma membrane comes close to the underlying substrates.[238] Actin microfilaments terminate in vinculin contained in adhesion plaques or focal contacts.[240] Human skin collagenase expression is stimulated by PDGF *in vitro*.[241]

C. RNA AND PROTEIN SYNTHESIS

Changes at the transcriptional level may be exerted by PDGF, and it has been estimated that between 0.1 and 1.0% of murine fibroblast genes are regulated by PDGF.[242] Three distinct mRNAs induced in BALB/c 3T3 cells stimulated by PDGF are also induced by other mitogenic agents, such as LPS.[243] The functions of PDGF-inducible genes are little understood, but one of the genes directly induced by PDGF in BALB/c 3T3 fibroblasts is that of the glucose transporter.[244] PDGF increases the rate at which the glucose transporter gene is transcribed and decreases the rate at which its mRNA is degraded. Since expression of the glucose transporter mRNA is associated with cellular proliferation, these results suggest that the glucose transporter gene is a member of the class of PDGF-inducible genes known as competence genes.

The levels of expression of a set of cellular genes (*JE, KC,* and *JB*) were found to be are altered in mouse fibroblasts exposed to PDGF.[242,245] The *JE* gene encodes a 148-amino acid residue basic secretory protein which exhibits striking similarity to the products of a family of small inducible genes and to several of the proteins secreted from platelet α-granules, including platelet factor 4.[246] PDGF and platelet factor 4 are stored together in the platelet α-granules and are released during platelet aggregation at a site of injury. PDGF and platelet factor 4 are chemotactic for monocytes, macrophages, neutrophils, and fibroblasts. Glucocorticoids inhibit the transcriptional induction of the *JE* gene.[247]

The levels of a species of RNA (28H6 RNA) are increased when resting cultured mouse cells are either infected with SV40 or stimulated with PDGF.[248] A 29-kDa nuclear protein is also induced in BALB/c 3T3 fibroblasts in response to PDGF.[249] Spontaneously transformed BALB/c 3T3 fibroblasts show constitutive synthesis of this protein and do not have a requirement for PDGF. In cultured human skin fibroblasts, c-Sis/PDGF-B stimulates fibronectin gene expression.[250] The synthesis of fibronectin and collagen is a function of differentiated dermal fibroblasts, and these proteins are assembled into an extracellular matrix network. Transformed mesenchymal cells usually show reduced fibronectin synthesis, which may be associated with the expression of an anchorage-independent phenotype and diminished cell adhesion.

PDGF induces the expression of genes encoding specific types of proteases.[251] Transcription of the gene coding for the matrix-degrading secreted metalloproteinase, transin, is stimulated by PDGF. As demonstrated with the use of c-*fos* antisense RNA, PDGF-induced expression of the transin gene in NIH/3T3 mouse fibroblasts requires endogenous expression of the c-*fos* proto-oncogene.[252] In contrast, EGF-induced expression of the transin gene is independent of c-*fos* gene expression. The stimulatory effect of both PDGF and EGF on transin gene transcription involves factors recognizing the nucleotide sequence TGAGTCA, which is found in the transin promoter and is known to be a binding site for Jun-Fos/AP-1 protein complexes.

Transcription of genes for other growth factors or their receptors may be modulated by PDGF. Expression of the IL-1 receptor gene is stimulated by PDGF in mouse cells by a mechanism which involves the products of immediate early genes.[253,254] PDGF stimulates the expression of the genes for IFN-β and (2′-5′)-oligoadenylate synthetase.[255] PDGF, EGF, and other growth factors may contribute to the regulation of IFN-γ production.[256] In turn, IFN-γ may inhibit the expression of certain genes regulated by PDGF.[257]

D. PROTO-ONCOGENE EXPRESSION

The mitogenic action of PDGF is mediated, at least in part, by changes in the expression of specific cellular genes, including proto-oncogenes. Expression of c-*fos* and a c-*fos*-related gene in mouse fibroblasts is stimulated in a rapid and transient manner by PDGF.[258-261] PDGF induces expression of c-*fos* and other genes (*JE, KC,* and *JB*) almost exclusively in dense cell cultures when the cells are in the G_0/G_1 phase of the cycle.[245] Expression of the c-*fos* gene induced in mouse fibroblasts by treatment with PDGF is superinduced by cycloheximide.[258] The transient induction of c-*fos* mRNA and protein induced by PDGF is both increased and prolonged by inhibitors of calmodulin, which may be due to alterations in the degradation of c-*fos* mRNA.[260] PDGF-induced expression of c-*fos* is associated with phospholipid breakdown and the ensuing activation of protein kinase C and release of Ca^{2+}. However, increases in the $[Ca^{2+}]_i$ are not required for the stimulation of c-*fos* and c-*myc* mRNA expression in various types of cells.[262,263] Studies with forskolin (a direct activator of adenylate cyclase) and with the cAMP analog, 9-bromo-cAMP, suggest that PDGF-induced c-*fos* gene expression in Swiss 3T3 mouse fibroblasts may be mediated by activation of the adenylate cyclase system.[264] The growth-promoting effects of PDGF on mouse 3T3 cells depend not only on the transcriptional expression of the c-*fos* gene, but also on the increased posttranslational stability of the nascent c-Fos protein.[265]

PDGF-induced c-*fos* gene expression is suppressed in NIH/3T3 cells transformed by a mutated c-H-*ras* oncogene.[266] These cells exhibit diminished PDGF-stimulated phospholipase C activity, which results in decreased levels of inositol trisphosphate and diacylglycerol and diminished intracellular mobilization of Ca^{2+}. In spite of the inhibition of PDGF-induced c-*fos* expression, the *ras*-transformed cells still respond mitogenically to PDGF. The proliferative action of PDGF in rat vascular smooth muscle (VSM) cells involves mechanisms that are independent of both protein kinase C activation and c-*fos* induction.[267] Thus, it is clear that the mitogenic effects of PDGF may be associated with the activation of different metabolic pathways in different types of cells.

Expression of the c-*myc* gene may be regulated by PDGF.[268-271] Quiescent BALB/c and NIH/3T3 cells show a rapid, 40-fold increase in c-*myc* mRNA levels subsequent to stimulation with calf serum or purified PDGF, but not with either EGF or insulin.[268,272,273] In contrast to c-*fos* expression, PDGF-induced expression of c-*myc* occurs preferentially when the mouse fibroblasts are in sparse cell culture.[245] The PDGF-induced activation of c-*myc* expression (as determined by the accumulation of c-*myc* mRNA) occurs subsequent to the activation of c-*fos* gene expression.[274]

The molecular mechanism of c-*myc* gene induction by PDGF are little understood, but the murine c-*myc* gene contains in the first exon, between the P1 and P2 promoters, a segment of 81 bp that functions as a PDGF-responsive element.[275] The mechanism responsible for the activation of this element is unknown. Pretreatment of BALB/c 3T3 fibroblasts with the protein synthesis inhibitor, anisomycin, results in a marked increase in the accumulation of c-*fos* and c-*myc* mRNA, indicating that protein synthesis is not required for this induction. PDGF has been shown to stimulate phosphoinositide turnover to produce inositol trisphosphate, which then mobilizes intracellular Ca^{2+} and activates protein kinase C,[196] and this mechanism may be responsible for the increase of c-*myc* and c-*fos* expression induced by PDGF in Swiss 3T3 mouse fibroblasts.[207,276] The calcium ionophores, A23187 and ionomycin, mimic the actions of PDGF and increase c-*myc* mRNA levels. These results suggest that Ca^{2+} may serve as an intracellular messenger for PDGF-induced expression of the c-*myc* gene. Enhanced c-*myc* expression is also induced very rapidly following the activation of T lymphocytes with LPS.[268] In general, c-*myc* expression is stimulated by agents that activate protein kinase C.[277] However, in cells other than murine fibroblasts PDGF-induced c-*myc* expression may occur by a pathway independent of increased phosphoinositide turnover. PDGF-induced accumulation of c-*myc* mRNA in MG-63 human osteosarcoma cells is independent of protein kinase C activation and increased $[Ca^{2+}]_i$.[278]

At least in some cellular systems, the c-Myc protein would act as an intracellular competence factor, i.e., as a factor rendering cells competent for undergoing the G_0-S phase transition in the cell cycle. Microinjection of c-Myc into mouse cells (Swiss 3T3 fibroblasts) stimulates DNA synthesis when the cells are exposed to platelet-poor plasma.[279] The presence in the medium of an antibody specific to PDGF abolishes PDGF-induced DNA synthesis, but the microinjected c-Myc protein stimulates DNA synthesis even when its own antibody is present in the medium. Expression of the c-*myc* gene, however, may not account for the mitogenic effect of PDGF, which depends on other mechanisms.[277] Treatment of MG-63 cells with PDGF results in a severalfold increase in the concentration of c-*myc* mRNA, but this change is not followed by DNA replication and cellular proliferation.[271] Furthermore, PDGF does not potentiate the mitogenic response of MG-63 cells to IGF-I. PDGF-modulated accumulation of c-*myc* transcripts and protein in MG-63 cells may not be sufficient to stimulate DNA synthesis and cell proliferation.

Expression of the c-Src protein is modified during the cellular response to PDGF.[280] Stimulation of chicken and mouse fibroblasts with PDGF or other agents (FGF, serum, ADH/vasopressin, sodium orthovanadate, or prostaglandin F) results in phosphorylation of c-Src at Ser-12.[281,282] This reaction is probably mediated by protein kinase C activation. PDGF also induces phosphorylation of one or two additional serine residues and one tyrosine residue located on the amino-terminal region of the c-Src molecule, and this is accompanied by both increased kinase activity of c-Src and increased phosphorylation of a 36-kDa cellular protein substrate *in vivo*.[280] The results are compatible with the hypothesis that c-Src may play a role in the mitogenic response to PDGF.

The ligand-activated PDGF receptor is capable of activating the serine/threonine-specific protein kinase activity of the c-*raf*-1 proto-oncogene product through phosphorylation on tyrosine residues.[283] Phosphorylation of the c-Raf-1 protein on tyrosine and activation of its specific kinase activity is increased by PDGF in CHO cells expressing wild-type PDGF receptors, but not in those with mutant receptors defective in stimulating mitogenesis. Most importantly, there is a correlation between PDGF-induced proliferative response and activation of c-Raf-1 kinase activity, suggesting that the transmission of signals from the PDGF receptor to the c-Raf-1 protein may be involved in mitogenic responses.

IX. ROLE OF PDGF IN MITOGENIC PROCESSES

PDGF may contribute to the regulation of genes involved in the control of cellular proliferation. However, PDGF alone may not optimally stimulate DNA synthesis, and other growth factors are required for the fulfillment of the complex biochemical events involved in cell cycle control. The prereplicative phase of mouse fibroblasts growing in a defined medium *in vitro* requires the operation of two growth-factor-controlled cell cycle events, namely, competence and progression.[101,102] A brief exposure to PDGF renders BALB/c 3T3 cells competent to DNA replication, but such cells do not progress through the prereplicative phase unless exposed to plasma or a second set of growth factors, called progression factors. In the BALB/c 3T3 system, PDGF acts as a competence factor and EGF or IGF-I may act as progression factors.

This simple scheme, however, may not be valid for other cellular systems, in particular for complex *in vivo* systems. In cultured human foreskin fibroblasts, PDGF and EGF are interchangeable in the prereplicative phase: a subliminal pulse of one factor, followed by a subliminal pulse of the other factor leads to stimulation of DNA synthesis.[284] These results suggest that in the prereplicative phase of cultured human skin fibroblasts, PDGF and EGF may act through the induction of similar or identical intracellular signals. Since both the activated PDGF receptor and the EGF receptor are tyrosine kinases, one possibility is that both factors phosphorylate a common substrate(s) that is involved in the transmission of the mitogenic signals. Alternatively, PDGF and EGF may initiate different early events which converge to a common pathway in the prereplicative phase. Activation of proto-oncogenes may be involved in the final pathway leading to the mitogenic action of growth factors.

The mechanisms responsible for the PDGF-induced competence state are unknown. cAMP may mediate some cellular actions of PDGF, especially those related to cellular proliferation. PDGF induces cAMP accumulation in quiescent mouse 3T3 cells, which is probably mediated by increased synthesis of E-type prostaglandins.[285] Induction of ODC activity and the resultant putrescine synthesis may play an important role in the mitogenic action of PDGF, as shown with growth-arrested arterial smooth muscle cells.[286,287] Other possible mechanisms of PDGF-induced mitogenesis are represented by the induction of specific proteins such as the pI protein,[288] or some proto-oncogene product(s). The c-Myc protein, whose expression is induced by PDGF,[268,272] may mediate the competence state induced by PDGF. This possibility is reinforced by the fact that microinjected c-Myc protein can act as a competence factor.[279] Constitutive expression of a cloned c-*myc* gene can increase the response of rodent cells to PDGF.[289] However, cells may remain competent in spite of expressing c-*myc* and c-*fos* genes at very low levels (i.e., at levels similar to those of quiescent cells), which suggests that c-Myc and c-Fos may not be directly involved in the maintenance of the competence state.[290]

In certain types of cells, PDGF or PDGF-related peptides may mediate the mitogenic action of other growth factors through the operation of autocrine loops. In human skin fibroblasts, stimulation of DNA synthesis by TGF-β would be exerted via an autocrine mechanism involving the induction of PDGF-A gene expression and the production of PDGF-related proteins.[291] PDGF-specific antibodies can block the TGF-β-induced DNA synthesis in cultured human fibroblasts. At low concentrations, TGF-β induces proliferation of human connective tissue cells (cultured smooth-muscle cells) by stimulating autocrine PDGF-AA secretion, which at higher concentrations of TGF-β is decreased by downregulation of PDGF receptor α-subunits and perhaps also by direct growth inhibition.[292] The mitogenic activity of IL-1 for smooth-muscle cells and fibroblasts would also be indirect and mediated by the induction of the PDGF-A gene and the subsequent synthesis and secretion of homodimeric PDGF-AA molecules.[293]

X. PDGF AND THE Sis ONCOPROTEIN

Unlike normal fibroblasts, simian sarcoma virus (SSV)-transformed mouse and human fibroblasts do not require exogenous PDGF for growth.[294] A region of virtual identity was found in the amino acid sequences of human PDGF and the SSV oncoprotein, v-Sis ($p28^{v-sis}$).[295-298] SSV have acquired primate cellular sequences which encode part of the PDGF molecule. Antisera to a synthetic peptide representing amino acid residues 139 to 155 of the v-Sis oncoprotein recognize human PDGF.[299] SSV-transformed cells secrete a PDGF-like product into conditioned media and the secreted protein has been identified as $p28^{v-sis}$/v-Sis or its cellular processed product.[300-302]

When normal cells are cocultured with SSV-transformed cells, the PDGF receptors of the normal cells are downregulated by factors released from the transformed cells, which suggests that SSV-transformed cells release a material that is functionally similar to PDGF.[303] SSV-transformed cells have no detectable PDGF receptors on the surface, but when they are exposed to suramin the receptors reappear on the cell surface and within 8 h are present at the same levels as in control cells. These results strongly suggest that the absence of PDGF receptors in SSV-transformed cells is due to downregulation of the receptor by an autocrine mechanism involving the endogenous production of PDGF or a PDGF-like compound represented by the v-sis oncoprotein. Antibodies against PDGF inhibit both cell proliferation and SSV-induced morphological transformation of human diploid fibroblasts,[304] suggesting that v-*sis*-induced transformation is due to the autocrine action of a PDGF agonist. The phenotypic characteristics of SSV-transformed human fibroblasts also suggest that the v-Sis oncoprotein acts as a PDGF receptor agonist in transformation.[305] However, the role of cell-surface PDGF receptors in v-Sis-induced neoplastic transformation is not clear. In contrast to the normal PDGF protein, the v-Sis oncoprotein induces a rapid degradation of the 160-kDa precursor forms of both the α and β PDGF receptors and prevents their subsequent processing to the mature cell-surface forms.[306] Internal autoactivation of PDGF receptors may be essential for v-*sis*-induced neoplastic transformation.

A. COMPARATIVE STRUCTURES OF PDGF AND v-Sis

Reduced forms of PDGF contain two polypeptides, PDGF A/PDGF-1 and PDGF-B/PDGF-2, and v-Sis has been shown to correspond in size and amino acid sequence to a monomer of the PDGF B-chain.[298] Moreover, v-Sis undergoes dimer formation and subsequent processing to a form analogous in structure to that of biologically active PDGF. While the entire PDGF-B sequence is encompassed within the v-*sis* gene product, there are three regions of the predicted v-Sis protein that are unrelated to PDGF.[307] These include the amino-terminal portion of the viral oncogene product, which is encoded by sequences derived from the *env* gene of the helper virus, and two v-*sis* cell-derived regions immediately flanking the PDGF-B homologous sequence.

The SSV-encoded oncoprotein v-Sis consists of 226 residues, and the amino-terminal 109 residues of PDGF-B are virtually identical to residues 67 to 175 of the v-Sis oncoprotein.[22,295,296] The region homologous to PDGF starts at Ser-67, which follows a double basic (Lys-Arg) sequence at positions 65-66 and appears to be the processing point yielding a 18,056-Da polypeptide of 160 residues, essentially the same size estimated for the PDGF-B chain on the basis of gel electrophoresis. In further studies, it was concluded that the biologically active v-Sis oncoprotein is a homodimer consisting of two PDGF-B chains linked together by disulfide bonds, and that its immunologic properties are identical to those of PDGF. The study of deletions in the carboxyl-terminal coding region of the v-*sis* oncogene indicates that dimerization of the oncoprotein is required for neoplastic transformation.[308] Biosynthesis of v-Sis was characterized with respect to signal sequence cleavage, glycosylation, and proteolytic processing.[309] Predictions were made on the conformation and antigenic determinants of the v-Sis protein homologous with human PDGF.[310]

The v-*sis* oncogene has been cloned in bacteria, where its product can be expressed with high efficiency under the control of phage transcriptional and translational signals.[311] Colonies of *Escherichia coli* expressing the v-Sis oncoprotein can be detected with monoclonal antibodies made against specific synthetic peptides from the v-Sis sequence.[312] The v-Sis oncoprotein produced by genetically manipulated bacteria inhibits PDGF binding to its receptor, presumably by directly competing for the binding sites.[313] The latter finding suggests that the predominant biological activity of v-Sis is the result of its interaction with the PDGF receptor, and it has been postulated that v-Sis stimulates autocrine cell growth through PDGF cell-surface receptors.[314] SSV-transformed NIH/3T3 mouse fibroblasts respond mitogenically to PDGF and have a limited number of PDGF receptors on the surface, which appear to recognize v-Sis as a ligand because the purified oncoprotein competes with labeled PDGF for receptor binding.[315] It has been demonstrated that v-*sis* translational products are capable of specifically binding PDGF receptors, stimulating tyrosine phosphorylation of the receptors, and inducing DNA synthesis in quiescent mouse fibroblasts.[316]

B. THE c-*sis* PROTO-ONCOGENE

The complete sequences of cDNA clones corresponding to the normal human c-*sis* gene and its 5' and 3' flanking cellular sequences have been reported.[317-320] In previous studies, nucleotide sequence analysis demonstrated that the human c-*sis* proto-oncogene contains five exons and is a structural gene for PDGF.[33] Recently, it has been shown that the human c-*sis*/PDGF-B gene contains seven exons, although the great majority of the first exon and the entire seventh exon are comprised of noncoding sequences.[318] DNA sequences of the isolated and cloned human c-*sis* gene are homologous to sequences present in five regions of the SSV v-*sis* oncogene.[22] The v-*sis* homologous sequences start at a position corresponding to the 5' border of the second exon of the human c-*sis*/PDGF-B gene.[318] The study of sequences of the regions within the human c-*sis* gene that corresponds to the entire v-*sis* oncogene indicates that the predicted protein products of v-*sis* and c-*sis* are 93% homologous, and suggest that c-*sis* would encode the B chain of PDGF.[321] Analysis of the B chain of PDGF demonstrated identity of amino acid sequences predicted for the human c-*sis* gene product through 109 residues, indicating that the human c-*sis* gene encodes a polypeptide precursor of the B chain of PDGF.[7]

Comparative analysis of the human and feline c-*sis* proto-oncogene indicates the existence of 5' human c-*sis* coding sequences that are not homologous to v-*sis*.[322,323] In both loci, similar unique DNA sequences were found upstream of the v-*sis* homologous region, and these sequences hybridized to a 4.2-kbp c-*sis* transcript in human lung tumor cells. Transcripts of 4.2 kbp related to *sis* sequences are present in a high proportion of sarcoma cell lines and, less frequently, in glioma cell lines.[324] Transcripts of c-*sis* are present in some normal human tissues. Activated human monocytes express the c-*sis* proto-oncogene and release a mediator showing PDGF-like activity.[92] The c-*sis* gene is actively transcribed in the first-trimester human placenta, especially in the highly proliferative and invasive cytotrophoblastic shell, where it parallels the distribution of c-*myc* transcripts.[325] The translation product of c-*sis* transcripts in human placenta is a PDGF-like protein, as shown by the release of a PDGF receptor-competing activity into media conditioned by fresh explants of first-trimester placenta. Moreover, cultured cytotrophoblasts display abundant high-affinity PDGF receptors and respond to exogenous PDGF by an activation of c-*myc* gene expression and induction of DNA synthesis. These results suggest that the developing human placenta represents a case of autocrine growth regulation in a normal tissue.

The c-*sis* gene is also normally expressed in human and bovine endothelial cells.[326] Cultured human endothelial cells express c-*sis*/PDGF-related transcripts whose levels are increased in conditions favoring proliferation and decreased in conditions favoring differentiation.[60] The functions of c-Sis/PDGF-B gene products in endothelial cells are unknown, but might have some role in the normal development of the vessel wall and in physiological processes related to vascularization, as well as in the pathogenesis of vascular lesions such as atherosclerosis. Purified human PDGF and recombinant human c-Sis/PDGF-B polypeptide homodimers are equally effective in stimulating fibroblast mitogenesis and chemotaxis of polymorphonuclear leukocytes, monocytes, and fibroblasts *in vitro* and in augmenting wound healing in a rat linear incision model *in vivo*.[327]

C. Sis-INDUCED TRANSFORMATION

The question as to whether the transforming ability of the v-Sis oncoprotein, as compared with the apparent lack of such an ability in the PDGF-B chain (PDGF-2) molecule, is due to qualitative or quantitative differences between the two molecules cannot be answered as yet. The v-Sis protein differs in several structural aspects from PDGF-B, and such differences could be important for its oncogenic potential. The v-Sis oncoprotein differs from PDGF by the presence of a short amino-terminal sequence derived from the viral *env* gene, by a number of amino acid substitutions, and by the lack of the PDGF-A chain. Essential regions for v-*sis*-induced transformation are those encoding the amino-terminal hydrophobic sequence, which is a signal sequence for insertion into or across the plasma membrane, and the region of predicted homology with PDGF.[317] Removal of the signal sequence from the v-Sis protein results in loss of biological activity,[136,328] which could be attributed to the impossibility for localization of the protein at the cell membrane and interaction with the PDGF receptor.

In contrast to PDGF, which is a classical secretory protein, the vast majority of the v-Sis oncoprotein is not secreted by the cell and remains cell associated.[329] It has been proposed that v-*sis*-induced transformation may occur through internal activation of the PDGF receptor before expression of the v-Sis oncoprotein or the PDGF receptor at the cell surface.[330] However, it has been demonstrated that exogenous PDGF can induce cell growth alterations that mimic the v-*sis*-transformed state and that a PDGF-neutralizing antibody inhibits cell proliferation.[331] The results from several studies indicate that v-Sis can bind and activate its receptors internally, but the autocrine mechanism for v-*sis*-induced transformation requires cell surface localization of the internally activated receptors in order to functionally couple with intracellular mitogenic signaling pathways.

Expression of the normal human c-*sis*/PDGF-B coding sequence can induce cellular transformation in experimental conditions.[332,333] A recombinant vector containing the PDGF-B chain sequence is capable of inducing transformation of NIH/3T3 cells in contrast to the inability of PDGF itself to transform cells when applied externally, which may be due to the intracellular overproduction of PDGF-B chain as a consequence of transcriptional activation by the SV40 promoter contained in the vector.[332] The expression of PDGF-B chain sequences in abnormal sites or tissues could contribute to the induction of malignant transformation. On the other hand, expression of the c-*sis*/PDGF-B gene may be associated with differentiation of neoplastic cells induced by chemical agents. Expression of the c-*sis* proto-oncogene and synthesis of PDGF occurs in HL-60 human myeloid leukemia cells during induced monocytic differentiation.[334]

The mechanisms of SSV-induced transformation is not understood. Transformation induced by v-*sis* may not involve alterations in the tyrosine phosphorylation of cellular proteins.[335] It has been suggested that processing of the PDGF receptor is altered in v-*sis*-transformed cells, and that a persistent ligand-receptor interaction at intracellular sites results in the abnormal generation of mitogenic signals capable of leading to a transformed state through an autocrine type of mechanism.[336] Further work is needed to elucidate the factors responsible for the oncogenic activity of the v-Sis protein and the apparent lack of this activity in the normal c-Sis/PDGF-B protein under natural conditions. In any case, the oncogenic potential of v-Sis depends on the susceptibility of the particular cell where it is expressed. Diploid human skin fibroblasts can be transformed with a recombinant plasmid carrying the v-*sis* oncogene, but the transformed cells do not acquire all the characteristics of malignant cells and are not tumorigenic in athymic mice.[337]

XI. PDGF AND PDGF-LIKE FACTORS IN RELATION TO NEOPLASIA

PDGF-like factors may have an important role in neoplastic transformation *in vitro* as well as in malignant diseases *in vivo*. In particular, these growth factors are involved in autocrine transformation.[338-340] The induction of a transformed phenotype in carcinogen-treated murine fibroblastic cell lines depends primarily on PDGF, which suggests that some PDGF-induced cellular events are essential for neoplastic transformation.[341] However, PDGF may be necessary, but not sufficient for transformation, and the interaction of other growth factors, including EGF and TGF-β, is required for the efficient induction of transformation in carcinogen-initiated cells. These growth factors may be produced by other cells such as platelets or by the neoplastic cells themselves; they may exert a growth-stimulatory action on these cells through an autocrine type of mechanism. This mechanism may operate not only by interaction between c-Sis/PDGF-B and surface PDGF receptors, but apparently also by interaction with the PDGF receptors located in intracellular compartments, which would result in functional activation of the receptors.[342]

A. PDGF-INDUCED NEOPLASTIC TRANSFORMATION

PDGF, as well as basic FGF or a combination of EGF and TGF-β, is capable of inducing anchorage-independent growth of nontransformed human fibroblasts.[343] Incubation of human synoviocytes in a medium supplemented with 20% serum or in basal media supplemented with PDGF, results in expression of a transformed phenotype with formation of colonies in soft agar.[344] The PDGF-induced changes are inhibited by TGF-β and retinoids. Overexpression of a c-*sis*/PDGF-B gene introduced in human diploid fibroblasts by transfection or electroporation may result in the acquisition of a partially transformed, anchorage-independent phenotype.[345] The transforming capability of c-*sis* and v-*sis* products in human cells is restricted, however. Expression of a transfected c-*sis*/PDGF-B proto-oncogene or a v-*sis* oncogene in normal, diploid human fibroblasts is capable of inducing a partially transformed phenotype, but is not capable of conferring an infinite life span or making such cells tumorigenic.[346]

B. ROLE OF PDGF AND PDGF-LIKE FACTORS IN NEOPLASTIC DISEASES

Optimal tumor growth *in vivo* probably requires the concerted action of many hormones and growth factors. PDGF itself may have a role in stimulating tumor cell proliferation. PDGF receptors are expressed by a diversity of tumor cells, and an interaction between PDGF and other growth factors or some hormones may be important for tumor cell proliferation. For example, coexpression of functionally active receptors for PDGF and TSH may facilitate the growth of human thyroid carcinoma cells in a selective environment.[347] Moreover, growth factors involved in tumor development could mediate their action through the production of PDGF or PDGF-related proteins. However, the precise role of PDGF-related factors in tumor development is little understood. Certain types of tumor cells require the presence of exogenous PDGF for their growth *in vitro* and probably also *in vivo*. The tumor cells from CML, for example, require increased amounts of PDGF for the stimulation of proliferation *in vitro* when compared to normal bone marrow progenitors.[348] PDGF and other growth factors may be required not only for the growth of tumor cells themselves, but also for neovascularization of the tumor tissue and for the growth of mesenchymal cells which may constitute a considerable portion of the tumor.[349] PDGF or PDGF-like mitogens may also have a role in the development of proliferative lesions of the arterial wall associated with the pathogenesis of atherosclerosis.[350]

Platelets probably have an important role in the growth of both primary and metastatic tumors.[1,2] Several types of antiplatelet substances have been tested in experimental model systems as possible agents for the prevention of metastasis.[351] PDGF-related factors are present in tumor tissues and may be released by human tumor cell lines. The suggestion has been advanced that "an autocrine activation of the PDGF receptor may be operational in the growth of human tumors of mesenchymal or glial origin."[352] PDGF may have important effects on the behavior of either normal or transformed cells and is capable of inducing the soft agar (anchorage-independent) growth of nontransformed cell lines.[353]

Complex interactions with other growth factors may determine the final effects of PDGF on different types of cells. TGF-β has an inhibitory effect on the response of NRK cells to PDGF.[353] PDGF alone does not induce transformation in nonneoplastic, contact-inhibited NRK fibroblasts, but it is capable of inducing such transformation when it acts, in the presence of plasma, in concert with two other growth factors derived from platelets (TGF-β and EGF-like peptides).[354] Treatment of G_0-arrested mouse embryo-derived AKR-2B cells with TGF-β results in the induction of c-*sis*/PDGF mRNA within 20 min, and the levels of this mRNA remain elevated for at least 24 h.[355] Furthermore, PDGF-regulated protooncogenes such as c-*fos* and c-*myc* are induced by TGF-β with delayed kinetics.

C. PRODUCTION OF PDGF AND PDGF-LIKE PROTEINS BY TRANSFORMED CELLS

Cultured neoplastic cells may require less exogenous PDGF to grow to high saturation densities.[356] A possible cause for this lower requirement is the endogenous production of PDGF or PDGF-like substances by the transformed cells. Although many types of normal cells can produce PDGF, their transformed counterparts may secrete higher amounts of this factor. Both PDGF-A and PDGF-B chain mRNAs are expressed at higher levels in human mesothelioma cell lines than in normal human mesothelial cells.[357,358] Transcripts of the PDGF-A and c-*sis*/PDGF-B gene, as well as transcripts of the PDGF receptor gene, are frequently expressed in human hepatoma cell lines.[359] These cell lines also express transcripts of the IGF-I and IGF-I receptor genes, suggesting that autocrine regulation may be an important mechanism in the maintenance of hepatoma cell lines. PDGF, or proteins similar to PDGF, are produced by many human mammary carcinoma cell lines.[349,360] In addition to PDGF, some of these cell lines produce other growth factor, for example, TGF-α and IGF-II. The exact role of each growth factor in the growth of a particular cell line is difficult to determine, however. The MeWo metastatic human melanoma cell line secretes a potent mitogenic activity that can reinitiate DNA replication in quiescent rodent fibroblasts and which is identical or closely related to PDGF. However, MeWo cells do not have PDGF-binding sites and are not sensitive to suramin for growth inhibition, suggesting that the secreted PDGF does not act as an autocrine factor for the growth of MeWo cells.[361] Instead, the autonomous proliferation of MeWo cells may result from the concerted action of basic FGF and a melanoma growth-stimulating activity (MGSA), which are mostly cell-associated. Human malignant epithelial cell lines derived from breast, lung, gastric, and ovarian carcinomas frequently express both PDGF-A and PDGF-B genes.[362] As PDGF receptors are not present on these malignant epithelial cells, the production of PDGF or PDGF-like proteins may affect other cells in the *in vivo* microenvironment by paracrine mechanisms and may contribute to the excessive cell proliferation, inflammatory reactions, and connective tissue remodeling seen in certain carcinomas.

Human tumor cell lines may express the genes for either PDGF-A, PDGF-B, both PDGF-A and PDGF-B, or none of them.[26] Melanoma cell lines of primary and metastatic origin express the genes encoding the A and B chains of PDGF and produce a PDGF-like factor.[363] Secretion of 31-kDa PDGF-like proteins correlates with expression of PDGF-A, but not PDGF-B mRNA. The PDGF-A and PDGF-B genes are located on different human chromosomes and can be expressed independently in tumor cells. TPA-induced megakaryoblastic differentiation of the human hematopoietic cell line K562 is associated with expression of RNAs for both PDGF-A and PDGF-B polypeptides as well as with secretion of PDGF, whereas erythroid differentiation induced in these cells with sodium butyrate is accompanied by PDGF-B expression only.[364] The human HL-60 leukemia cell line does not express RNA for PDGF-A, whereas the line U-937, which is of a similar origin, expresses this type of RNA. TGF-β induces expression of the PDGF-A gene, but not the c-*sis*/PDGF-B gene, in several leukemia cell lines as well as in the fibrosarcoma cell line HT-1080.[365] It is not known whether expression of PDGF-A or PDGF-B is necessary for the differentiation of K562, U-937, and HL-60 cells, and the mechanisms associated with the expression of PDGF chains in TPA-treated leukemia cell lines are not understood. A severalfold increase in expression of PDGF-B mRNA is induced by phorbol ester (PMA), but not by DMSO, in the human hematopoietic cell line HEL, which was established from a patient with Hodgkin's disease who later developed erythroleukemia.[366] Since PMA does not induce expression of the PDGF-A-chain gene in HEL cells, these results reinforce the hypothesis that expression of the PDGF-A and PDGF-B genes is controlled by independent mechanisms.

1. Human Osteosarcoma Cells

A PDGF-like substance is produced by the human osteosarcoma cell line U-2 OS.[367,368] These cells do not respond to exogenous PDGF, but they possess PDGF receptors that can be unmasked by treatment with suramin, a polyanionic compound that displaces bound PDGF from its receptor. A 180- to 200-kDa surface glycoprotein present in U-2 OS cells is apparently identical to the PDGF receptor.[369,370]

It has been postulated that U-2 OS cells satisfy their requirement for PDGF by endogenous production of PDGF or similar factors,[146] which is consistent with the autocrine hypothesis of neoplasti transformation.[371]

Moreover, mRNA from the U-2 OS cells hybridize with cDNA probes corresponding to the v-*sis* oncogene sequence.[372] Efficient reversion of SSV-induced neoplastic transformation and inhibition of growth factor-induced mitogenesis can be obtained by using suramin.[373] These results suggest that the appearance and/or maintenance of a transformed phenotype in U-2 OS cells involves a transcriptional activation of the c-*sis* proto-oncogene which results in the production of biologically active PDGF. The factor produced by U-2 OS cells, purified to homogeneity, appeared to be a homodimer of PDGF-A,[374] but the sequence of a cDNA clone prepared from the same cells by hybridization to a v-*sis* probe indicated that the mitogen secreted by U-2 OS cells is probably a homodimer of PDGF-B.[375] It seems likely that U-2 OS cells express both PDGF-A and PDGF-B transcripts.[26] However, the fact that DNA synthesis is not reduced in U-2 OS cells by incubation with suramin and is not stimulated by exogenous PDGF makes unlikely the possibility that the PDGF-like mitogen produced and secreted by U-2 OS cells stimulates proliferation of the cells through an autocrine mechanism.[376] It may be concluded that DNA synthesis in U-2 OS cells is independent of PDGF binding to functional cell-surface receptors.

Production of PDGF or PDGF-like substances is not universal in human osteogenic sarcomas because cells from the MG-63 human osteosarcoma cell line do not show endogenous secretion of PDGF-like growth factors.[372] MG-63 cells produce mitogenic activity which is not PDGF-like, have membrane receptors for PDGF, and respond to exogenous PDGF by increasing amino acid transport, DNA synthesis, and cell proliferation. Moreover, the EGF receptor is phosphorylated on tyrosine after addition of exogenous PDGF to MG-63 cells. In the absence of PDGF, an alkali-stable phosphoprotein of 116 kDa is detected in MG-63 cells, but the origin of this protein and its possible relationship to the activity of non-Sis-related proteins remain uncharacterized. Studies with somatic mouse cell hybrids indicate that responsiveness to PDGF may be dissociated from cell transformation and that cells may be transformed by mechanisms which are independent of PDGF.[377]

2. Human Neural Tumors

The growth of various types of human neural tumors may be associated with autocrine or paracrine mechanisms involving the synthesis and secretion of PDGF or PDGF-like molecules. Human malignant glioma (glioblastoma) cell lines frequently express PDGF transcripts. All of the 21 human glioblastoma cell lines examined expressed PDGF-A mRNA, and 16 of the 21 cell lines expressed c-*sis*/PDGF-B mRNA; these expressions occurred independently of each other.[378] PDGF receptors were present in 15 of the 21 glioblastoma cell lines, suggesting the operation of an autocrine mechanism of growth control in these cells. In addition to PDGF chains and PDGF receptors, the glioblastoma cells frequently expressed EGF transcripts as well as EGF receptors, which suggests that two autocrine loops may occur concomitantly in the malignant cells. In another study, five out of eight human glioblastoma cell lines expressed c-*sis*/PDGF-B mRNA, and in the cell line with the highest levels there were four to ten molecules of this mRNA per cell.[379] The fact that c-*sis*/PDGF-B mRNA is expressed in the majority of glioblastoma cell lines, compared to its absence in normal glial cells, suggests that constitutive synthesis of PDGF-B may contribute to either the formation or the maintenance of glioblastomas. On the other hand, the absence of such transcripts in other glioblastomas argues that expression of PDGF-B is not essential for glial cell transformation.

Cells of the line U-343 MGa, derived from a human malignant glioma biopsy, gave rise to clones with different amounts of PDGF-like activity secreted to the extracellular medium.[380] The cloned glioma cell lines exhibited a diversity of chromosome abnormalities, including a 12+ marker chromosome associated with late progression. Since the gene coding for the PDGF-A chain is located on human chromosome 7 and the c-*sis*/PDGF-B gene is on chromosome 22, a correlation could exist between the number of these chromosomes in the cloned tumor cells and the production of PDGF chains A and B. In fact, there was a slight correlation between the relative number of chromosomes 7 and the production of PDGF-like activity, but such correlation was not apparent for the number of chromosomes 22 and the production of PDGF-like activity. Proteins resembling PDGF, but with molecular weights ranging from 16 to 140 kDa, are synthesized and secreted by human glioblastoma A172 and fibrosarcoma HT-1080 cells in culture.[381] These two cell lines synthesize a mRNA that contains sequences from all exons of the human c-*sis* gene. Expression of c-*sis*/PDGF-B mRNA by the human glioblastoma cell line A172 is stimulated by phorbol ester or TGF-β.[382] Mouse neuroblastoma cells (Neuro-2A cells) express c-*sis* transcripts with concomitant production and secretion of a PDGF-like growth factor.[383] The factor produced by Neuro-2A cells is able to induce anchorage-independent growth of NRK cells in the presence of EGF.[384]

Studies on primary human glioblastomas have given some interesting results.[385] Hyperplasia of the vascular endothelium is a prominent characteristic of human glioblastoma multiform and v-*sis*

(SSV)-induced gliomas in primates (newborn marmosets). Analysis of the glioblastoma biopsies showed the presence of transcripts for PDGF-A and PDGF-B chains and the PDGF receptor. Overexpression of PDGF α receptor gene, associated or not with amplification of the gene, occurs in a number of primary human glioblastomas.[386] Tissue sections of the tumors examined by *in situ* hybridization revealed that the proliferating vascular endothelial cells contained large quantities of mRNA for both PDGF-B and its receptor and, to a lesser extent, for the PDGF-A chain. In contrast, the tumor cells expressed more mRNA for the PDGF-A chain than for the PDGF-B chain and PDGF receptor. These results suggest that autocrine stimulation by PDGF-B via its receptor, evoked by interaction with surrounding glioma cells, could be a mechanism involved in the proliferation of endothelial cells characteristically found in glioblastomas.

Primary human meningiomas coexpress the c-*sis*/PDGF-B gene and its receptor, whereas control pachymeninges derived from normal adult individuals express only the PDGF receptor mRNA, but not the c-*sis*/PDGF-B mRNA.[387] Human meningioma cells, as well as normal arachnoidal cells, express PDGF receptors almost exclusively of the β type, which bind PDGF-B homodimers with high affinity.[388] An autocrine mechanism may contribute to the growth and maintenance of some human meningiomas.[389]

Brain cells cultured from mice treated transplacentally with *N*-ethyl-*N*-nitrosourea (ENU) undergo morphological alterations characteristic of malignant transformation. Transformed glioma cells from these cultures differ from premalignant glial cells by containing high levels of c-*sis* transcripts and by synthesizing functional PDGF.[390] Since glial cells have PDGF receptors, an autocrine mechanism may play an important role in ENU-induced tumorigenesis in mice.

3. Other Human Tumors

Expression of PDGF A and/or B chains occurs in various types of primary human tumors and tumor cell lines, including breast cancer and lung cancer.[391,392] The malignant epithelial cells in primary human lung cancer coexpress *in vivo* PDGF and PDGF receptor mRNA and protein.[393] A close relationship exists between the expression of PDGF and TGF genes in human non-small cell lung-cancer cell lines and the presence of a prominent fibrous stroma reaction in mice inoculated with these cells.[394] In primary human gastric carcinomas, expression of PDGF-A mRNA may not differ in the tumor cells and cells from normal gastric mucosa, but PDGF receptor mRNA is expressed at higher levels in the gastric cancer cells than in normal gastric mucosa, and enhanced expression of these transcripts is frequently found in scirrhous gastric cancers.[395] Coexpression of PDGF-B and PDGF β-receptor mRNA and protein occurs in gastric cancer cells, but not in the adjacent nonmalignant gastric mucosa.[396] Cultured Kaposi's sarcoma-derived cells express functional PDGF A-type and B-type receptors.[397] Expression of PDGF and its receptor in AIDS-related Kaposi's sarcoma *in vivo* suggests paracrine and autocrine mechanisms of tumor maintenance.[398]

4. Embryonal Carcinoma Cells

Human embryonal carcinoma cells express PDGF receptors of the B type.[399] PDGF-like growth factors are produced by mouse embryonal carcinoma cells.[400] However, the murine cells do not bind to exogenously added PDGF, which could be attributed to either a lack of expression of PDGF receptors on the cell surface or to the occupancy and downregulation of the receptors by the PDGF-like growth factors produced by the same cells in an autocrine fashion. In contrast, endoderm-like cells derived from embryonal carcinoma cells do not release PDGF-like growth factors into the medium, but their process of differentiation is accompanied by a marked increase in ability to bind exogenously added PDGF. However, induction of F9 embryonal carcinoma cell differentiation into endoderm cells by treatment with retinoic acid is accompanied by the secretion of a factor into the medium which possesses PDGF-like activity for smooth muscle cells.[401] These results suggest that a mitoattractant PDGF-like factor may contribute to the regulation of cell growth and migration during the early stages of embryogenesis.

5. Virus-Transformed Cells

Cells transformed by oncogenic viruses may produce PDGF-like proteins. SV40-transformed NIH/3T3 cells produce one such protein.[402] A PDGF-like protein is produced in cells transformed by acute retroviruses (K-MuSV, M-MuSV, and SSV) and DNA viruses (SV40 and adenovirus). The protein is also present in cells spontaneously transformed in culture as well as in some human carcinoma cell lines (bladder carcinoma T24 and hepatoma HepG2), but is absent in MCA-transformed mouse cells.[403] A marked decrease in the number of PDGF receptors is observed in the same cells. Human T lymphocytes immortalized by the human retroviruses HTLV-I and HTLV-II express genes encoding both chains of

PDGF.[404] However, HTLV-infected lymphocytes do not express PDGF receptors, and the possible role of PDGF in their growth is not understood.

D. ROLE OF PROTO-ONCOGENES IN v-*Sis*-INDUCED TRANSFORMATION

Proto-oncogenes may cooperate with viral oncogenes, including v-*sis,* for the expression of a fully transformed phenotype. Mouse fibroblasts (NIH/3T3 cells) transformed by the v-*sis* oncogene are known to be stimulated in an autocrine fashion by PDGF-like molecules (PDGF-B homodimers) and these cells have elevated levels of c-*fos* proto-oncogene expression in relation to nontransformed controls. The transfection and integration of a plasmid vector directing the synthesis of antisense RNA to the c-*fos* gene leads to restoration of density-dependent growth arrest in monolayer cultures of the v-*sis*-transformed cells, although colony formation in soft agar is not inhibited.[405] NRK cells infected with K-MuSV retrovirus expressing v-K-Ras protein, but not cells expressing a v-Src oncoprotein, produce PDGF or PDGF-like mitogenic factors.[406]

E. ROLE OF PDGF IN ONCOGENE-INDUCED TRANSFORMATION

Murine NIH/3T3 fibroblasts transformed by the EJ c-H-*ras* oncogene display reduced PDGF-stimulated phospholipase C and phospholipase A_2 activities as measured by inositol 1,4,5-trisphosphate and Ca^{2+} mobilization.[215] Treatment of the transformed cells with cholera toxin or the cAMP analog, 8-bromo-cAMP, results in increased mobilization of intracellular Ca^{2+} and an almost complete recovery of PGE_2 synthesis.[407] These data suggest that oncogene-mediated inhibition of PDGF-stimulated intracellular events can be partially and transiently reversed by cAMP.

XII. NON-PDGF-LIKE FACTORS PRODUCED BY PLATELETS

In addition to PDGF and PDGF-like substances, other growth factors are present in platelets, including EGF, TGF-β, a hepatocyte growth factor, an endothelial growth factor, and other factors which remain poorly identified.[408-412] Platelet-derived factors may play an essential role in the neoplastic transformation of carcinogen-treated cells *in vitro* as well as in tumor development *in vivo*.[338] The primary structure of a platelet factor, called platelet factor 4 (PF-4), has been reported.[413] PF-4 is a 9.5-kDa protein of 88 amino acids and has a diversity of functions, including inhibition of LDL binding to its receptor and inhibition of PTH-stimulated calcium release from bone. An acid-sensitive melanoma growth factor activity was also purified from human platelets.[414] This factor is apparently a protein of 60 kDa with mitogenic properties for both human melanoma and bovine aortic endothelial cells.

A number of growth-inhibiting factors have been isolated from platelets.[415,416] One of these inhibitors may be identical to TGF-β, but other growth inhibitors isolated from platelets are apparently represented by distinct proteins. An inhibitor of endothelial-cell DNA synthesis and growth contained in human platelets is a 37-kDa polypeptide.[417] This inhibitor could have a role in the regulation of endothelial growth following injury. Platelets also contain factors capable of producing specific inhibition of proliferation and induction of differentiation of certain human carcinoma cells under the conditions of *in vitro* culture.[418]

REFERENCES

1. **Mehta, P.,** Potential role of platelets in the pathogenesis of tumor metastasis, *Blood,* 63, 55, 1984.
2. **Gasic, G.J.,** Role of plasma, platelets, and endothelial cells in tumor metastasis, *Cancer Metast. Rev.,* 3, 99, 1984.
3. **Ross, R. and Vogel, A.,** The platelet-derived growth factor, *Cell,* 14, 203, 1978.
4. **Scher, C.D., Shepard, R.C., Antoniades, H.N., and Stiles, C.D.,** Platelet-derived growth factor and the regulation of the mammalian fibroblast cell cycle, *Biochim. Biophys. Acta,* 560, 217, 1979.
5. **Antoniades, H.N. and Williams, L.T.,** Human platelet-derived growth factor: structure and function, *Fed. Proc.,* 42, 2630, 1983.
6. **Stiles, C.D.,** The molecular biology of platelet-derived growth factor, *Cell,* 33, 653, 1983.
7. **Deuel, T.F. and Huang, J.S.,** Platelet-derived growth factor: structure, function, and roles in normal and transformed cells, *J. Clin. Invest.,* 74, 669, 1984.
8. **Cochran, B.H.,** The molecular action of platelet-derived growth factor, *Adv. Cancer Res.,* 45, 183, 1985.

9. Ross, R., Raines, E.W., and Bowen-Pope, D.F., The biology of platelet-derived growth factor, *Cell*, 46, 155, 1986.
10. Williams, L.T., The *sis* gene and PDGF, *Cancer Surv.*, 5, 233, 1986.
11. Deuel, T.F., Pierce, G.F., Yeh, H.-J., Shawver, L.K., Milner, P.G., and Kimura, A., Platelet-derived growth factor/sis in normal and neoplastic cell growth, *J. Cell. Physiol.*, Suppl. 5, 95, 1987.
12. Ross, R., Platelet-derived growth factor, *Annu. Rev. Med.*, 38, 71, 1987.
13. Heldin, C.-H. and Westermark, B., Platelet-derived growth factor: three isoforms and two receptor types, *Trends Genet.*, 5, 108, 1989.
14. Heldin, C.-H. and Westermark, B., Platelet-derived growth factor: mechanism of action and possible in vivo function, *Cell Regul.*, 1, 555, 1990.
15. Pantazis, P., Goustin, A.S., and Nixon, J., Platelet-derived growth factor and its receptor in blood cell differentiation and neoplasia, *Eur. J. Haematol.*, 45, 127, 1990.
16. Deuel, T.F., Kawahara, R.S., Mustoe, T.A., and Pierce, G.F., Growth factors and wound healing. Platelet-derived growth factor as a model cytokine, *Annu. Rev. Med.*, 42, 567, 1991.
17. Heldin, C.-H., Structural and functional studies on platelet-derived growth factor, *EMBO J.*, 11, 4251, 1992.
18. Heldin, C.H., Westermark, B., and Wasteson, Å., Platelet-derived growth factor: purification and partial characterization, *Proc. Natl. Acad. Sci. U.S.A.*, 76, 3722, 1979.
19. Johnsson, A., Heldin, C.-H., Westermark, B., and Wasteson, Å., Platelet-derived growth factor. Identification of constituent polypeptide chain, *Biochem. Biophys. Res. Commun.*, 104, 66, 1982.
20. Antoniades, H.N. and Hunkapiller, M.W., Human platelet-derived growth factor (PDGF): amino-terminal amino acid sequence, *Science*, 220, 963, 1983.
21. Heldin, C.-H. and Westermark, B., Growth factors: mechanism of action and relation to oncogenes, *Cell*, 37, 9, 1984.
22. Johnsson, A., Heldin, C.-H., Wasteson, Å., Westermark, B., Deuel, T.F., Huang, J.S., Seeburg, P.H., Gray, A., Ullrich, A., Scrace, G., Stroobant, P., and Waterfield, M.D., The c-*sis* gene encodes a precursor of the B chain of platelet-derived growth factor, *EMBO J.*, 3, 921, 1984.
23. Östman, A., Rall, L., Hammacher, A., Wormstead, M.A., Coit, D., Valenzuela, P., Betsholtz, C., Westermark, B., and Heldin, C.-H., Synthesis and assembly of a functionally active recombinant platelet-derived growth factor AB heterodimer, *J. Biol. Chem.*, 263, 16202, 1988.
24. Hammacher, A., Hellman, U., Johnson, A., Östman, A., Gunnarsson, K., Westermark, B., Wasteson, A., and Heldin, C.-H., A major part of platelet-derived growth factor purified from human platelets is a heterodimer of one A and one B chain, *J. Biol. Chem.*, 263, 16493, 1988.
25. Clements, J.M., Bawden, L.J., Bloxidge, R.E., Catlin, G., Cook, A.L., Craig, S., Drummond, A.H., Edwards, R.M., Fallon, A., Green, D.R., Hellewell, P.G., Kirwin, P.M., Nayee, P.D., Richardson, S.J., Brown, D., Chahwala, S.B., Snarey, M., and Winslow, D., Two PDGF-B chain residues, arginine 27 and isoleucine 30, mediate receptor binding and activation, *EMBO J.*, 10, 4113, 1991.
26. Betsholtz, C., Johnsson, A., Heldin, C.-H., Westermark, B., Lind, P., Urdea, M.S., Eddy, R., Shows, T.B., Philpott, K., Mellor, A.L., Knott, T.J., and Scott, J., cDNA sequence and chromosomal localization of human platelet-derived growth factor A-chain and its expression in tumour cell lines, *Nature*, 320, 695, 1986.
27. Bonthron, D.T., Morton, C.C., Orkin, S.H., and Collins, T., Platelet-derived growth factor A chain: gene structure, chromosomal location, and basis for alternative mRNA splicing, *Proc. Natl. Acad. Sci. U.S.A.*, 85, 1492, 1988.
28. Steinman, G., Rorsman, F., and Betsholtz, C., Sublocalization of the human PDGF-A chain gene to chromosome 7, band q11.23 by *in situ* hybridization, *Exp. Cell Res.*, 178, 180, 1988.
29. Bonthron, D., Collins, T., Grzeschik, K.H., Van Roy, N., and Speleman, F., Platelet-derived growth factor A chain. Confirmation of localization of *PDGFA* to chromosome 7p22 and description of an unusual minisatellite, *Genomics*, 13, 257, 1992.
30. Stenman, G., Rorsman, F., Huebner, K., and Betsholtz, C., The human platelet-derived growth factor α chain *(PDGFA)* gene maps to chromosome 7p22, *Cytogenet. Cell Genet.*, 60, 206, 1992.
31. Takimoto, Y., Wang, Z.Y., Kobler, K., and Deuel, T.F., Promoter region of the human platelet-derived growth factor A-chain gene, *Proc. Natl. Acad. Sci. U.S.A.*, 88, 1686, 1991.
32. Gashler, A.L., Bonthron, D.T., Madden, S.L., Rauscher, F.J., Collins, T., and Sukhatme, V.P., Human platelet-derived growth factor-A chain is transcriptionally repressed by the Wilms tumor suppressor gene WT1, *Proc. Natl. Acad. Sci. U.S.A.*, 89, 10984, 1992.

33. **Chiu, I.-M., Reddy, E., Givol, D., Robbins, K.C., Tronick, S.R., and Aaronson, S.A.,** Nucleotide sequence analysis identifies the human c-*sis* proto-oncogene as a structural gene for platelet-derived growth factor, *Cell,* 37, 123, 1984.
34. **Jhanwar, S.C., Neel, B.G., Hayward, W.S., and Chaganti, R.S.K.,** Localization of the cellular oncogenes *ABL, SIS,* and *FES* on human germ-line chromosomes, *Cytogenet. Cell Genet.,* 38, 73, 1984.
35. **Tong, B.D., Levine, S.E., Jaye, M., Ricca, G., Droyan, W., Maaciag, T., and Deuel, T.F.,** Isolation and sequencing of a cDNA clone homologous to the v-*sis* oncogene from human endothelial cells, *Mol. Cell. Biol.,* 6, 3018, 1986.
36. **Sariban, E. and Kufe, D.,** Expression of the platelet-derived growth factor 1 and 2 genes in human myeloid cell lines and monocytes, *Cancer Res.,* 48, 4498, 1988.
37. **Hoppe, J., Schumacher, L., Eichner, W., and Weich, H.A.,** The long 3′-untranslated regions of the PDGF-A and -B mRNAs are only distantly related, *FEBS Lett.,* 223, 243, 1987.
38. **Deuel, T.F., Huang, J.S., Profitt, R.T., Baenziger, J.U., Chang, D., and Kennedy, B.B.,** Human platelet-derived growth factor: purification and resolution into two active fractions, *J. Biol. Chem.,* 256, 8896, 1981.
39. **Raines, E. and Ross, R.,** Platelet-derived growth factor. I. High yield purification and evidence for multiple forms, *J. Biol. Chem.,* 257, 5154, 1982.
40. **Niman, H.L., Houghten, R.A., and Bowen-Pope, D.F.,** Detection of high molecular weight forms of platelet-derived growth factor by sequence-specific antisera, *Science,* 226, 701, 1984.
41. **Collins, T., Pober, J.S., Gimbrone, M.A., Jr., Hammacher, A., Betsholtz, C., Westermark, B., and Heldin, C.-H.,** Cultured human endothelial cells express platelet-derived growth factor A chain, *Am. J. Pathol.,* 127, 7, 1987.
42. **Sejersen, T., Betsholtz, C., Sjölund, M., Heldin, C.-H., Westermark, B., and Thyberg, J.,** Rat skeletal myoblasts and arterial smooth muscle cells express the gene for the A chain but not the gene for the B chain (c-*sis*) of platelet-derived growth factor (PDGF) and produce a PDGF-like protein, *Proc. Natl. Acad. Sci. U.S.A.,* 83, 6844, 1986.
43. **Winkles, J.A., O'Connor, M.L., and Friesel, R.,** Altered regulation of platelet-derived growth factor A-chain and c-fos gene expression in senescent progeria fibroblasts, *J. Cell. Physiol.,* 144, 313, 1990.
44. **Tong, B.D., Auer, D.E., Jaye, M., Kaplow, J.M., Ricca, G., McConathy, E., Drohan, W., and Deuel, T.F.,** cDNA clones reveal differences between human glial and endothelial cell platelet-derived growth factor A-chains, *Nature,* 328, 619, 1987.
45. **Senior, R.M., Huang, J.S., Griffin, G.L., and Deuel, T.F.,** Dissociation of the chemotactic and mitogenic activities of platelet-derived growth factor by human neutrophil elastase, *J. Cell Biol.,* 100, 351, 1985.
46. **Poggi, A., Rucinski, B., James, P., Holt, J.C., and Niewiarowski, S.,** Partial purification and characterization of porcine platelet-derived growth factor (PDGF), *Exp. Cell Res.,* 150, 436, 1984.
47. **Stroobant, P. and Waterfield, M.D.,** Purification and properties of porcine platelet-derived growth factor, *EMBO J.,* 3, 2963, 1984.
48. **Igarashi, H., Rao, C.D., Siroff, M., Leal, F., Robbins, K.C., and Aaronson, S.A.,** Detection of PDGF-2 homodimers in human tumor cells, *Oncogene,* 1, 79, 1987.
49. **Escobedo, J.A., Navankasatussas, S., Coussens, L.S., Coughlin, S.R., Bell, G.I., and Williams, L.T.,** A common PDGF receptor is activated by homodimeric A and B forms of PDGF, *Science,* 240, 1532, 1988.
50. **Nistér, M., Hammacher, A., Mellström, K., Siegbahn, A., Rönnstrand, L., Westermark, B., and Heldin, C.-H.,** A glioma-derived PDGF A chain homodimer has different functional activities from PDGF AB heterodimer purified from human platelets, *Cell,* 52, 791, 1988.
51. **Reilly, C.F. and Broski, J.E.,** Differential effects of PDGF and PDGF-BB on vascular smooth muscle cells, *Biochem. Biophys. Res. Commun.,* 160, 1047, 1989.
52. **Keck, P.J., Hauser, S.D., Krivi, G., Sanzo, K., Warren, T., Feder, J., and Connolly, D.T.,** Vascular permeability factor, an endothelial cell mitogen related to PDGF, *Science,* 246, 1309, 1989.
53. **Witte, D.P., Stambrook, P.J., Feliciano, E., Jones, C.L.A., and Lieberman, M.A.,** Growth factor production by a human megakaryocytic tumor cell line, *J. Cell. Physiol.,* 136, 86, 1988.
54. **Shaw, R.J., Doherty, D.E., Ritter, A.G., Benedict, S.H., and Clark, R.A.F.,** Adherence-dependent increase in human monocyte PDGF(B) mRNA is associated with increases in c-*fos,* c-*jun,* and EGR2 mRNA, *J. Cell Biol.,* 111, 2139, 1990.

55. **Golden, M.A., Au, Y.P.T., Kirkman, T.R., Wilcox, J.N., Raines, E.W., Ross, R., and Clowes, A.W.**, Platelet-derived growth factor activity and mRNA expression in healing vascular grafts in baboons. Association in vivo of platelet-derived growth factor mRNA and protein with cellular proliferation, *J. Clin. Invest.*, 87, 406, 1991.
56. **Gay, C.G. and Winkles, J.A.**, Heparin-binding growth factor-1 stimulation of human endothelial cells induces platelet-derived growth factor A-chain gene expression, *J. Biol. Chem.*, 265, 3284, 1990.
57. **Majeski, M.W., Benditt, E.P., and Schwartz, S.M.**, Expression and development control of platelet-derived growth factor A-chain and B-chain/*sis* genes in rat aortic smooth muscle cells, *Proc. Natl. Acad. Sci. U.S.A.*, 85, 1524, 1988.
58. **Mendoza, A.E., Young, R., Orkin, S.H., and Collins, T.**, Increased platelet-derived growth factor A-chain expression in human uterine smooth muscle cells during the physiologic hypertrophy of pregnancy, *Proc. Natl. Acad. Sci. U.S.A.*, 87, 2177, 1990.
59. **Sakariassen, K.S., Powell, J.S., Raines, E.W., and Ross, R.**, Selective expression of mRNA encoding platelet growth factor B chain following transfection of foreign genes into cell lines derived from baby hamster kidney, *J. Cell. Biochem.*, 39, 87, 1989.
60. **Jaye, M., McConathy, E., Drohan, W., Tong, B., Deuel, T., and Maciag, T.**, Modulation of the *sis* gene transcript during endothelial cell differentiation in vitro, *Science*, 228, 882, 1985.
61. **Starksen, N.F., Harsh, G.R., IV, Gibbs, V.C., and Williams, L.T.**, Regulated expression of the platelet-derived growth factor A chain gene in microvascular endothelial cells, *J. Biol. Chem.*, 262, 14381, 1987.
62. **Daniel, T.O., Gibbs, V.C., Milfay, D.F., and Williams, L.T.**, Agents that increase cAMP accumulation block endothelial c-*sis* induction by thrombin and transforming growth factor-β, *J. Biol. Chem.*, 262, 11893, 1987.
63. **Kavanaugh, W.M., Harsh, G.R., IV, Starksen, N.F., Rocco, C.M., and Williams, L.T.**, Transcriptional regulation of the A and B chain genes of platelet-derived growth factor in microvascular endothelial cells, *J. Biol. Chem.*, 263, 8470, 1988.
64. **Daniel, T.O. and Fen, Z.**, Distinct pathways mediate transcriptional regulation of platelet-derived growth factor B/c-*sis* expression, *J. Biol. Chem.*, 263, 19815, 1988.
65. **Suzuki, H., Shibano, K., Okane, M., Kono, I., Matsui, Y., Yamane, K., and Kashiwagi, H.**, Interferon-γ modulates messenger RNA levels of c-*sis* (PDGF-B chain), PDGF-A chain, and IL-1β genes in human vascular endothelial cells, *Am. J. Pathol.*, 134, 35, 1989.
66. **Kourembanas, S. and Faller, D.V.**, Platelet-derived growth factor production by human umbilical vein endothelial cells is regulated by basic fibroblast growth factor, *J. Biol. Chem.*, 264, 4456, 1989.
67. **Silver, B.J., Jaffer, F.E., and Abboud, H.E.**, Platelet-derived growth factor synthesis in mesangial cells: induction by multiple peptide mitogens, *Proc. Natl. Acad. Sci. U.S.A.*, 86, 1056, 1989.
68. **Paulsson, Y., Austgulen, R., Hofsli, E., Heldin, C.-H., Westermark, B., and Nissen-Meyer, J.**, Tumor necrosis factor-induced expression of platelet-derived growth factor A-chain messenger RNA in fibroblasts, *Exp. Cell Res.*, 180, 490, 1989.
69. **Bowen-Pope, D.F., Malpass, T.W., Foster, D.M., and Ross, R.**, Platelet-derived growth factor in vivo: levels, activity, and rate of clearance, *Blood*, 64, 458, 1984.
70. **Huang, J.S., Huang, S.S., and Deuel, T.F.**, Specific covalent binding of platelet-derived growth factor to human plasma α_2-macroglobulin, *Proc. Natl. Acad. Sci. U.S.A.*, 81, 342, 1984.
71. **Raines, E.W., Bowen-Pope, D.F., and Ross, R.**, Plasma binding proteins for platelet-derived growth factor that inhibit its binding to cell-surface receptors, *Proc. Natl. Acad. Sci. U.S.A.*, 81, 3424, 1984.
72. **Brown, K.D. and Blakeley, D.M.**, Partial purification and characterization of a growth factor present in goat's colostrum, *Biochem. J.*, 219, 609, 1984.
73. **Tischer, E., Gospodarowicz, D., Mitchell, R., Silva, M., Schilling, J., Lau, K., Crisp, T., Fiddes, J.C., and Abraham, J.A.**, Vascular endothelial growth factor: a new member of the platelet-derived growth factor gene family, *Biochem. Biophys. Res. Commun.*, 165, 1198, 1989.
74. **Conn, G., Bayne, M.L., Soderman, D.D., Kwok, P.W., Sullivan, K.A., Palisi, T.M., Hope, D.A., and Thomas, K.A.**, Amino acid and cDNA sequences of a vascular endothelial cell mitogen that is homologous to platelet-derived growth factor, *Proc. Natl. Acad. Sci. U.S.A.*, 87, 2628, 1990.
75. **Di Corleto, P.E. and Bowen-Pope, D.F.**, Cultured endothelial cells produce a platelet-derived growth factor-like protein, *Proc. Natl. Acad. Sci. U.S.A.*, 80, 1919, 1983.
76. **Abboud, H.E., Poptic, E., and DiCorleto, P.**, Production of platelet-derived growth factorlike protein by rat mesangial cells in culture, *J. Clin. Invest.*, 80, 675, 1987.

77. **Kartha, S., Bradham, D.M., Grotendorst, G.R., and Toback, F.G.,** Kidney epithelial cells express c-*sis* protooncogene and secrete PDGF-like protein, *Am. J. Physiol.,* 255, F800, 1988.
78. **Daniel, T.O., Gibbs, V.C., Milfay, D.F., Garovoy, M.R., and Williams, L.T.,** Thrombin stimulates c-*sis* gene expression in microvascular endothelial cells, *J. Biol. Chem.,* 261, 9579, 1986.
79. **Collins, T., Bonthron, D.T., and Orkin, S.H.,** Alternative RNA splicing affects function of encoded platelet-derived growth factor A chain, *Nature,* 328, 621, 1987.
80. **Fox, P.L. and DiCorleto, P.E.,** Modified low density lipoproteins suppress production of a platelet-derived growth factor-like protein by cultured endothelial cells, *Proc. Natl. Acad. Sci. U.S.A.,* 83, 4774, 1986.
81. **Seifert, R.A., Schwartz, S.M., and Bowen-Pope, D.F.,** Developmentally regulated production of platelet-derived growth factor-like molecules, *Nature,* 311, 669, 1984.
82. **Nilsson, J., Sjölund, M., Palmberg, L., Thyberg, J., and Heldin, C.-H.,** Arterial smooth muscle cells in primary culture produce a platelet-derived growth factor-like protein, *Proc. Natl. Acad. Sci. U.S.A.,* 82, 4418, 1985.
83. **Sjölund, M., Hedin, U., Sejersen, T., Heldin, C.-H., and Thyberg, J.,** Arterial smooth muscle cells express platelet-derived growth factor (PDGF) A chain mRNA, secrete a PDGF-like mitogen, and bind exogenous PDGF in a phenotype- and growth factor-dependent manner, *J. Cell Biol.,* 106, 403, 1988.
84. **Valente, A.J., Delgado, R., Metter, J.D., Cho, C., Sprague, E.A., Schwartz, C.J., and Graves, D.T.,** Cultured primate aortic smooth muscle cells express both the PDGF-A and PDGF-B genes but do not secrete mitogenic activity or dimeric platelet-derived growth factor protein, *J. Cell. Physiol.,* 136, 479, 1988.
85. **Walker, L.N., Bowen-Pope, D.F., and Reidy, M.A.,** Production of platelet-derived growth factor-like molecules by cultured arterial smooth muscle cells accompanies proliferation after arterial injury, *Proc. Natl. Acad. Sci. U.S.A.,* 83, 7311, 1986.
86. **Barrett, T.B. and Benditt, E.P.,** The *sis* (platelet-derived growth factor B chain) gene transcript levels are elevated in human atherosclerotic lesions compared to normal artery, *Proc. Natl. Acad. Sci. U.S.A.,* 84, 1099, 1987.
87. **Barrett, T.B. and Benditt, E.P.,** Platelet-derived growth factor gene expression in human atherosclerotic plaques and normal artery wall, *Proc. Natl. Acad. Sci. U.S.A.,* 85, 2810, 1988.
88. **Libby, P., Warner, S.J.C., Salomon, R.N., and Birinyi, L.K.,** Production of platelet-derived growth factor-like mitogen by smooth-muscle cells from human atheroma, *N. Engl. J. Med.,* 318, 1493, 1988.
89. **Matsuoka, J. and Grotendorst, G.R.,** Two peptides related to platelet-derived growth factor are present in human wound fluid, *Proc. Natl. Acad. Sci. U.S.A.,* 86, 4416, 1989.
90. **Shimokado, K., Raines, E.W., Madtes, D.K., Barrett, T.B., Benditt, E.P., and Ross, R.,** A significant part of macrophage-derived growth factor consists of a least two forms of PDGF, *Cell,* 43, 277, 1985.
91. **Mornex, J.-F., Martinet, Y., Yamauchi, K., Bitterman, P.B., Grotendorst, G.R., Chytil-Weir, A., Martin, G.R., and Crystal, R.G.,** Spontaneous expression of the c-*sis* gene and release of a platelet-derived growth factorlike molecule by human alveolar macrophages, *J. Clin. Invest.,* 78, 61, 1986.
92. **Martinet, Y., Bitterman, P.B., Mornex, J.-F., Grotendorst, G.R., Martin, G.R., and Crystal, R.G.,** Activated human monocytes express the c-*sis* proto-oncogene and release a mediator showing PDGF-like activity, *Nature,* 319, 158, 1986.
93. **Yeh, H.J., Ruit, K.G., Wang, Y.X., Parks, W.C., Snider, W.D., and Deuel, T.F.,** PDGF A-chain gene is expressed by mammalian neurons during development and in maturity, *Cell,* 64, 209, 1991.
94. **Sasahara, M., Fries, J.W.U., Raines, E.W., Gown, A.M., Westrum, L.E., Frosch, M.P., Bonthrow, D.T., Ross, R., and Collins, T.,** PDGF B-chain in neurons of the central nervous system, posterior pituitary, and in a transgenic model, *Cell,* 64, 217, 1991.
95. **Welsh, M., Claesson-Welsh, L., Hallberg, A., Welsh, N., Arkhammar, P., Nilsson, T., Heldin, C. H., and Berggren, P.-O.,** Coexpression of the platelet-derived growth factor (PDGF) B chain and the PDGF β receptor in isolated pancreatic islet cells stimulates DNA synthesis, *Proc. Natl. Acad. Sci. U.S.A.,* 87, 5807, 1990.
96. **Rhudy, R.W. and McPherson, J.M.,** Influence of the extracellular matrix on the proliferative response of human skin fibroblasts to serum and purified platelet-derived growth factor, *J. Cell. Physiol.,* 137, 185, 1988.
97. **Lynch, S.E., Nixon, J.C., Colvin, R.B., and Antoniades, H.N.,** Role of platelet-derived growth factor in wound healing: synergistic effects with other growth factors, *Proc. Natl. Acad. Sci. U.S.A.,* 84, 7696, 1987.

98. **Pierce, G.F., Mustoe, T.A., Lingelbach, J., Masakowski, V.R., Griffin, G.L., Senior, R.M., and Deuel, T.F.,** Platelet-derived growth factor and transforming growth factor-β enhance tissue repair activities by unique mechanisms, *J. Cell Biol.,* 109, 429, 1989.
99. **Shure, D., Senior, R.M., Griffin, G.L., and Deuel, T.F.,** PDGF-AA homodimers are potent chemoattractants for fibroblasts and neutrophils, and for monocytes activated by lymphocytes or cytokines, *Biochem. Biophys. Res. Commun.,* 186, 1510, 1992.
100. **Soma, Y., Dvonch, V., and Grotendorst, G.R.,** Platelet-derived growth factor AA homodimer is the predominant isoform in human platelets and acute human wound fluid, *FASEB J.,* 6, 2996, 1992.
101. **Pledger, W.J., Stiles, C.D., Antoniades, H.N., and Scher, C.D.,** Induction of DNA synthesis in BALB/c-3T3 cells by serum components: re-evaluation of the commitment process, *Proc. Natl. Acad. Sci. U.S.A.,* 74, 4481, 1977.
102. **Pledger, W.J., Stiles, C.D., Antoniades, H.N., and Scher, C.D.,** An ordered sequence of events is required before BALB/c-3T3 cells become committed to DNA synthesis, *Proc. Natl. Acad. Sci. U.S.A.,* 75, 2839, 1978.
103. **Scher, C.D., Whipple, A.P., Singh, J.P., and Pledger, W.J.,** Modulation of the platelet-derived growth factor induced replicative response, *J. Cell. Physiol.,* 123, 10, 1985.
104. **Dupuy, E., Rohrlich, P.-S., and Tobelem, G.,** Heparin stimulates fibroblasts growth induced by platelet derived growth factor, *Cell Biol. Int. Rep.,* 12, 17, 1988.
105. **Bauer, E.A., Silverman, N., Busier, D.F., Kronberger, A., and Deuel, T.F.,** Diminished response of Werner's syndrome to growth factors PDGF and FGF, *Science,* 234, 1240, 1986.
106. **Deuel, T.F., Senior, R.M., Huang, J.S., and Griffin, G.L.,** Chemotaxis of monocytes and neutrophils to platelet-derived growth factor, *J. Clin. Invest.,* 69, 1046, 1982.
107. **Wilson, E., Laster, S.M., Gooding, L.R., and Lambeth, J.D.,** Platelet-derived growth factor stimulates phagocytosis and blocks agonist-induced activation of the neutrophil oxidative burst: a possible cellular mechanism to protect against oxygen radical damage, *Proc. Natl. Acad. Sci. U.S.A.,* 84, 2213, 1987.
108. **Higgy, N.A., Davidoff, A.W., Grothman, G.T., Hollenberg, M.D., Benediktsson, H., and Paul, L.C.,** Expression of platelet-derived growth factor receptor in rat heart allografts, *J. Heart Lung Transplant.,* 10, 1012, 1991.
109. **Ferns, G.A.A., Raines, E.W., Sprugel, K.H., Motani, A.S., Reidy, M.A., and Ross, R.,** Inhibition of neointimal smooth muscle accumulation after angioplasty by an antibody to PDGF, *Science,* 253, 1129, 1991.
110. **Williams, L.T., Escobedo, J.A., Keating, M.T., and Coughlin, S.R.,** Signal transduction by the platelet-derived growth factor receptor, *Cold Spring Harbor Symp. Quant. Biol.,* 53, 455, 1988.
111. **Heldin, C.H., Westermark, B., and Wasteson, Å.,** Specific receptors for platelet-derived growth factor on cells derived from connective tissue and glia, *Proc. Natl. Acad. Sci. U.S.A.,* 78, 3664, 1981.
112. **Bowen-Pope, D.F. and Ross, R.,** Platelet-derived growth factor. II. Specific binding to cultured cells, *J. Biol. Chem.,* 257, 5161, 1982.
113. **Ek, B., Westermark, B., and Heldin, C.-H.,** Stimulation of tyrosine-specific phosphorylation of platelet-derived growth factor, *Nature,* 295, 419, 1982.
114. **Ek, B. and Heldin, C.-H.,** Characterization of a tyrosine-specific kinase activity in human fibroblast membranes stimulated by platelet-derived growth factor, *J. Biol. Chem.,* 257, 10486, 1982.
115. **Nishimura, J., Huang, J.S., and Deuel, T.F.,** Platelet-derived growth factor stimulates tyrosine-specific protein kinase activity in Swiss mouse 3T3 cell membranes, *Proc. Natl. Acad. Sci. U.S.A.,* 79, 4303, 1982.
116. **Cooper, J.A., Bowen-Pope, D.F., Raines, E., Ross, R., and Hunter, T.,** Similar effects of platelet-derived growth factor and epidermal growth factor on the phosphorylation of tyrosine in cellular proteins, *Cell,* 31, 263, 1982.
117. **Heldin, C.-H., Ernlund, A., Rorsman, C., and Rönnstrand, L.,** Dimerization of B-type platelet-derived growth factor receptors occurs after ligand binding and is closely associated with receptor kinase activation, *J. Biol. Chem.,* 264, 8905, 1989.
118. **Fretto, L.J., Snape, A.J., Tomlinson, J.E., Seroogy, J.J., Wolf, D.L., LaRochelle, W.J., and Giese, N.A.,** Mechanisms of platelet-derived growth factor (PDGF) AA, AB, and BB binding to α and β PDGF receptor, *J. Biol. Chem.,* 268, 3525, 1993.
119. **Graves, D.T., Antoniades, H.N., Williams, S.R., and Owen, A.J.,** Evidence for functional platelet-derived growth factor receptors on MG-63 human osteosarcoma cells, *Cancer Res.,* 44, 2966, 1984.

120. **Alpers, C.E., Seifert, R.A., Hudkins, K.L., Johnson, R.J., and Bowen-Pope, D.F.,** PDGF receptor localizes to mesangial, parietal epithelial, and interstitial cells in human and primate kidney, *Kidney Int.,* 43, 286, 1993.
121. **Beitz, J.G., Kim, I.S., Calabrese, P., and Frackelton, A.R.,** Human microvascular endothelial cells express receptors for platelet-derived growth factor, *Proc. Natl. Acad. Sci. U.S.A.,* 88, 2021, 1991.
122. **Graves, D.T., Owen, A.J., and Antoniades, H.N.,** Demonstration of receptors for a PDGF-like mitogen on human osteosarcoma cells, *Biochem. Biophys. Res. Commun.,* 129, 56, 1985.
123. **Rosenfeld, M., Keating, A., Bowen-Pope, D.F., Singer, J.W., and Ross, R.,** Responsiveness of the *in vitro* hematopoietic microenvironment to platelet-derived growth factor, *Leukemia Res.,* 9, 427, 1985.
124. **Heldin, N.-E., Gustavsson, B., Claesson-Welsh, L., Hammacher, A., Mark, J., Heldin, C.-H., and Westermark, B.,** Aberrant expression of receptors for platelet-derived growth factor in an anaplastic thyroid carcinoma cell line, *Proc. Natl. Acad. Sci. U.S.A.,* 85, 9302, 1988.
125. **Andersen, H.A., Flodgaard, H., Klenow, H., and Leick, V.,** Platelet-derived growth factor stimulates chemotaxis and nucleic acid synthesis in the protozoan *Tetrahymena*, *Biochim. Biophys. Acta,* 782, 437, 1984.
126. **Yarden, Y., Escobedo, J.A., Kuang, W.-J., Yang-Feng, T.L., Daniel, T.O., Tremble, P.M., Chen, E.Y., Ando, M.E., Harkins, R.N., Francke, U., Fried, V.A., Ullrich, A., and Williams, L.T.,** Structure of the receptor for platelet-derived growth factor helps define a family of closely related growth factor receptors, *Nature,* 323, 226, 1986.
127. **Claesson-Welsh, L., Eriksson, A., Morén, A., Severinsson, L., Ek, B., Östman, A., Betsholtz, C., and Heldin, C.-H.,** cDNA cloning and expression of a human platelet-derived growth factor (PDGF) receptor for B-chain-containing PDGF molecules, *Mol. Cell. Biol.,* 8, 3476, 1988.
128. **Roberts, W.M., Look, A.T., Roussel, M.F., and Sherr, C.J.,** Tandem linkage of human CSF-1 receptor (c-*fms*) and PDGF receptor genes, *Cell,* 55, 655, 1988.
129. **Kobilka, B.K., Dixon, R.A.F., Frielle, T., Dohlman, H.G., Bolanowski, M.A., Sigal, I.S., Yang-Feng, T.L., Francke, U., Caron, M.G., and Lefkowitz, R.J.,** cDNA for the human β_2-adrenergic receptor: a protein with multiple membrane spanning domains and encoded by a gene whose chromosomal location is shared with that of the receptor for platelet-derived growth factor, *Proc. Natl. Acad. Sci. U.S.A.,* 84, 46, 1987.
130. **Hammacher, A., Nistér, M., and Heldin, C.-H.,** The A-type receptor for platelet-derived growth factor mediates protein tyrosine phosphorylation, receptor transmodulation and a mitogenic response, *Biochem. J.,* 264, 15, 1989.
131. **Matsui, T., Heideran, M., Miki, T., Popescu, N., La Rochelle, W., Kraus, M., Pierce, J., and Aaronson, S.A.,** Isolation of a novel receptor cDNA establishes the existence of two PDGF receptor genes, *Science,* 243, 800, 1989.
132. **Gronwald, R.G.K., Adler, D.A., Kelly, J.D., Disteche, C.M., and Bowen-Pope, D.F.,** The human PDGF receptor α-subunit gene maps to chromosome 4 in close proximity to c-*kit*, *Hum. Genet.,* 85, 383, 1990.
133. **Yarden, Y., Kuang, W.-J., Yang-Feng, T., Coussens, L., Munemitsu, S., Dull, T.J., Chen, E., Schlessinger, J., Francke, U., and Ullrich, A.,** Human proto-oncogene c-kit: a new cell surface receptor tyrosine kinase for an unidentified ligand, *EMBO J.,* 6, 3341, 1987.
134. **Hart, C.E., Seifert, R.A., Ross, R., and Bowen-Pope, D.F.,** Synthesis, phosphorylation, and degradation of multiple forms of the platelet-derived growth factor receptor studied using a monoclonal antibody, *J. Biol. Chem.,* 262, 10780, 1987.
135. **Claesson-Welsh, L., Rönnstrand, L., and Heldin, C.-H.,** Biosynthesis and intracellular transport of the receptor for platelet-derived growth factor, *Proc. Natl. Acad. Sci. U.S.A.,* 84, 8796, 1987.
136. **Claesson-Welsh, L., Hammacher, A., Westermark, B., Heldin, C.-H., and Nistér, M.,** Identification and structural analysis of the A type receptor for platelet-derived growth factor. Similarities with the B type receptor, *J. Biol. Chem.,* 264, 1742, 1989.
137. **Seifert, R.A., Hart, C.E., Phillips, P.E., Forstrom, J.W., Ross, R., Murray, M.J., and Bowen-Pope, D.F.,** Two different subunits associate to create isoform-specific platelet-derived growth factor receptors, *J. Biol. Chem.,* 264, 8771, 1989.
138. **Claesson-Welsh, L., Eriksson, A., Westermark, B., and Heldin, C.-H.,** cDNA cloning and expression of the human A-type platelet-derived growth factor (PDGF) receptor establishes structural similarity to the B-type PDGF receptor, *Proc. Natl. Acad. Sci. U.S.A.,* 86, 4917, 1989.

139. **Williams, L.T., Escobedo, J.A., Keating, M.T., and Coughlin, S.R.,** The stimulation of paracrine and autocrine mitogenic pathways by the platelet-derived growth factor receptor, *J. Cell. Physiol.,* Suppl. 5, 27, 1987.
140. **Keating, M.T. and Williams, L.T.,** Processing of the platelet-derived growth factor receptor: biosynthetic and degradation studies using antireceptor antibodies, *J. Biol. Chem.,* 262, 7932, 1987.
141. **Daniel, T.O., Tremble, P.M., Frackelton, A.R., Jr., and Williams, L.T.,** Purification of the platelet-derived growth factor receptor by using an anti-phosphotyrosine antibody, *Proc. Natl. Acad. Sci. U.S.A.,* 82, 2684, 1985.
142. **Zippel, R., Sturani, E., Toschi, L., Naldini, L., Alberghina, L., and Comoglio, P.M.,** In vivo phosphorylation and dephosphorylation of the platelet-derived growth factor receptor studied by immunoblot analysis with phosphotyrosine antibodies, *Biochim. Biophys. Acta,* 881, 54, 1986.
143. **Daniel, T.O., Milfay, D.F., Escobedo, J., and Williams, L.T.,** Biosynthetic and glycosylation studies of cell surface platelet-derived growth factor receptors, *J. Biol. Chem.,* 262, 9778, 1987.
144. **Rönnstrand, L., Beckmann, M.P., Faulders, B., Östman, A., Ek, B., and Heldin, C.-H.,** Purification of the receptor for platelet-derived growth factor from porcine uterus, *J. Biol. Chem.,* 262, 2929, 1987.
145. **Huang, J.S., Nishimura, J., Huang, S.S., and Deuel, T.F,** Protamine inhibits platelet derived growth factor receptor activity but not epidermal growth factor activity, *J. Cell. Biochem.,* 26, 205, 1984.
146. **Betsholtz, C., Westermark, B., Ek, B., and Heldin, C.-H.,** Coexpression of a PDGF-like growth factor and PDGF receptors in a human osteosarcoma cell line: implications for autocrine receptor activation, *Cell,* 39, 447, 1984.
147. **Hosang, M.,** Suramin binds to platelet-derived growth factor and inhibits its biological activity, *J. Cell. Biochem.,* 29, 265, 1985.
148. **Coffey, R.J., Jr., Leof, E.B., Shipley, G.D., and Moses, H.L.,** Suramin inhibition of growth factor receptor binding and mitogenicity in AKR-2B cells, *J. Cell. Physiol.,* 132, 143, 1987.
149. **Heldin, C.-H., Bäckström, G., Östman, A., Hammacher, A., Rönnstrand, L., Rubin, K., Nistér, M., and Westermark, B.,** Binding of different dimeric forms of PDGF to human fibroblasts: evidence for two separate receptor types, *EMBO J.,* 7, 1387, 1988.
150. **Hart, C.E., Forstrom, J.W., Kelly, J.D., Seifert, R.A., Smith, R.A., Ross, R., Murray, M.J., and Bowen-Pope, D.F.,** Two classes of PDGF receptor recognize different isoforms of PDGF, *Science,* 240, 1529, 1988.
151. **Bowen-Pope, D.F., Hart, C.E., and Seifert, R.A.,** Sera and conditioned media contain different isoforms of platelet-derived growth factor (PDGF) which bind to different classes of PDGF receptor, *J. Biol. Chem.,* 264, 2502, 1989.
152. **Do, M.S., Fitzerattas, C., Gubbay, J., Greenfeld, L., Feldman, M., and Eisenbach, L.,** Mouse platelet-derived growth factor-α receptor. Sequence, tissue-specific expression and correlation with metastatic phenotype, *Oncogene,* 7, 1567, 1992.
153. **Pringle, N.P., Mudhar, H.S., Collarini, E.J., and Richardson, W.D.,** PDGF receptors in the rat CNS. During late neurogenesis, PDGF α-receptor expression appears to be restricted to glial cells of the oligodendrocyte lineage, *Development,* 115, 535, 1992.
154. **Eriksson, A., Siegbahn, A., Westermark, B., Heldin, C.-H., and Claesson-Welsh, L.,** PDGF α- and β-receptors activate unique and common signal transduction pathways, *EMBO J.,* 11, 543, 1992.
155. **Young, R.M., Mendoza, A.E., Collins, T., and Orkin, S.H.,** Alternatively spliced platelet-derived growth factor A-chain transcripts are not tumor specific but encode normal cellular proteins, *Mol. Cell. Biol.,* 10, 6051, 1990.
156. **Stephenson, D.A., Mercola, M., Anderson, E., Wang, C., Stiles, C.D., Bowen-Pope, D.F., and Chapman, V.M.,** Platelet-derived growth factor receptor α-subunit gene *(Pdgfra)* is deleted in the mouse patch *(Ph)* mutation, *Proc. Natl. Acad. Sci. U.S.A.,* 88, 6, 1991.
157. **Ek, B. and Heldin, C.-H.,** Use of an antiserum against phosphotyrosine for the identification of phosphorylated components in human fibroblasts stimulated by platelet-derived growth factor, *J. Biol. Chem.,* 259, 11145, 1984.
158. **Frackelton, A.R., Jr., Tremble, P.M., and Williams, L.T.,** Evidence for the platelet-derived growth factor-stimulated tyrosine phosphorylation of the platelet-derived growth factor receptor *in vivo:* immunopurification using a monoclonal antibody to phosphotyrosine, *J. Biol. Chem.,* 259, 7909, 1984.
159. **Rönnstrand, L., Terracio, L., Claesson-Welsh, L., Heldin, C.-H., and Rubin, K.,** Characterization of two monoclonal antibodies reactive with the external domain of the platelet-derived growth factor receptor, *J. Biol. Chem.,* 263, 10429, 1988.

160. Fantl, W.J., Escobedo, J.A., and Williams, L.T., Mutations of the platelet-derived growth factor receptor that cause a loss of ligand-induced conformational change, subtle changes in kinase activity, and impair ability to stimulate DNA synthesis, *Mol. Cell. Biol.,* 9, 4473, 1989.
161. Bishayee, S., Ross, A.H., Womer, R., and Scher, C.D., Purified human platelet-derived growth factor receptor has ligand-stimulated tyrosine kinase activity, *Proc. Natl. Acad. Sci. U.S.A.,* 83, 6756, 1986.
162. Courtneidge, S.A., Kypta, R.M., Cooper, J.A., and Kazlauskas, A., Platelet-derived growth factor receptor sequences important for binding of *src* family tyrosine kinases, *Cell Growth Differ.,* 2, 483, 1991.
163. Valius, M., Bazenet, C., and Kazlauskas, A., Tyrosines 1021 and 1009 are phosphorylation sites in the carboxy terminus of the platelet-derived growth factor receptor β subunit and are required for binding of phospholipase Cγ and a 64-kilodalton protein, respectively, *Mol. Cell. Biol.,* 13, 133, 1993.
164. Eide, B.L., Krebs, E.G., Ross, R., Pike, L.J., and Bowen-Pope, D.F., Tumor promoter enhances mitogenesis by PDGF with little effect on PDGF binding, *J. Cell. Physiol.,* 126, 254, 1986.
165. Sturani, E., Vicentini, L.M., Zippel, R., Toshi, L., Pandiella-Alonso, A., Comoglio, P.M., and Meldolesi, J., PDGF-induced receptor phosphorylation and phosphoinositide hydrolysis are unaffected by protein kinase C activation in mouse Swiss 3T3 and human skin fibroblasts, *Biochem. Biophys. Res. Commun.,* 137, 343, 1986.
166. Gronwald, R.G.K., Seifert, R.A., and Bowen-Pope, D.F., Differential regulation of expression of two platelet-derived growth factor receptor subunits by transforming growth factor-β, *J. Biol. Chem.,* 264, 8120, 1989.
167. Bonner, C., Badgett, A., Osornio-Vargas, A.R., Hoffman, M., and Brody, A.R., PDGF-stimulated fibroblast proliferation is enhanced synergistically by receptor-recognized α_2-macroglobulin, *J. Cell. Physiol.,* 145, 1, 1990.
168. Weinmaster, G. and Lemke, G., Cell-specific cyclic AMP-mediated induction of the PDGF receptor, *EMBO J.,* 9, 915, 1990.
169. Diliberto, P.A., Gordon, G.W., Yu, C.-L., Earp, H.S., and Herman, B., Platelet-derived growth factor (PDGF) receptor activation modulates the calcium mobilizing activity of the PDGF β receptor in Balb/c3T3 fibroblasts, *J. Biol. Chem.,* 267, 11888, 1992.
170. Rosenfeld, M.E., Bowen-Pope, D.F., and Ross, R., Platelet-derived growth factor: morphologic and biochemical studies of binding, internalization, and degradation, *J. Cell. Physiol.,* 121, 263, 1984.
171. Satoh, T., Endo, M., Nakafuku, M., Nakamura, S., and Kariro, Y., Platelet-derived growth factor stimulates formation of active p21^{ras}-GTP complex in Swiss mouse 3T3 cells, *Proc. Natl. Acad. Sci. U.S.A.,* 87, 5993, 1990.
172. Lowenstein, E.J., Daly, R.J., Batzer, A.G., Li, W., Margolis, B., Lammers, R., Ullrich, A., Skolnik, E.Y., Bar-Sagi, D., and Schlessinger, J., The SH2 and SH3 domain-containing protein GRB2 links receptor tyrosine kinases to ras signaling, *Cell,* 70, 431, 1992.
173. Rozakis-Adcock, M., McGlade, J., Mbamalu, G., Pelicci, G., Daly, R., Li, W., Batzer, A., Thomas, S., Brugge, J., Pelicci, P.G., Schlessinger, J., and Pawson, T., Association of the Shc and Grb2/Sem5 SH2-containing proteins is implicated in activation of the Ras pathway by tyrosine kinases, *Nature,* 360, 689, 1992.
174. Egan, S.E., Giddings, B.W., Brooks, M.W., Buday, L., Sizeland, A.M., and Weinberg, R.A., Association of Sos Ras exchange protein with Grb2 is implicated in tyrosine kinase signal transduction and transformation, *Nature,* 363, 45, 1993.
175. Satoh, T., Fantl, W.J., Escobedo, J.A., Williams, L.T., and Kaziro, Y., Platelet-derived growth factor receptor mediates activation of Ras through different signaling pathways in different cell types, *Mol. Cell. Biol.,* 13, 3706, 1993.
176. Heldin, C.-H., Ek, B., and Rönnstrand, L., Characterization of the receptor for platelet-derived growth factor on human fibroblasts: demonstration of an intimate relationship with 185,000 dalton substrate for the PDGF receptor-kinase, *J. Biol. Chem.,* 258, 10054, 1983.
177. Kaplan, D.R., Whitman, M., Schaffhausen, B., Pallas, D.C., White, M., Cantley, L., and Roberts, T.M., Common elements in growth factor stimulation and oncogenic transformation: 85 kda phosphoprotein and phosphatidylinositol kinase activity, *Cell,* 50, 1021, 1987.
178. Wahl, M.I., Olashaw, N.E., Nishibe, S., Rhee, S.G., Pledger, W.J., and Carpenter, G., Platelet-derived growth factor induces rapid and sustained tyrosine phosphorylation of phospholipase C-γ in quiescent BALB/c 3T3 cells, *Mol. Cell. Biol.,* 9, 2934, 1989.
179. Kypta, R.M., Goldberg, Y., Ulug, E.T., and Courtneidge, S.A., Association between the PDGF receptor and members of the *src* family of tyrosine kinases, *Cell,* 62, 481, 1990.

180. **Brambilla, R., Zippel, R., Sturani, E., Morello, L., Peres, A., and Alberghina, L.,** Characterization of the tyrosine phosphorylation of calpactin-I (annexin-II) induced by platelet-derived growth factor, *Biochem. J.,* 278, 447, 1991.
181. **Rönnstrand, L., Sorokin, A., Engström, U., and Heldin, C.-H.,** Characterization of the platelet-derived growth factor β-receptor kinase activity by use of synthetic peptides, *Biochem. Biophys. Res. Commun.,* 167, 1333, 1990.
182. **Shawver, L.K. and Deuel, T.F.,** Nuclear pp64 is phosphorylated in both serine/threonine and tyrosine through complex pathways regulated by 12-*O*-tetradecanoylphorbol-13-acetate and platelet-derived growth factor, *Biochem. Biophys. Res. Commun.,* 167, 918, 1990.
183. **Escobedo, J.A. and Williams, L.T.,** A PDGF receptor domain essential for mitogenesis but not for many other responses to PDGF, *Nature,* 335, 85, 1988.
184. **Kazlauskas, A. and DiCorleto, P.E.,** A comparison of the platelet-derived growth factor-dependent tyrosine kinase activity in sparse and confluent fibroblasts, *J. Cell. Physiol.,* 126, 225, 1986.
185. **Suzuki-Sekimori, R., Matuoka, K., Nagai, Y., and Takenawa, T.,** Diacylglycerol, but not inositol 1,4,5-trisphosphate, accounts for platelet-derived growth factor-stimulated proliferation of BALB 3T3 cells, *J. Cell. Physiol.,* 140, 432, 1989.
186. **Fukami, K. and Takenawa, T.,** Quantitative changes in polyphosphoinositides 1,2-diacylglycerol and inositol 1,4,5-trisphosphate by platelet-derived growth factor and prostaglandin $F^2\alpha$, *J. Biol. Chem.,* 264, 14985, 1989.
187. **Kumjian, D.A., Wahl, M.I., Rhee, S.G., and Daniel, T.O.,** Platelet-derived growth factor (PDGF) binding promotes physical association of PDGF receptor with phospholipase C, *Proc. Natl. Acad. Sci. U.S.A.,* 86, 8232, 1989.
188. **Kim, U.H., Kim, H.S., and Rhee, S.G.,** Epidermal growth factor and platelet-derived growth factor promote translocation of phospholipase-C-γ from cytosol to membrane, *FEBS Lett.,* 270, 33, 1990.
189. **Sultzman, L., Ellis, C., Lin, L.-L., Pawson, T., and Knopf, J.,** Platelet-derived growth factor increases the in vivo activity of phospholipase C-γ_1 and phospholipase C-γ_2, *Mol. Cell. Biol.,* 11, 2018, 1991.
190. **Kim, H.K., Kim, J.W., Zilberstein, A., Margolis, B., Kim, J.G., Schlessinger, J., and Rhee, S.G.,** PDGF stimulation of inositol phospholipid hydrolysis requires PLC-γ1 phosphorylation on tyrosine residues 783 and 1254, *Cell,* 65, 435, 1991.
191. **Homma, Y., Sakamoto, H., Tsunoda, M., Aoki, M., Takenawa, T., and Ooyama, T.,** Evidence for involvement of phospholipase C-γ2 in signal transduction of platelet-derived growth factor in vascular smooth muscle cells, *Biochem. J.,* 290, 649, 1993.
192. **Hata, Y., Ogata, E., and Kojima, I.,** Platelet-derived growth factor stimulates synthesis of 1,2-diacylglycerol from monoacylglycerol in Balb/c 3T3 cells, *Biochem. J.,* 262, 947, 1989.
193. **Matuoka, K., Fukami, K., Nakanishi, O., Kawai, S., and Takenawa, T.,** Mitogenesis in response to PDGF and bombesin abolished by microinjection of antibody to PIP_2, *Science,* 239, 640, 1988.
194. **Blakeley, D.M., Corps, A.N., and Brown, K.D.,** Bombesin and platelet-derived growth factor stimulate formation of inositol phosphates and Ca^{2+} mobilization in Swiss 3T3 cells by different mechanisms, *Biochem. J.,* 258, 177, 1989.
195. **Pontbriant, C.M., Chen, J.-K., and Orlando, J.A.,** TGF-β inhibits the platelet-derived growth factor-induced formation of inositol trisphosphate in MG-63 human osteosarcoma cells, *J. Cell. Physiol.,* 145, 488, 1990.
196. **Berridge, M.J., Heslop, J.P., Irvine, R.F., and Brown, K.D.,** Inositol trisphosphate formation and calcium mobilization in Swiss 3T3 cells in response to platelet-derived growth factor, *Biochem. J.,* 222, 195, 1984.
197. **Chu, S.-H.W., Hoban, C.J., Owen, A.J., and Geyer, R.P.,** Platelet-derived growth factor stimulates polyphosphoinositide breakdown in fetal human fibroblasts, *J. Cell. Physiol.,* 124, 391, 1985.
198. **MacDonald, M.L., Mack, K.F., and Glomset, J.A.,** Regulation of phosphoinositide phosphorylation in Swiss 3T3 cells stimulated by platelet-derived growth factor, *J. Biol. Chem.,* 262, 1105, 1987.
199. **MacDonald, M., Mack, K.F., Richardson, C.N., and Glomset, J.A.,** Regulation of diacylglycerol kinase reaction in Swiss 3T3 cells: increased phosphorylation of endogenous diacylglycerol and decreased phosphorylation of didecanoylglycerol in response to platelet-derived growth factor, *J. Biol. Chem.,* 263, 1575, 1988.
200. **Margolis, B., Zilberstein, A., Franks, C., Felder, S., Kremer, S., Ullrich, A., Rhee, S.G., Skoricki, K., and Schlessinger, J.,** Effect of phospholipase C-γ overexpression on PDGF-induced second messengers and mitogenesis, *Science,* 248, 607, 1990.

201. **Hill, T.D., Dean, N.M., Mordan, L.J., Lau, A.F., Kanemitsu, M.Y., and Boynton, A.L.**, PDGF-induced activation of phospholipase C is not required for induction of DNA synthesis, *Science,* 248, 1660, 1990.
202. **Hawkins, P.T., Jackson, T.R., and Stephens, L.R.**, Platelet-derived growth factor stimulates synthesis of PtdIns(3,4,5)P3 by activating a PtdIns (4,5)P2 3-OH kinase, *Nature,* 358, 157, 1992.
203. **Ben-Av, P. and Liscovitch, M.**, Phospholipase D activation by the mitogens platelet-derived growth factor and 12-O-tetradecanoylphorbol 13-acetate in NIH-3T3 cells, *FEBS Lett.,* 259, 64, 1989.
204. **Susa, M., Keeler, M., and Varticovski, L.**, Platelet-derived growth factor activates membrane-associated phosphatidylinositol 3-kinase and mediates its translocation from the cytosol. Detection of enzyme activity in detergent-solubilized cell extracts, *J. Biol. Chem.,* 267, 22951, 1992.
205. **Fukami, K. and Takenawa, T.**, Phosphatidic acid that accumulates in platelet-derived growth factor-stimulated Balb/c 3T3 cells is a potential mitogenic signal, *J. Biol. Chem.,* 267, 10988, 1992.
206. **Frantz, C.N.**, Effects of platelet-derived growth factor on Ca^{2+} in 3T3 cells, *Exp. Cell Res.,* 158, 287, 1985.
207. **Tsuda, T., Kaibuchi, K., West, B., and Takai, Y.**, Involvement of Ca^{2+} in platelet-derived growth factor-induced expression of c-*myc* oncogene in Swiss 3T3 fibroblasts, *FEBS Lett.,* 187, 43, 1985.
208. **Roe, M.W., Hepler, J.R., Harden, T.K., and Herman, B.**, Platelet-derived growth factor and angiotensin II cause increases in cytosolic free calcium by different mechanisms in vascular smooth muscle cells, *J. Cell. Physiol.,* 139, 100, 1989.
209. **Ives, H.E. and Daniel, T.O.**, Interrelationship between growth factor-induced pH changes and intracellular Ca^{2+}, *Proc. Natl. Acad. Sci. U.S.A.,* 84, 1950, 1987.
210. **Tucker, R.W., Chang, D.T., and Maede-Cobun, K.**, Effects of platelet-derived growth factor and fibroblast growth factor on free intracellular calcium and mitogenesis, *J. Cell. Biochem.,* 39, 139, 1989.
211. **Benjamin, C.W., Tarpley, W.G., and Gorman, R.R.**, The lack of PDGF-stimulated PGE_2 release from *ras*-transformed NIH-3T3 cells results from reduced phospholipase C but not phospholipase A_2 activity, *Biochem. Biophys. Res. Commun.,* 145, 1254, 1987.
212. **Benjamin, C.W., Connor, J.A., Tarpley, W.G., and Gorman, R.R.**, NIH-3T3 cells transformed by the EJ-*ras* oncogene exhibit reduced platelet-derived growth factor-mediated Ca^{2+} mobilization, *Proc. Natl. Acad. Sci. U.S.A.,* 85, 4345, 1988.
213. **Larrodera, P., Cornet, M.E., Diaz-Meco, M.T., Lopez-Barrahona, M., Diaz-Laviada, I., Guddal, P.H., Johansen, T., and Moscat, J.**, Phospholipase C-mediated hydrolysis of phosphatidylcholine is an important step in PDGF-stimulated DNA synthesis, *Cell,* 61, 1113, 1990.
214. **Besterman, J.M., Duronio, V., and Cuatrecasas, P.**, Rapid formation of diacylglycerol from phosphatidylcholine: a pathway for generation of a second messenger, *Proc. Natl. Acad. Sci. U.S.A.,* 83, 6785, 1986.
215. **Benjamin, C.W., Tarpley, W.G., and Gorman, R.R.**, Loss of platelet-derived growth factor-stimulated phospholipase activity in NIH-3T3 cells expressing the EJ-*ras* oncogene, *Proc. Natl. Acad. Sci. U.S.A.,* 84, 546, 1987.
216. **Olinger, P.L. and Gorman, R.R.**, NIH-3T3 cells expressing high levels of the c-*ras* proto-oncogene display reduced platelet-derived growth factor-stimulated phospholipase activity, *Biochem. Biophys. Res. Commun.,* 150, 937, 1988.
217. **Whiteley, B., Deuel, T., and Glaser, L.**, Modulation of the activity of the platelet-derived growth factor receptor by phorbol myristate acetate, *Biochem. Biophys. Res. Commun.,* 129, 854, 1985.
218. **Zagari, M., Stephens, M., Earp, H.S., and Herman, B.**, Relationship of cytosolic ion fluxes and protein kinase C activation to platelet-derived growth factor induced competence and growth in BALB/c 3T3 cells, *J. Cell. Physiol.,* 139, 167, 1989.
219. **Frace, A.M. and Gargus, J.J.**, Activation of single-channel currents in mouse fibroblasts by platelet-derived growth factor, *Proc. Natl. Acad. Sci. U.S.A.,* 86, 2511, 1989.
220. **Domin, J. and Rozengurt, E.**, Platelet-derived growth factor stimulates a biphasic mobilization of arachidonic acid in Swiss 3T3 cells. The role of phospholipase A2, *J. Biol. Chem.,* 268, 8927, 1993.
221. **Moncada, S. and Vane, J.R.**, Pharmacology and endogenous roles of prostacyclin endoperoxides, thromboxane A_2, and prostacyclin, *Pharmacol. Rev.,* 30, 293, 1979.
222. **Callahan, K.S., Schorer, A., and Harlan, J.M.**, Platelet-derived growth factor does not stimulate prostacyclin synthesis by cultured endothelial cells, *Blood,* 67, 131, 1986.
223. **Williams, L.T., Antoniades, H.N., and Goetzl, E.J.**, Platelet-derived growth factor stimulates mouse 3T3 cell mitogenesis and leukocyte chemotaxis through different structural determinants, *J. Clin. Invest.,* 72, 1759, 1983.

224. **Wharton, W., Leof, E., Olashaw, N., O'Keefe, E.J., and Pledger, W.J.,** Mitogenic response to epidermal growth factor (EGF) modulated by platelet-derived growth factor in cultured fibroblasts, *Exp. Cell Res.,* 147, 443, 1983.
225. **Pledger, W.J., Hart, C.A., Locatell, K.L., and Scher, C.D.,** Platelet-derived growth factor-modulated proteins: constitutive synthesis by a transformed cell line, *Proc. Natl. Acad. Sci. U.S.A.,* 78, 4358, 1981.
226. **Davis, R.J. and Czech, M.P.,** Platelet-derived growth factor mimics phorbol diester action on epidermal growth factor receptor phosphorylation at threonine-654, *Proc. Natl. Acad. Sci. U.S.A.,* 82, 4080, 1985.
227. **Decker, S.J. and Harris, P.,** Effects of platelet-derived growth factor on phosphorylation of the epidermal growth factor receptor in human skin fibroblasts, *J. Biol. Chem.,* 264, 9204, 1989.
228. **Wrann, M., Fox, C.F., and Ross, R.,** Modulation of epidermal growth factor receptors on 3T3 cells by platelet-derived growth factor, *Science,* 210, 1363, 1980.
229. **Heldin, C.-H., Wasteson, Å., and Westermark, B.,** Interaction of platelet-derived growth factor with its fibroblast receptor: demonstration of ligand degradation and receptor modulation, *J. Biol. Chem.,* 257, 4216, 1982.
230. **Olashaw, N.E., O'Keefe, E.J., and Pledger, W.J.,** Platelet-derived growth factor modulates epidermal growth factor receptors by a mechanism distinct from that of phorbol esters, *Proc. Natl. Acad. Sci. U.S.A.,* 83, 3834, 1986.
231. **Kelly, J.D., Raines, E.W., Ross, R., and Murray, M.J.,** The B chain of PDGF alone is sufficient for mitogenesis, *EMBO J.,* 4, 3399, 1985.
232. **Reed, B.Y., King, M.T., Gitomer, W.L., and Veech, R.L.,** Early metabolic effects of platelet-derived growth factor and transforming growth factor-β in rat liver *in vitro, J. Biol. Chem.,* 262, 8712, 1987.
233. **Nakamura, K.D., Martinez, R., and Weber, M.J.,** Tyrosine phosphorylation of specific proteins after mitogen stimulation of chicken embryo fibroblasts, *Mol. Cell. Biol.,* 3, 380, 1983.
234. **Harrington, M.A., Estes, J.E., Leof, E., and Pledger, W.J.,** PDGF stimulates transient phosphorylation of 180,000 dalton protein, *J. Cell. Biochem.,* 27, 67, 1985.
235. **Nishimura, J. and Deuel, T.F.,** Stimulation of protein phosphorylation in Swiss mouse 3T3 cells by human platelet-derived growth factor, *Biochem. Biophys. Res. Commun.,* 103, 355, 1981.
236. **Shawver, L.K., Behrens, C.B., and Deuel, T.F.,** Characterization of pp64, a nuclear phosphoprotein induced by platelet-derived growth factor, *Biochem. Biophys. Res. Commun.,* 161, 1118, 1989.
237. **Bockus, B.J. and Stiles, C.D.,** Regulation of cytoskeletal architecture by platelet-derived growth factor, insulin and epidermal growth factor, *Exp. Cell Res.,* 153, 186, 1984.
238. **Herman, B. and Pledger, W.J.,** Platelet-derived growth factor-induced alterations in vinculin and actin distribution in BALB/c-3T3 cells, *J. Cell. Biol.,* 100, 1031, 1985.
239. **Herman, B., Roe, M.W., Harris, C., Wray, B., and Clemmons, D.,** Platelet-derived growth factor-induced alterations in vinculin distribution in porcine vascular smooth muscle cells, *Cell Motil. Cytoskel.,* 8, 91, 1987.
240. **Geiger, B.,** Membrane-cytoskeletal interaction, *Biochim. Biophys. Acta,* 737, 305, 1983.
241. **Bauer, E.A., Cooper, T.W., Huang, J.S., Altman, J.A., and Deuel, T.F.,** Stimulation of *in vitro* human skin collagenase expression by platelet-derived growth factor, *Proc. Natl. Acad. Sci. U.S.A.,* 82, 4132, 1985.
242. **Cochran, B.H., Reffel, A.C., and Stiles, C.D.,** Molecular cloning of gene sequences regulated by platelet-derived growth factor, *Cell,* 33, 939, 1983.
243. **Tannenbaum, C.S., Major, J., Poptic, E., DiCorleto, P.E., and Hamilton, T.A.,** Lipopolysaccharide-inducible macrophage early genes are induced in Balb/c 3T3 cells by platelet-derived growth factor, *J. Biol. Chem.,* 264, 4052, 1989.
244. **Rollins, B.J., Morrison, E.D., Usher, P., and Flier, J.S.,** Platelet-derived growth factor regulates glucose transporter expression, *J. Biol. Chem.,* 263, 16523, 1988.
245. **Rollins, B.J., Morrison, E.D., and Stiles, C.D.,** A cell-cycle constraint on the regulation of gene expression by platelet-derived growth factor, *Science,* 238, 1269, 1987.
246. **Kawahara, R.S. and Deuel, T.F.,** Platelet-derived growth factor-inducible gene *JE* is a member of a family of small inducible genes related to platelet factor 4, *J. Biol. Chem.,* 264, 679, 1989.
247. **Kawahara, R.S., Deng, Z.W., and Deuel, T.F.,** Glucocorticoids inhibit the transcriptional induction of JE, a platelet-derived growth factor-inducible gene, *J. Biol. Chem.,* 266, 13261, 1991.
248. **Linzer, D.I.H. and Nathans, D.,** Growth-related changes in specific mRNAs of cultured mouse cells, *Proc. Natl. Acad. Sci. U.S.A.,* 80, 4271, 1983.
249. **LoBue, J. and LoBue, P.A.,** Control of cell growth, *Transplant. Proc.,* 16, 341, 1984.

250. **Allen-Hoffmann, L.A., Schlosser, S.J., Brondyk, W.H., and Fahl, W.E.,** Fibronectin levels are enhanced in human fibroblasts overexpressing the c-*sis* proto-oncogene, *J. Biol. Chem.,* 265, 5219, 1990.
251. **Rabin, M.S., Doherty, P.J., and Gottesman, M.M.,** The tumor promoter phorbol 12-myristate 13-acetate induces a program of altered gene expression similar to that induced by platelet-derived growth factor and transforming oncogenes, *Proc. Natl. Acad. Sci. U.S.A.,* 83, 357, 1986.
252. **Kerr, L.D., Holt, J.T., and Matrisian, L.M.,** Growth factors regulate transin gene expression by c-*fos*-dependent and c-*fos*-independent pathways, *Science,* 242, 1424, 1988.
253. **Bonin, P.D. and Singh, J.P.,** Modulation of interleukin-1 receptor expression and interleukin-1 response in fibroblasts by platelet-derived growth factor, *J. Biol. Chem.,* 263, 11052, 1988.
254. **Chiou, W.J., Bonin, P.D., Harris, P.K.W., Carter, D.R., and Singh, J.P.,** Platelet-derived growth factor induces interleukin-1 receptor gene expression in Balb/c 3T3 fibroblasts, *J. Biol. Chem.,* 264, 21442, 1989.
255. **Zullo, J.N., Cochran, B.H., Huang, A.S., and Stiles, C.D.,** Platelet-derived growth factor and double-stranded ribonucleic acids stimulate expression of the same genes in 3T3 cells, *Cell,* 43, 793, 1985.
256. **Johnson, H.M. and Torres, B.A.,** Peptide growth factors PDGF, EGF, and FGF regulate interferon-γ production, *J. Immunol.,* 134, 2824, 1985.
257. **Einat, M., Resnitzky, D., and Kimchi, A.,** Inhibitory effects of interferon on the expression of genes regulated by platelet-derived growth factors, *Proc. Natl. Acad. Sci. U.S.A.,* 82, 7608, 1985.
258. **Cochran, B.H., Zullo, J., Verma, I.M., and Stiles, C.D.,** Expression of the c-*fos* gene and of a *fos*-related gene is stimulated by platelet-derived growth factor, *Science,* 226, 1080, 1984.
259. **Kruijer, W., Cooper, J.A., Hunter, T., and Verma, I.M.,** Platelet-derived growth factor induces rapid but transient expression of the c-*fos* gene and protein, *Nature,* 312, 711, 1984.
260. **Bravo, R., Neuberg, M., Burckhardt, J., Almendral, J., Wallich, R., and Müller, R.,** Involvement of common and cell type-specific pathways in c-*fos* gene control: stable induction by cAMP in macrophages, *Cell,* 48, 251, 1987.
261. **Cheung, H.S., Mitchell, P.G., and Pledger, W.J.,** Induction of expressions of c-*fos* and c-*myc* protooncogenes by basic calcium phosphate crystal: effect of β-interferon, *Cancer Res.,* 49, 134, 1989.
262. **Diliberto, P.A., Bernacki, S.H., and Herman, B.,** Interrelationships of platelet-derived growth factor isoform-induced changes in c-*fos* expression, intracellular free calcium, and mitogenesis, *J. Cell. Biochem.,* 44, 39, 1990.
263. **Nishimura, J., Kobayashi, S., Shikasho, T., and Kanaide, H.,** Platelet derived growth factor induces c-*fos* and c-*myc* mRNA in rat aortic smooth muscle cells in primary culture without elevation of intracellular Ca^{2+} concentration, *Biochem. Biophys. Res. Commun.,* 188, 1198, 1992.
264. **Kacich, R.L., Williams, L.T., and Coughlin, S.R.,** Arachidonic acid and cyclic adenosine monophosphate stimulation of c-*fos* expression by a pathway independent of phorbol ester-sensitive protein kinase C, *Mol. Endocrinol.,* 2, 73, 1988.
265. **Jackson, J.A., Holt, J.T., and Pledger, W.J.,** Platelet-derived growth factor regulation of Fos stability correlates with growth induction, *J. Biol. Chem.,* 267, 17444, 1992.
266. **Lin, A.H., Groppi, V.E., and Gorman, R.R.,** Platelet-derived growth factor does not induce c-*fos* in NIH 3T3 cells expressing the EJ-*ras* oncogene, *Mol. Cell. Biol.,* 8, 5052, 1988.
267. **Sharma, R.V. and Bhalla, R.C.,** PDGF-induced mitogenic signaling is not mediated through protein kinase C and c-*fos* pathway in VSM cells, *Am. J. Physiol.,* 264, C71, 1993.
268. **Kelly, K., Cochran, B.H., Stiles, C.D., and Leder, P.,** Cell-specific regulation of the c-*myc* gene by lymphocyte mitogens and platelet-derived growth factor, *Cell,* 35, 603, 1983.
269. **Armelin, H.A., Armelin, M.C.S., Kelly, K., Stewart, T., Leder, P., Cochran, B.H., and Stiles, C.D.,** Functional role for c-*myc* in mitogenic response to platelet-derived growth factor, *Nature,* 310, 655, 1984.
270. **Letterio, J.J., Coughlin, S.R., and Williams, L.T.,** Pertussis toxin-sensitive pathway in the stimulation of c-*myc* expression and DNA synthesis by bombesin, *Science,* 234, 1117, 1986.
271. **Womer, R.B., Frick, K., Mitchell, C.D., Ross, A.H., Bishayee, S., and Scher, C.D.,** PDGF induces c-*myc* mRNA expression in MG-63 human osteosarcoma cells but does not stimulate cell replication, *J. Cell. Physiol.,* 132, 65, 1987.
272. **Kelly, K. and Siebenlist, U.,** The role of c-myc in the proliferation of normal and neoplastic cells, *J. Immunol.,* 5, 65, 1985.

273. Greenberg, M.E., Hermanowski, A.L., and Ziff, E.B., Effect of protein synthesis inhibitors on growth factor activation of c-*fos*, c-*myc*, and actin gene transcription, *Mol. Cell. Biol.*, 6, 1050, 1986.
274. Müller, R., Bravo, R., Burckhardt, J., and Curran, T., Induction of c-*fos* gene and protein by growth factors precedes activation of c-*myc*, *Nature*, 312, 716, 1984.
275. Sacca, R. and Cochran, B.H., Identification of a PDGF-responsive element in the murine c-*myc* gene, *Oncogene*, 5, 1499, 1991.
276. McCaffrey, P.G. and Rosner, M.R., Growth state-dependent regulation of protein kinase C in normal and transformed murine cells, *Cancer Res.*, 47, 1081, 1987.
277. Coughlin, S.R., Lee, W.M.F., Williams, P.W., Giels, G.M., and Williams, L.T., The c-*myc* gene expression is stimulated by agents that activate protein kinase C and does not account for the mitogenic action of PDGF, *Cell*, 43, 243, 1985.
278. Frick, K.K., Womer, R.B., and Scher, C.D., Platelet-derived growth factor-induced c-*myc* RNA expression. Analysis of an inducible pathway independent of protein kinase C, *J. Biol. Chem.*, 263, 2948, 1988.
279. Kaczmarek, L, Hyland, J.K., Watt, R., Rosenberg, M., and Baserga, R., Microinjected c-*myc* as a competence factor, *Science*, 228, 1313, 1985.
280. Ralston, R. and Bishop, J.M., The product of the proto-oncogene c-*src* is modified during the cellular response to platelet-derived growth factor, *Proc. Natl. Acad. Sci. U.S.A.*, 82, 7845, 1985.
281. Tamura, T., Friis, R.R., and Bauer, H., pp60$^{c\text{-}src}$ is a substrate for phosphorylation when cells are stimulated to enter cycle, *FEBS Lett.*, 177, 151, 1984.
282. Gould, K.L. and Hunter, T., Platelet-derived growth factor induces multisite phosphorylation of pp60$^{c\text{-}src}$ and increases its protein-tyrosine kinase activity, *Mol. Cell. Biol.*, 8, 3345, 1988.
283. Morrison, D.K., Kaplan, D.R., Escobedo, J.A., Rapp, U.R., Roberts, T.M., and Williams, L.T., Direct activation of the serine/threonine kinase activity of Raf-1 through tyrosine phosphorylation by the PDGF β-receptor, *Cell*, 58, 649, 1989.
284. Westermark, B. and Heldin, C.-H., Similar action of platelet-derived growth factor and epidermal growth factor in the prereplicative phase of human fibroblasts suggests a common intracellular pathway, *J. Cell Physiol.*, 124, 43, 1985.
285. Rozengurt, E., Stroobant, P., Waterfield, M.D., Deuel, T.F., and Keehan, M., Platelet-derived growth factor elicits cyclic AMP accumulation in Swiss 3T3 cells: role of prostaglandin production, *Cell*, 34, 265, 1983.
286. Thyberg, J. and Fredholm, B.B., Modulation of arterial smooth muscle cells from contractile to synthetic phenotype requires induction of ornithine decarboxylase activity and polyamine synthesis, *Exp. Cell Res.*, 170, 153, 1987.
287. Thyberg, J. and Fredholm, B.B., Induction of ornithine decarboxylase activity and putrescine synthesis in arterial smooth muscle cells stimulated with platelet-derived growth factor, *Exp. Cell Res.*, 170, 160, 1987.
288. Olashaw, N.E. and Pledger, W.J., Association of platelet-derived growth factor-induced protein with nuclear material, *Nature*, 306, 272, 1983.
289. Sorrentino, V., Drozdoff, V., McKinney, M.D., Zeitz, L., and Fleissner, E., Potentiation of growth factor activity by exogenous c-*myc* expression, *Proc. Natl. Acad. Sci. U.S.A.*, 83, 8167, 1986.
290. Bravo, R., Burckhardt, J., and Müller, R., Persistence of the competent state in mouse fibroblasts is independent of c-*fos* and c-*myc* expression, *Exp. Cell Res.*, 160, 540, 1985.
291. Soma, Y. and Grotendorst, G.R., TGF-β stimulates primary human skin fibroblast DNA synthesis via an autocrine production of PDGF-related peptides, *J. Cell. Physiol.*, 140, 246, 1989.
292. Battegay, E.J., Raines, E.W., Seifert, R.A., Bowen-Pope, D.F., and Ross, R., TGF-β induces bimodal proliferation of connective tissue cells via complex control of an autocrine PDGF loop, *Cell*, 63, 515, 1990.
293. Raines, E.W., Dower, S.K., and Ross, R., Interleukin-1 mitogenic activity for fibroblasts and smooth muscle cells is due to PDGF-AA, *Science*, 243, 393, 1989.
294. Scher, C.D., Pledger, W.J., Martin, P., Antoniades, H.N., and Stiles, C.D., Transforming viruses directly reduce the cellular growth requirement for a platelet-derived growth factor, *J. Cell Physiol.*, 97, 371, 1978.
295. Waterfield, M.D., Scrace, G.T., Whittle, N., Stroobant, P., Johnsson, A., Wasteson, Å., Westermark, B., Heldin, C.-H., Huang, J.S., and Deuel, T.F., Platelet-derived growth factor is structurally related to the putative transforming protein p28^{sis} of simian sarcoma virus, *Nature*, 304, 35, 1983.

296. Doolittle, R.F., Hunkapiller, M.W., Hood, L.E., Devare, S.G., Robbins, K.C., Aaronson, S.A., and Antoniades, H.N., Simian sarcoma *onc* gene, v-*sis*, is derived from the gene (or genes) encoding a platelet-derived growth factor, *Science,* 221, 275, 1983.
297. Deuel, T.F., Huang, J.S., Huang, S.S., Stroobant, P., and Waterfield, M.D., Expression of a platelet-derived growth factor-like protein in simian sarcoma virus transformed cells, *Science,* 221, 1348, 1983.
298. Robbins, K.C., Antoniades, H.N., Devare, S.G., Hunkapiller, M.W., and Aaronson, S.A., Structural and immunological similarities between simian sarcoma virus gene product(s) and human platelet-derived growth factor, *Nature,* 305, 605, 1983.
299. Niman, H.L., Antisera to a synthetic peptide of the *sis* viral oncogene product recognize human platelet-derived growth factor, *Nature,* 307, 180, 1984.
300. Thiel, H.-J. and Hafenrichter, R., Simian sarcoma virus transformation-specific glycopeptide: immunological relationship to human platelet-derived growth factor, *Virology,* 136, 414, 1984.
301. Owen, A.J., Pantazis, P., and Antoniades, H.N., Simian sarcoma virus-transformed cells secrete a mitogen identical to platelet-derived growth factor, *Science,* 225, 54, 1984.
302. Johnsson, A., Betsholtz, C., von der Helm, K., Heldin, C.-H., and Westermark, B., Platelet-derived growth factor agonist activity of a secreted form of the v-*sis* oncogene product, *Proc. Natl. Acad. Sci. U.S.A.,* 82, 1721, 1985.
303. Garrett, J.S., Coughlin, S.R., Niman, H.L., Tremble, P.M., Giels, G.M., and Williams, L.T., Blockade of autocrine stimulation in simian sarcoma virus-transformed cells reverses down-regulation of platelet-derived growth factor receptors, *Proc. Natl. Acad. Sci. U.S.A.,* 81, 7466, 1984.
304. Johnsson, A., Betsholtz, C., Heldin, C.-H., and Westermark, B., Antibodies against platelet-derived growth factor inhibit acute transformation by simian sarcoma virus, *Nature,* 317, 438, 1985.
305. Johnsson, A., Betsholtz, C., Heldin, C.-H., and Westermark, B., The phenotypic characteristics of simian sarcoma virus-transformed human fibroblasts suggest that the v-*sis* gene product acts solely as a PDGF receptor agonist in cell transformation, *EMBO J.,* 5, 1535, 1986.
306. Bejcek, B.E., Hoffman, R.M., Lipps, D., Li, D.Y., Mitchell, C.A., Majerus, P.W., and Deuel, T.F., The v-*sis* oncogene product but not platelet-derived growth factor (PDGF) A homodimers activate PDGF α and β receptors intracellularly and initiate cellular transformation, *J. Biol. Chem.,* 267, 3289, 1992.
307. King, C.R., Giese, N.A., Robbins, K.C., and Aaronson, S.A., *In vitro* mutagenesis of the v-*sis* transforming gene defines functional domains of its growth factor-related product, *Proc. Natl. Acad. Sci. U.S.A.,* 82, 5295, 1985.
308. Hannink, M., Sauer, M.K., and Donoghue, D.J., Deletions in the C-terminal coding region of the v-*sis* gene: dimerization is required for transformation, *Mol. Cell. Biol.,* 6, 1304, 1986.
309. Hannink, M. and Donoghue, D.J., Biosynthesis of the v-*sis* gene product: signal sequence cleavage, glycosylation, and proteolytic processing, *Mol. Cell. Biol.,* 6, 1343, 1986.
310. Robson, B., Platt, E., Finn, P.W., Millard, P., Gibrat, J.-F., and Garnier, J., Predictions of the conformation and antigenic determinants of the v-sis viral oncogene product homologous with human platelet-derived growth factor, *Int. J. Peptide Protein Res.,* 25, 1, 1985.
311. Devare, S.G., Shatzman, A., Robbins, K.C., Rosenberg, M., and Aaronson, S.A., Expression of the PDGF-related transforming protein of simian sarcoma virus in *E. coli, Cell,* 36, 43, 1984.
312. Kennett, R.H., Leunk, R., Meyer, B., and Silenzio, V., Detection of *E. coli* colonies expressing the v-sis oncogene product with monoclonal antibodies made against synthetic peptides, *J. Immunol. Methods,* 85, 169, 1985.
313. Wang, J.Y.J. and Williams, L.T., A v-*sis* oncogene protein produced in bacteria competes for platelet-derived growth factor binding to its receptor, *J. Biol. Chem.,* 259, 10645, 1984.
314. Huang, J.S., Huang, S.S., and Deuel, T.F., Transforming protein of simian sarcoma virus stimulates autocrine growth of SSV-transformed cells through PDGF cell-surface receptors, *Cell,* 39, 79, 1984.
315. Deuel, T.F. and Huang, J.S., Roles of growth factor activities in oncogenesis, *Blood,* 64, 951, 1984.
316. Leal, F., Williams, L.T., Robbins, K.C., and Aaronson, S.A., Evidence that the v-*sis* gene product transforms by interaction with the receptor for platelet-derived growth factor, *Science,* 230, 327, 1985.
317. Ratner, L., Josephs, S.F., Jarrett, R., Reitz, M.S., Jr., and Wong-Staal, F., Nucleotide sequence of transforming human c-*sis* cDNA clones with homology to platelet-derived growth factor, *Nucleic Acids Res.,* 13, 5007, 1985.

318. Rao, C.D., Igarashi, H., Chiu, I.-M., Robbins, K.C., and Aaronson, S.A., Structure and sequence of the human c-*sis*/platelet-derived growth factor 2 *(SIS/PDGF2)* transcriptional unit, *Proc. Natl. Acad. Sci. U.S.A.,* 83, 2392, 1986.
319. Van den Ouweland, A.M.W., Van Groningen, J.J.M., Schalken, J.A., Van Neck, H.W., Bloemers, H.P.J., and Van de Ven, W.J.M., Genetic organization of the c-*sis* transcription unit, *Nucleic Acids Res.,* 15, 959, 1987.
320. Van den Ouweland, A.M.W., Van Groningen, J.J.M., Hendricksen, P.J.M., Bloemers, H.P.J., and Van de Ven, W.J.M., Nucleotide sequence of the DNA region immediately upstream of the human c-*sis* proto-oncogene, *Nucleic Acids Res.,* 15, 4349, 1987.
321. Josephs, S.F., Guo, C., Ratner, L., and Wong-Staal, F., Human proto-oncogene nucleotide sequences corresponding to the transforming region of simian sarcoma virus, *Science,* 223, 487, 1984.
322. van den Ouweland, A.M.W., Breuer, M.L., Steenbergh, P.H., Schalken, J.A., Bloemers, H.P.J., and Van de Ven, W.J.M., Comparative analysis of the human and feline c-*sis* proto-oncogenes. Identification of 5′ human c-*sis* coding sequences that are not homologous to the transforming gene of simian sarcoma virus, *Biochim. Biophys. Acta,* 825, 140, 1985.
323. Van den Ouweland, A.M.W., Roebroek, A.J.M., Schalken, J.A., Claesen, C.A.A., Bloemers, H.P.J., and Van de Ven, W.J.M., Structure and nucleotide sequence of the 5′ region of the human and feline c-*sis* proto-oncogenes, *Nucleic Acids Res.,* 14, 765, 1986.
324. Eva, A., Robbins, K.C., Andersen, P.R., Srinivasan, A., Tronick, S.R., Reddy, E.P., Ellmore, N.W., Galen, A.T., Lautenberger, J.A., Papas, T.S., Westin, E.H., Wong-Staal, F., Gallo, R.C., and Aaronson, S.A., Cellular genes analogous to retroviral *onc* genes are transcribed in human tumour cells, *Nature,* 295, 116, 1982.
325. Goustin, A.S., Betsholtz, C., Pfeifer-Ohlsson, S., Persson, H., Rydnert, J., Bywater, M., Holmgren, G., Heldin, C.-H., Westermark B., and Ohlsson, R., Coexpression of the *sis* and *myc* proto-oncogenes in developing human placenta suggests autocrine control of trophoblast growth, *Cell,* 41, 301, 1985.
326. Barrett, T.B., Gajdusek, C.M., Schwartz, S.M., McDougall, J.K., and Benditt, E.P., Expression of the *sis* gene by endothelial cells in culture and *in vivo, Proc. Natl. Acad. Sci. U.S.A.,* 81, 6772, 1984.
327. Pierce, G.F., Mustoe, T.A., Senior, R.M., Reed, J., Griffin, G.L., Thomason, A., and Deuel, T.F., In vivo incisional wound healing augmented by platelet-derived growth factor and recombinant c-*sis* gene homodimeric proteins, *J. Exp. Med.,* 167, 974, 1988.
328. Hannink, M. and Donoghue, D.J., Requirement for a signal sequence in biological expression of the v-*sis* oncogene, *Science,* 226, 1197, 1984.
329. Robbins, K.C., Leal, F., Pierce, J.H., and Aaronson, S.A., The v-*sis*/PDGF-2 transforming gene product localizes to cell membranes but is not a secretory protein, *EMBO J.,* 4, 1783, 1985.
330. Bejcek, B.E., Li, D.Y., and Deuel, T.F., Transformation by v-*sis* occurs by an internal autoactivation mechanism, *Science,* 245, 1496, 1989.
331. Fleming, T.P., Matsui, T., Molloy, C.J., Robbins, K.C., and Aaronson, S.A., Autocrine mechanism for v-*sis* transformation requires cell surface localization of internally activated growth factor receptors, *Proc. Natl. Acad. Sci. U.S.A.,* 86, 8063, 1989.
332. Josephs, S.F., Ratner, L., Clarke, M.F., Westin, E.H., Reitz, M.S., and Wong-Staal, F., Transforming potential of human c-*sis* nucleotide sequences encoding platelet-derived growth factor, *Science,* 225, 636, 1984.
333. Gazit, A., Igarashi, H., Chiu, I.-M., Srinivasan, A., Yaniv, A., Tronick, S.R., Robbins, K.C., and Aaronson, S.A., Expression of the normal human *sis*/PDGF-2 coding sequence induces cellular transformation, *Cell,* 39, 89, 1984.
334. Pantazis, P., Sariban, E., Kufe, D., and Antoniades, H.N., Induction of c-*sis* gene expression and synthesis of platelet-derived growth factor in human myeloid leukemia cells during monocytic differentiation, *Proc. Natl. Acad. Sci. U.S.A.,* 83, 6455, 1986.
335. Wang, J.Y.J., Isolation of antibodies for phosphotyrosine by immunization with a v-*abl* oncogene-encoded protein, *Mol. Cell. Biol.,* 5, 3640, 1985.
336. Huang, S.S. and Huang, J.S., Rapid turnover of the platelet-derived growth factor receptor in *sis*-transformed cells and reversal by suramin. Implications for the mechanism of autocrine transformation, *J. Biol. Chem.,* 263, 12608, 1988.

337. **Fry, D.G., Milam, L.D., Maher, V.M., and McCormick, J.J.,** Transformation of diploid human fibroblasts by DNA transfection with the v-*sis* oncogene, *J. Cell. Physiol.,* 128, 313, 1986.
338. **Heldin, C.-H. and Westermark, B.,** Platelet-derived growth factor and autocrine mechanisms of oncogenic processes, *Crit. Rev. Oncogenesis,* 2, 109, 1991.
339. **Westermark, B. and Heldin, C.-H.,** Platelet-derived growth factor in autocrine transformation, *Cancer Res.,* 51, 5087, 1991.
340. **Silver, B.J.,** Platelet-derived growth factor in human malignancy, *Biofactors,* 3, 217, 1992.
341. **Mordan, L.J.,** Induction by growth factors from platelets of the focus-forming transformed phenotype in carcinogen-treated C3H/10T1/2 fibroblasts, *Carcinogenesis,* 9, 1129, 1988.
342. **Keating, M.T. and Williams, L.T.,** Autocrine stimulation of intracellular PDGF receptors in v-*sis*-transformed cells, *Science,* 239, 914, 1988.
343. **Palmer, H., Maher, V.M., and McCormick, J.J.,** Platelet-derived growth factor or basic fibroblast growth factor induce anchorage-independent growth of human fibroblasts, *J. Cell. Physiol.,* 137, 588, 1988.
344. **Lafyatis, R., Remmers, E.F., Roberts, A.B., Yocum, D.E., Sporn, M.B., and Wilder, R.L.,** Anchorage-independent growth of synoviocytes from arthritic and normal joints. Stimulation by exogenous platelet-derived growth factor and inhibition by transforming growth factor-β and retinoids, *J. Clin. Invest.,* 83, 1267, 1989.
345. **Stevens, C.W., Brondyk, W.H., Burgess, J.A., Manoharan, T.H., Häne, B.G., and Fahl, W.E.,** Partially transformed, anchorage-independent human diploid fibroblasts result from overexpression of the c-*sis* oncogene: mitogenic activity of an apparent monomeric platelet-derived growth factor 2 species, *Mol. Cell. Biol.,* 8, 2089, 1988.
346. **Fry, D.G., Hurlin, P.J., Maher, V.M., and McCormick, J.J.,** Transformation of diploid human fibroblasts by transfection with the v-*sis, PDGF2/c-sis,* or T24 H-*ras* genes, *Mutat. Res.,* 199, 341, 1988.
347. **Heldin, N.E., Cvejic, D., Smeds, S., and Westermark, B.,** Coexpression of functionally active receptors for thyrotropin and platelet-derived growth factor in human thyroid carcinoma cells, *Endocrinology,* 129, 2187, 1991.
348. **Katz, F.E., Michalevicz, R., Lam, G., Hoffbrand, A., and Goldman, J.M.,** Effect of platelet-derived growth factor on enriched populations of haemopoietic progenitors from patients with chronic myeloid leukaemia, *Leukemia Res.,* 11, 339, 1987.
349. **Peres, R., Betsholtz, C., Westermark, B., and Heldin, C.-H.,** Frequent expression of growth factors for mesenchymal cells in human mammary carcinoma cell lines, *Cancer Res.,* 47, 3425, 1987.
350. **Nilsson, J.,** Growth factors and the pathogenesis of atherosclerosis, *Atherosclerosis,* 62, 185, 1986.
351. **Tsubura, E., Yamashita, T., and Sone, S.,** Inhibition of the arrest of hematogeneously disseminated tumor cells, *Cancer Metast. Rev.,* 2, 223, 1983.
352. **Nistér, M., Heldin, C.-H., Wasteson, Å., and Westermark, B.,** A glioma-derived analog to platelet-derived growth factor: demonstration of receptor competing activity and immunological cross reactivity, *Proc. Natl. Acad. Sci. U.S.A.,* 81, 926, 1984.
353. **Rizzino, A., Ruff, E., and Rizzino, H.,** Induction and modulation of anchorage-independent growth by platelet-derived growth factor, fibroblast growth factor, and transforming growth factor-β, *Cancer Res.,* 46, 2816, 1986.
354. **Assoian, R.K., Grotendorst, G.R., Miller, D.M., and Sporn, M.B.,** Cellular transformation by coordinated action of three peptide growth factors from human platelets, *Nature,* 309, 804, 1984.
355. **Leof, E.B., Proper, J.A., Goustin, A.S., Shipley, G.D., DiCorleto, P.E., and Moses, H.L.,** Induction of c-sis mRNA and activity similar to platelet-derived growth factor by transforming growth factor β: a proposed model for indirect mitogenesis involving autocrine activity, *Proc. Natl. Acad. Sci. U.S.A.,* 83, 2453, 1986.
356. **Powers, S., Fisher, P.B., and Pollack, R.,** Analysis of the reduced growth factor dependency of simian virus 40-transformed 3T3 cells, *Mol. Cell. Biol.,* 4, 1572, 1984.
357. **Gerwin, B.I., Lechner, J.F., Reddel, R.R., Roberts, A.B., Robbins, K.C., Gabrielson, E.W., and Harris, C.C.,** Comparison of production of transforming growth factor-β and platelet-derived growth factor by normal human mesothelial cells and mesothelioma cell lines, *Cancer Res.,* 47, 6180, 1987.
358. **Versnel, M.A., Hagemeijer, A., Bouts, M.J., van der Kwast, T.H., and Hoogsteden, H.C.,** Expression of c-*sis* (PDGF B-chain) and PDGF A-chain genes in ten human malignant mesothelioma cell lines derived from primary and metastatic tumors, *Oncogene,* 2, 601, 1988.

359. Tsai, T.-F., Yauk, Y.-K., Chou, C.-K., Ting, L.-P., Chang, C., Hu, C., Han, S.-H., and Su, T.-S., Evidence of autocrine regulation in human hepatoma cell lines, *Biochem. Biophys. Res. Commun.*, 153, 39, 1988.
360. Rozengurt, E., Sinnett-Smith, J., and Taylor-Papadimitriou, J., Production of PDGF-like growth factor by breast cancer cell lines, *Int. J. Cancer*, 36, 247, 1985.
361. Pichon, F. and Lagarde, A.E., Autoregulation of MeWo metastatic melanoma cell growth: characterization of intracellular (FGF, MGSA) and secreted (PDGF) growth factors, *J. Cell. Physiol.*, 140, 344, 1989.
362. Sariban, E., Sitaras, N.M., Antoniades, H.N., Kufe, D.W., and Pantazis, P., Expression of platelet-derived growth factor (PDGF)-related transcripts and synthesis of biologically active PDGF-like proteins by human malignant epithelial cell lines, *J. Clin. Invest.*, 82, 1157, 1988.
363. Westermark, B., Johnsson, A., Paulsson, Y., Betsholtz, C., Heldin, C.-H., Herlyn, M., Rodeck, U., and Koprowski, H., Human melanoma cell lines of primary and metastatic origin express the genes encoding the chains of platelet-derived growth factor (PDGF) and produce a PDGF-like growth factor, *Proc. Natl. Acad. Sci. U.S.A.*, 83, 7197, 1986.
364. Alitalo, R., Andersson, L.C., Betsholtz, C., Nilsson, K., Westermark, B., Heldin, C.-H., and Alitalo, K., Induction of platelet-derived growth factor gene expression during megakaryoblastic and monocytic differentiation of human leukemia cell lines, *EMBO J.*, 6, 1213, 1987.
365. Mäkelä, T.P., Alitalo, R., Paulsson, Y., Westermar, B., Heldin, C.-H., and Alitalo, K., Regulation of platelet-derived growth factor gene expression by transforming growth factor β and phorbol ester in human leukemia cell lines, *Mol. Cell. Biol.*, 7, 3656, 1987.
366. Weich, H.A., Herbst, D., Schairer, H.U., and Hoppe, J., Platelet-derived growth factor. Phorbol ester induces the expression of the B-chain but not of the A-chain in HEL cells, *FEBS Lett.*, 213, 89, 1987.
367. Heldin, C.H., Westermark, B., and Wasteson, Å., Chemical and biological properties of a growth factor from human cultured osteosarcoma cells, resembling PDGF, *J. Cell Physiol.*, 105, 235, 1980.
368. Graves, D.T., Owen, A.J., and Antoniades, H.N., Evidence that a human osteosarcoma cell line secretes a mitogen similar to platelet-derived growth factors present in platelet-poor plasma, *Cancer Res.*, 43, 83, 1983.
369. Graves, D.T., Owen, A.J., Williams, S.R., and Antoniades, H.N., Identification of processing events in the synthesis of platelet-derived growth factor-like proteins by human osteosarcoma cells, *Proc. Natl. Acad. Sci. U.S.A.*, 83, 4636, 1986.
370. Graves, D.T. and Antoniades, H.N., Characterization of a high-molecular-weight protein immunoprecipitated by platelet-derived growth factor antisera, *J. Cell. Physiol.*, 137, 263, 1988.
371. Sporn, M.B. and Todaro, G.J., Autocrine secretion and malignant transformation of cells, *N. Engl. J. Med.*, 303, 878, 1980.
372. Graves, D.T., Owen, A.J., Barth, R.K., Tempst, P., Winoto, A., Fors, L., Hood, L.E., and Antoniades, H.N., Detection of c-sis transcripts and synthesis of PDGF-like proteins by human osteosarcoma cells, *Science*, 226, 972, 1984.
373. Betsholtz, C., Johnsson, A., Heldin, C.-H., and Westermark, B., Efficient reversion of simian sarcoma virus-transformation and inhibition of growth factor-induced mitogenesis by suramin, *Proc. Natl. Acad. Sci. U.S.A.*, 83, 6440, 1986.
374. Heldin, C.-H., Johnsson, A., Wennergren, S., Wernstedt, C., Betsholtz, C., and Westermark, B., A human osteosarcoma cell line secretes a growth factor structurally related to a homodimer of PDGF A-chains, *Nature*, 319, 511, 1986.
375. Weich, H.A., Sebald, W., Schairer, H.-U., and Hoppe, J., The human osteosarcoma cell line U-2 OS expresses a 3.8 kilobase mRNA which codes for the sequence of the PDGF-B chain, *FEBS Lett.*, 198, 344, 1986.
376. Richter, M.R. and Graves, D.T., DNA synthesis in U-2 OS human osteosarcoma cells is independent of PDGF binding to functional cell surface receptors, *J. Cell. Physiol.*, 135, 474, 1988.
377. Scher, C.D., Engle, L.J., Eberenz, W.M., Ganguly, K., and Wharton, W., Dissociation of cellular transformation from platelet-derived growth factor independence, *J. Cell. Physiol.*, 126, 333, 1986.
378. Nistér, M., Libermann, T.A., Betsholtz, C., Petersson, M., Claesson-Welsh, L., Heldin, C.-H., Schessinger, J., and Westermark, B., Expression of messenger RNAs for platelet-derived growth factor and transforming growth factor-α and their receptors in malignant glioma cell lines, *Cancer Res.*, 48, 3910, 1988.

379. **Press, R.D., Samols, D., and Goldthwait, D.A.,** Expression and stability of c-sis mRNA in human glioblastoma cells, *Biochemistry,* 27, 5736, 1988.
380. **Nistér, M., Wedell, B., Betsholtz, C., Bywater, M., Pettersson, M., Westermark, B., and Mark, J.,** Evidence for progressional changes in the human malignant glioma line U-343 MGa: analysis of karyotype and expression of genes encoding the subunit chains of platelet-derived growth factor, *Cancer Res.,* 47, 4953, 1987.
381. **Pantazis, P., Pelicci, P.G., Dalla-Favera, R., and Antoniades, H.N.,** Synthesis and secretion of proteins resembling platelet-derived growth factor by human glioblastoma and fibrosarcoma cells in culture, *Proc. Natl. Acad. Sci. U.S.A.,* 82, 2404, 1985.
382. **Press, R.D., Misra, A., Gillaspy, G., Samols, D., and Goldthwait, D.A.,** Control of the expression of c-*sis* mRNA in human glioblastoma cells by phorbol ester and transforming growth factor β, *Cancer Res.,* 49, 2914, 1989.
383. **van Zoelen, E.J.J., van de Ven, W.J.M., Franssen, H.J., van Oostwaard, T.M.J., van der Saag, P.T., Heldin, C.-H., and de Laat, S.W.,** Neuroblastoma cells express c-*sis* and produce a transforming growth factor antigenically related to the platelet-derived growth factor, *Mol. Cell. Biol.,* 5, 2289, 1985.
384. **van Zoelen, E.J.J., van Oostward, T.M.J., and de Laat, S.W.,** PDGF-like growth factor induces EGF-potentiated phenotypic transformation of normal rat kidney cells in the absence of TGF β, *Biochem. Biophys. Res. Commun.,* 141, 1229, 1986.
385. **Hermansson, M., Nistér, M., Betsholtz, C., Heldin, C.-H., Westermark, B., and Funa, K.,** Endothelial cell hyperplasia in human glioblastoma: coexpression of mRNA for platelet-derived growth factor (PDGF) B chain and PDGF receptor suggests autocrine growth stimulation, *Proc. Natl. Acad. Sci. U.S.A.,* 85, 7748, 1988.
386. **Fleming, T.P., Saxena, A., Clark, W.C., Robertson, J.T., Oldfield, E.H., Aaronson, S.A., and Ali, I.U.,** Amplification and/or overexpression of platelet-derived growth factor receptors and epidermal growth factor receptor in human glial tumors, *Cancer Res.,* 52, 4550, 1992.
387. **Maxwell, M., Galanopoulos, T., Hedley-Whyte, E.T., Black, P. McL., and Antoniades, H.N.,** Human meningiomas co-express platelet-derived growth factor (PDGF) and PDGF-receptor genes and their protein products, *Int. J. Cancer,* 46, 16, 1990.
388. **Wang, J.-L., Nistér, M., Hermansson, M., Westermark, B., and Pontén, J.,** Expression of PDGF β-receptor in human meningioma cells, *Int. J. Cancer,* 46, 772, 1990.
389. **Adams, E.F., Todo, T., Schrell, U.M.H., Thierauf, P., White, M.C., and Fahlbusch, R.,** Autocrine control of human meningioma proliferation. Secretion of platelet-derived growth factor-like molecules, *Int. J. Cancer,* 49, 398, 1991.
390. **Lens, P.F., Altena, B., and Nusse, R.,** Expression of c-*sis* and platelet-derived growth factor in in vitro-transformed glioma cells from rat brain tissue transplacentally treated with ethylnitrosourea, *Mol. Cell. Biol.,* 6, 3537, 1986.
391. **Bronzert, D.A., Pantazis, P., Antoniades, H.N., Kasid, A., Davidson, N., Dickson, R.B., and Lippman, M.E.,** Synthesis and secretion of platelet-derived growth factor by human breast cancer cell lines, *Proc. Natl. Acad. Sci. U.S.A.,* 84, 5763, 1987.
392. **Söderdahl, G., Betsholtz, C., Johansson, A., Nilsson, K., and Bergh, J.,** Differential expression of platelet-derived growth factor and transforming growth factor genes in small- and non-small-cell human lung carcinoma cells, *Int. J. Cancer,* 41, 636, 1988.
393. **Antoniades, H.H., Galanopoulos, T., Neville-Golden, J., and O'Hara, C.J.,** Malignant epithelial cells in primary human lung carcinomas coexpress *in vivo* platelet-derived growth factor (PDGF) and PDGF receptor RNAs and their protein products, *Proc. Natl. Acad. Sci. U.S.A.,* 89, 3942, 1992.
394. **Bergh, J.,** The expression of the platelet-derived and transforming growth factor genes in human nonsmall lung cancer cell lines is related to tumor stroma formation in nude mice tumors, *Am. J. Pathol.,* 133, 434, 1988.
395. **Tsuda, T., Yoshida, K., Tsujino, T., Nakayama, H., Kajiyama, G., and Tahara, E.,** Coexpression of platelet-derived growth factor (PDGF) A-chain and PDGF receptor genes in human gastric carcinomas, *Jpn. J. Cancer Res.,* 80, 813, 1989.
396. **Chung, C.K. and Antoniades, H.N.,** Expression of c-*sis*/platelet-derived growth factor B, insulin-like growth factor I, and transforming growth factor α messenger RNAs and their respective receptor messenger RNAs in primary human gastric carcinomas: *in vivo* studies with *in situ* hybridization and immunocytochemistry, *Cancer Res.,* 52, 3454, 1992.

397. **Werner, S., Hofschneider, P.H., Heldin, C.-H., Östman, A., and Roth, W.K.,** Cultured Kaposi's sarcoma-derived cells express functional PDGF A-type and B-type receptors, *Exp. Cell Res.,* 187, 98, 1990.
398. **Sturzl, M., Roth, W.K., Brockmeyer, N.H., Zietz, C., Speiser, B., and Hofschneider, P.H.,** Expression of platelet-derived growth factor and its receptor in AIDS-related Kaposi sarcoma in vivo suggests paracrine and autocrine mechanisms of tumor maintenance, *Proc. Natl. Acad. Sci. U.S.A.,* 89, 7046, 1992.
399. **Weima, S.M., van Rooijen, M.A., Mummery, C.L, Feyen, A., de Laat, S.W., and van Zoelen, E.J.J.,** Identification of the type-β receptor for platelet-derived growth factor in human embryonal carcinoma cells, *Exp. Cell Res.,* 186, 324, 1990.
400. **Rizzino, A. and Bowen-Pope, D.F.,** Production of PDGF-like growth factors by embryonal carcinoma cells and binding of PDGF to their endoderm-like differentiated cells, *Develop. Biol.,* 110, 15, 1985.
401. **Grotendorst, G.R., Harvey, A.K., Nagarajan, L., Anderson, W.B., and Gatewood, E.,** Differentiation-dependent production of a platelet-derived growth factor-like mitoattractant by endoderm cells derived from embryonal carcinoma cells, *J. Cell. Physiol.,* 134, 437, 1988.
402. **Bleiberg, I., Harvey, A.K., Smale, G., and Grotendorst, G.R.,** Identification of a PDGF-like mitoattractant produced by NIH/3T3 cells after transformation with SV40, *J. Cell. Physiol.,* 123, 161, 1985.
403. **Bowen-Pope, D.F., Vogel, A., and Ross, R.,** Production of platelet-derived growth factor-like molecules and reduced expression of platelet-derived growth factor receptors accompany transformation by a wide spectrum of agents, *Cancer Res.,* 81, 2396, 1984.
404. **Pantazis, P., Sariban, E., Bohan, C.A., Antoniades, H.N., and Kalynaraman, V.S.,** Synthesis of PDGF by cultured human T cells transformed with HTLV-I and II, *Oncogene,* 1, 285, 1987.
405. **Mercola, D., Rundell, A., Westwick, J., and Edwards, S.A.,** Antisense RNA to the c-*fos* gene: restoration of density-dependent growth arrest in a transformed cell line, *Biochem. Biophys. Res. Commun.,* 147, 288, 1987.
406. **Durkin, J.P. and Whitfield, J.F.,** Evidence that the viral Ki-RAS protein, but not the pp60^{v-src} protein of ASV, stimulates proliferation through the PDGF receptor, *Biochem. Biophys. Res. Commun.,* 148, 376, 1987.
407. **Olinger, P.L., Benjamin, C.W., Gorman, R.R., and Connor, J.A.,** Cyclic AMP can partially restore platelet-derived growth factor-stimulated prostaglandin E$_2$ biosynthesis, and calcium mobilization in EJ-*ras*-transformed NIH-3T3 cells, *J. Cell. Physiol.,* 139, 335, 1989.
408. **Heldin, C.H., Wasteson, Å., and Westermark, B.,** Partial purification and characterization of platelet factors stimulating the multiplication of normal human glial cells, *Exp. Cell Res.,* 109, 429, 1977.
409. **Cowan, D.H. and Graham, J.,** Stimulation of human tumor colony formation by platelet lysate, *J. Lab. Clin. Med.,* 102, 973, 1983.
410. **Paul, D. and Piasecki, A.,** Rat platelets contain growth factor(s) distinct from PDGF which stimulate DNA synthesis in primary adult rat hepatocyte cultures, *Exp. Cell Res.,* 154, 95, 1984.
411. **Bauer, G., Birnbaum, U., Höfler, P., and Heldin, C.-H.,** EBV-inducing factor from platelets exhibits growth-promoting activity for NIH 3T3 cells, *EMBO J.,* 4, 1957, 1985.
412. **Miyazono, K. and Heldin, C.-H.,** High-yield purification of platelet-derived endothelial cell growth factor: structural characterization and establishment of a specific antiserum, *Biochemistry,* 28, 1704, 1989.
413. **Ciaglowski, R.E., Snow, J., and Walz, D.A.,** Isolation and amino acid sequence of bovine platelet factor 4, *Arch. Biochem. Biophys.,* 250, 249, 1986.
414. **Sipes, N.J., Meyskens, F.L., Jr., and Bregman, M.D.,** Biological characterization of an acid-sensitive growth factor from human platelets: role in the proliferation of human melanoma and bovine endothelial cells, *Biochem. Biophys. Res. Commun.,* 138, 795, 1986.
415. **Nakamura, T., Teramoto, H., Tomita, Y., and Ichihara, A.,** Two types of growth inhibitor in rat platelets for primary cultured rat hepatocytes, *Biochem. Biophys. Res. Commun.,* 134, 755, 1986.
416. **Ristow, H.-J.,** BSC-1 growth inhibitor/type β transforming growth factor is a strong inhibitor of thymocyte proliferation, *Proc. Natl. Acad. Sci. U.S.A.,* 83, 5531, 1986.

417. **Brown, M.T. and Clemmons, D.R.,** Platelets contain a peptide inhibitor of endothelial cell replication and growth, *Proc. Natl. Acad. Sci. U.S.A.,* 83, 3321, 1986.
418. **Lechner, J.F., McClendon, I.A., LaVeck, M.A., Shamsuddin, A.M., and Harris, C.C.,** Differential control by platelet factors of squamous differentiation in normal and malignant human bronchial epithelial cells, *Cancer Res.,* 43, 5915, 1983.

Chapter 8

Transferrins

I. INTRODUCTION

Iron is an essential element required for the synthesis of proteins including hemoglobin and myoglobin as well as enzymes such as the cytochromes and ribonucleotide reductase. The transferrins are a family of iron-binding proteins which carry ferric iron from the intestine, reticuloendothelial system, and liver parenchymal cells to all proliferating cells in the body.[1-3] The transferrin family includes serotransferrin (isolated from serum), ovotransferrin (from hen egg white), lactotransferrin (from human milk), and melanotransferrin (from melanocarcinoma cells). All members of the family are single-polypeptide-chain glycoproteins of approximately 80 kDa, and the amino acid sequences of different transferrins of human and nonhuman origin indicate a relatively high degree of structural homology.[4]

Transferrins are present in human serum and milk as well as in many embryonic and adult tissues.[5] Liver is the major source of serum transferrin but an identical molecule may be produced in other organs, including the testis and brain.[6] The synthesis of transferrin in different mammalian tissues depends on the interaction of specific nuclear proteins with enhancer DNA sequences contained in the transferrin gene.

Transferrin is synthesized in the chick oviduct and testis.[7] Ovotransferrin is the iron-binding protein found in avian egg white and is nearly identical to transferrin in its polypeptide structure, but both molecules differ in their carbohydrate moieties. Ovotransferrin is a substrate for protein kinase C-dependent phosphorylation *in vitro*.[8] The biological significance of this phosphorylation is unknown. Lactotransferrin is an iron-binding protein present in human exocrine secretions, including milk, and is also expressed in hematopoietic cells in late stages of granulocytic differentiation.[9] Transferrins are necessary components of almost all serum-free tissue culture media, acting as requisite factors. A growth-promoting factor for human myeloid leukemia cells purified to homogeneity from horse serum was identified as horse serum transferrin.[10]

Although transferrin-mediated iron delivery has generally been considered to be the only route for cellular iron accumulation, there is evidence indicating the existence of genes distinct from the transferrin gene that encode iron-binding proteins as well as transferrin-independent systems of iron uptake. A 56-kDa iron-binding protein, mobilferrin, which was identified in the duodenal mucosa of rats, participates in iron transport in the gut by some as yet unknown mechanism.[11] Studies performed on perfused rat liver and HeLa cells clearly demonstrated the operation of a transferrin-independent uptake system for iron.[12]

II. STRUCTURE AND SYNTHESIS OF TRANSFERRINS

All transferrins are glycoproteins composed of a single polypeptide chain of about 700 amino acid residues and with a molecular weight of approximately 80 kDa.[13] Each transferrin reversibly binds two iron ions (as Fe^{3+}), concomitantly with two carbonate or bicarbonate ions. X-ray diffraction studies provided accurate data about the composition and spatial conformation of the iron-binding sites of transferrin molecules. The characteristics of the carbohydrate moiety of transferrins are specific to each of them on the basis of the primary structure of glycans and/or their number, but there is an unexplainable microheterogeneity of the glycan moieties and no relationship can be established *a priori* between primary structure and function of transferrin glycans.[14] The relative proportions of transferrin carbohydrate variants are altered in the serum of pregnant women.[15] The members of the transferrin family are the result of evolutionary intragenic duplication followed by a series of independent gene duplications. Human and rat transferrins have been studied in detail.

A. HUMAN TRANSFERRIN

The major transferrin gene is located on human chromosome region 3q15-q25, and chromosome region 3q26.2 contains the gene for the transferrin cellular receptor.[16,17] The same region contains the gene for human melanoma-associated antigen p97.[18] The lactotransferrin gene is also located on human chromosome 3, in the region 3q21-qter.[19] Genes encoding members of the transferrin family, including transferrin, lactotransferrin, and p97 antigen, are products of an ancient intragenic duplication that occurred 300 to 500 million years ago, and the presence of these genes, as well as that of the transferrin receptor, on human chromosome 3q suggests that they have remained together since that time.

The complete nucleotide sequence of a cDNA derived from the human transferrin gene has been determined.[17] The human gene is composed of 2324 bp and contains a 19-residue leader sequence followed by the homologous amino-terminal and carboxy-terminal domains of the protein. During evolution three areas of the homologous domains have been strongly conserved, possibly reflecting functional constraints associated with iron binding. The transferrin gene contains at least 12 exons, ranging from 33 to 181 bp, separated by introns of 0.7- to 4.9-kbp.[20] The gene can be divided into two unequal parts corresponding to the known domains of the protein. The organization of the transferrin gene family can be easily explained on the basis of gene duplication during evolution. The 5' regulatory region of the transferrin gene is composed of multiple positive and negative cis-acting elements which interact with DNA-binding proteins.[21,22] The segment of the transferrin gene between −620 and −45 bp contains sequences that allow transcription regulation in a tissue-specific manner. Analysis of the expression of chimeric human transferrin genes in transgenic mice indicate that DNA sequences within a region between −152 and −622 bp of the 5'-flanking region of the gene contain direct liver and brain expression more than 1000-fold greater than in tissues such as the heart and kidney.[23] The sequence from −622 to +46 bp of the human transferrin gene is adequate for response to iron administration.

Amino acid sequence analysis demonstrated that the human transferrin polypeptide is composed of two homologous regions (residues 1–336 and 337–679), which is reflected in the presence of two discrete structural domains in the transferrin molecule.[24] Transferrin and albumin are both synthesized in the liver, but have marked differences in their secretion kinetics. Transferrin is a glycoprotein while albumin is not, and mammalian transferrin has a more complex tertiary structure and disulfide bond arrangement than does albumin. An adequate tertiary structure may be required for transferrin secretion, but the mechanisms responsible for the relatively delayed transferrin secretion are not understood.[25] A possibility is that some form of rate-limiting receptor-associated transfer mechanism may be involved in transferrin transport and release.

Altered transferrin molecules have been detected in cancer patients. Altered glycosylation of serum transferrin is commonly found in patients with hepatocellular carcinoma.[26] Tumor cells may produce transferrin-like molecules. A transferrin-related molecule of 41 kDa, which reacts with transferrin antibodies, is released by HL-60 human leukemia cells.[27] Physiological levels of iron salts completely abolish the requirement of exogenous transferrin, suggesting that the endogenous transferrin-related polypeptide(s), in the presence of iron salts, is sufficient for the growth of HL-60 cells provided insulin or related growth factors are present in the medium. The addition of transferrin receptor antibodies inhibits the stimulatory action of endogenous transferrin-related activity, indicating that this protein may act as an autocrine promotor of cell proliferation.

B. RAT TRANSFERRIN

The rat transferrin gene is transcribed into a single mRNA species of 2400 bp which is present at a high level in the liver and at a lower concentration in various other fetal and adult rat tissues.[5] In most extrahepatic rat tissues (lung, heart, spleen, kidney, and muscle) transferrin mRNA content increases progressively during fetal development and reaches a maximum between day 3 and 1 before birth, then drops quickly after birth and remains stable at a very low level during adult life. In the brain, however, the concentration of transferrin mRNA is very low during fetal life and then increases after birth to reach a maximum in the adult, where it remains constant at 1:10 of the value found in adult liver.[5] Transferrin mRNA is found in the rat testis by 5 days of age and reach maximum levels in the adult animal. The mRNA is little induced in rat Sertoli cells by treatment with gonadotropin (FSH), but a combined treatment of FSH, insulin, retinol, and testosterone results in a maximal level of induction.[28] The transcriptional activity of the transferrin gene may be transiently inhibited by cAMP.[29] Rat transferrin has been synthesized in *Escherichia coli* by means of a recombinant phage constructed from a cDNA library derived from rat liver mRNA.[30]

C. TRANSFERRINS AND THE B-Lym-1 PROTEIN

The putative proto-oncogene B-*lym*-1 of human and chicken encodes a protein showing structural homology to the amino terminus of transferrins.[31-34] The predicted amino acid sequence of the chicken B-Lym-1 protein exhibits 36% homology to sequences of proteins of the transferrin family. The human B-Lym-1 protein is composed of 58 amino acid residues, with 6 identities of 39 aligned from the amino-terminal region of the protein and 10 residues of the human B-Lym-1 proteins conserved in at least one of the sequences of the transferrin family.[20] These results suggest the existence of a common ancestry for the B-*lym*-1 gene and genes of the transferrin family. They also suggest that the B-Lym-1 protein may function via a pathway related to transferrin.

D. LACTOTRANSFERRIN

Lactotransferrin (lactoferrin) is an iron-binding protein of 80 kDa which is found in human exocrine secretions. The milk and other exocrine secretions of most mammals contain transferrin, lactotransferrin, or both. Milk transferrins are not derived from serum but are synthesized in the mammary gland. The synthesis and secretion of milk transferrins are regulated in pregnancy.[35] Prolactin can stimulate lactotransferrin secretion in explants of mammary tissue from midpregnancy mice.[36] Lactotransferrin is the major estrogen-inducible protein of mouse uterine secretions.[37,38] Estrogen regulates lactotransferrin synthesis and secretion in the uterus but not in the mammary gland, suggesting that regulation of lactotransferrin expression is tissue specific.[39] The factors involved in the regulation of lactotransferrin expression in other mouse tissues such as ovary, lung, kidney, and submaxillary glands are unknown. Lactotransferrin is expressed in hematopoietic cells in late granulocytic differentiation.[9] A cDNA clone coding for human neutrophil transferrin has been constructed.[40] Transferrin or lactotransferrin could be involved in downregulation of myelopoiesis,[41,42] but their possible function in this process *in vivo* remains controversial.[43] It was proposed that lactotransferrin is involved in a negative regulation of CSF production by macrophages, but other results suggest that lactotransferrin stimulates granulocyte production both *in vitro* and *in vivo*.[44]

Human myeloid cell populations containing cell precursors more mature than promyelocytes synthesize lactotransferrin mRNA.[40] Circulating leukocytes from CML patients contain lactotransferrin transcripts. In contrast, lactotransferrin transcripts are not detected in the peripheral white cells of chronic granulocytic leukemia during blast crisis, or in acute myeloblastic leukemia or acute promyelocytic leukemia cells. Lactotransferrin transcripts are absent in undifferentiated HL-60 and PLB-85 human myeloid leukemia cell lines. Chemically induced differentiation of these cell lines with DMSO, TPA, or dibutyryl cAMP fails to induce lactoferrin transcripts, which indicates that *in vitro* maturation of these neoplastic cells is defective.

E. MELANOTRANSFERRIN

Transferrin-like proteins are present in some tumors. A protein identified as the human melanoma surface antigen p97 is a member of the transferrin family.[45] Antigen p97, also called melanotransferrin, was detected in 90% of different human melanoma cell lines, but was also present in more than half of the cell lines established from a wide diversity of other human tumors.[46] Melanotransferrin was not detected in B-lymphoblastoid cell lines or in cultivated fibroblasts from human donors. The primary structure of the human melanoma-associated melanotransferrin has been deduced from the mRNA sequence.[47]

F. HORMONAL REGULATION OF TRANSFERRIN GENE EXPRESSION

The steroid-regulated expression of the transferrin gene was studied in intact chickens and transgenic mice.[48,49] In chickens, the transferrin gene is expressed in a highly specific manner in the liver and oviduct. Transcription of the transferrin gene is stimulated by estrogen in both tissues and by iron deficiency in the liver. Induction of the chicken transferrin gene expression by estrogen persists even in the transgenic mouse liver, which indicates that the elements responsible for the control of transferrin gene expression have been conserved between species that diverged more than 150 million years ago. Moreover, the estrogen induction of the transferrin gene is observed in different cell lines from the transgenic animal, demonstrating that the response to inducers can function independently of the chromosomal environment when introduced into whole animals.

Transferrin is secreted by malignant human cells such as the breast cancer cell line MCF-7.[50] Secretion of transferrin by MCF-7 cells is stimulated by estradiol and reduced by the antiestrogen, 4-hydroxy tamoxifen. Transferrin synthesized by cancer cells could act as an autocrine growth factor and may confer selective advantages for tumor cell growth.

III. THE TRANSFERRIN RECEPTOR

The cellular metabolism of iron is regulated in a precise fashion through iron-dependent changes in the abundance of ferritin, which sequesters excess iron, and transferrin receptors, which control iron uptake. Transferrin receptors are crucially involved in the control of cell proliferation and differentiation in different types of tissues.[51,52] The receptors are widely distributed in various types of cells, including both normal cells and tumor cells, but are not expressed by mature resting lymphocytes. The receptors are involved in iron uptake by a process consisting of iron-mediated endocytosis and the subsequent recycling of the receptor to the cell surface. During internalization, iron is released from transferrin and apotransferrin is dissociated from the receptor upon its return to the cell surface.[53,54] Intracellular iron is thus rendered available for the synthesis of heme-containing proteins such as hemoglobin and myoglobin and oxidative enzymes such as the cytochromes, and for other iron-requiring enzymes, including ribonucleotide reductase.

Transferrin-polycation conjugates have been used as carriers for the introduction of DNA into hematopoietic cells through a process of transferrin receptor-mediated endocytosis.[55,56] By coupling transferrin to the DNA-binding cations, polylysine or protamine conjugates can be created that bind nucleic acids and carry them into the cell during the normal transferrin cycle. Advantages of this procedure, referred to as "transferrinfection", are that there is no overt limit to the size of the transfected DNA molecules and that they may be expressed in the majority of the treated cells.

A. THE TRANSFERRIN RECEPTOR GENE

The transferrin receptor gene was cloned, by a gene transfer approach, from human cell lines expressing the receptor.[57,58] The cloned genomic DNA of the receptor is close to 31 kbp and contains 19 distinct exons. With the exception of the exon at the 3' end, these exons are each less than 200 bp long. A large nontranslated, but transcribed region at the 3' end of the gene may be involved in the regulation of transferrin receptor expression.[59]

A 365-bp DNA fragment containing the 5' region of the human transferrin receptor gene has been cloned and sequenced.[60] This region represents the transferrin receptor gene promoter and contains four repeats of the sequence GGGGC, which are probably involved in recognizing transcription regulation signals and are also found in the genes coding for dihydrofolate reductase and IL-3. A protein-blotting procedure and a specific DNA probe have been used to identify nuclear proteins that recognize the promoter region of the transferrin receptor gene.[61]

B. STRUCTURE OF THE TRANSFERRIN RECEPTOR

The transferrin receptor on the plasma membrane is a 180-kDa phosphorylated glycoprotein in its nonreduced homodimeric form.[62,63] The receptor is composed of two identical subunits of 90 kDa, linked as a dimer by a disulfide bridge.[64] As deduced from the sequence of the respective mRNA, the human transferrin receptor is composed of 760 amino acid residues and contains a stretch of 26 predominantly nonpolar amino acids with a sequence of 9 hydrophobic residues in the center (residues 66–88), which would correspond to the transmembrane region of the receptor molecule.[58,64] Since the latter sequence resides at the amino-terminal end of the protein and no hydrophobic stretch is detected at the carboxy-terminal portion, it can be deduced that the receptor must be unusually oriented, with its amino-terminus on the cytoplasmic side and with a large carboxy-terminal extracellular domain of 672 amino acids. No strong sequence homology was detected between the transferrin receptor and any known protein.

The chicken transferrin receptor has been characterized.[65] The receptor is represented by a glycoprotein of 95 kDa that exists, albeit only partially, as a disulfide-linked dimer on the cell surface. Although biochemical evidence indicates that the chicken transferrin receptor resembles the mammalian homologous receptor, immunological analysis suggests dissimilarities. An estrogen-inducible transferrin receptor present in the chicken oviduct appears to be structurally distinct from the iron-modulated red cell transferrin receptor of the chicken.[66] The biological significance of this difference remains to be evaluated.

C. POSTTRANSLATIONAL MODIFICATION OF THE TRANSFERRIN RECEPTOR

The transferrin receptor protein undergoes posttranslational modifications consisting of glycosylation, fatty acid acylation, and phosphorylation.[67] Little is known of the functional role of these modifications, but there is evidence that biosynthesis of the receptor is associated with the acquisition of its functional properties.[68] Glycosylation is not necessary for specific binding of transferrin to its receptor, but the affinity of this binding can be influenced greatly by the presence or absence of carbohydrate residues.[69] Fatty acid acylation may be important for the association of the receptor with the plasma membrane.

The functional role of transferrin receptor phosphorylation is not clear. In contrast to the receptors of hormones and growth factors, phosphorylation of the transferrin receptor occurs not on tyrosine, but on serine and threonine residues. Transferrin binding to the receptor does not alter the extent of basal receptor phosphorylation. However, hemin rapidly inhibits the incorporation of transferrin iron into reticulocytes, and phosphorylation of transferrin receptors is increased by hemin treatment of the cells in the presence of transferrin.[70] These results suggest that a cycle of phosphorylation and dephosphorylation may have a role in transferrin receptor internalization.[71] However, at least in certain neoplastic cells (A431 and KB human epidermoid carcinoma cell lines), phosphorylation of the transferrin receptor does not contribute to the regulation of its expression on the cell surface.[72]

Protein kinase is involved in phosphorylation of the transferrin receptor.[73,74] Ser-24 is the unique site on the transferrin receptor phosphorylated by protein kinase C.[75] Treatment of mouse 3T3 fibroblasts with phorbol ester or PDGF causes phosphorylation of the transferrin receptor by protein kinase C at Ser-24 and increase the cell-surface expression of the receptor.[76] Protein kinase C-induced phosphorylation of the transferrin receptor can act as a trigger to stimulate receptor internalization whether or not the physiologic ligand is present.[77] However, the regulation of transferrin receptor cycling by protein kinase C is independent of phosphorylation at Ser-24.[78]

Downregulation of the transferrin receptor is induced by phorbol ester, which is associated with hyperphosphorylation of the receptor by the action of protein kinase C.[73,74] Intracellular activation of protein kinase C and regulation of the surface transferrin receptor by 1,2-diacylglycerol is a spontaneously reversible process that is associated with rapid formation of phosphatidic acid.[79] In addition, transferrin may induce an increase in the synthesis or expression of protein kinase C in cells such as the human lymphoblastoid cell line CCRF-CEM.[80]

D. TRANSFERRIN RECEPTOR EXPRESSION

Expression of the transferrin receptor at the cell surface may represent a specific marker for rapidly growing cells. In general, transferrin receptor expression is closely linked to the proliferative state of the cell. Stimulation of cell proliferation is generally associated with increased expression of transferrin receptors on the cell surface. For example, partial hepatectomy, which induces regeneration of the remaining liver cells, produces a marked increase in the ability of these cells to bind transferrin to receptors on the cell surface, which is due to the translocation of intracellular transferrin receptors to the surface.[81] In contrast, resting or differentiated cells usually have a reduced level of surface transferrin receptors. Inhibition of cell growth is frequently, but not always, associated with decreased levels of transferrin receptor expression. Treatment of Daudi and HL-60 cells with IFN-a results in inhibition of cell growth, but this effect does not depend on changes in the expression of transferrin receptors.[82] At least in certain types of cells, the levels of expression of transferrin receptors are not constant during the cell cycle. In synchronized murine M1 myeloid leukemia cells, expression of transferrin receptors is lowest in the early G_1 phase of the cycle and highest in the late G_1 phase, whereas the reverse is true for c-*myc* gene expression.[83]

Transferrin receptor synthesis is enhanced when stationary human erythroleukemia cells are subcultured at low density in fresh medium, which may be due to a depletion in their intracellular iron pool.[84] The transferrin receptor gene is hyperexpressed in differentiating erythroid cells, which is associated with its regulation at the transcriptional level.[85]

Transferrin receptors are expressed by both immature and activated normal lymphocytes as well as by lymphoblastoid cells, but are not expressed by mature resting lymphocytes.[86,87] Expression of the transferrin receptor may have a crucial role in lymphocyte activation. Intact transferrin receptors complexed with transferrin are found in human plasma.[88] The plasma receptors exhibit a constant relationship to the tissue receptors, and their number may reflect the rate of erythropoiesis. Decreased concentrations of plasma transferrin receptors are found in patients with erythroid hypoplasia, whereas increased concentrations occur in patients with erythroid hyperplasia.

1. Regulation of Transferrin Receptor Expression

Many factors contribute to the regulation of the number of transferrin receptors expressed on the cell surface. Hemin, iron, and protoporphyrin IX may represent the main molecules involved in the regulation of transferrin receptors.[89] In particular, the expression of transferrin receptors depends on the amount of iron accumulated into the cells. When cells accumulate large amounts of iron, they reduce the number of transferrin receptors expressed on the surface in order to prevent further accumulation of iron; in contrast, when the intracellular iron concentration is low and the cells need more iron, they express an increased number of transferrin receptors on the cell surface to permit rapid accumulation of iron.[89] Transferrin receptor regulation is coupled to intracellular ferritin in proliferating and differentiating HL-60 human promyelocytic leukemia cells.[90] These cells display transferrin receptors, but exhibit a decrease in receptor expression on the surface after differentiation, induction, or accumulation of intracellular iron. Iron salts modulate the synthesis of transferrin receptors and ferritin in human erythroleukemia cell lines via different molecular mechanisms of the transcriptional and translational type, respectively.[91] Phorbol esters modulate expression of the transferrin receptor gene at the transcriptional level in cultured lymphoblastoid T cells.[92]

Serum, as well as purified hormones and growth factors and other extracellular agents, including insulin, IGFs, EGF, PDGF, TNF-α, erythropoietin, phorbol esters, and viruses can exert regulatory effects on the expression of transferrin receptors on the cell surface.[93-97] Exposure of certain cells to insulin results in a relatively slow and prolonged stimulation of transferrin binding. Treatment of isolated fat cells with insulin stimulates diferric transferrin uptake and causes redistribution of transferrin receptors from an internal microsomal compartment to the plasma membrane.[75] This effect of insulin is due to an increase in the rate of transferrin receptor externalization.[98] The enhancing effects of PDGF, IGF-I, EGF, and TNF-α on transferrin receptor expression at the cell surface are very rapid, with maximal effects being observed within 5 min of BALB/c 3T3 fibroblast treatment with these mitogens.[93,97] The speed of this response indicates that the increase in the expression of the transferrin receptors at the cell surface cannot be accounted for by increased synthesis of the receptor, but should be attributed to a redistribution of transferrin receptors within the cell.

The addition of EGF to human fibroblasts results in induction of a rapid but transient increase in cell surface transferrin receptors, which is apparently due to a translocation of intracellular transferrin receptors to the surface without a change in the total cellular transferrin receptor content.[99] EGF and TNF-α may generate similar or identical intracellular signals for cellular growth and the regulation of transferrin receptor expression.[97] An increase in the expression of transferrin receptors on the surface may be an obligatory requirement for the DNA synthesis and mitogenic effects elicited by EGF and TNF-α in certain cell types. Both IFN-α and IFN-γ inhibit the expression of transferrin receptors in human lymphoblastoid cells and mitogen-induced lymphocytes.[100] The larger the number of cell transferrin receptors before IFN-α treatment, the weaker the cell sensitivity to the antigrowth effects of IFN-α. The inhibitory effect of IFNs on transferrin receptor expression may be at least one of the mechanisms by which they inhibit cell proliferation. IL-2 can regulate transferrin receptor mRNA expression at both the transcriptional and posttranscriptional levels.[101]

An increase in the number of transferrin receptors is observed during erythropoietin-induced differentiation of Friend virus-infected erythroid cells.[94] Upon culture of the cells with erythropoietin, the synthesis of transferrin receptors increases severalfold and the number of transferrin binding sites per cell is doubled after 24 h, but the rate of iron uptake from transferrin remains constant during this period and the amount of transferrin internalized does not change.

Estrogen-induced sexual maturation in the chicken is accompanied by the synthesis of serum transferrin in the liver and the egg-white protein, conalbumin (ovotransferrin), in the oviduct, as well as by the expression of transferrin receptors in the oviduct.[102] Since conalbumin binds iron and its secretion serves as a food reserve for the developing embryo, the observed changes induced by estrogen in the oviduct may contribute not only to cover the metabolic needs of this organ but also to replace the significant losses of iron which accompany conalbumin secretion.

Inhibition of calcium influx in both normal and malignant human T cells by the tertiary amino compound, diltiazem, results in inhibition of transferrin receptor synthesis and expression, cell cycle arrest in the G_1 phase, and inhibition of DNA synthesis.[103] However, this effect does not alter c-*myc* or c-*myb* gene expression nor IL-2 receptor gene expression, indicating that expression of these genes is not sufficient to support G_1 traversal when Ca^{2+} influx is blocked and that expression of transferrin receptors is crucial for traversal of the G_1/S boundary and initiation of DNA synthesis in normal and malignant cells.

2. Mechanism of Regulation of Transferrin Receptor mRNA

Iron regulates the synthesis of ferritin and the transferrin receptor through mRNA/protein interactions.[104] The effect of alteration in intracellular iron concentrations is mainly exerted on mature mRNA rather than on DNA transcription or protein degradation. When iron is in excess, cells use stored ferritin mRNA to synthesize more ferritin for iron storage and, at the same time, the stability of transferrin receptor mRNA decreases, which diminishes receptor synthesis and iron uptake. Conversely, when iron levels are low transferrin receptor mRNA is stabilized, more receptor is synthesized, and iron uptake increases. At the same time, ferritin mRNA is masked, ferritin synthesis declines, and iron storage decreases. A regulatory sequence, termed iron-responsive element (IRE), occurs in the 5′-untranslated region of all ferritin mRNAs and is repeated as five variations in the 3′-untranslated region of transferrin receptor mRNA.[104] The location of a common sequence in different regions of the two mRNAs may be related to the opposite effects exerted by iron on these mRNAs. When the IRE is in the 5′-untranslated region of ferritin mRNA, translation is enhanced by excess iron, whereas the presence of IREs in the 3′-untranslated region of the transferrin receptor mRNA leads to its iron-dependent degradation. A soluble 90-kDa regulatory protein binds to IRE sequences, although it is not an iron-binding protein. This protein is the first specific mRNA regulatory protein identified in any eukaryotic system.

3. Internalization of the Transferrin Receptor

Transferrin receptor-diferric transferrin complexes are internalized by endocytosis, which requires the action of a specific trigger.[105] Internalization of the transferrin receptor depends on the structure of its cytoplasmic domain and is not associated with its phosphorylation by protein kinase C.[77,106,107] The cytoplasmic domain of the human transferrin receptor contains a specific signal sequence located within amino acid residues 19–28 that determines high-efficiency endocytosis of the receptor molecule, and the Tyr-20 residue is an important element of this sequence.[108] Whether the receptor undergoes a conformational change during this process is not yet known. After release of iron from transferrin, both apotransferrin and the transferrin receptor recirculate back to the cell surface. They are not degraded in lysosomes, as usually occurs with other ligand-receptor complexes.[109,110] A rapid endocytosis of the transferrin receptor may also occur in the absence of bound transferrin, and it has been suggested that binding of the ligand may not be required for an endocytic/exocytic cycle of the transferrin receptor.[111,112] It is possible that transferrin receptors, and perhaps also other types of receptors, are recognized as being ligand-occupied, not at the cell surface, but at some other site in the recycling pathway within the cell. Downregulation of the receptors would occur not by speeding up the entry of receptors from the cell surface, but by slowing down, or abolishing, the return of internalized receptors to the cell surface. Expression of transferrin receptors on the surface of BeWo human choriocarcinoma cells stimulated to form syncytia similar to syncytiotrophoblasts by treatment with forskolin or theophylline is maintained by an increased externalization rate constant.[113]

Intracellular calcium and protein kinase C are involved in the regulation of transferrin receptor expression.[114] The cytoskeleton may be involved in regulating the expression and downregulation of transferrin receptors on the cell surface. However, disruption of the microtubular system in the human leukemia cell line CCRF-CEM by treatment with the stathmokinetic agent, vincristine, has little effect on transferrin receptor turnover, which suggests that microtubules do not play a major role in the recycling of transferrin receptors.[115] Lymphoblastoid T cells modulate expression of transferrin receptors through two independent mechanisms: a cytoskeleton-dependent pathway triggered by binding of iron-saturated transferrin and a cytoskeleton-independent pathway that may be triggered by treatment of cells with phorbol esters.[116] In addition to receptor internalization events, lymphoblastoid cells may modulate transferrin receptor expression on the cell surface by other mechanisms, possibly including an alteration in the cell surface orientation of the receptor molecule.[117]

The endocytosis and recycling of the human transferrin receptor have been evaluated in K562 human leukemia cells perturbed with monensin, a carboxylic ionophore that causes major disruption of membrane vesicular transport from the Golgi complex to the plasma membrane and which is also lysosomotropic.[118] The results suggest the existence of two distinct transferrin receptor recycling pathways, one monensin-sensitive and the other monensin-resistant. The monensin-sensitive pathway would be Golgi-dependent, whereas the monensin-resistant pathway would be independent of the Golgi apparatus. In addition, the evidence indicates that transferrin receptor internalization can occur independently of ligand binding and that trafficking of receptors into either pathway is not highly dependent upon transferrin.

Treatment of K562 cells with trifluoroperazine, a drug that inhibits both calmodulin-dependent and calcium-activated phospholipid-dependent kinases, results in reduction in the number of transferrin receptors on the cell surface with no change in the affinity of the remaining receptors.[119] The receptors that remain at the surface in trifluoperazine-treated cells continue to internalize transferrin and to recycle apotransferrin to the cell surface, albeit more slowly than in untreated cells. Bovine transferrin binds specifically to the human transferrin receptor in K562 cells, but with approximately 2000-fold less affinity than human transferrin. However, bovine transferrin is internalized thereafter, which demonstrates interspecies transferrin receptor recognition and internalization.[120]

E. TRANSFERRIN RECEPTORS IN NORMAL AND NEOPLASTIC CELLS

Transferrin receptors are especially abundant in hemoglobin-synthesizing cells and in the placental trophoblast cells. They are generally detectable on dividing cells, including tumor cells and established cell lines, but are usually undetectable in fully differentiated, nondividing cells and tissues.[121] Studies on the effects of phorbol ester on normal and RSV-transformed myogenic cells suggest that there are functional differences between the transferrin receptors of normal and transformed cells.[122]

1. Testicular Transferrin Receptors

Transferrin may have an important role in the regulation and maintenance of spermatogenesis. High amounts of transferrin are secreted by Sertoli cells, which may be crucial for the delivery of iron to developing germinal cells. The synthesis of transferrin mRNA and the secretion of transferrin by rat Sertoli cells is regulated by hormones.[28] Transferrin receptor mRNA is expressed in all testicular cell types of the rat, except spermatids, and the highest amounts of this mRNA are found in the Sertoli cells.[123] The expression of transferrin receptors in rat Sertoli cells maintained in culture are regulated by iron availability and not by hormones. However, chronic administration of testosterone or FSH to hypophysectomized rats results in increased levels of transferrin receptor mRNA in the testes. Both transferrin mRNA and transferrin receptor mRNA are regulated throughout the cycle of the seminiferous epithelium.

2. Placental Transferrin Receptors

In the human placental syncytiotrophoblast, transferrin receptors are present in both the apical microvillous plasma membrane, which faces maternal blood circulation, and the basal plasma membrane, which faces the fetal circulation.[124] Although these two receptors are apparently identical, they must serve different functions: in the microvillous membrane the receptor mediates the uptake of iron from maternal blood for transcellular transfer, whereas in the basal membrane the receptor functions in iron uptake for internal use. In any case, placental transferrin receptors must accomplish the crucial function of transferring the essential nutrient, iron, from the mother to the fetus.

3. Transferrin Receptors in Lymphocyte Activation

Transferrin receptor induction is required for human B-lymphocyte activation but not for Ig secretion.[125] After stimulation of resting (G_0) peripheral blood mononuclear cells with mitogens, T cells enter the G_1 phase of the cell cycle where they produce and express receptors for IL-2.[126] Interaction of IL-2 with IL-2 receptors on activated T cells is then required for expression of transferrin receptors.[127] The subsequent binding of transferrin to its receptor during late-phase G_1 of the cell cycle allows T cells to make the G_1 to S transition. Expression of c-*myc* is regulated at several points of the cycle in normal lymphocytes and may contribute to the control of lymphocyte proliferation.[128] Incubation of human lymphocytes with purified IL-2 results in increased expression of both c-*myc* and transferrin receptor mRNAs.[129]

4. Effect of Antitransferrin Receptor Antibodies

Transferrin is a critical component of serum-free media, being required for supporting the proliferation of both normal and neoplastically transformed cells.[130] Antitransferrin receptor antibodies may inhibit growth of a variety of normal and malignant human hematopoietic cells through mechanisms involving both transferrin receptor degradation and cross-linking of the receptors at the cell surface.[130] Monoclonal antitransferrin receptor antibodies of the IgM type, but not of the IgG type, are able to induce a complete inhibition of growth in most cell lines.[132,133] However, a rat IgG monoclonal antibody (C2F2) against the murine transferrin receptor produced highly selective inhibition of T and B lymphocyte activation protocols.[134] The IgA antitransferrin receptor monoclonal antibody 42/6 is capable of inducing a profound inhibition of the growth of cultured normal and malignant human hematopoietic cells, but is a relatively inefficient inhibitor of solid tumor cell growth.[135] The resistance of tumor cells to 42/6 antibody may be due, in part, to a greater heterogeneity of transferrin receptor display by proliferating cells, as well as to differences in transferrin processing or iron requirements. The results indicate that the profound effects of the IgM antitransferrin receptor antibodies on cell growth are due to extensive cross-linking of cell-surface transferrin receptors which may interfere in some way with transferrin receptor function of iron delivery into the cell. Some cell types, however, may escape from the growth-inhibitory effect of antitransferrin receptor antibodies by a mechanism involving increased iron uptake.[136]

5. Transferrin Receptors in Neoplastic Cells

Transferrin receptor expression may be important for the growth and malignant behavior or transformed cells. Appearance and internalization of transferrin receptors is frequently observed at the margins of spreading human tumor cells.[137] A marked reduction of the surface transferrin receptors was observed in the A431 human epidermoid carcinoma cell line when the cells enter mitosis, and this situation persisted until telophase when receptors reappear to a level that exceeds the original interphase value.[138]

Transferrin receptors are present in a diversity of human hematopoietic cell lines, and relatively high levels of expression of these receptors have been detected in cells from human leukemia and lymphoproliferative disorders.[89,139,140] Transferrin receptor expression in differentiating HL-60 human leukemia cells may occur by regulation at the transcriptional level.[141] Using the transferrin receptor-specific monoclonal antibody OKT9 to study cryostat sections of 267 human non-Hodgkin's lymphomas and related neoplasms, it was found that 70% of the tumors (67% of the B-cell type and 85% of the T-cell type) were stained by OKT9.[142] However, there was considerable heterogeneity with respect to the incidence and intensity of cellular staining among the various subtypes of lymphomas, and transferrin receptor expression by certain histologic subtypes of lymphomas did not correlate with their morphologic grade. Clinical follow-up of patients with chronic lymphocytic leukemia/small-cell lymphocytic lymphoma or difuse large-cell and immunoblastic lymphoma showed that transferrin receptor expression in these two groups does not correlate with survival. Using a specific immunoglobulin antibody (IgG2a), it was found that a unique epitope of the transferrin receptor is exposed on the cell surface of high-grade, aggressive human lymphomas, but not on low-grade indolent lymphomas.[143] Biochemical studies on blast cells from acute human T-cell leukemia showed constitutive expression in these cells of transferrin receptors with reduced molecular weight, which is due to abnormal glycosylation of the receptors.[144]

A correlation between the proliferation rate of normal or malignant cells and the expression of transferrin receptors is not always apparent. Variation in the expression of transferrin receptors is observed in both malignant and nonmalignant human breast tissue.[145] Analysis of the expression of transferrin receptors in human colon cancer cell lines by flow cytometry using the OKT-9 monoclonal antibody, which is specific for the receptor, did not show any difference in transferrin receptor expression between the fast- and slow-growing lines.[146] Moreover, the cell lines did not change the proportion of transferrin receptor-positive cells in their transit from the exponential into the stationary phase of growth. Direct measurements of transferrin receptor expression in malignant cells may not provide a clinically useful marker to distinguish highly proliferative tumors from those with a slower growth resulting from a larger proportion of quiescent cells. Association between the transferrin receptor and Ras protein was detected in extracts of a human bladder carcinoma cell line.[147] This association, however, was recognized later as an artifact of the immunoprecipitation technique.[148]

6. Neoplastic Cell Differentiation and Transferrin Receptor Expression

Modulation of transferrin receptor expression on the cell surface may be important for the process of differentiation of neoplastic cells. Differentiation HL-60 human leukemia cells and other neoplastic hematopoietic cell lines induced by phorbol esters, retinoic acid, DMSO, or aclacinomycin A is associated with inhibition of transferrin binding and iron uptake and decreased numbers of transferrin receptors on the surface.[149-152] Downregulation of transferrin receptor expression in the treated HL-60 cells is due, at least in part, to decreased transcriptional expression of the receptor gene and would mediate the cessation of proliferation in the differentiating cells. Treatment of human erythroleukemia or HL-60 cells with phorbol esters results in hyperphosphorylation and internalization of transferrin receptors.[71-74,153] Transferrin receptor phosphorylation occurs on serine and threonine residues and may be a direct effect of protein kinase C activation. TPA causes a decrease in the number of transferrin receptors on the surface of K562 leukemia cells and HepG2 hepatoma cells.[154,155] This decrease is due to both reduced biosynthesis and accelerated degradation of the receptors, and the changes occur in spite of the fact that TPA does not induce differentiation of K562 cells. In other human tumor cell lines (A431 and KB epidermoid carcinoma cells), phorbol ester may cause phosphorylation of transferrin receptors but has little and variable effects on the expression of these receptors on the cell surface.[72]

Differentiation induced in neoplastic cells by compounds other than phorbol esters may be accompanied by similar changes in transferrin receptor expression. Differentiation of HL-60 cells induced by treatment with DMSO is associated with a significant decrease in the expression of transferrin receptors, which is regulated at the transcriptional level.[141] Transcriptional inactivation of transferrin receptor expression is also observed when HL-60 cells are induced to differentiate along the monocytic pathway by treatment with dibutyryl cAMP.[156] Differentiation of cultured Friend erythroleukemia cells induced to hemoglobin synthesis by treatment with DMSO is accompanied by changes in the number of transferrin receptors and in the efficiency of iron release from internalized transferrin.[157] However, the exact relationship between the expression of transferrin receptors and the process of differentiation of neoplastic cells in general is not understood, since the reduction of transferrin receptor mRNA level and surface receptor protein observed in HL-60 cells occurs well before the expression of the mature phenotype. Moreover, it remains unclear whether transcriptional regulation of transferrin receptor expression is required for the differentiation of HL-60 cells.

IV. EFFECTS OF TRANSFERRIN ON CELL PROLIFERATION AND DIFFERENTIATION

Transferrins are requisite factors for almost all serum-free tissue culture media. Using serum-free assay conditions, it was demonstrated that transferrin represents a major source of the mitogenic activity present in pituitary extracts and is required for the growth of normal and malignant cells *in vitro*.[158] Transferrin is one of the factors that promotes the clonal growth of granulocyte and macrophage precursors in serum-free cultures *in vitro*.[159] It may act as a competence or progression factor in the proliferation of epithelial cells. The nontumorigenic and anchorage-dependent hepatic cell line WB-F344, which produces IGF-II and TGF-β constitutively, grows in serum-free medium supplemented only with transferrin.[160] In the absence of transferrin, the proliferation of WB-F-344 cells is arrested in serum-free medium at the G_0/G_1 phase, and a period of protein synthesis after the addition of transferrin is necessary before the cells can proceed to S phase and initiate DNA synthesis.

In addition to its important effects on the regulation of cell proliferation, transferrin is involved in regulating the differentiation of some types of cells. Transferrin has an inhibitory effect on the differentiation of rat granulosa cells *in vitro*.[161] Transferrin is a progression factor for the differentiation of ML1 human myelocytic leukemia cells.[162]

A. MECHANISMS OF THE GROWTH-PROMOTING ACTION OF TRANSFERRIN

The mechanism by which transferrin promotes cell growth crucially depends on the expression of transferrin receptor and is intimately associated with iron transport into the cell. However, additional mechanisms may be involved in the growth-promoting action of transferrin. Activation of the Na^+/H^+ antiport by diferric transferrin may provide an additional basis for diferric transferrin stimulation of growth.[163]

B. TUMOR-PROMOTING EFFECTS OF TRANSFERRIN

Transferrin may have tumor-promoting effects under certain conditions, for example, in the heterotopically transplanted rat urinary bladder system.[164] The possible role of urinary transferrin in the normal growth and tumorigenic processes of the urothelial system is unknown. Transferrin selectively stimulates the growth of prostatic carcinoma cells.[165]

REFERENCES

1. **Huebers, H.A. and Finch, C.A.**, Transferrin: physiologic behavior and clinical implications, *Blood*, 64, 763, 1984.
2. **Pré, J.**, Transferrin, *Pathol. Biol.*, 37, 222, 1989.
3. **De Jong, G., Van Dijk, J.P., and Van Eijk, H.G.**, The biology of transferrin, *Clin. Chim. Acta*, 190, 1, 1990.
4. **Bowman, B.H., Yang, F., and Adrian, G.S.**, Transferrin: evolution and genetic regulation of expression, *Adv. Genet.*, 25, 1, 1988.
5. **Levin, M.J., Tuil, D., Uzan, G., Dreyfus, J.-C., and Kahn, A.**, Expression of the transferrin gene during development of nonhepatic tissues, *Biochem. Biophys. Res. Commun.*, 122, 212, 1984.
6. **Zakin, M.M.**, Regulation of transferrin gene expression, *FASEB J.*, 6, 3253, 1992.
7. **Skinner, M.K., Cosand, W.L., and Griswold, M.D.**, Purification and characterization of testicular transferrin secreted by rat Sertoli cells, *Biochem. J.*, 218, 313, 1984.
8. **Horn, F., Gschwendt, M., and Marks, F.**, Partial purification and characterization of the calcium-dependent and phospholipid-dependent protein kinase C from chick oviduct, *Eur. J. Biochem.*, 148, 533, 1985.

9. **Pryzwansky, K.B., Martin, L.E., and Spitznagel, J.K.,** Immunocytochemical localization of myeloperoxidase lactoferrin, lysozyme and neutral proteases in human monocytes and neutrophilic granulocytes, *J. Reticuloendothel. Soc.,* 24, 295, 1978.
10. **Yoshinari, K., Yuasa, K., Iga, F., and Mimura, A.,** A growth-promoting factor for human myeloid leukemia cells from horse serum identified as horse serum transferrin, *Biochim. Biophys. Acta,* 1010, 28, 1989.
11. **Conrad, M.E., Umbreit, J.N., Moore, E.G., Peterson, R.D.A., and Jones, M.B.,** A newly identified iron binding protein in duodenal mucosa of rats. Purification and characterization of mobilferrin, *J. Biol. Chem.,* 265, 5273, 1990.
12. **Sturrock, A., Alexander, J., Lamb, J., Craven, C.M., and Kaplan, J.,** Characterization of a transferrin-independent uptake system for iron in HeLa cells, *J. Biol. Chem.,* 265, 3139, 1990.
13. **Legrand, D., Mazurier, J., Montreuil, J., and Spik, G.,** Structure and spatial conformation of the iron-binding sites of transferrins, *Biochimie,* 70, 1185, 1988.
14. **Spik, G., Coddeville, B., and Montreuil, J.,** Comparative study of the primary structures of sero-, lacto-, and ovotransferrin glycans from different species, *Biochimie,* 70, 1459, 1988.
15. **Léger, D., Campion, B., Decottignies, J.-P., Montreuil, J., and Spik, G.,** Physiological significance of the marked increased branching of the glycans of human serotransferrin during pregnancy, *Biochem. J.,* 257, 231, 1989.
16. **Huerre, C., Uzan, G., Grzeschik, K.H., Weil, D., Levin, M., Hors-Cayla, M.-C., Boué, J., Kahn, A., and Junien, C.,** The structural gene for transferrin (TF) maps to 3q21-3qter, *Ann. Genét.,* 27, 5, 1984.
17. **Yang, F., Lum, J.B., McGill, J.R., Moore, C.M., Naylor, S.L., van Bragt, P.H., Baldwin, W.D., and Bowman, B.H.,** Human transferrin: cDNA characterization and chromosomal localization, *Proc. Natl. Acad. Sci. U.S.A.,* 81, 2752, 1984.
18. **Plowman, G.D., Brown, J.P., Enns, C.A., Schröder, J., Nikinmaa, B., Sussman, H.H., Hellström, K.E., and Hellström, I.,** Assignment of the gene for human melanoma-associated antigen p97 to chromosome 3, *Nature,* 303, 70, 1983.
19. **Teng, C.T., Pentecost, B.T., Marshall, A., Solomon, A., Bowman, B.H., Lalley, P.A., and Naylor, S.L.,** Assignment of the lactotransferrin gene to human chromosome 3 and to mouse chromosome 9, *Somat. Cell Mol. Genet.,* 13, 689, 1987.
20. **Park, I., Schaeffer, E., Sidoli, A., Baralle, F.E., Cohen, G.N., and Zakin, M.M.,** Organization of the human transferrin gene: direct evidence that it originated by gene duplication, *Proc. Natl. Acad. Sci. U.S.A.,* 82, 3149, 1985.
21. **Brunel, F., Ochoa, A., Schaeffer, E., Boissier, F., Guillou, Y., Cereghini, S., Cohen, G.N., and Zakin, M.M.,** Interactions of DNA-binding proteins with the 5' region of the human transferrin gene, *J. Biol. Chem.,* 263, 10180, 1988.
22. **Schaeffer, E., Boissier, F., Py, M.-C., Cohen, G.N., and Zakin, M.M.,** Cell type-specific expression of the human transferrin gene. Role of promoter, negative, and enhancer elements, *J. Biol. Chem.,* 264, 7153, 1989.
23. **Adrian, G.S., Bowman, B.H., Herbert, D.C., Weaker, F.J., Adrian, E.K., Robinson, L.K., Walter, C.A., Eddy, C.A., Riehl, R., Pauerstein, C.J., and Yang, F.,** Human transferrin. Expression and iron modulation of chimeric genes in transgenic mice, *J. Biol. Chem.,* 265, 13344, 1990.
24. **MacGillivray, R.T.A., Mendes, E., Shewale, J.G., Sinha, S.K., Lineback-Zins, J., and Brew, K.,** The primary structure of human serum transferrin, *J. Biol. Chem.,* 258, 3543, 1983.
25. **Morgan, E.H. and Peters, T., Jr.,** The biosynthesis of rat transferrin: evidence for rapid glycosylation, disulfide bond formation, and tertiary folding, *J. Biol. Chem.,* 260, 14793, 1985.
26. **Yamashita, K., Koide, N., Endo, T., Iwaki, Y., and Kobata, A.,** Altered glycosylation of serum transferrin of patients with hepatocellular carcinoma, *J. Biol. Chem.,* 264, 2415, 1989.
27. **Dittmann, K.H. and Petrides, P.E.,** A 41 kDa transferrin related molecule acts as an autocrine growth factor for HL-60 cells, *Biochem. Biophys. Res. Commun.,* 176, 473, 1991.
28. **Huggenvik, J.I., Idzerda, R.L., Haywood, L., Lee, D.C., McKnight, G.S., and Griswold, M.D.,** Transferrin messenger ribonucleic acid: molecular cloning and hormonal regulation in rat Sertoli cells, *Endocrinology,* 120, 332, 1987.
29. **Tuil, D., Vaulont, S., Levin, M.J., Munnich, A., Moguilewsky, M., Bouton, M.M., Brissot, P., Dreyfus, J.-C., and Kahn, A.,** Transient transcriptional inhibition of the transferrin gene by cyclic AMP, *FEBS Lett.,* 189, 310, 1985.

30. **Aldred, A.R., Howlett, G.J., and Schreiber, G.,** Synthesis of rat transferrin in *Escherichia coli* containing a recombinant bacteriophage, *Biochem. Biophys. Res. Commun.,* 122, 960, 1984.
31. **Goubin, G., Goldman, D.S., Luce, J., Neiman, P.E., and Cooper, G.M.,** Molecular cloning and nucleotide sequence of a transforming gene detected by transfection of chicken B-cell lymphoma DNA, *Nature,* 302, 114, 1983.
32. **Diamond, A., Cooper, G.M., Ritz, J., and Lane, M.-A.,** Identification and molecular cloning of the human *Blym* transforming gene activated in Burkitt's lymphomas, *Nature,* 305, 112, 1983.
33. **Devine, J.M., Diamond, A., Lane, M.-A., and Cooper, G.M.,** Characterization of the Blym-1 transforming genes of chicken and human B-cell lymphomas, *J. Cell. Physiol.,* Suppl. 3, 193, 1984.
34. **Neiman, P.,** The *BLYM* oncogenes, *Adv. Cancer Res.,* 45, 107, 1985.
35. **Lee, E.Y.-H., Barcellos-Hoff, M.H., Chen, L.-H., Parry, G., and Bisell, M.J.,** Transferrin is a major mouse milk protein and is synthesized by mammary epithelial cells, *In Vitro Cell. Dev. Biol.,* 23, 221, 1987.
36. **Green, M.R. and Pastewka, J.V.,** Lactoferrin is a marker for prolactin response in mouse mammary explants, *Endocrinology,* 103, 1510, 1989.
37. **Teng, C.T., Walker, M.P., Bhattacharyya, S.N., Klapper, D.G., DiAugustine, R.P., and McLachlan, J.A.,** Purification and properties of an oestrogen-stimulated mouse uterine glycoprotein (approx. 70 kDa), *Biochem. J.,* 240, 413, 1986.
38. **Pentecost, B.T. and Teng, C.T.,** Lactotransferrin is the major estrogen inducible protein of mouse uterine secretions, *J. Biol. Chem.,* 262, 10134, 1987.
39. **Teng, C.T., Pentecost, B.T., Chen, Y.H., Newbold, R.R., Eddy, E.M., and McLachlan, J.A.,** Lactotransferrin gene expression in the mouse uterus and mammary gland, *Endocrinology,* 124, 992, 1989.
40. **Rado, T.A., Wei, X., and Benz, E.J., Jr.,** Isolation of lactoferrin cDNA from a human myeloid library and expression of mRNA during normal and leukemic myelopoiesis, *Blood,* 70, 989, 1987.
41. **Broxmeyer, H.E., Smithyman, A., Eger, R.R., Meyers, P.A., and de Sousa, M.,** Identification of lactoferrin as the granulocyte-derived inhibitor of colony-stimulating activity production, *J. Exp. Med.,* 148, 1052, 1978.
42. **Fletcher, J. and Willars, J.,** The role of lactoferrin released by phagocytosing neutrophils in the regulation of colony-stimulating activity production by human mononuclear cells, *Blood Cells,* 11, 447, 1986.
43. **Delforge, A., Stryckmans, P., Prieels, J.P., Bieva, C., Ronge-Collard, E., Schlusselberg, J., and Efira, A,** Lactoferrin: its role as a regulator of human granulopoiesis?, *Ann. N.Y. Acad. Sci.,* 459, 85, 1985.
44. **Sawatzki, G. and Rich, I.N.,** Lactoferrin stimulates colony stimulating factor production in vitro and in vivo, *Blood Cells,* 15, 371, 1989.
45. **Brown, J.P., Hewick, R.M., Hellström, K.E., Doolittle, R.F., and Dreyer, W.J.,** Human melanoma-associated antigen p97 is structurally and functionally related to transferrin, *Nature,* 296, 171, 1982.
46. **Woodbury, R.G., Brown, J.P., Yeh, M.-Y., Hellström, I., and Hellström, K.E.,** Identification of a cell surface protein, p97, in human melanomas and certain other neoplasms, *Proc. Natl. Acad. Sci. U.S.A.,* 77, 2183, 1980.
47. **Rose, T.M., Plowman, G.D., Teplow, D.B., Dreyer, W.J., Hellström, K.E., and Brown, J.P.,** Primary structure of the human melanoma-associated antigen p97 (melonotransferrin) deduced from the mRNA sequence, *Proc. Natl. Acad. Sci. U.S.A.,* 83, 1261, 1986.
48. **McKnight, G.S., Lee, D.C., and Palmiter, R.D.,** Transferrin gene expression: regulation of mRNA transcription in chick liver by steroid hormones and iron deficiency, *J. Biol. Chem.,* 255, 148, 1980.
49. **Hammer, R.E., Idzerda, R.L., Brinster, R.L., and McKnight, G.S.,** Estrogen regulation of the avian transferrin gene in transgenic mice, *Mol. Cell. Biol.,* 6, 1010, 1986.
50. **Vandewalle, B., Hornez, L., Revillion, F., and Lefebvre, J.,** Secretion of transferrin by human breast cancer cells, *Biochem. Biophys. Res. Commun.,* 163, 149, 1989.
51. **Neckers, L.M.,** Regulation of transferrin receptor expression and control of cell growth, *Pathobiology,* 59, 11, 1991.
52. **Testa, U., Pelosi, E., and Peschle, C.** The transferrin receptor, *Crit. Rev. Oncogenesis,* 4, 241, 1993.
53. **Morgan, E.H., Smith, G.D., and Peters, T.J.,** Uptake and subcellular processing of ^{59}Fe-^{125}I-labelled transferrin by rat liver, *Biochem. J.,* 237, 163, 1986.
54. **Testa, U., Testa, E.P., Mavilio, F., Petrini, M., Sposi, N.M., Petti, S., Samoggia, P., Montesoro, E., Giannella, G., Bottero, L., Camagna, A., Salvo, G., Isacchi, G., Habetswaller, D., and Peschle, C.,** Differential regulation of transferrin receptor gene expression in human hemopoietic cells: molecular and cellular aspects, *J. Receptor Res.,* 7, 355, 1987.

55. **Wagner, E., Zenke, M., Cotten, M., Beug, H., and Birnstiel, M.L.,** Transferrin-polycation conjugates as carriers for DNA uptake into cells, *Proc. Natl. Acad. Sci. U.S.A.,* 87, 3410, 1990.
56. **Cotten, M., Längle-Rouault, F., Kirlappos, H., Wagner, E., Mechtler, K., Zenke, M., Beug, H., and Birnstiel, M.L.,** Transferrin-polycation-mediated introduction of DNA into human leukemic cells: stimulation by agents that affect the survival of transfected DNA or modulate transferrin receptor levels, *Proc. Natl. Acad. Sci. U.S.A.,* 87, 4033, 1990.
57. **Kühn, L.C., McClelland, A., and Ruddle, F.H.,** Gene transfer, expression, and molecular cloning of the human transferrin receptor gene, *Cell,* 37, 95, 1984.
58. **McClelland, A., Kühn, L.C., and Ruddle, F.H.,** The human transferrin receptor gene: genomic organization, and the complete primary structure of the receptor deduced from a cDNA sequence, *Cell,* 39, 267, 1984.
59. **Owen, D. and Kühn, L.C.,** Noncoding 3′ sequences of the transferrin receptor gene are required for mRNA regulation by iron, *EMBO J.,* 6, 1287, 1987.
60. **Miskimins, W.K., McClelland, A., Roberts, M.P., and Ruddle, F.H.,** Cell proliferation and expression of the transferrin receptor gene: promoter sequence homologies and protein interactions, *J. Cell Biol.,* 103, 1781, 1988.
61. **Miskimins, W.K., Roberts, M.P., McClelland, A., and Ruddle, F.H.,** Use of a protein-blotting procedure and a specific DNA probe to identify nuclear proteins that recognize the promoter region of the transferrin receptor gene, *Proc. Natl. Acad. Sci. U.S.A.,* 82, 6741, 1985.
62. **Sutherland, R., Delia, D., Schneider, C., Newman, R., Kemshead, J., and Greaves, M.,** Ubiquitous cell-surface glycoprotein on tumor cells is proliferation-associated receptor for transferrin, *Proc. Natl. Acad. Sci. U.S.A.,* 78, 4515, 1981.
63. **Schneider, C., Sutherland, R., Newman, R., and Greaves, M.,** Structural features of the cell surface receptor for transferrin that is recognized by the monoclonal antibody OKT9, *J. Biol. Chem.,* 257, 8516, 1982.
64. **Schneider, C., Owen, M.J., Banville, D., and Williams, J.G.,** Primary structure of human transferrin receptor deduced from the mRNA sequence, *Nature,* 311, 675, 1984.
65. **Schmidt, J.A., Marshall, J., and Hayman, M.J.,** Identification and characterization of the chicken transferrin receptor, *Biochem. J.,* 232, 735, 1985.
66. **Poola, I., Mason, A.B., and Lucas, J.J.,** The chicken oviduct and embryonic red blood cell transferrin receptors are distinct molecules, *Biochem. Biophys. Res. Commun.,* 171, 26, 1990.
67. **Adam, M.A. and Johnstone, R.M.,** Protein kinase C does not phosphorylate the externalized form of the transferrin receptor, *Biochem. J.,* 242, 151, 1987.
68. **Enns, C.A., Clinton, E.M., Reckhow, C.L., Root, B.J., Si, D.O., and Cook, C.,** Acquisition of the functional properties of the transferrin receptor during its biosynthesis, *J. Biol. Chem.,* 266, 13272, 1991.
69. **Hunt, R.C., Riegler, R., and Davis, A.A.,** Changes in glycosylation alter the affinity of the human transferrin receptor for its ligand, *J. Biol. Chem.,* 264, 9643, 1989.
70. **Cox, T.M., O'Donnell, M.W., Aisen, P., and London, I.M.,** Hemin inhibits internalization of transferrin by reticulocytes and promotes phosphorylation of the membrane transferrin receptor, *Proc. Natl. Acad. Sci. U.S.A.,* 82, 5170, 1985.
71. **May, W.S., Jacobs, S., and Cuatrecasas, P.,** Association of phorbol ester-induced hyperphosphorylation and reversible regulation of transferrin membrane receptors in HL60 cells, *Proc. Natl. Acad. Sci. U.S.A.,* 81, 2016, 1984.
72. **Castagnola, J., MacLeod, C., Sunada, H., Mendelsohn, J., and Taetle, R.,** Effects of epidermal growth factor on transferrin receptor phosphorylation and surface expression in malignant epithelial cells, *J. Cell. Physiol.,* 132, 492, 1987.
73. **Kohno, H., Taketani, S., and Tokunaga, R.,** Tumor-promoting, phorbol ester-induced phosphorylation of cell-surface transferrin receptors in human erythroleukemia cells, *Cell Struct. Funct.,* 10, 95, 1985.
74. **May, W.S., Sahyoun, N., Jacobs, S., Wolf, M., and Cuatrecasas, P.,** Mechanism of phorbol diester-induced regulation of surface transferrin receptor involves the action of activated protein kinase C and an intact cytoskeleton, *J. Biol. Chem.,* 260, 9419, 1985.
75. **Davis, R.J., Corvera, S., and Czech, M.P.,** Insulin stimulates cellular iron uptake and causes the redistribution of intracellular transferrin receptors to the plasma membrane, *J. Biol. Chem.,* 261, 8708, 1986.
76. **Davis, R.J. and Meisner, H.,** Regulation of transferrin receptor cycling by protein kinase C is independent of receptor phosphorylation at serine 24 in Swiss 3T3 fibroblasts, *J. Biol. Chem.,* 262, 16041, 1987.

77. **May, W.S. and Tyler, G.,** Phosphorylation of the surface transferrin receptor stimulates receptor internalization in HL-60 leukemic cells, *J. Biol. Chem.,* 262, 16710, 1987.
78. **McGraw, T.E., Dunn, K.W., and Maxfield, F.R.,** Phorbol ester treatment increases the exocytic rate of the transferrin receptor recycling pathway independent of serine-24 phosphorylation, *J. Cell Biol.,* 106, 1061, 1988.
79. **May, W.S., Lapetina, E.G., and Cuatrecasas, P.,** Intracellular activation of protein kinase C and regulation of the surface transferrin receptor by diacylglycerol is a spontaneously reversible process that is associated with rapid formation of phosphatidic acid, *Proc. Natl. Acad. Sci. U.S.A.,* 83, 1281, 1986.
80. **Phillips, J.L., Boldt, D.H., and Harper, J.,** Iron-transferrin-induced increase in protein kinase C activity in CCRF-CEM cells, *J. Cell. Physiol.,* 132, 349, 1987.
81. **Hirose-Kumagai, A. and Akamatsu, N.,** Change in transferrin receptor distribution in regenerating rat liver, *Biochem. Biophys. Res. Commun.,* 164, 1105, 1989.
82. **Meadows, L.M., George, D.J., and Kaufman, R.E.,** Dissociation of thymidine incorporation and transferrin receptor expression from cell growth and c-myc accumulation in α-interferon-treated cells, *J. Biol. Response Modif.,* 9, 212, 1990.
83. **Neckers, L.M., Tsuda, H., Weiss, E., and Pluznik, D.H.,** Differential expression of *c-myc* and the transferrin receptor in G_1 synchronized M1 myeloid leukemia cells, *J. Cell. Physiol.,* 135, 339, 1988.
84. **Testa, E.P., Testa, U., Samoggia, P., Salvo, G., Camagna, A., and Peschle, C.,** Expression of transferrin receptors in human erythroleukemic lines: regulation in the plateau and exponential phase of growth, *Cancer Res.,* 46, 5330, 1986.
85. **Chen, L.N.L. and Gerhardt, E.M.,** Transferrin receptor gene is hyperexpressed and transcriptionally regulated in differentiating erythroid cells, *J. Biol. Chem.,* 267, 8254, 1992.
86. **Larrick, J.W. and Cresswell, P.,** Transferrin receptors on human B and T lymphoblastoid cell lines, *Biochim. Biophys. Acta,* 583, 483, 1979.
87. **Mazurier, J., Legrand, D., Hu, W.L., Montreuil, J., and Spik, G.,** Expression of human lactotransferrin receptors in phytohemagglutinin-stimulated human peripheral blood lymphocytes. Isolation of the receptors by antiligand-affinity chromatography, *Eur. J. Biochem.,* 179, 481, 1989.
88. **Huebers, H.A., Beguin, Y., Pootrakul, L.P., Einspahr, D., and Finch, C.A.,** Intact transferrin receptors in human plasma and their relation to erythropoiesis, *Blood,* 75, 102, 1990.
89. **Louache, F., Testa, U., Pelicci, P., Thomopoulos, P., Titeux, M., and Rochant, H.,** Regulation of transferrin receptors in human hematopoietic cell lines, *J. Biol. Chem.,* 259, 11576, 1984.
90. **Rhyner, K., Taetle, R., Bering, H., and To, D.,** Transferrin receptor regulation is coupled to intracellular ferritin in proliferating and differentiating HL60 leukemia cells, *J. Cell. Physiol.,* 125, 608, 1985.
91. **Louache, F., Pelosi, E., Titeux, M., Peschle, C., and Testa, U.,** Molecular mechanisms regulating the synthesis of transferrin receptors and ferritin in human erythroleukemic cell lines, *FEBS Lett.,* 183, 223, 1985.
92. **Alcantara, O., Denham, C.A., Phillips, J.L., and Boldt, D.H.,** Transcriptional regulation of transferrin receptor expression by cultured lymphoblastoid T cells treated with phorbol diesters, *J. Immunol.,* 142, 1719, 1989.
93. **Davis, R.J. and Czech, M.P.,** Regulation of transferrin receptor expression at the cell surface by insulin-like growth factors, epidermal growth factor and platelet-derived growth factor, *EMBO J.,* 5, 653, 1986.
94. **Sawyer, S.T. and Krantz, S.B.,** Transferrin receptor number, synthesis, and endocytosis during erythropoietin-induced maturation of Friend virus-infected erythroid cells, *J. Biol. Chem.,* 261, 9187, 1986.
95. **Ward, D.M. and Kaplan, J.,** Mitogenic agents induce redistribution of transferrin receptors from internal pools to the cell surface, *Biochem. J.,* 238, 721, 1986.
96. **Testa, E.P., Testa, U., Samoggia, P., Salvo, G., Camagna, A., and Peschle, C.,** Expression of transferrin receptors in human erythroleukemic lines: regulation in the plateau and exponential phase of growth, *Cancer Res.,* 45, 5330, 1986.
97. **Hori, T., Kashiyama, S., Oku, N., Hayakawa, M., Shibamoto, S., Tsujimoto, M., Nishihara, T., and Ito, F.,** Effects of tumor necrosis factor on cell growth and expression of transferrin receptors in human fibroblasts, *Cell Struct. Funct.,* 13, 425, 1988.

98. **Tanner, L.I. and Lienhard, G.E.,** Insulin elicits a redistribution of transferrin receptors in 3T3-L1 adipocytes through an increase in the rate constant for receptor externalization, *J. Biol. Chem.,* 262, 8975, 1987.
99. **Wiley, H.S. and Kaplan, J.,** Epidermal growth factor rapidly induces a redistribution of transferrin receptor pools in human fibroblasts, *Proc. Natl. Acad. Sci. U.S.A.,* 81, 7456, 1984.
100. **Bourgeade, M.-F., Silbermann, F., Thang, M.N., and Besancon, F.,** Reduction of transferrin receptor expression by interferon γ in a human cell line sensitive to its antiproliferative effect, *Biochem. Biophys. Res. Commun.,* 153, 897, 1988.
101. **Seiser, C., Teixeira, S., and Kuhn, L.C.,** Interleukin-2-dependent transcriptional and post-transcriptional regulation of transferrin receptor messenger RNA, *J. Biol. Chem.,* 268, 13074, 1993.
102. **Poola, I. and Lucas, J.J.,** Purification and characterization of an estrogen-inducible membrane glycoprotein. Evidence that it is a transferrin receptor, *J. Biol. Chem.,* 263, 19137, 1988.
103. **Neckers, L.M., Bauer, S., McGlennen, R.C., Trepel, J.B., Rao, K., and Greene, W.C.,** Diltiazem inhibits transferrin receptor expression and causes G1 arrest in normal and neoplastic T cells, *Mol. Cell. Biol.,* 6, 4244, 1986.
104. **Theil, E.C.,** Regulation of ferritin and transferrin receptor mRNAs, *J. Biol. Chem.,* 265, 4771, 1990.
105. **Larrick, J.W., Enns, C., Raubitschek, A., and Weintraub, H.,** Receptor-mediated endocytosis of human transferrin and its cell surface receptor, *J. Cell. Physiol.,* 124, 283, 1985.
106. **Rothenberger, S., Iacopetta, B.J., and Kühn, L.C.,** Endocytosis of the transferrin receptor requires the cytoplasmic domain but not its phosphorylation site, *Cell,* 49, 423, 1987.
107. **Iacopetta, B.J., Rothenberger, S., and Kühn, L.C.,** A role for the cytoplasmic domain in transferrin receptor sorting and coated pit formation during endocytosis, *Cell,* 54, 485, 1988.
108. **Jing, S., Spencer, T., Miller, K., Hopkins, C., and Trowbridge, I.S.,** Role of the human transferrin receptor cytoplasmic domain in endocytosis: localization of a specific signal sequence for internalization, *J. Cell Biol.,* 110, 283, 1990.
109. **Dautry-Varsat, A., Ciechanover, A., and Lodish, H.F.,** pH and the recycling of transferrin during receptor-mediated endocytosis, *Proc. Natl. Acad. Sci. U.S.A.,* 90, 2258, 1983.
110. **Hopkins, C.R. and Trowbridge, I.S.,** Internalization and processing of transferrin and the transferrin receptor in human carcinoma A431 cells, *J. Cell Biol.,* 97, 508, 1983.
111. **Watts, C.,** Rapid endocytosis of the transferrin receptor in the absence of bound transferrin, *J. Cell Biol.,* 100, 633, 1985.
112. **Ajioka, R.S. and Kaplan, J.,** Intracellular pools of transferrin receptors result from constitutive internalization of unoccupied receptors, *Proc. Natl. Acad. Sci. U.S.A.,* 83, 6445, 1986.
113. **van der Ende, A., du Maine, A., Schwartz, A.L., and Strous, G.J.,** Modulation of transferrin-receptor activity and recycling after induced differentiation of BeWo choriocarcinoma cells, *Biochem. J.,* 270, 451, 1990.
114. **Iacopetta, B., Carpentier, J.-L., Pozzan, T., Lew, D.P., Gorden, P., and Orci, L.,** Role of intracellular calcium and protein kinase C in the endocytosis of transferrin and insulin by HL60 cells, *J. Cell Biol.,* 103, 851, 1986.
115. **Hedley, D.W. and Musgrove, E.A.,** Transferrin receptor cycling by human lymphoid cells: lack of effect from inhibition of microtubule assembly, *Biochem. Biophys. Res. Commun.,* 138, 1216, 1986.
116. **Alcantara, O., Phillips, J.L., and Boldt, D.H.,** Phorbol diesters and transferrin modulate lymphoblastoid cell transferrin receptor expression by two different mechanisms, *J. Cell. Physiol.,* 129, 329, 1986.
117. **Boldt, D.H., Phillips, J.L., and Alcantara, O.,** Disparity between expression of transferrin receptor ligand binding and nonligand binding domains on human lymphocytes, *J. Cell. Physiol.,* 132, 331, 1987.
118. **Stein, B.S. and Sussman, H.H.,** Demonstration of two distinct transferrin receptor recycling pathways and transferrin-independent receptor internalization in K562 cells, *J. Biol. Chem.,* 261, 10319, 1986.
119. **Hunt, R.C. and Marshall-Carlson, L.,** Internalization and recycling of transferrin and its receptor. Effect of trifluoperazine on recycling in human erythroleukemic cells, *J. Biol. Chem.,* 261, 3681, 1986.
120. **Tsavaler, L., Stein, B.S., and Sussman, H.H.,** Demonstration of the specific binding of bovine transferrin to the human transferrin receptor in K562 cells: evidence of interspecies transferrin internalization, *J. Cell. Physiol.,* 128, 1, 1986.
121. **Trowbridge, I.S. and Omary, M.B.,** Human cell surface glycoprotein related to cell proliferation is the receptor for transferrin, *Proc. Natl. Acad. Sci. U.S.A.,* 78, 3039, 1981.

122. **Sorokin, L.M., Morgan, E.H., and Yeoh, G.C.T.**, Differences in transferrin receptor function between normal developing and transformed myogenic cells as revealed by differential effects of phorbol ester on receptor distribution and rates of iron uptake, *J. Biol. Chem.*, 263, 14128, 1988.
123. **Roberts, K.P. and Griswold, M.D.**, Characterization of rat transferrin receptor cDNA: the regulation of transferrin receptor mRNA in testes and in Sertoli cells in culture, *Mol. Endocrinol.*, 4, 531, 1990.
124. **Vanderpuye, O.A., Kelley, L.K., and Smith, C.H.**, Transferrin receptors in the basal plasma membrane of the human placental syncytiotrophoblast, *Placenta*, 7, 391, 1986.
125. **Neckers, L.M., Yenokida, G., Trepel, J.B., Lipford, E., and James, S.**, Transferrin receptor induction is required for human B-lymphocyte activation but not for immunoglobulin secretion, *J. Cell. Biochem.*, 27, 377, 1985.
126. **Cantrell, D.A. and Smith, K.A.**, The interleukin-2 T-cell system: a new cell growth model, *Science*, 224, 1326, 1984.
127. **Neckers, L.M. and Cossman, J.**, Transferrin receptor induction in mitogen-stimulated human T lymphocytes is required for DNA synthesis and cell division and is regulated by interleukin 2, *Proc. Natl. Acad. Sci. U.S.A.*, 80, 3494, 1983.
128. **Reed, J.C., Nowell, P.C., and Hoover, R.G.**, Regulation of c-*myc* mRNA levels in normal human lymphocytes by modulators of cell proliferation, *Proc. Natl. Acad. Sci. U.S.A.*, 82, 4221, 1985.
129. **Depper, J.M., Leonard, W.J., Drogula, C., Krönke, M., Waldmann, T.A., and Greene, W.C.**, Interleukin 2 (IL-2) augments transcription of the IL-2 receptor gene, *Proc. Natl. Acad. Sci. U.S.A.*, 82, 4230, 1985.
130. **Zirvi, K.A., Chee, D.O., and Hill, G.J.**, Continuous growth of human tumor cell lines in serum-free media, *In Vitro Cell. Dev. Biol.*, 22, 369, 1986.
131. **Taetle, R., Castagnola, J., and Mendelsohn, J.**, Mechanisms of growth inhibition by anti-transferrin receptor monoclonal antibodies, *Cancer Res.*, 46, 1759, 1986.
132. **Trowbridge, I.S. and Lopez, F.**, Monoclonal antibody to transferrin receptor blocks transferrin binding and inhibits human tumor cell growth in vitro, *Proc. Natl. Acad. Sci. U.S.A.*, 79, 1175, 1982.
133. **Lesley, J.F. and Schulte, R.J.**, Inhibition of cell growth by monoclonal anti-transferrin receptor antibodies, *Mol. Cell. Biol.*, 5, 1814, 1985.
134. **Kemp, J.D., Thorson, J.A., McAlmont, T.H., Horowitz, M., Cowdery, J.S., and Ballas, Z.K.**, Role of the transferrin receptor in lymphocyte growth: a rat IgG monoclonal antibody against the murine transferrin receptor produces highly selective inhibition of T and B cell activation protocols, *J. Immunol.*, 138, 2422, 1987.
135. **Taetle, R. and Honeysett, J.M.**, Effects of monoclonal anti-transferrin receptor antibodies on *in vitro* growth of human solid tumor cells, *Cancer Res.*, 47, 2040, 1987.
136. **Leenen, P.J.M., Kroos, M.J., Melis, M., Slieker, W.A.T., van Ewijk, W., and van Eijk, H.G.**, Differential inhibition of macrophage proliferation by anti-transferrin receptor antibody ER-MP21: correlation to macrophage differentiation stage, *Exp. Cell Res.*, 189, 55, 1990.
137. **Hopkins, C.R.**, The appearance and internalization of transferrin receptors at the margins of spreading human tumor cells, *Cell*, 40, 199, 1985.
138. **Warren, G., Davoust, J., and Cockroft, A.**, Recycling of transferrin receptors in A431 cells is inhibited during mitosis, *EMBO J.*, 3, 2217, 1984.
139. **Larrick, J.W. and Logue, G.**, Transferrin receptors on leukaemia cells, *Lancet*, 2, 862, 1980.
140. **Barnett, D., Wilson, G.A., Lawrence, A.C.K., and Buckley, G.A.**, Transferrin receptor expression in the leukaemias and lymphoproliferative disorders, *Clin. Lab. Haematol.*, 9, 361, 1987.
141. **Ho, P.T.C., King, I., and Sartorelli, A.C.**, Transcriptional regulation of the transferrin receptor in differentiating HL-60 cells, *Biochem. Biophys. Res. Commun.*, 138, 995, 1986.
142. **Medeiros, L.J., Picker, L.J., Horning, S.J., and Warnke, R.A.**, Transferrin receptor expression by non-Hodgkin's lymphomas: correlation with morphologic grade and survival, *Cancer*, 61, 1844, 1988.
143. **Esserman, L., Takahashi, S., Rojas, V., Warnke, R., and Levy, R.**, An epitope of the transferrin receptor is exposed on the cell surface of high-grade but not low-grade human lymphomas, *Blood*, 74, 2718, 1989.
144. **Petrini, M., Pelosi-Testa, E., Sposi, N.M., Mastroberardino, G., Camagna, A., Bottero, L., Mavilio, F., Testa, U., and Peschle, C.**, Constitutive expression and abnormal glycosylation of transferrin receptor in acute T-cell leukemia, *Cancer Res.*, 49, 6989, 1989.
145. **Walker, R.A. and Day, S.J.**, Transferrin receptor expression in non-malignant and malignant human breast tissue, *J. Pathol.*, 148, 217, 1986.

146. **Drewinko, B., Moskwa, P., and Reuben, J.,** Expression of transferrin receptors is unrelated to proliferative status in cultured human colon cancer cells, *Anticancer Res.,* 7, 139, 1987.
147. **Finkel, T. and Cooper, G.M.,** Detection of a molecular complex between *ras* proteins and transferrin receptor, *Cell,* 36, 1115, 1984.
148. **Harford, J.,** An artefact explains the appaHut association of the transferrin receptor with a *ras* gene product, *Nature,* 311, 673, 1984.
149. **Pelicci, P.G., Testa, U., Thomopoulos, P., Tabilio, A., Vanchenker, W., Titeux, M., Gourdin, M.F., and Rochant, H.,** Inhibition of transferrin binding and iron uptake of hematopoietic cell lines by phorbol esters, *Leukemia Res.,* 8, 597, 1984.
150. **Rovera, G., Ferreo, D., Pagliardi, G.L., Vartikar, J., Pessano, S., Bottero, L., Abraham, S., and Lebman, D.,** Induction of differentiation of human myeloid leukemias by phorbol diesters: phenotypic changes and mode of action, *Ann. N.Y. Acad. Sci.,* 397, 211, 1982.
151. **Ho, P.T.C., Ishiguro, K., and Sartorelli, A.C.,** Regulation of transferrin receptor in myeloid and monocytic differentiation of HL-60 leukemia cells, *Cancer Res.,* 49, 1989, 1989.
152. **Barker, K.A. and Newburger, P.E.,** Relationships between the cell cycle and the expression of c-*myc* and transferrin receptor genes during induced myeloid differentiation, *Exp. Cell Res.,* 186, 1, 1990.
153. **Klausner, R.D., Harford, J., and van Renswoude, J.,** Rapid internalization of the transferrin receptor in K562 cells is triggered by ligand binding or treatment with a phorbol ester, *Proc. Natl. Acad. Sci. U.S.A.,* 81, 3005, 1984.
154. **Kohno, H., Taketani, S., and Tokunaga, R.,** Phobol ester-induced regulation of transferrin receptors in human leukemia K562 cells, *Cell Struct. Funct.,* 11, 181, 1986.
155. **Fallon, R.J. and Schwartz, A.L.,** Regulation by phorbol esters of a sialoglycoprotein and transferrin receptor distribution and ligand affinity in a hepatoma cell line, *J. Biol. Chem.,* 261, 15081, 1986.
156. **Trepel, J.B., Colamonici, O.R., Kelly, K., Schwab, G., Watt, R.A., Sausville, E.A., Jaffe, E.S., and Neckers, L.M.,** Transcriptional inactivation of c-*myc* and the transferrin receptor in dibutyryl cyclic AMP-treated HL-60 cells, *Mol. Cell. Biol.,* 7, 2644, 1987.
157. **Hradilek, A. and Neuwirt, J.,** Iron uptake from transferrin and transferrin endocytic cycle in Friend erythroleukemia cells, *J. Cell. Physiol.,* 133, 192, 1987.
158. **Riss, T.L. and Sirbasku, D.A.,** Purification and identification of transferrin as a major pituitary-derived mitogen for MTW9/PL2 rat mammary tumor cells, *In Vitro Cell. Dev. Biol.,* 23, 841, 1987.
159. **Iizuka, Y. and Murphy, M.J., Jr.,** Colony formation of granulocyte (CFU-g) and macrophage (CFU-m) precursors in serum- and albumin-free culture: effect of transferrin on clonal growth, *Exp. Cell Biol.,* 54, 275, 1986.
160. **Tsao, M.-S., Sanders, G.H.S., and Grisham, J.W.,** Regulation of growth of cultured hepatic epithelial cells by transferrin, *Exp. Cell Res.,* 171, 52, 1987.
161. **Jing, H.Y. and Findlay, J.K.,** An inhibitory effect of transferrin on differentiation of rat granulosa cells in vitro, *Endocrinology,* 128, 1841, 1991.
162. **Denstman, S., Hromchak, R., Guan, X.P., and Bloch, A.,** Identification of transferrin as a progression factor for ML1 human myelocytic leukemia cell differentiation, *J. Biol. Chem.,* 266, 14873, 1991.
163. **Sun, I.L., Garcia-Cañero, R., Liu, W., Toole-Simms, W., Crane, F.L., Morré, D.J., and Löw, H.,** Diferric transferrin reduction stimulates the Na^+/H^+ antiport of HeLa cells, *Biochem. Biophys. Res. Commun.,* 145, 467, 1987.
164. **Hayashi, O., Noguchi, S., and Oyasu, R.,** Transferrin as a growth factor for rat bladder carcinoma cells in culture, *Cancer Res.,* 47, 4560, 1987.
165. **Rossi, M.C. and Zetter, B.R.,** Selective stimulation of prostatic carcinoma cell proliferation by transferrin, *Proc. Natl. Acad. Sci. U.S.A.,* 89, 6197, 1992.

INDEX

A

Acetylcholine, 104
Acetylsalicylate, 259
Aclacinomycin A, 343
Acquired immune deficiency syndrome (AIDS), 9, 14, 45
  colony-stimulating factor-2 and, 191
  interleukin-2 and, 56, 61, 63, 67, 68, 77–79
  interleukin-6 and, 98
  interleukin-10 and, 103
  tumor necrosis factor and, 242
  tumor necrosis factor-α and, 259
Acquired immune deficiency syndrome (AIDS)-related complex (ARC), 45
ACTH, see Adrenocorticotropic hormone
Actin, 304
Actin-binding proteins, 73, see also specific types
Actinomycin D, 18, 258, 259
Activator of DNA replication (ADR), 75
Activin A, 285, 286
Acute lymphocytic leukemia (ALL), 6
  B-cell growth factors and, 89
  colony-stimulating factor-1 and, 181, 182, 184
  interferon and, 228, 230
  interleukin-2 and, 59, 67, 69, 70, 77
  interleukin-3 and, 86
  interleukin-7 and, 100
Acute monocytic leukemia (AML), 6–9, 15
  colony-stimulating factor-1 and, 182, 184, 185
  colony-stimulating factor-2 and, 188, 189
  colony-stimulating factor-3 and, 191, 195
  interleukin-1 and, 36, 52
  interleukin-3 and, 86
  interleukin-11 and, 103
Acute promyelocytic leukemia (APML), 192
Adenocarcinomas, 3, 36, see also specific types
Adenoviruses, 61, 255, see also specific types
Adenylate cyclase, 194
Adenylyl cyclase, 66, 71, 248
Adipocytes, 255
Adipogenesis inhibitory factor, 103
ADR, see Activator of DNA replication
Adrenocorticotropic hormone (ACTH), 40, 96, 253
Adriamycin, 259
Adult T-cell leukemia (ATL) cells, 38, 44, 69, 76–77
Aging, 62–63
Agranulocytosis, 195
AIDS, see Acquired immune deficiency syndrome
Alkaline phosphatase, 39, 186, 191, 195, 253
Alkalinization, 177, 303
ALL, see Acute lymphocytic leukemia
Allergic diseases, 93, see also specific types
Alveolar macrophages, 8
Amiloride, 49
AML, see Acute monocytic leukemia
Amyloid A, 251
Androstenedione, 253
Angiogenesis, 101, 252
Angiotensin II, 299
Anorexia, 255, 256

Antibodies, 82, see also specific types
  B-cell growth factors and, 87
  immunoglobulin, 93
  immunoglobulin E, 90
  immunoglobulin G, 342
  interleukin-4 and, 90, 93
  interleukin-12 and, 104
  monoclonal, see Monoclonal antibodies
  OKT11A, 16
  production of, 87
  to transferrin receptors, 342
Antiinflammatory drugs, 259, see also specific types
Antitumor immune response, 46
Aortic smooth muscle cells, 295
APML, see Acute promyelocytic leukemia
Apoptosis, 1, 255, 282
Apotransferrin, 338, 341
Arachidonic acid, 46, 50
  colony-stimulating factor-2 and, 188
  colony-stimulating factor-3 and, 194
  interferon and, 222
  interleukin-2 and, 55, 62
  interleukin-3 and, 84
  platelet-derived growth factor and, 302, 303
  tumor necrosis factor-α and, 248, 250
Arterial smooth muscle cells, 294, 296
Arthritis, 39, 45, 101
Ascites tumor cells, 104, 225
Astrocytes, 7, 44, 83, 187, 193
Astrocytoma, 96
Atherogenesis, 181
Atherosclerosis, 296, 297, 309
ATL, see Adult T-cell leukemia
Autocrine, 14, 181, 244
Autocrine growth factor, 35, 89
Autoimmune disorders, 40, 80, see also specific types
Autoimmune processes, 12
Autophosphorylation, 182, 299
Avridine, 230
Azacytidine, 45, 227

B

Bacillus Calmette-Guerin (BCG), 243, 244
Bacterial endotoxins, 4, 45, 81, 179, see also specific types
Bacterial infections, 68, 221, 243, 244, 252, 255
Bacterial interleukin-1 receptors, 48–49
BAF (B-cell activating factor), see Interleukin-1
Basophilic erythroblasts, 279
Basophils, 7, 93, 177
BCDF, see B-cell differentiation factor
B-cell activating factor (BAF), see Interleukin-1
B-cell chronic lymphocytic leukemia, 88, 89, 90, 259
B-cell-derived T-cell growth factor, see Interleukin-10
B-cell differentiation factor (BCDF), 87
B-cell growth factor (BCGF), 16, 87–89
B-cell growth factor I (BCGF-I), see Interleukin-4
B-cell growth factor II (BCGF-II), see Interleukin-5
B-cell hybridoma growth factor, see Interleukin-6
B-cell leukemias, 69, 77, 88–90, 259, see also specific types

B-cell lymphomas, 70, 86, 89, see also specific types
B-cells, 9, 16, 36, 37
   activation of, 88
   colony-stimulating factor-1 and, 179, 181
   colony-stimulating factor-2 and, 185, 187, 190
   differentiation of, 35, 87–88, 90, 93, 99, 190
   interferon and, 221, 223, 224, 228, 229
   interleukin-1 and, 37, 40, 41, 44, 51
   interleukin-2 and, 53, 55, 61
   interleukin-3 and, 80, 81, 86
   interleukin-5 and, 93, 94
   interleukin-6 and, 95–97
   interleukin-7 and, 99
   interleukin-10 and, 102, 103
   interleukin-11 and, 103
   interleukin-13 and, 104
   pancreatic, 51
   proliferation of, 87–88, 90, 93, 99
   resting, 93
   stimulation of, 15
   transferrin and, 342
B-cell stimulatory factor (BSF), 87, 88, 93, 198, 223
B-cell stimulatory factor 1 (BSF-1), see Interleukin-4
B-cell stimulatory factor 2 (BSF-2), see Interleukin-6
BCG, see Bacillus Calmette-Guerin
BCGF, see B-cell growth factor
BCGF-I (B-cell growth factor I), see Interleukin-4
BCGF-II (B-cell growth factor II), see Interleukin-5
BCHGF (B-cell hybridoma growth factor), see Interleukin-6
Beta-adrenergic receptor agonists, 67, see also specific types
BFU, see Burst-forming unit
Bicarbonate ions, 335
Biological effects
   of colony-stimulating factor-1, 177
   of colony-stimulating factor-2, 185–186, 191
   of colony-stimulating factor-3, 191–192
   of erythropoietin, 281–282
   of interleukin-1, 36–41, 43
   of interleukin-2, 53–55
   of interleukin-3, 80–81
   of interleukin-4, 90–92
   of interleukin-6, 95–96, 103
   of interleukin-7, 99
   of interleukin-8, 101
   of interleukin-11, 103
   of interleukin-12, 104
   of leukemia inhibitory factor, 105
   of tumor necrosis factor, 241
   of tumor necrosis factor-α, 241
   of tumor necrosis factor-β, 241
Biopterin, 72
Bladder carcinoma, 5, 187, 192, 227, 313
Blast cells, 181, 189, 195
Blastocysts, 105
Blood coagulation, 252–253
Bombesin, 302
Bone marrow, 1, 3, 5, 17, 18
   colony-stimulating factors and, 177
   fetal, 2
   interleukin-11 and, 103
   megakaryocyte colony-stimulating factors and, 196
   proto-oncogenes in, 4
Bone marrow stem cells, 7
Bone marrow stroma, 2
Bone marrow stromal cells, 4, 9, 36, 95

Bone metabolism, 105
Bone remodeling, 38, 253
Bone resorption, 38, 39, 92, 253
Bone tissue, 38–40, 253
BPA, see Burst-promoting activity
BPA-E (erythroid burst-promoting activity), see Interleukin-3
Brain tumors, 102
Breast cancer, 7, 52, 244
   colony-stimulating factor-2 and, 186
   interferon and, 229
   platelet-derived growth factor and, 311, 313
   transferrin and, 337
   tumor necrosis factor-α and, 246, 250
8-Bromo-cyclic AMP, 314
9-Bromo-cyclic AMP, 305
BSF, see B-cell stimulatory factor
BSF-1 (B-cell stimulatory factor 1), see Interleukin-4
BSF-2 (B-cell stimulatory factor 2), see Interleukin-6
B-TCGF (B-cell-derived T-cell growth factor), see Interleukin-10
Burkitt's lymphoma, 18, 92, 103
Burst-forming units (BFUs), 196, 279
Burst-promoting activity (BPA), 279

C

Cachectin, 243, 255–256
Cachexia, 105, 245, 251, 255, 256
Calcitriol, 18, 44, 62
   colony-stimulating factor-1 and, 182
   colony-stimulating factor-2 and, 186, 187
   interferon and, 226
   interleukin-3 and, 80
   interleukin-6 and, 97
   leukemia inhibitory factor and, 104
   tumor necrosis factor-α and, 260
Calcium, 45, 46, 49, 50
   B-cell growth factors and, 87, 88
   colony-stimulating factor-2 and, 188
   colony-stimulating factor-3 and, 194
   erythropoietic growth factor and, 284, 286
   extracellular, 72
   influx of, 92, 300
   interferon and, 222, 224, 225
   interleukin-2 and, 62, 72
   interleukin-3 and, 80, 82
   interleukin-4 and, 92
   interleukin-5 and, 94
   intracellular, 58, 248, 303
   intracellular mobilization of, 68, 74, 225, 248, 286, 301
   mobilization of, 68, 74, 222, 225, 248, 286, 301, 302
   phosphoinositide metabolism and translocation of, 301–302
   platelet-derived growth factor and, 300–303
   redistribution of, 94
   translocation of, 301–302
   tumor necrosis factor-α and, 248
Calcium ionophores, 16, 54, 62, 249, 302, 306, see also specific types
Cancer, 6, 9, 12, see also Tumors; specific types
   B-cell growth factors and, 89
   bladder, 5, 187, 192, 227, 313
   breast, see Breast cancer
   colon, 3, 188, 229, 259
   colony-stimulating factor-1 and, 182, 184–185
   colony-stimulating factor-2 and, 188–189, 191

colony-stimulating factor-3 and, 193, 195–196
endometrial, 185
epithelial, 185
erythropoietin and, 284–285
gastric, 93, 188, 227, 313
head and neck, 77
hematopoietic growth factors and, 14–15
hemotopoietic growth factors and, 14–15
interferon and, 221, 226, 228–230
interleukin-2 and, 76–77, 79
interleukin-2 receptors and, 76–77
interleukin-3 and, 86
interleukin-4 and, 91, 93
interleukin-6 and, 98–99
interleukin-7 and, 100
interleukin-8 and, 102
interleukin-9 and, 102
interleukin-10 and, 103
interleukin-11 and, 103
lung, see Lung cancer
non-small-cell lung, 188
ovarian, 52, 98, 185, 256, 259
platelet-derived growth factor and, 310–314
platelet-derived growth factor-like factors and, 310–314
stomach, 93, 188, 227, 313
systemic manifestations of, 98
transferrin and, 336, 337, 344
transferrin receptors and, 342–344
treatment of, 15, 79
tumor necrosis factor-α and, 250, 256–259
Cap-binding protein, 249
Carbonate ions, 335
Carcinomas, see also Cancer; specific types
bladder, 5, 187, 192, 227, 313
breast, see Breast cancer
cervical, 52, 245, 247, 249
colon, 229, 259
colony-stimulating factor-2 and, 186, 187, 191
colony-stimulating factor-3 and, 192, 194
embryonal, 313
epidermoid, 226, 339, 343
erythropoietic growth factor and, 284
gastric, 93, 227, 313
hepatocellular, 284
interferon and, 227, 229
interleukin-3 and, 80, 82, 86
interleukin-4 and, 93
laryngeal, 246
lung, see Lung cancer
nasopharyngeal, 45
ovarian, 256
pancreatic, 178
platelet-derived growth factor and, 297, 311, 313
prostatic, 98, 344
renal cell, 93
small-cell lung, 86, 194
squamous cell, 38, 80, 192, 227
stomach, 93, 227, 313
thyroid, 297
transferrin and, 339, 343, 344
tumor necrosis factor-α and, 244–247, 249, 253, 255, 256, 259
tumor necrosis factor-β and, 255
Cartilage, 38–40, 253
Castanospermine, 180

Catecholamines, 104, see also specific types
CBGF, see Colostrum basic growth factor
Cell-bound antigens, 56
Cell differentiation, 35, see also specific types of cells
inhibitors of, 260
interferon and, 227–229
interleukin-1 and, 52–53
interleukin-3 and, 86
regulation of, 221
transferrin and, 343–344
tumor necrosis factor-α and, 260
Cell proliferation, see also under specific types of cells
interferon and, 226–230, 252
interleukin-1 and, 52–53
platelet-derived growth factor and, 306
regulation of, 221
transferrin and, 339, 344
tumor necrosis factor and, 241
Cellular proteins, 71, see also specific types
Ceramide, 248, 249
Cervical carcinoma, 52, 245, 247, 249
CFUs, see Colony-forming units
Chemotherapy, 9, see also specific types
Cholera toxin, 314
Cholinergic neuronal differentiation factor (CNDF), see Leukemia inhibitory factor (LIF)
Chondrocytes, 39, 44, 45
Chondrosarcoma, 50
Choriocarcinoma, 179, 181, 183, 194
Chronic lymphocytic leukemia (CLL), 193
B-cell, 88–90, 259
B-cell growth factors and, 88, 89
interleukin-2 and, 59, 69
interleukin-4 and, 90
interleukin-7 and, 100
tumor necrosis factor-α and, 258
Chronic myeloid leukemia (CML), 5, 70, 257, 337
CIL, see Colony-inhibiting lymphokine
Ciliary neurotrophic factor (CNTF), 12, 103
CLL, see Chronic lymphocytic leukemia
CLMF (cytotoxic lymphocyte maturation factor), see Interleukin-12
CML, see Chronic myeloid leukemia
CNDF (cholinergic neuronal differentiation factor), see Leukemia inhibitory factor (LIF)
CNTF, see Ciliary neurotrophic factor
Cobalt chloride, 281
Collagen, 39, 252
Collagenase, 304
Colon cancer, 3, 188, 229, 259
Colony-forming units, 7, 13, 196, 251, 279, 281, 286
Colony-inhibiting lymphokine (CIL), 13
Colony-stimulating activity (CSA), 39, 197
megakaryocyte, see Megakaryocyte colony-stimulating factors (MK-CSFs)
multilineage, see Interleukin-3
Colony-stimulating factor (CSF), 5–10, 13, 15, 18, 177–198, see also specific types
B-cell growth factors and, 87
biological effects of, 177, 181, 185–186, 191–192
classification of, 7–8
eosinophil, see Interleukin-5
formation of, 198
hematopoiesis and, 1, 3
interleukin-1 and, 37, 40, 44, 52

interleukin-2 and, 53, 66, 75
interleukin-3 and, 81, 82, 85, 86
interleukin-6 and, 95
interleukin-12 and, 104
megakaryocyte, 196–197
multilineage, 3
multipotential, see Interleukin-3
production of, 95, 178–179, 187, 190, 193
regulation of, 8
structure of, 177–178, 186–187, 192–193
tumor necrosis factor-α and, 254
Colony-stimulating factor (CSF) receptors, 35, 81, see also specific types
Colony-stimulating factor-1 (CSF-1), 177–185, 228
  biological effects of, 177
  cancer and, 184–185
  deficiency of, 179
  gene expression by, 183
  genes of, 177–178
  genetic deficiency of, 179
  mechanisms of action of, 183
  postreceptor mechanisms of action of, 183
  production of, 178–179
  proto-oncogenes and, 181, 183–184
  structure of, 177–178
Colony-stimulating factor-1 (CSF-1) receptors, 179–183, 251
Colony-stimulating factor-2 (CSF-2), 185–191
  biological effects of, 185–186, 191
  cancer and, 188–189, 191
  colony-stimulating factor-3 and, 191
  erythropoietic growth factor and, 279
  genes of, 186–187, 190
  mechanisms of action of, 188
  megakaryocyte colony-stimulating factors and, 197
  postreceptor mechanisms of action of, 188
  production of, 187, 190
  proto-oncogenes and, 189–190
  structure of, 186–187
  tumor necrosis factor-α and, 244, 254
Colony-stimulating factor-2 (CSF-2) receptors, 187–188
Colony-stimulating factor-3 (CSF-3), 191–196
  biological effects of, 191–192
  cancer and, 193, 195–196
  colony-stimulating factor-2 and, 191
  erythropoietic growth factor and, 279
  formation of, 198
  genes of, 192–193
  in vivo administration of, 194–195
  mechanisms of action of, 194
  postreceptor mechanisms of action of, 194
  production of, 193
  proto-oncogenes and, 194
  structure of, 192–193
Colony-stimulating factor-3 (CSF-3) receptors, 193–194
Colostrum basic growth factor (CBGF), 295
Complement factor B, 95
Complement protein factors, 38
Con A, see Concanavalin A
Conalbumin, 340
Concanavalin A
  interleukin-1 and, 37, 45, 47
  interleukin-2 and, 53, 54, 66, 74
  interleukin-4 and, 92
  interleukin-6 and, 95
  interleukin-7 and, 99

macrophage-derived growth factors and, 198
tumor necrosis factor-α and, 247
Connective tissue, 38–40, 105
Connective tissue-activating peptide, 101
Converter proteins, 67, see also specific types
Corticosteroids, 223, see also specific types
Corticotropin releasing factor (CRF), 40, 253
CRF, see Corticotropin releasing factor
CRH, see Cytokine receptor homologous
CSA, see Colony-stimulating activity
CSF, see Colony-stimulating factor
CSIF (cytokine synthesis inhibitory factor), see Interleukin-10
Cyclic AMP, 71, 248, 253, 300, 314
Cyclic AMP-dependent protein kinase, 248
Cyclic GMP, 248
Cycloheximide, 258, 305
Cyclooxygenase, 50, 84
Cyclooxygenase inhibitors, 52
Cyclophosphamide, 9, 55, 259
Cyclosporin A, 16, 66, 68
Cyclosporine, 79
Cyclosporine A, 187
Cytochromes, 247, 335, see also specific types
Cytokine receptor homologous domain, 40, 96, 193
Cytokine receptors, 282, see also specific types
Cytokines, 4, 9–13, 35–36, 241, see also specific types
  bone resorption and, 38, 39
  cellular responses to, 12
  characterization of, 10
  hemotopoietic growth factors and, 5
  induction of, 105
  inflammatory, 241
  inhibitory activity of, 36
  interactions between, 251
  interleukin-2 and other, 68, 78
  leukemia inhibitory factor and, 105
  megakaryocyte colony-stimulating factors and, 196
  networks of, 35
  receptors of, 10, 12
  stromal cell-derived, see Interleukin-11
  synthesis of, 102
  transductional mechanisms of, 35
  tumor necrosis factor and other, 241
  tumor necrosis factor-α and other, 259
Cytokine synthesis inhibitory factor (CSIF), see Interleukin-10
Cytolysin, 241
Cytomegaloviruses, 68, see also specific types
Cytophoblasts, 309
Cytoplasmic alkalinization, 303
Cytoskeletal changes, 304
Cytotoxic lymphocyte maturation factor (CLMF), see Interleukin-12
Cytotoxins, 241, see also specific types

D

Daudi cells, 17, 18, 225, 226, 339
Decarboxylation, 252
Dendritic cells, 39, 43, 56
Dermal fibroblasts, 39
Dexamethasone, 16, 44, 62, 68, 187
D-factor (differentiation-inducing factor), see Leukemia inhibitory factor (LIF)
Diabetes, 12, 41, 96, 251

Diacylglycerol, 51, 68, 72
  interferon and, 224
  interleukin-3 and, 84
  platelet-derived growth factor and, 301, 302, 303
  transferrin and, 339
Differentiation-inducing activity (DIA), see Leukemia inhibitory factor (LIF)
Differentiation-inducing factor (D-factor), see Leukemia inhibitory factor (LIF)
Digestive tract, 38
Diltiazem, 340
Dimethyl sulfoxide (DMSO), 17, 182, 195, 311, 343, 344
DMSO, see Dimethyl sulfoxide
DNA-binding proteins, 336, see also specific types
DNA methylation, 227
DNA replication, 75, 228, 306
DNA synthesis, 40, 250, 284
  interleukin-2 and, 75
  platelet-derived growth factor and, 295–297, 302, 304, 306, 307, 309
  transferrin and, 344
DNA viruses, 241, 252, see also specific types

E

EBPA, see Erythroid burst-promoting activity
EBPA (erythroid burst-promoting activity), see Interleukin-3
EBV, see Epstein Barr virus
ECGF, see Endothelial cell growth factor
ECM, see Extracellular matrix
ECSF, see Erythroid cell-stimulating factor
EDF, see Erythroid differentiation factor
EGF, see Epidermal growth factor
Ehrlich ascites tumor cells, 225
Elastin, 249
Embryogenesis, 105, 313
Embryonal carcinoma, 313
Embryonic cells, 105, 197, 294
Encephalomyocarditis virus, 222
Endocrine system, 40–41, 55, 96, 253–254
Endocytosis, 223, 247, 341
Endogenous hormones, 4, see also specific types
Endometrial cancer, 185
Endometrium, 35
Endorphins, 40, 50, 51
Endothelial cell growth factor, 12, 98, 293, 295, 314
Endothelial cells, 4, 7, 9, 12, 35
  colony-stimulating factor-1 and, 179
  colony-stimulating factor-2 and, 187
  colony-stimulating factor-3 and, 193, 194
  erythropoietic growth factor and, 283
  interleukin-1 and, 39, 40, 44, 52
  interleukin-3 and, 80
  interleukin-6 and, 97
  interleukin-8 and, 101
  platelet-derived growth factor and, 294, 295, 309
  tumor necrosis factor-α and, 249, 252
Endothelium, 92
Endotoxic shock, 251
Endotoxins, see also specific types
  bacterial, 4, 45, 81, 179
  interleukin-10 and, 102
  tumor necrosis factor-α and, 243, 252, 253
Eo-CSF (eosinophil colony-stimulating factor), see Interleukin-5

Eosinophil colony-stimulating factor , see Interleukin-5
Eosinophils, 7, 63, 81, 93, 177, 185
EPA, see Erythroid-potentiating activity
Epidermal cell-derived thymocyte activating factor, 44
Epidermal growth factor (EGF), 7
  interferon and, 221
  interleukin-1 and, 38
  platelet-derived growth factor and, 295, 296, 303–304, 306, 307, 311, 314
  transferrin and, 340
  tumor necrosis factor-α and, 248, 254, 255
Epidermal growth factor receptors, 227, 228, 254, 303, 307
Epidermoid carcinoma, 226, 339, 343
Epithelial cancer, 185
Epithelial cells, 98, 258
Epithelial fungus infections, 40
Epstein Barr virus (EBV), 43, 44, 48, 88, 89
  colony-stimulating factor-1 and, 179
  interferon and, 223
  interleukin-5 and, 93
  interleukin-10 and, 102, 103
  tumor necrosis factor and, 242
  tumor necrosis factor-α and, 251
Erythroblastic leukemia, 284
Erythroblasts, 17, 279
Erythrocytes, 1
Erythrocytosis, 283
Erythroid burst-promoting activity (EBPA, BPA-E), see Interleukin-3
Erythroid cells, 37, 81
  colony-stimulating factor-2 and, 186, 191
  colony-stimulating factor-3 and, 191
  differentiation of, 280, 286
  erythropoietic growth factor and, 279, 280, 286
  interleukin-4 and, 91
  progenitor, 81, 102, 281, 282
  tumor necrosis factor-α and, 254
Erythroid cell-stimulating factor (ECSF), 279
Erythroid differentiation factor (EDF), 285–286
Erythroid-potentiating activity (EPA), 279–280
Erythroid progenitor cells, 81, 102, 281, 282
Erythroleukemias, 280, 283, 285, 286, 339, 344
Erythropoiesis, 1, 82, 279, 286
Erythropoietic growth factor, 279–286
Erythropoietin, 6
  biological effects of, 281–282
  cancer and, 284–285
  colony-stimulating factor-2 and, 186, 188
  colony-stimulating factor-3 and, 192
  defined, 281
  erythropoietic growth factor and, 281–285
  genes of, 282
  interleukin-1 and, 37
  interleukin-2 and, 66
  interleukin-3 and, 81
  interleukin-9 and, 102
  mechanisms of action of, 283–284
  megakaryocyte colony-stimulating factors and, 196, 197
  origin of, 281
  postreceptor mechanisms of action of, 283–284
  structure of, 282
  synthesis of, 281
  transferrin and, 340
Erythropoietin receptors, 35, 282–283, 285
Estradiol, 96

Estrogen, 96, 337, 340
Estrogen receptors, 279
Etoposide, 259
Eucosanoids, 84
Exotoxins, 93, see also specific types
Extracellular matrix (ECM), 39, 296

F

Factor P40, see Interleukin-9
FAF (fibroblast-activating factor), see Interleukin-1
Ferritin, 340
Fetal bone marrow, 2
FGF, see Fibroblast growth factor
Fibroblast-activating factor (FAF), see Interleukin-1
Fibroblast growth factor (FGF), 197
    erythropoietic growth factor and, 279
    interferon and, 221
    platelet-derived growth factor and, 295, 297
    tumor necrosis factor-α and, 254
Fibroblastoid cells, 37, 97
Fibroblasts, 4, 7, 9, 35
    colony-stimulating factor-1 and, 178
    colony-stimulating factor-2 and, 187
    colony-stimulating factor-3 and, 192, 193
    dermal, 39
    interferon and, 221, 222, 230
    interleukin-1 and, 38, 39, 43, 44, 48, 51
    interleukin-6 and, 95, 97
    interleukin-8 and, 101
    platelet-derived growth factor and, 295, 296, 298, 302, 303, 305, 306
    proliferation of, 43
    tumor necrosis factor-α and, 244, 248–250, 254
Fibronectin, 193, 305
Fibrosarcomas, see also specific types
    colony-stimulating factor-3 and, 192
    macrophage-derived growth factors and, 198
    platelet-derived growth factor and, 312
    tumor necrosis factor-α and, 253, 256–259
5-Fluorouracil, 259
Flutenamic acid, 39
Follicle-stimulating hormone (FSH), 286, 336, 342
Follistatin, 286
Forskolin, 97, 341
Friend erythroleukemias, 344
Friend murine leukemia virus, 285
FSH, see Follicle-stimulating hormone
Fungal infections, 40, 252
Fungoides, 76

G

GALV, see Gibbon ape leukemia virus
GAP, see Guanosine triphosphatase activating protein
Gastric cancer, 93, 188, 227, 313
GCF (granulocyte chemotactic factor), see Interleukin-8
G-CSF (granulocyte colony-stimulating factor), see Colony-stimulating factor-3 (CSF-3)
Gene expression
    colony-stimulating factor-1 and, 183
    erythropoietic growth factor and, 279, 284
    in hematopoiesis, 4
    interferon and, 224–227

    interleukin-1 and, 51
    interleukin-2 and, 74
    interleukin-3 and, 82
    interleukin-4 and, 92
    regulation of, 224
    transferrin and, 337
Genistein, 302
Germ cells, 6
Gibbon ape leukemia virus (GALV), 63
Gibbon leukemia virus (GLV), 61
Glial cells, 296, 298
Glioblastomas, 7, 96, 98, 225, 312
Glioma-derived growth factor, 294
Gliomas, 44, 83, 230, 299, 308, 312
Glucocorticoid receptors, 68
Glucocorticoids, 40, 44, 48, see also specific types
    colony-stimulating factor-3 and, 192
    interleukin-2 and, 55, 62
    interleukin-6 and, 98
    tumor necrosis factor-α and, 250, 255
Glucose, 40, 183, 249, 304
Glutathione, 252
Glycolysis, 304
Glycosylation, 57, 60, 94, 96, 105, 343
GM-CSF (granulocyte-macrophage colony-stimulating factor), see Colony-stimulating factor-2(CSF-2)
Gonadotropin, 96, 179, 253, 336
Gonads, 40–41, 55, 253
G protein-coupled receptor, 62
G proteins, 84, 101, 188, 194, 198, 248
Granulocyte chemotactic factor (GCF), see Interleukin-8
Granulocyte colony-stimulating factor (G-CSF), see Colony-stimulating factor-3 (CSF-3)
Granulocyte-macrophage colony-stimulating factor (GM-CSF), see Colony- stimulating factor-1 (CSF-1)
Granulocytes, 1, 7, 8, 17, 44
    colony-stimulating factor-1 and, 183
    colony-stimulating factor-2 and, 185
    colony-stimulating factor-3 and, 191
    interleukin-3 and, 80
    transferrin and, 337
    tumor necrosis factor-α and, 251, 252
Granulocytic leukemias, see Myeloid leukemias
Granulocytopoiesis, 37
Granulocytosis, 101
Granulopoiesis, 1, 191, 252
Granulosa cells, 41, 253, 344
Graves' disease, 40
Growth factors, see specific types
Growth hormone, 12, 40, 74, 194, 253
Growth hormone receptor, 35
GTP, see Guanosine triphosphate
Guanosine triphosphatase, 248
Guanosine triphosphatase activating protein, 12, 284, 302
Guanosine triphosphate (GTP) binding, 71, 248

H

Hairy-cell leukemia, 67, 69, 88, 89, 225, 229, 259
Haptoglobin, 95
HCGF, see Hepatocyte growth factor
Head and neck cancer, 77
Heart transplants, 297
HeLa cells, 52, 226, 229, 246, 247, 250

Hematopoiesis, 1–4
  colony-stimulating factors and, 177
  control of, 1–3
  gene expression in, 4
  growth factor regulation of, 2–3
  inhibitors of, 8
  interleukin-1 and, 36–38
  interleukin-6 and, 94
  interleukin-9 and, 102
  regulation of, 2–5, 13, 94, 251
  tumor necrosis factor-α and, 251–252
Hematopoietic cells
  colony-stimulating factor-1 and, 178
  erythropoietic growth factor and, 283
  interferon and, 225, 226, 229
  interleukin-1 effects on, 36–38
  platelet-derived growth factor and, 311
  transferrin and, 337, 343
  tumor necrosis factor-α and, 254
Hematopoietic growth factors (HGFs), 1–18, 59, 78, see also specific types
  cancer and, 14–15
  characterization of, 2
  colony-stimulating factors and, see Colony-stimulating factor
  cytokines and, 4, 9–13
  growth stimulating effects of, 13
  hematopoiesis and, 1–4
  hematopoietic inhibiting factors and, 13–14
  lineage-specific, 3
  multilineage, 3, 5
  oncogenes and, 15, 18
  pluripotent, 5–7
  proto-oncogenes and, 4–6, 10, 12, 16–18
  receptors of, 5
  tumor suppressor genes and, 4, 16–18
Hematopoietic inhibiting factors, 13–14
Hematopoietic progenitor cells, 2, 13
Hematopoietic stem cells, 1, 95, 191, 196
Hematopoietin-2, see Interleukin-3
Hematopoietins, 12, see also specific types
Hemin, 339
Hemoglobin, 286, 335, 342, 344
Hemopoiesis, see Hematopoiesis
Hemopoietins, 5, 42
Heparin, 279, 297
Hepatic adenocarcinoma, 36
Hepatitis, 68
Hepatocellular carcinoma, 284
Hepatocyte growth factor (HCGF), 3, 314
Hepatocytes, 38, 197, 344
Hepatocyte-stimulating factor (HSF), 95, 223, see also Interleukin-1
Hepatocyte-stimulating factor-III (HSF-III), see Leukemia inhibitory factor (LIF)
Hepatomas, 38, 281, 311, 313, 343
Hexamethylene biacetamide, 182
HGFs, see Hematopoietic growth factors
HGPRT, see Hypoxanthine-guanine phosphoribosyltransferase
HILDA (human interleukin for DA cells), see Leukemia inhibitory factor (LIF)
Histiocytic leukemia, 43
Histiocytic lymphomas, 13, 44, 246, 247
Histiocytosis, 44
HIV, see Human immunodeficiency virus
Hodgkin's disease, 44, 70, 98, 102, 311

Homing, 56
Hormones, see also specific types
  adrenocorticotropic, 40, 96, 253
  colony-stimulating factor-2 and, 188
  colony-stimulating factor-3 and, 194
  cytokines and, 35
  endogenous, 4
  erythropoietic growth factor and, 281
  follicle-stimulating, 286, 336, 342
  growth, 12, 35, 40, 74, 194, 253
  interferon and, 221
  luteinizing, 40
  luteinizing hormone releasing, 41
  melanocyte-stimulating, 46
  parathyroid, 38
  pituitary, 40
  steroid, 62
  thymic, 66
  thyroid, 281
  thyroid-stimulating, 40, 253
  transferrin and, 337, 340
  tumor necrosis factor-α and, 253
HSF, see Hepatocyte-stimulating factor
HTLV, see Human T-cell leukemia virus
Human immunodeficiency virus (HIV), see also Acquired immune deficiency syndrome (AIDS)
  B-cell growth factors and, 89
  interleukin-2 and, 56, 67–68, 77, 78
  tumor necrosis factor and, 242
  tumor necrosis factor-α and, 259
Human interleukin for DA cells (HILDA), see Leukemia inhibitory factor (LIF)
Human T-cell leukemia virus (HTLV), 47
  interleukin-2 and, 61, 67, 69, 70, 76–78
  interleukin-3 and, 83
  platelet-derived growth factor and, 313–314
  tumor necrosis factor and, 242
Human umbilical vein endothelial (HUVE) cells, 179
Hutchinson-Gilford syndrome, 294
HUVE, see Human umbilical vein endothelial
6-Hydroxymethylpterin, 72
Hypoxanthine-guanine phosphoribosyltransferase (HGPRT), 85

I

IAP, see Intracisternal A particle
Idiopathic hypereosinophilic syndrome, 93
IgA-EF (immunoglobulin A-enhancing factor), see Interleukin-5
IGF, see Insulin growth factor
Immune system, 9, 12
  antitumor, 46
  deficiencies in, 78
  development of, 56
  interleukin-2 and, 53, 56, 59
  interleukin-4 and, 89
  interleukin-6 and, 94, 96
  interleukin-7 and, 99
  interleukin-13 and, 104
  leukemia inhibitory factor and, 105
  T-cells and, 36, 53, 89
  tumor necrosis factor-α and, 257
Immunoblastic lymphomas, 76
Immunoglobulin A, 93
Immunoglobulin A-enhancing factor (IgA-EF), see Interleukin-5

Immunoglobulin antibodies, 93, see also specific types
Immunoglobulin E, 90, 104
Immunoglobulin E antibodies, 90
Immunoglobulin G, 90, 104, 342
Immunoglobulin M, 49, 90, 342
Immunoglobulins, 57, 87, 90, 93, see also specific types
Immunoregulatory mechanisms, 177
Immunostimulatory signal, 66
Immunotherapy, 46, see also specific types
Indomethacin, 39, 46, 50, 253, 259
Inflammatory cytokines, 241, see also specific types
Inositol, 72, 224
Inositol trisphosphate, 68, 286, 302
Inositol 1,4,5-trisphosphate, 68
Insulin
    colony-stimulating factor-2 and, 188
    erythropoietic growth factor and, 279
    glucose-induced secretion of, 40
    interleukin-1 and, 38, 40
    interleukin-2 and, 66
    interleukin-6 and, 96
    secretion of, 40, 51
    transferrin and, 340
    tumor necrosis factor-α and, 254
Insulin growth factor (IGF), 3, 4, 41, 279
    erythropoietic growth factor and, 281
    platelet-derived growth factor and, 296, 306, 311
    transferrin and, 340
Insulin growth factor (IGF) receptors, 311
Integrins, 39
Interferon, 9, 10, 12, 221–230, see also specific types
    B-cell growth factors and, 87, 88
    cancer and, 221, 226, 228–230
    cell differentiation and, 227–229
    cell proliferation and, 226–230, 252
    colony-stimulating factor-1 and, 177, 183
    colony-stimulating factor-2 and, 191
    colony-stimulating factor-3 and, 191, 195
    cytostatic effects of, 229–230
    defined, 221
    gene expression and, 224–227
    genes of, 222–223
    hemotopoietic growth factors and, 13, 16, 18
    interleukin-1 and, 40, 46, 50, 52
    interleukin-2 and, 55, 59, 61, 62, 67, 68, 72, 74, 79
    interleukin-4 and, 92
    interleukin-6 and, 96, 97
    interleukin-10 and, 102
    interleukin-12 and, 104
    interleukin-13 and, 104
    macrophage-derived growth factors and, 197
    mechanisms of action of, 223–224
    megakaryocyte colony-stimulating factors and, 197
    oncogenes and, 230
    oncosuppressor activity of, 230
    postreceptor mechanisms of action of, 223–224
    production of, 221–222
    proto-oncogenes and, 225–227, 229
    resistance to, 226
    structure of, 222–223
    tumoricidal effects of, 229–230
    tumor necrosis factor-α and, 251
    vascular cells and, 40
    viruses and, 252
Interferon-α, 244, 339, 340
Interferon-β, 244, 254, 305
Interferon-β2, see Interleukin-6
Interferon-γ
    platelet-derived growth factor and, 293, 305
    transferrin and, 340
    tumor necrosis factor-α and, 243, 244, 247, 251, 254, 257–260
Interferon inducers, 221, 230, see also specific types
Interferon receptors, 223
Interferon-regulatory element (IRE), 100
Interferon-responsive sequence (IRS), 224
Interferon-stimulatable response element, 221, 224
Interferon-stimulated gene factor (ISGF), 224
Interleukin-1, 35–53
    biological effects of, 36–41, 43
    bone tissue and, 38–40
    cartilage and, 38–40
    cell differentiation and, 52–53
    cell proliferation and, 52–53
    colony-stimulating factor-1 production and, 179
    connective tissue and, 38–40
    digestive tract and, 38
    endocrine system and, 40–41
    gene expression and, 51
    generation of, 251
    genes of, 41–43
    gonads and, 40–41
    hematopoiesis and, 36–38
    hematopoietic cells and, 36–38
    hemotopoietic growth factors and, 4–6, 8, 10, 12
    interferon and, 221, 223, 225
    leukemia inhibitory factor and, 105
    macrophage-derived, 59
    mechanisms of action of, 49–51
    mitogenesis and, 35
    neural tissues and, 41
    polyamines and, 49
    postreceptor mechanisms of action of, 49–51
    production of, 43–46
    proteins related to, 43
    protein synthesis and, 51
    secretion of, 42–46
    skin and, 40
    structure of, 41–43
    tumor necrosis factor and, 242
    tumor necrosis factor-α and, 251–253
    urine-derived inhibitors of, 46
    vascular cells and, 40
Interleukin-1 inhibitors, 46–47
Interleukin-1 receptor antagonist, 47
Interleukin-1 receptor antagonist protein, 47, 49, 91
Interleukin-1 receptors, 42–43, 47–49, 305
    bacterial, 48–49
    colony-stimulating factor-3 and, 192
    nuclear, 48
Interleukin-2, 12, 35, 44, 53–80, 185
    age-related changes in, 62–63
    AIDS and, 56, 61, 63, 67, 68, 77–79
    B-cells and, 53, 55
    biological effects of, 53–55
    biosynthesis of, 61
    calcium and, 62
    cancer and, 76–77, 79
    cyclic AMP and, 71

DNA synthesis and, 75
endocrine cells and, 55
glycosylation of, 57, 60
gonads and, 55
guanosine triphosphate binding and, 71
hemotopoietic growth factors and, 5, 8–10, 12, 16
inhibitors of, 63, 68, 80
interferon and, 221, 222
large granular lymphocytes and, 54, 56
mechanisms of action of, 71–75
mitogenesis and, 35
monocytes and, 53, 55
myelopoiesis and, 55
natural killer cells and, 53, 54
oncoproteins and, 55
other cytokines and, 78
other lymphokines and, 54–55
phorbol esters and, 54, 62
phosphoinositide metabolism and, 71–72
phosphoinositide turnover and, 62
platelet-activating factor and, 62
polyamines and, 72
postreceptor mechanisms of action of, 71–75
production of, 61–63, 95
protein phosphorylation and, 71, 73–74
proto-oncogenes and, 69, 73–75
pteridines and, 72
secretion of, 62–63
serum inhibitors of, 63
solid tumors and, 77
structure of, 60
T-cell activating protein and, 58
T-cell antigen receptor complex and, 56–59
T-cell receptor genes and, 58–59
transcriptional expression of genes of, 60–61
transferrin and, 340
tumor necrosis factor-α and, 244, 251, 259
Interleukin-2 receptors, 16, 35, 51, 53, 59, 63–66, 99, 228
aging and, 63
altered expression of, 70–71
cancer and, 76–77
degradation of, 67
expression of, 54, 66–68
genes of, 224
inducers of, 68
induction of, 66–67
interferon and, 221, 222, 224
internalization of, 67
leukemias and, 69–71
low-affinity, 67
lymphomas and, 69–71
phosphorylation of, 65–66
regulation of expression of, 68–69
soluble, 67–68, 78
Interleukin-3, 5–6, 12, 80–86, 280–281, 284
biological effects of, 80–81
cancer and, 86
degradation of, 80
erythropoietic growth factor and, 279, 282
genes of, 82–83
hemotopoietic growth factors and, 3, 4, 6, 8, 18
mechanisms of action of, 84
megakaryocyte colony-stimulating factors and, 196, 197
oncogene expression and, 85
physiological effects of, 86

postreceptor mechanisms of action of, 84
protein phosphorylation and, 83, 84
proto-oncogenes and, 85, 86
release of, 55
structure of, 82–83
tumor necrosis factor-α and, 244
Interleukin-3 receptors, 35, 83
Interleukin-4, 53, 89–93
biological effects of, 90–92
cancer and, 93
genes of, 90
hemotopoietic growth factors and, 8, 10
mechanisms of action of, 92–93
mitogenesis and, 35
postreceptor mechanisms of action of, 92–93
signal generated by, 54
structure of, 90
Interleukin-4 receptors, 35, 92
Interleukin-5, 10, 35, 87, 93–94
Interleukin-5 receptors, 35, 93, 94
Interleukin-6, 94–99
biological effects of, 95–96, 103
cancer and, 98–99
genes of, 96
growth-inhibitory effects, 99
hemotopoietic growth factors and, 3–5, 10, 14
mechanisms of action of, 98
megakaryocyte colony-stimulating factors and, 197
mitogenesis and, 35
postreceptor mechanisms of action of, 98
production of, 96–99, 104
structure of, 96
Interleukin-6 receptors, 35, 98
Interleukin-7, 99–100
Interleukin-7 receptors, 35, 100
Interleukin-8, 100–102, 198
Interleukin-8 receptors, 101
Interleukin-9, 102
Interleukin-9 receptors, 102
Interleukin-10, 102–103
Interleukin-11, 103
Interleukin-11 receptors, 103
Interleukin-12, 103–104
Interleukin-12 receptors, 104
Interleukin-13, 104
Interleukin receptors, 35, see also specific types
Interleukins, 5, 9, 10, 35–36, see also specific types
Intimal smooth muscle cells, 296
Intracisternal A particle (IAP), 80
Ion channels, 92
Ion fluxes, 49, 183
Ionizing radiation, 244
Ionomycin, 16, 62, 66, 302, 306
IRAP, see Interleukin-1 receptor antagonist protein
IRE, see Interferon-regulatory element; Iron-responsive element
Iron, 335, 339, 340, 344
Iron-binding proteins, 335, see also specific types
Iron-responsive element (IRE), 341
IRS, see Interferon-responsive sequence
ISGF, see Interferon-stimulated gene factor
ISRE, see Interferon-stimulatable response element

J

Joint diseases, 39, see also specific types
Jurkat cells, 51, 58, 60, 90

K

Kaposi's sarcoma, 14, 79, 98
KD-TCGF (keratinocyte-derived T-cell growth factor), see Interleukin-1
Keratinocyte-derived T-cell growth factor (KD-TCGF), see Interleukin-1
Keratinocytes, 40, 44, 102, 187, 229
Killer-helper factor, see Interleukin-5
Kinases, 12, 16, see also specific types
    erythropoietic growth factor and, 284
    interleukin-7 and, 100
    microtubule-associated, 188
    phosphatidylinositol, 51
    phosphatidylinositol 4-phosphate, 101
    protein, see Protein kinases
    secondary activation of, 73
    serine/threonine, 12, 73, 75, 84
    serine/threonine-specific protein, 50
    tyrosine, see Tyrosine kinases
Kostmann's syndrome, 195
Krebs ascites tumor cells, 104
Kupffer cells, 38

L

Lactoferrin, 337
Lactotransferrin, 335, 337
LAF (lymphocyte-activating factor), see Interleukin-1
LAI (leukocyte adhesion inhibitor), see Interleukin-8
LAK, see Lymphokine-activated killer
Large-cell anaplastic lymphoma, 102
Large granular lymphocytes, 13, 54, 56, 59, 65, 77
    interleukin-8 and, 101
    interleukin-13 and, 104
    tumor necrosis factor and, 241
    tumor necrosis factor-α and, 244
Laryngeal carcinoma, 246
Lectins, 45, 53, see also specific types
Leukemia inhibitory factor (LIF), 3, 14, 97, 104–105
    biological effects of, 105
    cellular mechanisms of action of, 105
    interleukin-6 and, 98
    interleukin-11 and, 103
    structure of, 105
Leukemia inhibitory factor (LIF) receptors, 105
Leukemias, 1, 5, 8, 14, 15, 18, 50, see also specific types
    acute lymphocytic, see Acute lymphocytic leukemia
    acute monocytic, see Acute monocytic leukemia
    B-cell, 69, 77, 88–90, 259
    B-cell growth factors and, 89
    chronic lymphocytic, 59, 69, see Chronic lymphocytic leukemia
    chronic myeloid, 5, 70, 257, 337
    colony-stimulating factor-1 and, 179, 181, 182, 184
    colony-stimulating factor-2 and, 185, 188, 189
    colony-stimulating factor-3 and, 191–196
    erythroblastic, 284
    erythropoietic growth factor and, 284
    granulocytic, see Myeloid leukemias
    hairy-cell, 67, 69, 88, 89, 225, 229, 259
    histiocytic, 43
    interferon and, 224–226, 228–230
    interleukin-1 and, 44, 52
    interleukin-2 and, 58, 61, 67, 69, 70
    interleukin-2 receptors and, 69–71
    interleukin-3 and, 84, 86
    interleukin-6 and, 97–99
    interleukin-7 and, 100
    interleukin-9 and, 102
    interleukin-11 and, 103
    myeloblastic, 229, 260
    myeloid, see Myeloid leukemias
    myelomonocytic, 3, 96, 193
    proliferation of, 70
    promyelocytic, see Promyelocytic leukemias
    Sezary's, 69
    T-cell, 38, 44, 58, 69, 70, 343
    transferrin and, 335, 337, 339, 341, 343, 344
    tumor necrosis factor and, 241
    tumor necrosis factor-α and, 244, 248, 250, 254, 256, 258, 260
Leukemogenesis, 100
Leukocyte adhesion inhibitor (LAI), see Interleukin-8
Leukocytes, 185, 221
Leukocytosis, 38
Leukotrienes, 62, 244
Leydig cells, 41, 45, 55, 253
LGLs, see Large granular lymphocytes
LH, see Luteinizing hormone
LHRH, see Luteinizing hormone releasing hormone
LIF, see Leukemia inhibitory factor
Lineage-specific hematopoietic growth factors, 3
Lipases, 92, 103, 255, see also specific types
Lipooxygenase, 84
Lipoprotein lipase, 103, 255
LP-1 (lymphopoietin 1), see Interleukin-7
Lung cancer, 7, 52, 86, 188, 193
    interferon and, 226, 229
    platelet-derived growth factor and, 313
    small-cell, 194
Lupus, 63, 79, 80, 89
Luteal cells, 41
Luteinizing hormone (LH), 40
Luteinizing hormone releasing hormone (LHRH), 41
Lymphoblastoid cells, 43, 88, 241, 242, 244, 339
Lymphoblasts, 104, 196
Lymphocyte-activating factor (LAF), see Interleukin-1
Lymphocyte mitogenic factors, 35
Lymphocytes, 1, 4, 9, 35, see also specific types
    activation of, 16, 73, 342
    B-, see B-cells
    colony-stimulating factor-1 and, 177, 179, 181
    colony-stimulating factor-2 and, 185
    interferon and, 221, 228
    interleukin-2 and, 54, 63, 65, 73
    interleukin-3 and, 80, 81
    interleukin-6 and, 97
    interleukin-13 and, 104
    large granular, see Large granular lymphocytes (LGLs)
    PHA-stimulated, 16
    T-, see T-cells
    transferrin and, 339, 342
    tumor necrosis factor and, 242
    tumor necrosis factor-α and, 244, 247

Lymphoid cells, 9, 35, 59, 80, see also specific types
   B-cell growth factors and, 87
   colony-stimulating factor-1 and, 179
   interferon and, 227
   interleukin-6 and, 95
   interleukin-9 and, 102
   interleukin-12 and, 104
Lymphokine-activated killer cells, 12, 54, 76, 79, 103, 104
Lymphokines, 9, 10, 241, see also specific types
   colony-inhibiting, 13
   colony-stimulating factor-2 and, 187
   interleukin-2 and other, 54–55
   secretion of, 10
   synthesis of, 10
   T-leukemia-derived suppressor, 13
Lymphomagenesis, 100
Lymphomas, 1, 5, 15, see also specific types
   B-cell, 70, 86, 89
   Burkitt's, 18, 92, 103
   colony-stimulating factor-3 and, 193, 195
   histiocytic, 13, 44, 246, 247
   immunoblastic, 76
   interferon and, 228
   interleukin-2 and, 58, 61, 62, 76
   interleukin-2 receptors and, 69–71
   interleukin-3 and, 86
   interleukin-6 and, 98
   interleukin-7 and, 100
   interleukin-9 and, 102
   interleukin-10 and, 103
   large-cell anaplastic, 102
   lymphocytic, 69
   non-Hodgkin's, 58, 70, 77, 228
   T-cell, 70
   transferrin and, 343
   tumor necrosis factor-α and, 246, 247
Lymphopoiesis, 9, 35, 81, 99
Lymphopoietin 1 (LP-1), see Interleukin-7
Lymphoproliferative disorders, 343, see also specific types
Lymphotoxins, 12, see also Tumor necrosis factor; specific types

M

Macroglobulin, 295
Macrophage-activating factors (MAFs), 197–198
Macrophage colony-stimulating activity, 197
Macrophage colony-stimulating factor (M-CSF), see Colony-stimulating factor-1 (CSF-1)
Macrophage-derived factor, 12
Macrophage-derived growth factors (MDGFs), 197–198
Macrophage-derived growth inhibitor, 14
Macrophage inflammatory protein (MIP), 10, 14, 101
Macrophage migration factors, 198
Macrophage migration inhibition factor (MIF), 198
Macrophage migration stimulation factor (MSF), 198
Macrophage proinflammatory proteins (MIPs), 198, see also specific types
Macrophages, 4, 7, 8, 12, 17, 36, 91, 241, see also specific types
   alveolar, 8
   B-cell growth factors and, 87
   colony-stimulating factor-1 and, 177, 179, 181, 184, 185
   colony-stimulating factor-2 and, 185, 187, 188
   differentiation of, 251
   interferon and, 225, 226, 228, 229
   interleukin-1 and, 38, 41, 43, 46
   interleukin-2 and, 53, 56, 59, 66
   interleukin-3 and, 80
   interleukin-7 and, 100
   interleukin-10 and, 102
   leukemia inhibitory factor and, 105
   macrophage-derived growth factors and, 197
   tumor-killing factor and, 260
   tumor necrosis factor and, 241
   tumor necrosis factor-α and, 243, 244, 251, 257, 258
Madin-Darby cells, 227
MAFs, see Macrophage-activating factors
Major histocompatibility complex (MHC), 12
   interferon and, 229
   interleukin-2 and, 56, 57
   interleukin-10 and, 102, 103
   tumor necrosis factor and, 242
   tumor necrosis factor-α and, 244, 249, 251
Malaria, 252
MAP, see Microtubule-associated protein
Mast cell growth enhancing activity (MEA, MCGEA), see Interleukin-9
Mast cell growth factor (MCGF), see Interleukin-3
Mast cells, 6, 80, 86, 90, 91, 102
Mastocytoma, 229
MCA, see Methylcholanthrene
MCAF, see Monocyte chemotactic and cell activating factor
MCGEA (mast cell growth enhancing activity), see Interleukin-9
MCGF (mast cell growth factor), see Interleukin-3
MCPs (monocyte chemoattractant proteins), see Macrophage inflammatory proteins (MIPs)
M-CSF (macrophage colony-stimulating factor), see Colony-stimulating factor-1 (CSF-1)
MDCF, see Monocyte-derived cytotoxic factor
MDGFs, see Macrophage-derived growth factors
MDNCF (monocyte-derived neutrophil chemotactic factor), see Interleukin-8
MEA (mast cell growth enhancing activity), see Interleukin-9
Megakaryoblast growth factor (MKBGF), see Interleukin-9
Megakaryoblasts, 196, 197
Megakaryocyte colony-stimulating activity (MK-CSA), see Megakaryocyte colony-stimulating factors (MK-CSFs)
Megakaryocyte colony-stimulating factors (MK-CSFs), 196–197
Megakaryocyte potentiator, 197
Megakaryocytes, 1, 8, 91, 196, 197
   burst-forming unit, 196
   colony-stimulating factor-2 and, 186
   colony-stimulating factor-3 and, 191
   erythropoietic growth factor and, 282, 283
   interleukin-11 and, 103
   leukemia inhibitory factor and, 105
   platelet-derived growth factor and, 293, 294
Megakaryocytopoiesis, 81, 95, 103, 186, 196, 197
Megakaryopoiesis, 1
MEL, see Mouse erythroleukemia
Melanocyte growth-stimulatory activity, 101
Melanocyte-stimulating hormone (MSH), 40, 46
Melanoma growth-stimulating activity (MGSA), 101, 311
Melanomas, 45, 52, 77, see also specific types
   colony-stimulating factor-2 and, 185
   interferon and, 225, 226
   interleukin-1 and, 49
   interleukin-2 and, 54
   interleukin-4 and, 93
   interleukin-6 and, 99

interleukin-7 and, 100
interleukin-8 and, 101
platelet-derived growth factor and, 311
transferrin and, 337
tumor necrosis factor and, 241
tumor necrosis factor-α and, 248, 253, 256, 257, 259
Melanotransferrin, 335, 337
Melanoma growth-stimulatory activity, 225
Membrane-associated protein, 36
Meningiomas, 313
Mesangial cells, 44, 248, 295
Mesenchymal cells, 178
Mesothelial cells, 5, 7
Mesothelioma, 5
Mesotheliomas, 7, 311
Metalloproteinase, 305
Metallothionein, 98
Methylcholanthrene (MCA), 243, 256
MGSA, see Melanoma growth-stimulating activity
MHC, see Major histocompatability complex
Microtubule-associated protein (MAP) kinase, 188
MIF, see Macrophage migration inhibition factor
MIP, see Macrophage inflammatory protein
MIPs, see Macrophage proinflammatory proteins
Mitogenesis, 35, 73, 302, 306–307
Mitogens, 244, see also specific types
MKBGF (megakaryoblast growth factor), see Interleukin-9
MK-CSA (megakaryocyte colony-stimulating activity), see Megakaryocyte colony-stimulating factors (MK-CSFs)
MK-CSFs, see Megakaryocyte colony-stimulating factors
Mobilferrin, 335
Monensin, 341
Monoacylglycerol, 302
Monoclonal antibodies, 6, 16
    colony-stimulating factor-1 and, 177
    interleukin-2 and, 54, 58, 63, 69, 75
    transferrin and, 342, 343
Monocyte chemoattractant proteins (MCPs), see Macrophage inflammatory proteins (MIPs)
Monocyte chemotactic and cell activating factor (MCAF), 38, 249
Monocyte-derived cytotoxic factor (MDCF), 251
Monocyte-derived growth factors, 95
Monocyte-derived neutrophil chemotactic factor (MDNCF), see Interleukin-8
Monocytes, 1, 7, 12, 17, 35, 36
    colony-stimulating factor and, 177
    colony-stimulating factor-1 and, 177, 178, 181, 185
    colony-stimulating factor-2 and, 185, 186, 188, 191
    interferon and, 227, 228
    interleukin-1 and, 41, 43, 45–47, 51
    interleukin-2 and, 53, 55, 66, 67
    interleukin-4 and, 93
    interleukin-6 and, 96, 97
    interleukin-8 and, 100, 101
    interleukin-13 and, 104
    leukemia inhibitory factor and, 104, 105
    macrophage-derived growth factors and, 197, 198
    platelet-derived growth factor and, 296, 309
    tumor necrosis factor and, 241
    tumor necrosis factor-α and, 243–245, 249
Monokines, 9, 10, 35
Mononuclear cells, 12, 17
Mononucleosis, 68
Mouse erythroleukemia (MEL) cells, 17

MPLV, see Myeloproliferative leukemia virus
MSF, see Macrophage migration stimulation factor
MSH, see Melanocyte-stimulating hormone
Multicytokine-resistant phenotype, 14
Multilineage colony-stimulating activity (multi-CSA), see Interleukin-3
Multilineage colony-stimulating factors, 3
Multilineage hematopoietic growth factors, 3, 5
Multiple myeloma, 178
Multiple sclerosis, 79, 83
Multipotential colony-stimulating factors (Multi-CSFs), see Interleukin-3
Multipotential hematopoietic progenitors, 95
Multipotential stem cells, 1
Murine growth inhibitory factor, 14
Mutagenesis, 180, 192
Muteins, 245
Myeloblastic cells, 194, 226
Myeloblastic leukemia, 229, 260
Myeloblasts, 84
Myelodysplastic syndromes, 98, 193, 195, see also specific types
Myeloid cells
    colony-stimulating factor-1 and, 180, 181
    colony-stimulating factor-2 and, 190
    colony-stimulating factor-3 and, 194, 195
    interferon and, 229
    interleukin-3 and, 84, 86
    interleukin-4 and, 91
    interleukin-6 and, 97, 99
    interleukin-7 and, 99
    interleukin-9 and, 102
Myeloid growth factors, see Colony-stimulating factor
Myeloid leukemias, 3, 7, 8, 18, 44, 52, 90, see also specific types
    chronic, 5, 70, 257, 337
    colony-stimulating factor-2 and, 185
    colony-stimulating factor-3 and, 194
    transferrin and, 335, 337, 344
    tumor necrosis factor and, 241
    tumor necrosis factor-α and, 260
Myelomas, 178
Myelomonocytic leukemia, 3, 96, 193
Myelopoiesis, 55, 82, 252
Myeloproliferative leukemia virus (MPLV), 10
Myelosuppression, 15
Myoblasts, 296
Myoglobin, 335

N

NAP-1 (neutrophil-activating peptide 1), see Interleukin-8
Nasopharyngeal carcinoma, 45
Natural killer (NK) cells, 13
    activation of, 72
    interferon and, 228
    interleukin-1 and, 41
    interleukin-2 and, 53, 54, 72
    interleukin-3 and, 81
    interleukin-6 and, 95
    interleukin-12 and, 104
    proliferation of, 104
    tumor necrosis factor and, 241
Natural killer (NK) cell stimulating factor (NKCSF, NKSF), see Interleukin-12

Natural killer (NK) cytotoxicity factor (NKCF), 13
Neopterin, 72
Nerve growth factor (NGF), 9, 41, 254
Neural tissues, 41
Neural tumors, 312–313
Neuroblastomas, 259, 312
Neuroleukin, 89
Neutropenia, 183
Neutrophil-activating peptide, 101
Neutrophil-activating peptide 1 (NAP-1), see
    Interleukin-8
Neutrophil elastase, 303
Neutrophilopoiesis, 193
Neutrophil oxidative burst, 297
Neutrophils, 7, 37
    colony-stimulating factor and, 177
    colony-stimulating factor-2 and, 185, 186, 191
    colony-stimulating factor-3 and, 191, 193, 195
    interleukin-1 and, 40
    interleukin-3 and, 81
    interleukin-6 and, 95
    interleukin-8 and, 100, 101
    macrophage-derived growth factors and, 198
    platelet-derived growth factor and, 294, 297, 303
    tumor necrosis factor and, 241
    tumor necrosis factor-α and, 252
Nevovascularization, 12
NGF, see Nerve growth factor
NK, see Natural killer
NKCF, see Natural killer (NK) cytotoxicity factor
NKCSF (natural killer cell stimulating factor), see Interleukin-12
NKSF (natural killer cell stimulating factor), see Interleukin-12
Non-Hodgkin's lymphoma, 58, 70, 77, 228
Non-small-cell lung cancer, 188
Nonsteroidal antiinflammatory drugs, 259, see also specific types
Nuclear interleukin-1 receptors, 48
Nuclear proteins, 4, see also specific types

O

OAF (osteoclast-activating factor), see Interleukin-1
OKT11A antibody, 16
Oligoadenylate synthetase, 305
Oncogenes, 15, 18
    colony-stimulating factor-1 and, 180, 182
    colony-stimulating factor-2 and, 189, 190
    erythropoietic growth factor and, 285
    interferon and, 227, 230
    interleukin-3 and, 85, 86
    platelet-derived growth factor and, 302, 308, 314
    proto-, see Proto-oncogenes
    tumor necrosis factor-α and, 255
Oncoproteins, 12, 15, 16, see also specific types
    colony-stimulating factor-1 and, 180
    interleukin-2 and, 55, 63
    interleukin-3 and, 85, 86
    interleukin-6 and, 98
    platelet-derived growth factor and, 307–310
Oncostatin M, 13–14, 103, 105
Oncosuppressor genes, 4, 230
Ornithine, 252
Osteoblasts, 39, 186, 248
Osteocalcin, 186
Osteoclast-activating factor (OAF), see Interleukin-1

Osteoclastogenesis, 96
Osteoclasts, 39, 80, 181
Osteogenic sarcoma, 186
Osteopenia, 96
Osteopetrosis, 179
Osteoporosis, 96
Osteosarcomas, 39, 188
    colony-stimulating factor-2 and, 187
    interferon and, 227, 230
    interleukin-3 and, 80
    interleukin-6 and, 97
    platelet-derived growth factor and, 306, 311–312
Ovarian cancer, 52, 98, 185, 256, 259
Ovotransferrin, 335, 340
Oxygen sensors, 281

P

PAF, see Platelet-activating factor
PAIs, see Plasminogen activator inhibitors
Pancreatic carcinoma, 178
Paracrine, 181, 244
Parasites, 221, 252
Parathyroid hormone (PTH), 38
PBP, see Platelet basic protein
PD-ECGF, see Platelet-derived endothelial cell growth
    factor
PDGF, see Platelet-derived growth factor
Pepsin, 38
Peritoneal cells, 193
PFs, see Platelet factors
Phagocytes, 17, 40, 177, 179, 187
Phagocytosis, 177, 185, 297
Phenylbutazone, 259
Pheochromocytoma, 96
Phorbol esters, 3, 16, see also specific types
    colony-stimulating factor-1 and, 182
    interleukin-1 and, 47, 50, 62
    interleukin-2 and, 54, 62, 66, 68, 70–73
    interleukin-3 and, 84
    platelet-derived growth factor and, 295, 303, 304, 311
    transferrin and, 339, 340, 343
    tumor necrosis factor-α and, 244
Phosphatidic acid, 188, 302, 339
Phosphatidic acid phosphohydrolase, 302
Phosphatidylcholine, 51, 84, 302
Phosphatidylethanolamine, 51
Phosphatidylinositol, 68, 179
Phosphatidylinositol 4,5-biphosphate, 301, 303
Phosphatidylinositol hydrolysis, 58, 62
Phosphatidylinositol kinase, 51
Phosphatidylinositol 3-kinase, 299
Phosphatidylinositol 4-phosphate kinase, 101
Phosphatidylinositol 3,4,5-trisphosphate, 302
Phosphatidylserine, 51
Phosphohydrolase, 302
Phosphoinositide, 50–51
    breakdown of, 286
    hydrolysis of, 72
    metabolism of, 71–72, 84
        colony-stimulating factor-2 and, 188
        interferon and, 224
        interleukin-5 and, 94
        interleukin-7 and, 100

interleukin-8 and, 101
  platelet-derived growth factor and, 301–302
 turnover of, 62, 71, 84, 87, 92, 183
Phospholipase A, 50, 248, 302, 303
Phospholipase B, 101
Phospholipase C, 40, 51, 56, 58
 colony-stimulating factor-1 and, 180, 183
 colony-stimulating factor-2 and, 188
 colony-stimulating factor-3 and, 194
 platelet-derived growth factor and, 301
Phospholipase D, 188, 224, 248, 302
Phospholipid metabolism, 248–249
Phosphorylation, 57, 72
 of cellular proteins, 71
 of colony-stimulating factor-1 receptors, 182
 of epidermal growth factor receptors, 303
 interleukin-6 and, 96
 of interleukin-2 receptors, 65–66
 of platelet-derived growth factor receptor, 299–300
 protein, see Protein phosphorylation
 serine, 43
 of T-cell receptor, 63, 71
 of transferrin receptors, 338, 339
 tyrosine, see Tyrosine phosphorylation
Physiologic effects, 86, 241, 250–254
Pituitary gland, 35, 96, 296
Pituitary hormone, 40
PKC, see Protein kinase C
Placenta, 35, 40, 62
 colony-stimulating factor-1 and, 179, 181
 colony-stimulating factor-3 and, 194
 erythropoietic growth factor and, 282
 platelet-derived growth factor and, 309
 transferrin and, 342
 tumor necrosis factor-α and, 243
Placental cells, 80
Plasmacytoma growth factor, 185
Plasmacytomas, 98, 103
Plasma proteins, 36, 38, see also specific types
Plasmin, 253
Plasminogen, 253
Plasminogen activator genes, 225
Plasminogen activator inhibitors (PAIs), 253
Platelet-activating factor (PAF), 62, 177
Platelet-activating factor (PAF) antagonists, 62, see also specific types
Platelet basic protein (PBP), 198
Platelet-derived endothelial cell growth factor, 293
Platelet-derived growth factor (PDGF), 293–314
 binding of, 301
 cancer and, 310–314
 cellular responses to, 303
 colony-stimulating factor-1 and, 181
 cytoplasmic alkalinization and, 303
 cytoskeletal changes and, 304
 epidermal growth factor and, 303–304
 functions of, 296–297
 genes of, 293–294
 interferon and, 221, 228
 interleukin-1 and, 39, 48, 51
 interleukin-2 and, 66
 interleukin-3 and, 82
 interleukin-6 and, 98
 macrophage-derived growth factors and, 197
 mechanisms of action of, 300–306
 in mitogenesis, 306–307
 molecular forms of, 293–294, 298–299
 oncogenes and, 314
 oncoproteins and, 307–310
 posttransductional mechanisms of action of, 304–306
 production of, 294–296
 proto-oncogenes and, 293, 294, 296, 298, 305–306, 308–309, 314
 sodium-hydrogen antiport and, 303
 structure of, 293–294, 308
 transductional mechanisms of action of, 300–303
 transferrin and, 339, 340
 tumor necrosis factor-α and, 254
 viruses and, 313–314
Platelet-derived growth factor (PDGF)-like factors, 310–314
Platelet-derived growth factor (PDGF)-like polypeptides, 294–296, see also specific types
Platelet-derived growth factor (PDGF) receptors, 82, 181, 297–300, 308, 309
Platelet-derived growth factor (PDGF)-related peptides, 307
Platelet-derived growth factor (PDGF)-related proteins, 298
Platelet factors (PFs), 198, 225, 293, 305
Pluripotent hemotopoietic growth factors, 5–7
Polyamines, 49, 72, 248, see also specific types
Polycytidylic acid, 221
Polyinosinic acid, 221
Porphobilinogen deaminase, 284
Postreceptor mechanisms of action
 of colony-stimulating factor-1, 183
 of colony-stimulating factor-2, 188
 of colony-stimulating factor-3, 194
 of erythropoietin, 283–284
 of interferon, 223–224
 of interleukin-1, 49–51
 of interleukin-2, 71–75
 of interleukin-3, 84
 of interleukin-4, 92–93
 of interleukin-5, 94
 of interleukin-6, 98
 of interleukin-7, 100
 of interleukin-8, 101
 of tumor necrosis factor-α, 247–250
Pre-B-cell growth factor (pre-BCGF), see Interleukin-7
Pre-BCGF (pre-B-cell growth factor), see Interleukin-7
Preleukemia, 179
Progenitor cells, see also specific types
 colony-stimulating factor-1 and, 177
 colony-stimulating factor-2 and, 186
 colony-stimulating factor-3 and, 191
 erythroid, 81, 102, 281, 282
 erythropoietic growth factor and, 281, 282
 hematopoietic, 2, 13
 interleukin-4 and, 91
 interleukin-9 and, 102
 interleukin-11 and, 103
 megakaryocyte colony-stimulating factors and, 196
 tumor necrosis factor-α and, 254
Progesterone, 253
Proinflammatory peptides, 198, see also specific types
Prolactin, 12, 35, 40, 96, 337
Prolactin receptors, 35
Promyelocytic leukemias, 17, 99, see also specific types
 acute, 192
 colony-stimulating factor-1 and, 182

interferon and, 229
transferrin and, 339
tumor necrosis factor-α and, 244, 250, 260
Prostacyclins, 50, 303
Prostaglandin E, 39, 48, 50, 71
   colony-stimulating factor-2 and, 187
   interleukin-4 and, 91
   synthesis of, 46
   tumor necrosis factor-α and, 244, 248, 251–253
Prostaglandins, 48, see also specific types
   interleukin-1 and, 50
   platelet-derived growth factor and, 302, 304
   production of, 50, 248
   release of, 302
   synthesis of, 39, 302, 304
   tumor necrosis factor-α and, 244, 248, 253
Prostatic carcinoma, 98, 344
Protamine sulfate, 298
Proteases, 305, see also specific types
Protein kinase A, 97
Protein kinase C, 16, 45, 46, 50, 51
   activation of, 3, 56, 62, 87, 92, 222, 303
   B-cell growth factors and, 87
   colony-stimulating factor-1 and, 182
   colony-stimulating factor-2 and, 188
   colony-stimulating factor-3 and, 194
   erythropoietic growth factor and, 284
   interferon and, 222, 224, 225
   interleukin-1 and, 40
   interleukin-2 and, 56, 58, 62, 68, 71, 72, 74
   interleukin-3 and, 84, 86
   interleukin-4 and, 92
   interleukin-8 and, 101
   platelet-derived growth factor and, 300, 301, 302, 303, 306
   transferrin and, 335, 339, 341
   tumor necrosis factor-α and, 247, 248
Protein kinase P, 84
Protein kinases, 50, see also specific types
   ceramide-activated, 249
   cyclic AMP-dependent, 248
   interleukin-2 and, 56
   interleukin-4 and, 92
   platelet-derived growth factor and, 301
   serine/threonine-specific, 50
   tumor necrosis factor-α and, 249
Protein phosphorylation, 3, 35–36
   B-cell growth factors and, 87
   colony-stimulating factor-1 and, 183
   colony-stimulating factor-2 and, 188
   erythropoietic growth factor and, 284
   interleukin-2 and, 50, 71, 73–74
   interleukin-3 and, 83, 84
   interleukin-4 and, 92
   interleukin-5 and, 94
   interleukin-7 and, 100
   interleukin-11 and, 103
   platelet-derived growth factor and, 301, 304
   transferrin and, 335
   tumor necrosis factor-α and, 247, 249
Proteins, see also specific types
   actin-binding, 73
   cap-binding, 249
   cellular, 71
   converter, 67
   DNA-binding, 336
   G, 84, 101, 188, 194, 198, 248
   guanosine triphosphatase activating, 12, 284, 302
   interleukin-1-related, 43
   iron-binding, 335
   macrophage inflammatory, 10, 14, 101
   macrophage proinflammatory, 198
   membrane-associated, 36
   microtubule-associated, 188
   monocyte chemoattractant, see Macrophage inflammatory proteins (MIPs)
   nuclear, 4
   onco-, see Oncoproteins
   phosphorylation of, see Protein phosphorylation
   plasma, 36, 38
   platelet basic, 198
   platelet-derived growth factor-related, 298
   steroidogenesis-inducing, 41
   synthesis of, 51, 224, 250, 304–305
   T-cell activating, 58
   tumor necrosis factor-α-induced, 250
Protein-tyrosine phosphatase, 84
Proteoglycans, 39, 253, see also specific types
Proto-oncogenes, 36, see also specific types
   B-cell growth factors and, 88–89
   colony-stimulating factor-1 and, 181, 183–184
   colony-stimulating factor-2 and, 189–190
   colony-stimulating factor-3 and, 194
   erythropoietic growth factor and, 279, 284
   hemotopoietic growth factors and, 4–6, 10, 12, 16–18
   interferon and, 225–229
   interleukin-1 and, 51
   interleukin-2 and, 69, 73–75
   interleukin-3 and, 85, 86
   interleukin-4 and, 92
   interleukin-5 and, 94
   interleukin-6 and, 98
   megakaryocyte colony-stimulating factors and, 196
   platelet-derived growth factor and, 293, 294, 296, 298, 305–306, 308–309, 314
   transferrin and, 336–337
   tumor necrosis factor-α and, 249–250
Protoporphyrins, 339
Psoriasis, 40
Pteridines, 72
PTH, see Parathyroid hormone
Putrescine, 49, 248, 252, 307
Pyrogens, 36, 255, see also specific types

R

Radiation, 9, 244, 252, see also specific types
Rat tracheal epithelial (RTE) cells, 182
Rauscher erythroleukemia, 285
Reed-Sternberg cells, 44, 91, 102
Renal cell carcinoma, 93
Renal failure, 68
Reproductive system, 253–254
Reticuloendothelial system, 177
Retinoblastomas, 230
Retinoic acid, 17, 18, 195, 229, 260, 343
Retroviruses, 15, 16, 47, see also specific types
   erythropoietic growth factor and, 284
   interferon and, 227

platelet-derived growth factor and, 313, 314
  tumor necrosis factor-α and, 259
Rheumatoid arthritis, 39, 45, 101
RNA synthesis, 297, 304–305
RNA viruses, 252, see also specific types
RTE, see Rat tracheal epithelial

S

Saramin, 298, 307
Sarcoidosis, 68, 243
Sarcomas, see also specific types
  colony-stimulating factor-2 and, 186, 191
  interleukin-6 and, 98
  Kaposi's, 14, 79, 98
  osteogenic, 186
  platelet-derived growth factor and, 307, 308, 309, 313
  tumor necrosis factor-α and, 244, 252, 256, 258, 259
Sarcoma viruses, 180, 307, 309, 313, see also specific types
SCDC (stromal cell-derived cytokine), see Interleukin-11
SCF, see Stem cell growth factor
SCGF, see Stem cell growth factor
Schwann cells, 300
SCI, see Stem-cell inhibitor
Sendai virus, 244
Serine, 83, 84, 94, 301
Serine phosphorylation, 43
Serine/threonine kinase, 12, 73, 75, 84
Serine/threonine-specific protein kinase, 50
Serotransferrin, 335
Sertoli cells, 6, 96, 336, 342
Sezary's syndrome, 69, 76
SFFV, see Spleen focus-forming virus
Sialylation, 96
Signal transduction, 92, 188
Simian sarcoma virus (SSV), 307, 309, 313
SIP, see Steroidogenesis-inducing protein
Skin diseases, 40, see also specific types
SLE, see Systemic lupus erythematosus
Small-cell lung carcinoma, 86, 194
Smooth muscle cells, 40, 44, 97
  aortic, 295
  arterial, 294, 296
  colony-stimulating factor-1 and, 181
  colony-stimulating factor-3 and, 193
  intimal, 296
  platelet-derived growth factor and, 294–296
  tumor necrosis factor-α and, 252
  vascular, 40, 97, 181, 193, 252, 296
Sodium acetate, 44
Sodium-hydrogen antiport, 303, 344
Sodium influx, 49
Sodium orthovanadate, 84
Solid tumors, 77, 86, 189, see also specific types
Spermatogenesis, 96, 342
Sphingolipid metabolism, 248–249
Sphingomyelin, 248
Sphingomyelinase, 249
Spleen focus-forming virus (SFFV), 285
Splenocytes, 35
Squamous cell carcinoma, 38, 80, 192, 227
SSV, see Simian sarcoma virus
Stem cell growth factor (SCGF), 5–7, 99
Stem-cell inhibitor (SCI), 14

Stem cells, 1, 2, 6, see also specific types
  bone marrow, 7
  colony-stimulating factor-3 and, 191
  differentiation of, 35, 104, 105
  embryonic, 105
  hematopoietic, 1, 95, 191, 196
  interleukin-2 and, 55
  interleukin-6 and, 95
  leukemia inhibitory factor and, 104, 105
  megakaryocyte colony-stimulating factors and, 196
  multipotential, 1
  proliferation of, 55
  renewal of, 35
Steroidogenesis, 55, 253
Steroidogenesis-inducing protein (SIP), 41
Steroids, 62, see also specific types
Stomach cancer, 93, 188, 227, 313
Stromal cell-derived cytokine (SCDC), see Interleukin-11
Stromal cells, 9
  bone marrow, 4, 9, 36, 95
  colony-stimulating factor-2 and, 187
  colony-stimulating factor-3 and, 193
  interleukin-1 and, 39, 52
  interleukin-7 and, 99
Superoxide anions, 177, 195, 252
Suramin, 311
Surface glycoprotein antigens, 54
Synovial cells, 45, 101, 248
Systemic lupus erythematosus (SLE), 63, 79, 80, 89

T

TAF (T-cell activating factor), see Interleukin-6
Talin, 50
TAP, see T-cell activating protein
T-cell activating factor (TAF), see Interleukin-6
T-cell activating protein (TAP), 58
T-cell antigen receptor complex, 56–59
T-cell-derived growth inhibitors, 13
T-cell growth factor (TCGF), see also Interleukin-2
  B-cell-derived, see Interleukin-10
  keratinocyte-derived, see Interleukin-1
T-cell growth factor (TCGF)-III, see Interleukin-9
T-cell immune response, 36
T-cell leukemias, 58, 70, see also specific types
  adult, 38, 44, 69, 76–77
  transferrin and, 343
T-cell lymphomas, 70, see also specific types
T-cell mitogenic factor (TCMF), see Interleukin-2
T-cell receptors, 53, 56, 58–59, 63, 71
T-cell replacing factor (TCRF), see Interleukin-5
T-cells, 7, 9, 10, 16, 37
  activation of, 59, 72, 80, 89, 90
  aging and, 62–63
  B-cell growth factors and, 87
  clones of, 15
  colony-stimulating factor-2 and, 185, 188
  cytotoxic effector, 13
  differentiation of, 35, 56, 59
  growth of, 53
  helper, 54, 56, 77, 87, 91
  hemotopoietic growth factors and, 5
  immune responses mediated by, 53
  immunosuppressive functions of, 37

interferon and, 221, 222, 228
interleukin-1 and, 37, 44, 47, 51
interleukin-2 and, 53–57, 59, 61
Interleukin-2 and, 62
interleukin-2 and, 65, 66, 71, 72
interleukin-3 and, 80, 82
interleukin-4 and, 89–91
interleukin-5 and, 93
interleukin-6 and, 95
interleukin-7 and, 99
interleukin-8 and, 100, 101
interleukin-9 and, 102
interleukin-10 and, 102
interleukin-11 and, 103
interleukin-12 and, 103
macrophage-derived growth factors and, 197, 198
megakaryocyte colony-stimulating factors and, 196
peripheral, 37
platelet-derived growth factor and, 306, 313
progression of cycle of, 53
proliferation of, 16, 62
subsets of, 56–57
suppressor, 68
transferrin and, 340, 343
tumor necrosis factor and, 241, 242
tumor necrosis factor-α and, 251
TCGF (T-cell growth factor), see Interleukin-2
TCGF-III (T-cell growth factor III), see Interleukin-9
TCMF (T-cell mitogenic factor), see Interleukin-2
Teniposide, 259
Testosterone, 284, 342
Tetrapyrrole, 284
TGF, see Transforming growth factor
Theophylline, 341
Threonine, 12, 50, 73, 75, 84, 301
Thrombin, 295
Thrombocytopoiesis, 196
Thrombocytopoiesis-stimulating factor (TSF), 197
Thromboglobulin, 198
Thromboplastin, 177
Thrombopoietin, see Thrombocytopoiesis-stimulating factor
Thymic hormones, 66
Thymic stroma-derived T-cell growth factor, 4, 53
Thymocyte activating factor, 44
Thymocytes, 4, 35, 43
　interleukin-1 and, 47
　interleukin-2 and, 53, 56
　interleukin-4 and, 91
　interleukin-5 and, 93
　interleukin-7 and, 100
　leukemia inhibitory factor and, 105
Thymomas, 47, 49, 62, 68
Thyrocytes, 40
Thyroid carcinoma, 297
Thyroid disease, 40
Thyroid gland, 40
Thyroid hormone, 281
Thyroid-stimulating hormone (TSH), 40, 253
TIF, see Tumor-inhibitory factor
TIF-2 (tumor-inhibitory factor 2), see Interleukin-1
TIMPs, see Tissue inhibitor of metalloproteinases
Tissue inhibitor of metalloproteinases (TIMPs), 280
Tissue repair, 198, 296
TKF, see Tumor-killing factor
TLCF (T-lymphocyte chemotactic factor), see Interleukin-8

T-leukemia-derived suppressor lymphokine (TLSL), 13
TLSL, see T-leukemia-derived suppressor lymphokine
T-lymphocyte chemotactic factor (TLCF), see Interleukin-8
TMIF, see Tumor migration inhibition factor
TNF, see Tumor necrosis factor
Transferrin, 335–344, see also specific types
　cancer and, 336, 337, 344
　cell differentiation and, 344
　cell proliferation and, 344
　growth-promoting action of, 344
　mechanisms of action of, 344
　structure of, 335–337
　synthesis of, 335–337
　tumor-promoting effects of, 344
"Transferrinfection", 338
Transferrin glycans, 335
Transferrin receptors, 227, 254, 284, 286, 337
　cancer and, 342–344
　expression of, 339–341
　internalization of, 341
　in normal cells, 342–344
　posttranslational modification of, 338–339
Transforming growth factor (TGF), 5, 39, 54, 196, 197, 251, 254, 296
Transforming growth factor (TGF)-α receptors, 279
Transforming growth factor (TGF)-β, 300, 307, 310, 311, 314
Transin, 305
Transmembrane signaling, 68
Trifluoroperazine, 341
Trophoblasts, 40, 97, 105, 194, 342
TSF, see Thrombocytopoiesis-stimulating factor
TSH, see Thyroid-stimulating hormone
Tumor-inhibitory factor 2 (TIF-2), see Interleukin-1
Tumor-killing factor (TKF), 260–261
Tumor-killing factor (TKF) receptors, 261
Tumor migration inhibition factor (TMIF), 241, 260
Tumor necrosis factor (TNF), 9, 10, 12, 241–261, see also specific types
　biological effects of, 241
　bone resorption and, 38
　colony-stimulating factor-1 and, 177, 179, 181
　colony-stimulating factor-2 and, 186, 187, 191
　colony-stimulating factor-3 and, 194
　genes of, 244–245
　hemotopoietic growth factors and, 8, 13
　interferon and, 223, 225, 228, 229
　interleukin-1 and, 36, 38, 39, 45, 48, 50, 52
　interleukin-2 and, 53, 54, 68, 78
　interleukin-3 and, 81
　interleukin-4 and, 91
　interleukin-6 and, 95–97
　physiologic effects of, 241
　production of, 243–244
　structure of, 244–245
Tumor necrosis factor (TNF) receptors, 53, 245, 247, see also specific types
Tumor necrosis factor (TNF)-α, 241, 242, 243–260
　biological effects of, 241
　cachectin and, 255–256
　cancer and, 256–259
　cell differentiation and, 260
　cell-killing effects of, 254–255
　cytotoxic effects of, 250
　endocrine system and, 253–254
　genes of, 244–245

growth-inhibiting effects of, 254–255
mechanisms of action of, 247–250
physiologic effects of, 250–254
platelet-derived growth factor and, 295
postreceptor mechanisms of action of, 247–250
production of, 243–244
proteins induced by, 250
proto-oncogenes and, 249–250
reproductive system and, 253–254
resistance to, 258
sensitivity to, 258
side effects of, 258–259
structure of, 244–245
transferrin and, 340
tumor cell growth and, 256–260
tumor cell sensitivity to, 258
tumor-promoting effects of, 259
tumor regression and, 256–257
undesirable effects of, 258–259
viruses and, 254, 255
Tumor necrosis factor (TNF)-α inhibitors, 247
Tumor necrosis factor (TNF)-α receptors, 245–247, 258
Tumor necrosis factor (TNF)-β, 241, 242, 244, 255
  biological effects of, 241
  functions of, 242
  genes of, 242
  platelet-derived growth factor and, 295
  structure of, 242
Tumor promoters, 182–183, see also specific types
Tumor regression, 256–257
Tumors, see also Cancer; specific types
  brain, 102
  neural, 312–313
  solid, 77, 86, 189
  tumor necrosis factor-α and, 244
Tumor suppressor genes, 4, 16–18, 86, 228
Tyrosine, 83, 94, 249
Tyrosine kinases, 4, 5, 12, 16, 36
  colony-stimulating factor-1 and, 179, 180
  colony-stimulating factor-2 and, 188, 190
  interferon and, 224, 227
  interleukin-2 and, 55, 56, 65, 66, 73
  interleukin-3 and, 84
  interleukin-7 and, 100
  platelet-derived growth factor and, 297, 299, 304
Tyrosine phosphatase, 56
Tyrosine phosphorylation, 6, 56, 87, 92, 103, 179
  colony-stimulating factor-1 and, 182, 183
  colony-stimulating factor-2 and, 188

  erythropoietic growth factor and, 284
  interferon and, 224
  platelet-derived growth factor and, 299, 301
  tumor necrosis factor-α and, 249

U

Ukeroferrin, 7
Urokinase, 225, 253

V

Vascular cells, 40
Vascular endothelial cell growth factor (VEGF), 295
Vascular smooth muscle cells, 40, 97, 181, 193, 252, 296
VEGF, see Vascular endothelial cell growth factor
Vincristine, 341
Vinculin, 304
Viruses, see also specific types
  adeno-, 61, 255
  cytomegalo-, 68
  DNA, 241, 252
  encephalomyocarditis, 222
  Epstein Barr, see Epstein Barr virus (EBV)
  Friend murine leukemia, 285
  gibbon ape leukemia, 63
  gibbon leukemia, 61
  human immunodeficiency, see Human immunodeficiency virus (HIV)
  human T-cell leukemia, see Human T-cell leukemia virus
  interferon and, 221, 222, 252
  myeloproliferative leukemia, 10
  platelet-derived growth factor and, 313–314
  retro-, see Retroviruses
  RNA, 252
  sarcoma, 180, 307, 309, 313
  Sendai, 244
  simian sarcoma, 307, 309, 313
  spleen focus-forming, 285
  transferrin and, 340
  tumor necrosis factor and, 241
  tumor necrosis factor-α and, 252, 254, 255

W

Werner's syndrome, 297
Wound healing, 101, 197, 198, 296
  cancer and, 336, 337, 344